Atlas of Dermatologic Diseases in Solid Organ Transplant Recipients

Jane Tomimori
Walmar Roncalli Pereira de Oliveira
Carla Ferrándiz-Pulido • Marilia Marufuji Ogawa
Editors

Atlas of Dermatologic Diseases in Solid Organ Transplant Recipients

Springer

Editors
Jane Tomimori
Department of Dermatology
Universidade Federal de São Paulo
São Paulo, São Paulo, Brazil

Carla Ferrándiz-Pulido
Department of Dermatology
Hospital Universitari Vall d'Hebron
Universitat Autònoma de Barcelona
Barcelona, Spain

Walmar Roncalli Pereira de Oliveira
Department of Dermatology
University of São Paulo
São Paulo, São Paulo, Brazil

Marilia Marufuji Ogawa
Department of Dermatology
Universidade Federal de São Paulo
São Paulo, São Paulo, Brazil

ISBN 978-3-031-13334-3 ISBN 978-3-031-13335-0 (eBook)
https://doi.org/10.1007/978-3-031-13335-0

This Springer imprint is published by the registered company Springer Nature Switzerland AG
The registered company address is: Gewerbestrasse 11, 6330 Cham, Switzerland

Preface

The number of solid organ transplant recipients is increasing worldwide every year, which has meant a significant improvement of recipient's survival and quality of life. On the other hand, immunosuppression maintenance is required for long-term graft survival; however, at the same time it has facilitated the appearance of complications derived from chronic immunosuppression in these patients, highlighting by its frequency and severity, the development of skin cancer and opportunistic infections. During the induction phase of immunosuppression, herpetic, fungal, and bacterial infections are the most common cutaneous complications; while in the chronic phase, opportunistic infections and cutaneous neoplasms may appear, with the characteristic of being more aggressive and difficult to treat than in the immunocompetent patient.

The role of dermatologists in the follow-up of solid organ transplant recipients relies on minimizing the deleterious effects of iatrogenic immunosuppression, not only contributing to the treatment of skin cancer or cutaneous infections, but also in the prevention and diagnosis of these complications. A careful and periodic cutaneous clinical examination after receiving a transplanted organ should be part of the comprehensive patient's care.

The Atlas of Dermatologic Diseases in Solid Organ Transplant Recipients includes the experience of worldwide dermatologists who conduct research and follow this population through the post-transplant period. The main objective of this Atlas is to share this knowledge through clinical descriptions, illustrated by pictures collected over the years of the authors' experience. This work presents the particularities of dermatological diseases in solid organ transplant recipients and how to deal with them. In a single publication, you will find the extensive collaboration of researchers in this field working in several countries, giving a holistic vision of the individual who received a solid organ transplantation.

In this Atlas, the reader will also obtain a better understanding of immunosuppressant therapy through a chapter that includes the mechanism of action of immunosuppressive drugs and the strategies used to avoid graft rejection in different transplanted organs. It is a concise and complete publication in this essential subject.

The knowledge on cutaneous complications in solid organ transplant recipients is a growing challenge on us all.

São Paulo, SP, Brazil — Jane Tomimori
São Paulo, SP, Brazil — Walmar Roncalli Pereira de Oliveira
Barcelona, Spain — Carla Ferrándiz-Pulido
São Paulo, SP, Brazil — Marilia Marufuji Ogawa

Acknowledgments

We are indebted to all coauthors for their extraordinary contribution to this monograph and for their interest in the field of dermatologic diseases in solid organ transplant recipients.

We also would like to thank:

Adriana Maria Porro, MD, PhD, Associate professor, Department of Dermatology, Escola Paulista de Medicina, for providing pictures of hospitalized patients.

Álvaro Gómez-Tomás, Vall d'Hebron University Hospital, Barcelona, for providing dermatoscopic pictures.

Berta Ferrer Fàbregas, MD, Dermatopathologist, Vall d'Hebron Hospital, Barcelona, for providing histopathological pictures.

Christoph Höller, Department of Dermatology, Medical University of Vienna, for providing clinical pictures.

Julia Maria Ressler, Department of Dermatology, Medical University of Vienna, for providing clinical pictures.

Maria Teresa Martín-Gómez, MD, PhD, Vall d'Hebron Hospital, Barcelona, for providing fungal colonies pictures.

Maria Ubals, MD, Vall d'Hebron University Hospital, Barcelona, for providing clinical pictures.

Milvia Maria Simões e Silva Enokihara, MD, PhD, Adjunct professor, Department of Pathology, Escola Paulista de Medicina, for providing histopathological pictures.

Pabro Castro-Garcia, MD, Vall d'Hebron University Hospital, Barcelona, for providing dermatoscopic pictures.

Patricio Christian Godoy Martinez, PhD, Universidad Austral de Chile, for providing fungal colonies pictures.

Vicente García-Patos, MD, PhD, Vall d'Hebron Hospital, Barcelona, for providing clinical pictures.

Contents

Part III Neoplasic Diseases

Part I
Immunosuppression and Iatrogeny

Immunosuppression and Solid Organ Transplantation

Helio Tedesco Silva Jr.

1 Introduction

Significant advancements in solid organ transplantation immunosuppressive medications and regimens have resulted in improved short- and long-term outcomes over the last 20 years. Generally, patients receive induction therapy with depleting or non-depleting antibody agents followed by a combination of medications with complimentary mechanisms of action to inhibit cell activation and proliferation. Typically, a calcineurin inhibitor, an anti-metabolite agent, and a corticosteroid are used as the initial triple medication regimen. Reduction of the impact of long-term toxicities, such as chronic nephrotoxicities, cardiovascular diseases, infections, and malignancies is an unmet medical need. Alternative drug combinations seeking to avoid or spare the use of calcineurin inhibitors and corticosteroids have been investigated with inconsistent results. The target of rapamycin inhibitors has been used as an adjuvant treatment to reduce the incidence and progression of certain types of cancer, particularly those associated with oncoviruses. Relative success has been achieved in patients with non-melanoma skin cancer, Kaposi sarcoma, mantle cell lymphoma, and papillomavirus-associated skin lesions. Novel agents such as costimulatory blockers are under development and may allow a more personalized strategy for each recipient of solid organ transplant in the future.

H. T. Silva Jr. (✉)
Division of Nephrology, Hospital do Rim, Escola Paulista de Medicina,
Universidade Federal de São Paulo, São Paulo, SP, Brazil
e-mail: heliotedesco@medfarm.com.br

J. Tomimori et al. (eds.), *Atlas of Dermatologic Diseases in Solid Organ Transplant Recipients*, https://doi.org/10.1007/978-3-031-13335-0_1

2 The Immunobiology of Rejection

The innate and adaptive immunity comprise complex and redundant pathways with substantial functional overlap that are involved in the process of allograft rejection. These pathways integrate signals derived from antigen-independent and -dependent mechanisms leading to cellular activation, production of inflammatory chemokines and cytokines, cellular proliferation, and differentiation [1].

To understand the key mechanism of action of each immunosuppressive drug and the rational for the drug combinations used to prevent or treat acute allograft rejection, an oversimplification of the key phases of the alloimmune response is required. Dendritic cells of the allograft and the recipient origin become activated and move to secondary lymphoid organs to activate T cells via cognate T-cell receptors (Signal 1). Dendritic cells also provide various costimulatory signals, primarily by the interaction of CD80 (cluster of differentiation 80) and CD86 on the surface of dendritic cells with CD28 on T cells (Signal 2). The combination of Signals 1 and 2 provides maximal activation of three downstream transduction pathways (calcium–calcineurin, RAS–mitogen-activated protein kinase, and nuclear factor-kB). These pathways activate gene transcription of several interleukins and interleukin receptors, classically represented by the interleukin-2 and its receptor. The binding of interleukins to the respective receptors activates the mechanistic target of rapamycin, a protein complex system that coordinates several downstream pathways leading to nucleotide synthesis, cell growth, and proliferation and clonal expansion (Signal 3). Proliferation and differentiation lead to a large number of effector cytotoxic T cells [2] (Fig. 1a–e).

B-cell activation is predominantly through T-cell-dependent mechanisms. T-cell activation of B cells occurs by a three-stage pathway. Naive mature B cells recognize both membrane-bound and soluble alloantigens via B-cell receptor, providing an activation signal via CD19 complex (Signal 1). Primed B cells translocate into the T-cell-rich area, interacting with cognate follicular T helper (Tfh) cells to receive further activation signals. In addition to antigen recognition through the B cell receptor, the second signal for B cell activation is costimulation (Signal 2). A cognate interaction between helper T (Th) cells and B cells provides multiple costimulation signals for B-cell activation. CD40L from T cells signaling via CD40 on B cells drives B-cell proliferation, antibody affinity maturation, and class switch recombination. After alloantigen recognition and costimulation, B-cell activation requires cytokines (Signal 3), produced by various Th cells including Th1, Th2, and Th17. These Tfh cells provide IL-21 and costimulation and induce the proliferation of cognate B cells, isotype switching, and somatic mutation. This B cell expansion and differentiation lead to the formation of hyperplastic germinal centers in the B cell follicle. The germinal center response induces the differentiation of isotype-switched affinity mature B cells into memory B cells or into long-lived plasma cells [3].

Ultimately, without the use of immunosuppressive drugs, the integrated immune response rapidly generates the chemokines, interleukins, effector T cells, activated B cells, and alloantibodies required to produce irreversible allograft rejection.

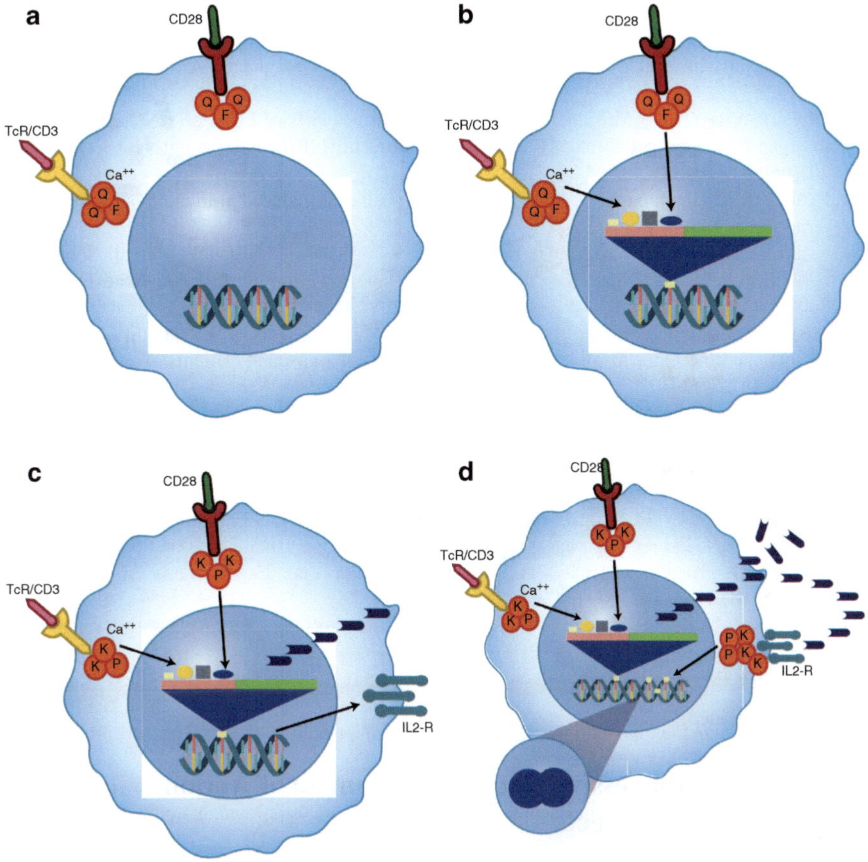

Fig. 1 (**a**) Activation of T cells via cognate T-cell receptors (Signal 1) and costimulatory signals, CD80 and CD86 on the surface of dendritic cells with CD28 on T cells (Signal 2). (**b**) The combination of Signals 1 and 2 provides maximal activation of three downstream transduction pathways (calcium–calcineurin, RAS–mitogen-activated protein kinase, and nuclear factor-kB). (**c**) These pathways activate gene transcription of several interleukins and interleukin receptors, classically represented by the interleukin-2 and its receptor. (**d**) The binding of interleukins to the respective receptors activates the mechanistic target of rapamycin, a protein complex system that coordinates several downstream pathways leading to nucleotide synthesis, cell growth, and proliferation and clonal expansion (Signal 3). (**e**) Proliferation and differentiation lead to a large number of effector cytotoxic T cells

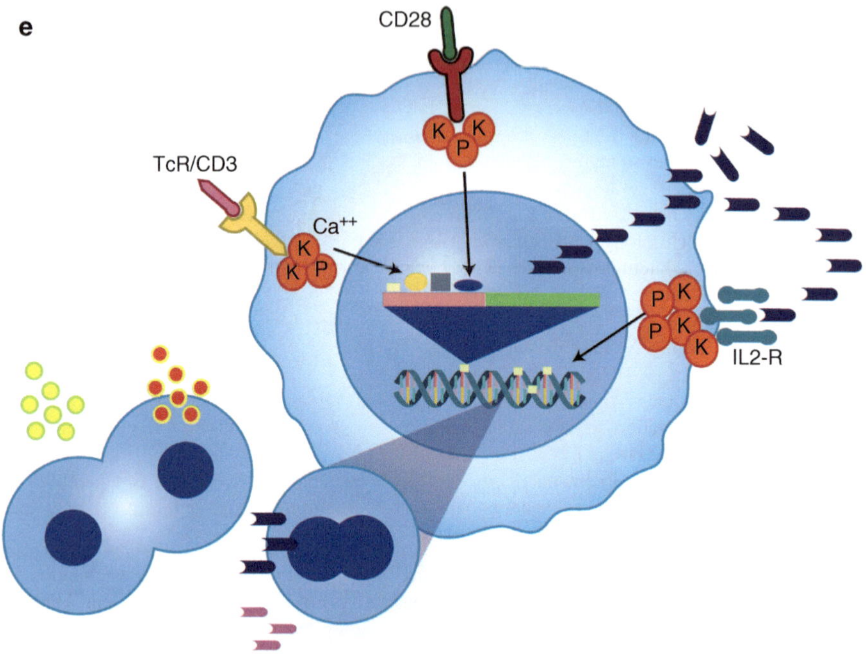

Fig. 1.1 (continued)

3 Immunosuppressive Drugs: Mechanism of Action and Adverse Effects

3.1 Monoclonal Antibodies

3.1.1 Anti-Interleukin-2 Receptor Blockers (Fig. 2)

Basiliximab (chimeric human/murine) and daclizumab (humanized) are non-depleting, monoclonal antibodies directed against the alpha chain of the IL-2 receptor (IL-2R) CD25, which is selectively expressed on the surface of activated T-lymphocytes. IL-2R is a heterotrimeric protein with alpha (CD25), beta (CD122), and gamma (CD132) subunit chains, expressed on the surface of lymphocytes. Binding to the three IL-2R chains triggers three intracellular signaling pathways, the mammalian mitogen-activated protein kinase, the phosphatidylinositol-3-kinase (PI3K), and the JAK-Signal (Janus kinase-Signal) Transducer and Activator of Transcription pathways, leading to cell proliferation and differentiation [4].

Basiliximab and daclizumab inhibit T-cell proliferation and differentiation but does not cause T-cell depletion [5, 6]. Daclizumab is no longer available for clinical use after solid organ transplantation. After its administrations as induction therapy, the pharmacodynamic effect of basiliximab, as measured by the presence of CD25-positive T cells in peripheral blood, lasts up to 2 months. Basiliximab is indicated

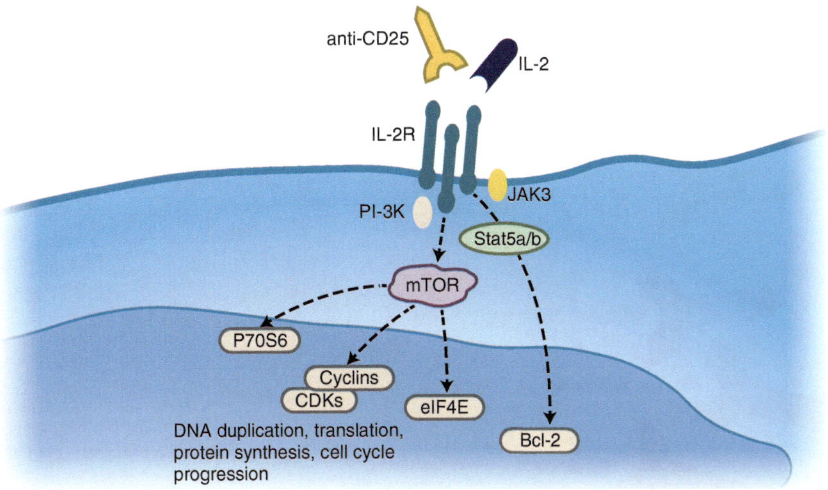

Fig. 2 Basiliximab, an anti-CD25 monoclonal antibodies bind to the α-chain of the interleukin (IL)-2R preventing transduction of IL-2R mediated proliferating signals. Bcl-2 = antiapoptotic protein that controls the intrinsic cell death pathway; CDKs = cyclin-dependent kinases; eIF4E = eukaryotic initiation factor 4E (required for initiation of translation); JAK3 = Janus kinase 3; mTOR = mammalian target of rapamycin; P70S6 = 70 kDa ribosomal S6 kinase; PI-3K = phosphatidylinositol-3-kinase; STAT5a/b = signal transducer and activator of transcription

for the prophylaxis of acute organ rejection in patients receiving renal transplantation when used as part of an immunosuppressive regimen that includes cyclosporine and corticosteroids. In adult patients, the recommended regimen is two doses of 20 mg given within 2 h prior to transplantation surgery and 4 days after transplantation, via central or peripheral line over the course of 20–30 min, without premedication or special monitoring during the infusion. Adverse effects and hypersensitivity reactions are uncommon [6].

3.1.2 **Alemtuzumab** (Fig. 3)

Alemtuzumab is a humanized, rat IgG1k monoclonal antibody directed against the CD52 cell surface antigen, producing depletion of T and B lymphocytes, NK (natural killer) cells, dendritic cells, granulocytes, and monocytes. Depletion occurs by complement-dependent cytotoxicity, antibody-dependent NK cells and macrophages cytotoxicity through their IgG fragment C receptor, and by induction of apoptosis. CD52 is one of the most abundant membrane glycoproteins on T and B lymphocytes and is also expressed on NK cells, monocytes, macrophages, dendritic cells, and eosinophilic granulocytes and to a lesser extent on neutrophilic granulocytes. The exact function of CD52 is unknown, but it is suggested that the molecule may be involved in T-lymphocyte co-stimulation, the induction of regulatory T lymphocytes, and T-lymphocyte migration and adhesion. Depletion occurs within 1 h

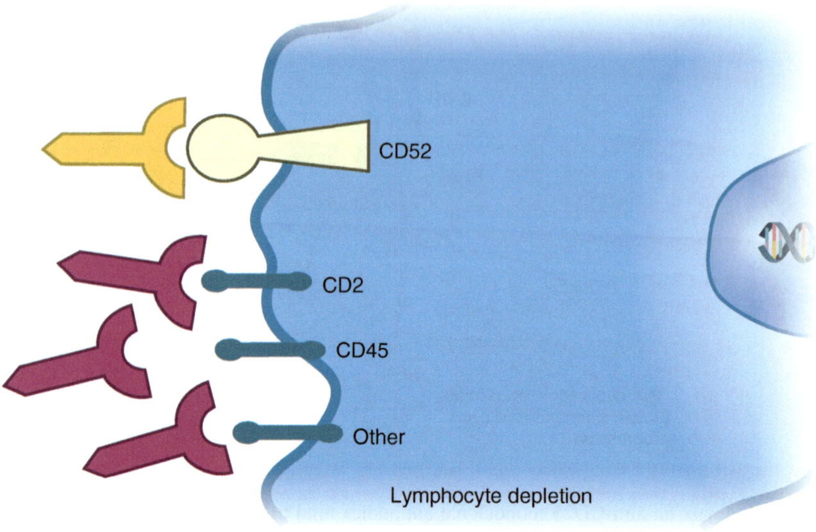

Fig. 3 Anti-CD52 monoclonal antibodies and anti-thymocyte polyclonal antibodies induce lymphocyte depletion

from peripheral lymphocytes and 3–5 days from secondary lymphoid tissues occurs over 3–5 days, lasting between 6 and 36 months depending on the cell line.

Alemtuzumab is approved for B-cell chronic lymphocytic leukemia, but it has been used off-label for both the prevention and treatment of acute allograft rejection in kidney, pancreas, intestinal, and lung transplantation. The recommended dose of alemtuzumab is 30 mg administered subcutaneously or intravenously over 2 h. When alemtuzumab is administered, vital signs should be monitored every 15–30 min until the infusion is complete. Complete blood counts (CBCs), which include platelet levels, should be monitored weekly during alemtuzumab therapy. Acute infusion-related reactions occur in 70–80% of patients and are caused by cytokine release from lysed immune cells. These reactions are mostly mild to moderate and include headache, rash, nausea, hypotension, rigors, and pyrexia. Following subcutaneous administration, infusion-related reactions occur less frequently, although local injection-site reactions do occur [7].

3.2 Polyclonal Antibodies

3.2.1 Anti-Thymocyte Globulin (Fig. 3)

Anti-thymocyte globulins (ATGs) are immunoglobulin G (IgG) preparations containing antibodies against T-cell markers such as CD2, CD3, CD4, CD8, CD11a, CD18, CD25, CD44, CD45, HLA-DR, HLA Class I heavy chains, and ß2 micro-globulin. ATG interacts with a large range of antigens on immune and non-immune cell types, inducing apoptosis of B cells, peripheral T cells and NK cells, and modulates leukocyte/endothelium interactions, homing and cytotoxic activities [8].

ATGs are produced from horses (hATG) or rabbits (rATG) immunized with human thymocytes. rATG is preferred over hATG because of increased potency and tolerability. In addition, rATG is superior to hATG in reversing and preventing rejection. rATG is dosed at 1.5 mg/kg and hATG is dosed at 10–15 mg/kg, adjusted based on platelet and white blood cell counts. However, dosing is often individualized based on patient-specific and center-specific protocols. In patients, T-cell depletion is usually observed within a day after initiating rATG therapy. rATG is approved by the FDA (Food and Drug Administration) for this the prevention and treatment of acute rejection [9].

The administration of rATG should be into a high-flow vein over the course of 6–8 h to minimize phlebitis, thrombosis, and systemic side effects. Antibodies in the ATG preparation may bind to the T-cell receptor, causing T-cell activation, producing the known cytokine release syndrome, which includes symptoms such as fever, chills, hypotension, and pulmonary edema and is most pronounced with the first dose. Acetaminophen, diphenhydramine, and a corticosteroid are administered prior to the ATG infusion to prevent the symptoms of cytokine release syndrome; however, cytokine release syndrome may occur despite administration of premedications. Frequent monitoring of vital signs is important during the administration of ATG [9, 10].

3.3 Calcineurin Inhibitors (Fig. 4)

Cyclosporine (CsA) and tacrolimus (TAC) are calcineurin inhibitors (CNI) that exert immunomodulatory effects by blocking T-cell infiltration, activation, and the subsequent release of inflammatory cytokines. After reaching the cytoplasm of T cells, cyclosporine binds to cyclophilin, forming a cyclosporine/cyclophilin complex while tacrolimus binds to FKBP12, forming a tacrolimus/FKBP12 complex. These two complexes have the ability to prevent calcineurin-mediated dephosphorylation of the nuclear factor of activated T cells and the consequent transcription of cytokine genes, including those of IL-2 and IL-4 [11]. Cyclosporine additionally inhibits p38 activation and JNK (c-Jun N-terminal kinase) activation, which leads to IL-2 production. The subsequent reduction in IL-2 levels further reduces the function of effector T cells.

Cyclosporine is approved for the prophylaxis of acute rejection after kidney, liver, and heart transplantation in conjunction with corticosteroids. Cyclosporine microemulsion is available as 10, 25, 50, and 100 mg soft gelatin capsules and as an oral solution containing 100 mg/ml. Cyclosporine dosing ranges from 4 to 12 mg/kg/day orally divided into two equal doses. Doses are adjusted based on whole blood through concentrations (C0), between 100 and 300 ng/mL, or 2 h whole blood concentrations (C2), between 600 and 2000 ng/mL [12].

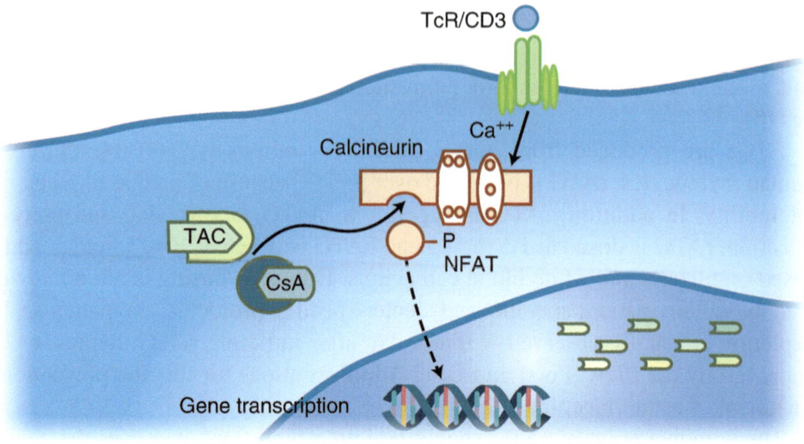

Fig. 4 Cyclosporine (cyclosporine [CsA])/cyclophilin and tacrolimus (TAC)/FKBP12 inhibit calcineurin phosphatase, preventing the nuclear migration of nuclear factor of activated T cell (NFAT) to initiate gene transcription

Tacrolimus is approved by the FDA for organ rejection prophylaxis in liver, kidney, and heart transplants. It is available as capsules of 0.5, 1, and 5 mg, or an intravenous (IV) formulation. Initial dosing is 0.075–0.2 mg/kg/day orally divided into two equal doses depending on the type of transplant. In 2013, a modified release tacrolimus product became available, allowing for once-daily dosing [13, 14]. Target therapeutic whole blood tacrolimus through concentrations vary depending on the type of organ transplant, time since transplant, concomitant immunosuppression, typically between 5 and 15 ng/mL [15].

Calcineurin inhibitors display an array of clinically relevant adverse effects. These adverse effects may be idiosyncratic or concentration dependent, acute and chronic, and eventually irreversible. Nephrotoxicity and hypertension, neurotoxicity, electrolyte abnormalities include hypomagnesemia, hyperkalemia, hyperlipidemia, hyperglycemia, post-transplant diabetes, and cosmetic changes such as alopecia, hirsutism, and gingival hyperplasia are the most prevalent reported adverse effects [16].

3.4 Anti-Metabolites

3.4.1 Azathioprine (Fig. 5)

The thioguanine derivative, azathioprine (AZA), is a prodrug of 6-mercaptopurine (6-MP), that is further metabolized into thiopurine active forms, sulfur analogs of the naturally occurring purine adenine, by various enzymes present in the liver and gut. 6-MP metabolites have been shown to inhibit de novo purine ribonucleotide

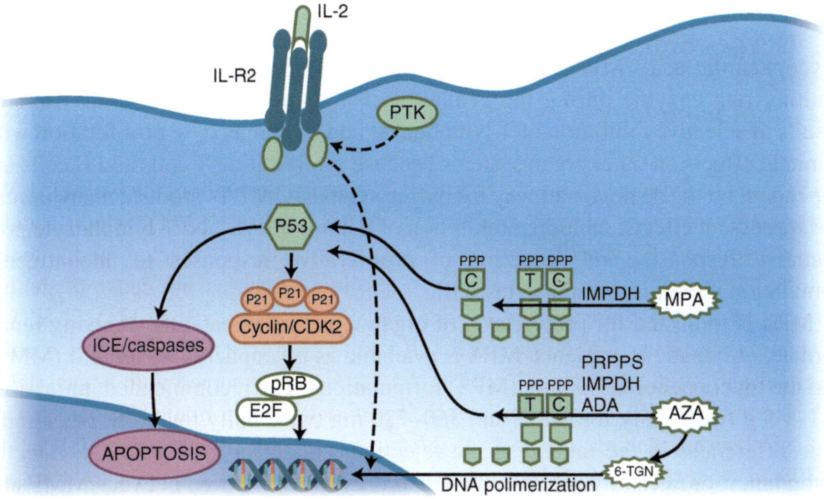

Fig. 5 Azathioprine (AZA) inhibits adenosine (A) and guanosine triphosphate (GTP) nucleotide synthesis; mycophenolic acid (MPA) selectively inhibits GTP nucleotide synthesis. Nucleotide imbalance induces receptor-mediated p53-dependent apoptotic cell death; 6-thioguanine nucleotide (6-TGN) inhibits DNA polymerization. *6-TGN* 6-thioguanine nucleotide, *A* adenosine, *ADA* adenosine deaminase, *CDK2* cyclin-dependent kinase 2, *C* cytidine, *E2F* E2 promoter-binding factor-1, *ICE* IL-1β converting enzyme, *IMPDH* inosine monophosphate dehydrogenase, *pRB* retinoblastoma protein, *PRPPS* phosphoribosyl pyrophosphate synthetase, *PTK* protein tyrosine kinase, *T* thymidine

synthesis and purine ribonucleotide interconversion to be incorporated into cellular RNA and DNA. The key mechanism of action may vary according to different cell types. For instance, incorporation of thioguanylate into cellular RNA may have a large inhibitory effect on a bone marrow cell but only a small effect on a circulating T-lymphocyte. While the incorporation of thiopurine nucleotides into cellular nucleic acids is a mechanism of cytotoxicity, inhibition of de novo purine ribonucleotide synthesis and interconversion is the predominant mechanism for growth inhibition [17]. 6-MP is metabolized via two major pathways, one of which is thiopurine S-methyltransferase (TPMT). Since TPMT activity is controlled by genetic polymorphisms that are present in 10% of the population, genotyping and phenotyping can identify patients at higher risk of developing azathioprine-associated toxicities [18].

Azathioprine is available as an oral formulation and is indicated for the prevention of rejection in renal transplantation. Azathioprine maintenance dosing, between 1 and 3 mg/kg/day, have been empirically selected to avoid overt toxicities.

The main adverse effects of azathioprine are hematologic and gastrointestinal. Dose-dependent myelosuppression can occur and can be reversed by dose reduction or discontinuation. Liver impairment, including cholestatic jaundice and hepatic veno-occlusive disease, has also been reported [19].

3.4.2 **Mycophenolate** (Fig. 5)

Mycophenolic acid (MPA) inhibits the inosine monophosphate dehydrogenase, a limiting rate enzyme during the synthesis of guanine nucleotide synthesis. This results in selective inhibition of T-lymphocyte and B-lymphocyte proliferation with minimal effects on other organ systems because proliferating T cells and B cells are dependent on the de novo pathway for purine synthesis. MPAs produce many immunosuppressant effects, including inhibition of B-lymphocyte and T-lymphocyte proliferative responses and reduction of proliferative responses to alloantigenic stimulation in human lymphocytes [20].

MPA is indicated for prophylaxis of organ rejection in patients receiving renal, cardiac, or hepatic transplants. MPA is available as mycophenolate mofetil (MMF) and the mycophenolate sodium (MPS) formulations. The recommended initial dose is 1–1.5 g twice daily for MMF and 360–720 mg twice daily for MPS. No significant differences in the rates of acute rejection, patient or graft survival, rates of malignancy, or rates of gastrointestinal disorders were observed between MMF and MPA [21].

The key adverse effects are gastrointestinal or hematological. MPA is administered as a fixed dose regimen, with dose reductions based on signs of toxicity. There is no consensus regarding the clinical utility of using plasma concentration monitoring to guide dose adjustments [22]. Women of childbearing age should be counseled on pregnancy prevention and planning due to the risk of first trimester pregnancy loss and congenital malformations with the use of mycophenolate [23].

3.5 Mammalian Target of Rapamycin Inhibitors (mTORi) (Fig. 6)

Sirolimus (SRL) and everolimus (EVR), once in the cytoplasm of the cells, form complexes with the 12 kDa immunophilin FK506-binding proteins (FKBP12/FKBP1A). These complexes bind to the (FKBP-rapamycin binding) FRB domain of one serine/threonine kinase, the mechanistic target of rapamycin (mTOR), ultimately cell proliferation [24]. mTOR controls cell growth, cell size, organ shape, and body plan. Mammals exhibit one mTOR protein, which represents the core component of two multi-subunit complexes. The TOR complex 1 (TORC1) integrates signals that sense the availability of amino acids, oxygen, growth factors as well as the cellular energy or stress levels. As a result, TORC1 promotes cell growth via its support of protein biosynthesis, cell cycle, and cellular metabolism as well as the inhibition of autophagy. The TOR complex 2 (TORC2) functions controls mainly the organization of the cytoskeleton. While the activity of TORC1 is blocked by SRL and EVR, TORC2 is insensitive [25].

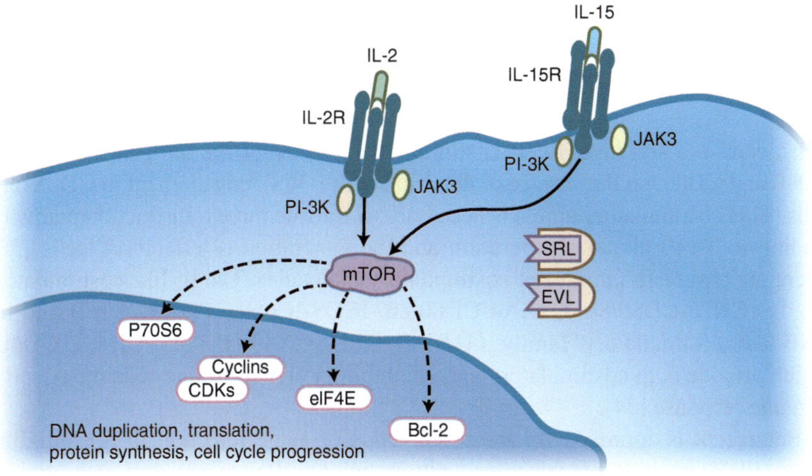

Fig. 6 Sirolimus (SRL)/FKBP12 and everolimus (EVL)/FKBP12 inhibit mammalian target of rapamycin (mTOR) pathway, which regulates G(1) cell cycle progression and translation initiation. Bcl-2 = antiapoptotic protein that controls the intrinsic cell death pathway; CDKs = cyclin-dependent kinases; eIF4E = eukaryotic initiation factor 4E (required for initiation of translation); JAK3 = Janus kinase 3; PI-3K = phosphatidylinositol-3-kinase; P70S6 = 70 kDa ribosomal S6 kinase

Sirolimus is approved for the prophylaxis of acute rejection after kidney transplantation. After an initial loading dose, the maintenance dosing of sirolimus is 2–5 mg once daily, adjusted to maintain through concentrations between 5 and 10 ng/mL in combination with CNIs. There are no well-defined target ranges in combination with other immunosuppressive drugs [26].

Everolimus is approved for the prevention of acute rejection in kidney, liver, and heart transplant recipients. Everolimus initial dosing is 0.75 mg twice daily in combination with cyclosporine or 1.5 mg twice daily in combination with tacrolimus. Doses should be adjusted to maintain a target whole through level of 3–8 ng/mL [27].

Sirolimus and everolimus produce a variety of adverse events. Their most important adverse effects are thrombocytopenia, leukopenia, hypercholesterolemia, stomatitis, diarrhea, and, although rare, interstitial pneumonitis. Adverse events particular for these immunosuppressive drug class are delayed wound healing, lymphoceles, recovery from ischemia reperfusion injury, and proteinuria [28, 29]. The use of sirolimus and everolimus increases the risk of developing venous thromboembolism after kidney, lung, heart, and liver transplant [30]. Treatment with an mTORi leads to increased endothelial activation, thrombin formation, and impaired fibrinolysis in renal transplant recipients [31]. Most adverse events are associated with whole blood drug concentration, and there are well-defined recommendations for the management of these adverse reactions [32].

3.6 *Costimulation Blockers*

3.6.1 **Belatacept** (Fig. 7)

Belatacept is a selective T-cell costimulation blocker of the antigen-independent CD80 and CD86, on the surface of dendritic cells (DCs), engagement to CD28 on T cells. This costimulatory signal is necessary to activate three transduction pathways leading to T-cell clonal proliferation and the generation of effector T cells [33]. There are two main families of costimulatory molecules. The Ig-like costimulatory family (CD28-CD80/86, CTLA4-CD80/86, ICOS-ICOSL, PD1-PDL1/2) and the TNF-like costimulatory family (41BB-41BBL, OX40-OX40L, CD40L-CD40), which provide both costimulatory and coinhibitory signals to fine-tune the adaptive immune response [34].

Belatacept is approved for the prophylaxis of acute rejection in Epstein–Barr virus (EBV)-positive kidney transplants recipients. Belatacept dosing is divided into two phases. In the initial phase, a dose of 10 mg/kg is administered intravenously on day 1 (day of transplant, prior to implantation), day 5, and at the end of weeks 2, 4, 8, and 12. The maintenance phase follows with an IV dose of 5 mg/kg at the end of week 16 and every 4 weeks thereafter [35].

Safety analysis indicates that the drug is well tolerated and there few and mild infusion-related adverse events. Patients who are EBV-negative have a higher risk of developing post-transplant lymphoproliferative disease (PTLD), including central nervous system PTLD. Most cases occurred in the first 24 months after transplantation. Risk factors for PTLD were EBV-status, T-cell depleting therapy, and

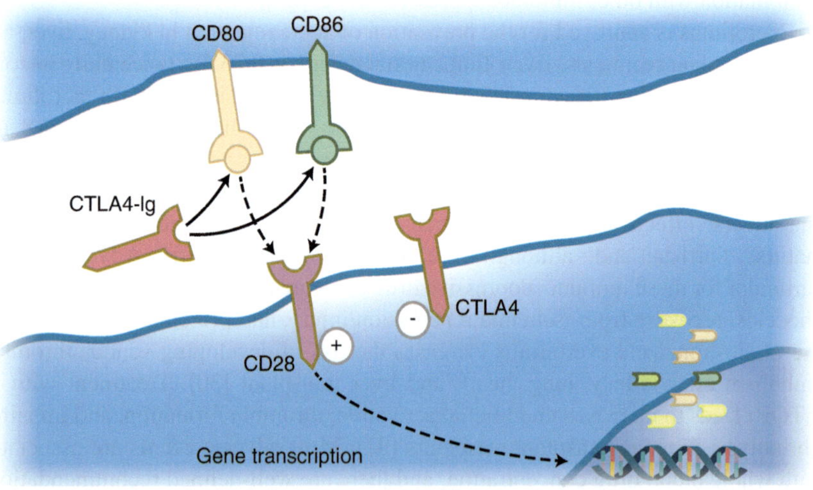

Fig. 7 Cytotoxic-T-lymphocyte (CTL)A4-Ig fusion protein (belatacept) blocks costimulation inhibiting gene transcription and lymphocyte activation

CMV infection. There was a higher incidence of central nervous system PTLD in belatacept groups, and even higher in the more intensive regimen, perhaps associated with the immunosuppressive [36]. There is no evidence of increased incidence of viral, bacterial, or fungal infections compared to patients receiving CNIs [37] although increased risk of tuberculosis has been observed in endemic countries [38].

3.7 Corticosteroids (Fig. 8)

Corticosteroids exhibit anti-inflammatory and immunosuppressive activity by inhibiting several stages of the T-cell activation cascade, including the synthesis of lipocortins which, by inhibiting phospholipase A2 activity, prevent arachidonic acid release from membrane-bound stores, blockade of select elements of the signal transduction pathways that operate as a consequence of T-cell activation, inhibition of leukocyte adhesion to target tissue, by down modulating leukocyte adhesion molecule expression and suppression of T-cell-derived and antigen-presenting cell-derived cytokine production and expression. However, it is likely that the glucocorticoids (GCs) may exert their effects by a multitude of mechanisms depending on the cell type and activation state [39].

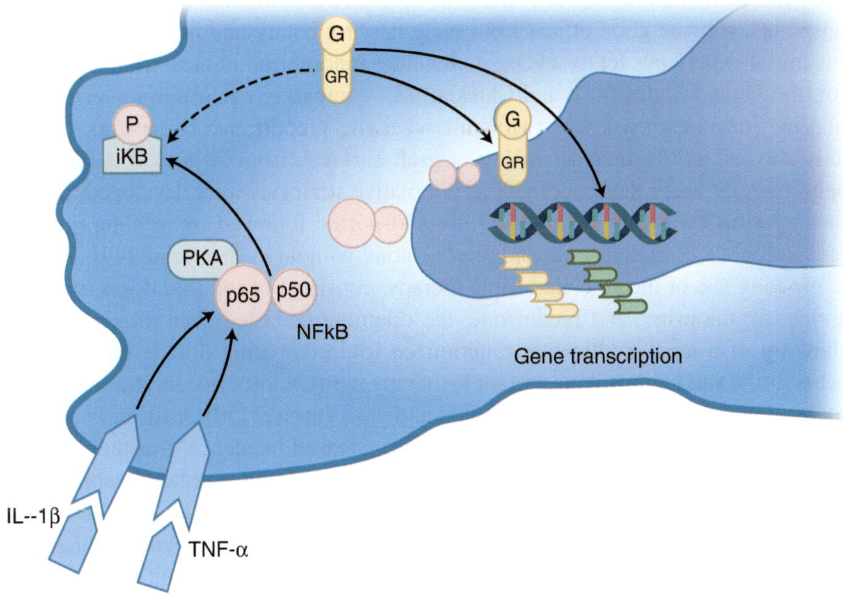

Fig. 8 Glucocorticoid/receptor binds directly to glucocorticoid (GC) responsive element or interferes with the binding of nuclear factor (NF)-κB inhibiting gene transcription. *GR* glucocorticoid receptor, *iκB* inhibitory NF-κB protein, *P* phosphate, *PKA* protein kinase A, *TNFα* tumor necrosis factor-α

Corticosteroids are available in several formulations including tablets, liquid, and injection. Most common used formulations are methylprednisolone for intravenous and prednisone or prednisolone for oral administration. GCs are associated to increased risk of post transplant diabetes mellitus (PTDM), osteopenia, osteoporosis and fractures, cardiovascular events, and cataracts [40].

4 Immunosuppressive Drug Regimens

4.1 Kidney

Azathioprine was first used as an immunosuppressive drug in 1961 [41]. During the first decade, the combination of azathioprine and corticosteroids was used to prevent acute rejection after kidney transplantation [42]. At this time, the 1-year deceased donor kidney graft survival was 53% [43]. In the late 1960s, induction therapy started with the use of horse anti-thymocyte globulin (ALG) preparations, allowing the reduction of the doses of azathioprine and prednisone. Interestingly, in the usual case, daily injections were started 5 days before surgery, continued each day for 10–17 days afterwards, then every other day for 2 weeks, twice a week for 2 months and once a week for 1 month, a dosing regimen far higher than the current use [44].

In 1978, a pilot study using cyclosporine as the sole immunosuppressant, at an astonishing initial 25 mg/kg daily dose, in 7 recipients of first deceased donor kidney transplants, showed good efficacy but early nephrotoxicity and hepatotoxicity [45]. This initial experience let to several multicenter randomized clinical trials in Europe [46], the United States [47], and Canada [48], comparing cyclosporine versus azathioprine in kidney transplant recipients receiving prednisone. These trials consistently showed a 20% increase in 1 year graft survival, from 50% to 70%. Because nephrotoxicity was a key issue, several alternative strategies were developed, including long-term cyclosporine, short-term cyclosporine followed by azathioprine and prednisolone, and azathioprine and prednisolone without cyclosporine [49]. Despite the growing use of the so-called triple therapy, consisted of reduced doses of cyclosporine, azathioprine, and prednisone, the dilemma persisted even after long-term follow-up of a large multicenter randomized trial comparing double therapy with cyclosporine and prednisolone and triple therapy with cyclosporine, azathioprine, and prednisolone showing comparable patient and graft survival [50]. Also, early elective cyclosporine withdrawal was associated with increased incidence of acute rejection without influencing short-term graft or patient survivals after renal transplantation [51]. Notwithstanding these initial dosing dilemmas, perhaps the critical role of cyclosporine was to confirm organ transplantation as the best therapeutic strategy for patients with end-stage chronic kidney, liver, heart, pancreas, and lung diseases.

In 1990, a new drug initially called FK506, currently tacrolimus, showed high efficacy for the prevention of acute rejection of kidneys, livers, and hearts [52]. Given that tacrolimus belongs to the same class of cyclosporine, similar concerns regarding nephrotoxicity emerged and alternative regimens were evaluated [53].

In 1995, three multicenter randomized trials showed that mycophenolate was associated with higher efficacy for the preservation of acute rejection compared to azathioprine or placebo in kidney transplant recipients receiving cyclosporine [54–56]. The combination of cyclosporine, mycophenolate, and corticosteroids became then the standard of care immunosuppressive regimen for kidney transplant recipients.

In 1997, multicenter randomized comparative trials conducted in the United States [57] and Europe [58] confirmed the higher efficacy of tacrolimus for the prevention of acute rejection compared to cyclosporine, suggesting that tacrolimus would be the preferred CNI to be used after solid organ transplantation. Eventually tacrolimus became the preferred calcineurin inhibitor choice in most of the transplant centers.

Early in 2000, anti-IL2R blockers were introduced in clinical practice. Between 1997 and 2000, two multicenter trails showed that induction therapy with basiliximab was associated with reduced incidence of acute rejection in kidney transplant recipients receiving cyclosporine and prednisone [59, 60] or cyclosporine, azathioprine, and prednisone [61]. Similar results were observed with daclizumab, another anti-IL2R blocker that is no longer used in transplant recipients [62, 63].

In parallel, the mTORi were developed, first as a substitute for the CNIs. In 2000 and 2001, two prospective, multicenter, randomized, double-blind trials showed that the addition of sirolimus, compared with azathioprine [64] or placebo [65] to a cyclosporine and prednisone regimen was associated with reduced incidence of acute rejection episodes. Because of the potential nephrotoxic drug-to-drug interaction between mTORi and CNI, a further study investigated the efficacy of cyclosporine withdrawal from a sirolimus CsA-steroid regimen at 3 months, showing improvement in renal function but a slight increase in the incidence of acute rejection after CsA discontinuation [66]. Subsequently, several studies demonstrated that mTORi did not have sufficient efficacy for the prevention of acute rejection without the concomitant use of CNI [67]. For almost 20 years, several studies investigated the efficacy and safety of the combination of the CNIs with the mTORi, from the day of the transplant or as a conversion strategy, either early, within the first 6 months after transplantation, or late, after the first year [67–69].

Given the growing number of possible drug combinations, it became difficult to determine the best regime. For regulatory purposes, the combination of cyclosporine, mycophenolate, and prednisone was considered the standard of care regimen although accumulating data suggested that tacrolimus was associated with improved efficacy for the prevention of acute rejection compared to cyclosporine.

While the use of anti-IL2R blockers, tacrolimus, mycophenolate, and corticosteroids increased over time, it was only after the landmark clinical trial Symphony that this drug combination became the new standard of care regimen after kidney transplantation. The Symphony trial addressed this issue [70], confirming that induction therapy with anti-IL2R receptor blocker combined with reduced doses of tacrolimus, mycophenolate, and prednisone was associated with lower incidence of acute rejection, better renal function, and graft survival 1 year after kidney transplantation, ultimately becoming the current standard of care immunosuppressive regimen.

Later, in 2010, the combination of anti-IL2R receptor blocker with reduced doses of cyclosporine, everolimus, and prednisone were approved by the FDA [71]. More recently, everolimus showed comparable efficacy for the prevention of acute rejection and similar kidney function compared to mycophenolate in kidney transplant recipients receiving induction therapy with anti-IL2R receptor blocker or anti-thymocyte globulin, cyclosporine or tacrolimus, and prednisone [72].

Finally, the interest in induction therapy with depleting agents, anti-thymocyte globulin or alemtuzumab, reemerged, with several objectives, including induction of tolerance, corticosteroid or CNI avoidance of sparring regimens, and prevention of acute rejection in high risk patients such as sensitized patients, retransplants, and patients with delayed graft function [9].

There were several CNI avoidance and sparing studies to minimize the cardiovascular, metabolic, and nephrotoxic effects. These studies combined mycophenolate and mTORi without CNI [73, 74], and early (<6 months) [75–78] or late (>6 months) [79, 80] conversion from CNIs to mTORi after transplantation. Yet, the majority of these studies showed increased incidence of acute rejection and toxic adverse events with small benefit in kidney function [67].

Belatacept is the first costimulatory blocker approved for the prevention of acute rejection after kidney transplantation [81]. In two prospective multicenter trials in recipients of kidneys from standard [82] or extended criteria donor [83], the use of belatacept was associated with superior renal function and similar patient and graft survival compared to cyclosporine at 1-year post-transplant, despite a higher rate of early acute rejection. Seven years after transplantation, patient and graft survival and the mean eGFR were significantly higher with belatacept than with cyclosporine [35]. A meta-analysis including five studies that compared belatacept and CNIs concluded that there is no evidence of any difference in the effectiveness of belatacept and CNI in preventing acute rejection, graft loss and death, but treatment with belatacept is associated with less chronic kidney scarring and better kidney transplant function. Treatment with belatacept is also associated with better blood pressure and lipid profile and a lower incidence of diabetes mellitus versus treatment with CNI. Important side effects (particularly PTLD) remain poorly reported and so the relative benefits and harms of using belatacept remain unclear [84]. Finally, in a recent trial, kidney transplant recipients were randomized to receive alemtuzumab/belatacept, rabbit anti-thymocyte globulin (rATG)/belatacept, or rATG/tacrolimus. The composite primary endpoint consisted of patient death, renal allograft loss, or a modification of diet in renal disease-calculated eGFR of <45 mL/min/1.73 m^2 at 12 months. Belatacept-based CNI avoidance with early steroid withdrawal regimens did not prove to be superior for the primary or secondary endpoints. Belatacept-treated patients demonstrated an increase in biopsy-proved acute cellular rejection and reduced neurologic and metabolic adverse events [85].

4.2 Liver

Liver transplantation became an effective and safe therapy after the development of the cyclosporine-based immunosuppressive regimens. In one of the first randomized clinical trials in liver transplant recipients, the efficacy and safety of the conventional cyclosporine-based was compared to tacrolimus-based immunosuppressive regimen in 545 liver transplant recipients from eight European centers. The use of tacrolimus was associated with a significant reduction in acute rejection episodes, from 49.8% to 40.5% [86]. A follow-up open-label, randomized, multicenter trial showed similar results [87].

In another multicenter randomized trial involving 606 patients, a reduction in the composite endpoint of death, retransplantation, or treatment failure for immunological reasons was observed in patients receiving tacrolimus (21%) compared to cyclosporine microemulsion formulation (32%) [88]. Subsequently, in a multicenter, randomized, open-label study involving 495 liver transplant recipients, the incidence of acute rejection at 3 months was comparable between patients receiving cyclosporine microemulsion, with cyclosporine doses adjusted based on 2 h blood concentrations, or tacrolimus (26% vs. 24%) [89].

The use of induction therapy with basiliximab was associated with lower incidence of biopsy-confirmed acute rejection (35.1% vs. 43.5%) and the composite endpoint of death, graft loss, or first biopsy-confirmed acute rejection (44.1% vs. 52.8%) compared to placebo at 6 months in 381 recipients of liver transplants receiving cyclosporine and steroids [90].

In a randomized, double-blind comparative study the use of MMF was associated with reduced incidence of acute rejection or graft loss compared to azathioprine in 565 liver transplant recipients receiving cyclosporine and corticosteroids (38.5% vs. 47.7%) [91].

A follow-up study showed that, compared to the standard-dose tacrolimus, reduced-dose tacrolimus with MMF was not associated with increased incidence of acute graft rejection (30% vs. 46%) but with reduced incidence of renal dysfunction or arterial hypertension or diabetes mellitus (64% vs. 80%) [92].

In a prospective, open-label, multicenter study, conversion from CNI/MMF to SRL/MMF 4–12 weeks after liver transplantation was associated with improvement in renal function but with increased incidence of biopsy confirmed acute rejection (12.2% vs. 4.1%) and graft loss (8.3% vs. 3.4%) compared to patients maintained with CNI/MMF [93]. In another study in liver transplant recipients receiving basiliximab induction, tacrolimus and MPS, with or without steroids, conversion from tacrolimus to everolimus 4 weeks after transplantation showed similar results [94]. A subsequent study confirmed the higher incidence of acute rejection in patients converted from tacrolimus to everolimus 4 weeks after liver transplantation. On the other hand, everolimus combined with reduced TAC concentrations was noninferior to standard tacrolimus concentration for the primary efficacy endpoint, treated biopsy confirmed acute rejection, graft loss, or death at 12 months (6.7% vs. 9.7%) and was associated with superior renal function [95].

In summary, induction therapy with basiliximab followed by tacrolimus and mycophenolate, with or without corticosteroids, is the current standard of care treatment for liver transplant recipients. The use of everolimus combined with reduced concentrations of tacrolimus is an alternative that is associated with comparable efficacy and superior renal function.

4.3 Heart

The introduction of cyclosporine stimulated the development of several clinical trials in heart transplant recipients. The first study included 32 patients randomized to receive pretransplant transfusion, prednisone, azathioprine, and rabbit anti-thymocyte globulin ($n = 14$) or cyclosporine and prednisone ($n = 18$). There were no differences in mortality or number of rejection episodes per patient. The initial concern was renal dysfunction and hypertension in patients treated with cyclosporine [96].

A subsequent study in 82 heart transplant recipients compared the use of tacrolimus- ($n = 54$) or cyclosporine-based therapy ($n = 28$). No significant differences were evident between the two treatment groups in either rejection (26.3% vs. 18.5%) or survival rates (79.6% vs. 92.9%) at 1 year [97].

In a double-blind, active-controlled, randomized trial including 650 patients receiving cyclosporine and corticosteroids, the use of MMF was associated with reduction in mortality (6.2% vs. 11.4%) and in the requirement for rejection treatment (65.7% vs. 73.7%) compared to azathioprine [98].

In a single-blind, multicenter trial including 154 de novo heart transplant patients who were treated with cyclosporine microemulsion and corticosteroids, the incidence of treated biopsy-proven acute rejection, graft loss or death was comparable among patients receiving MPS compared to MMF (57.7% vs. 60.5%), with similar overall safety profile [99].

In a small study, the use induction therapy with rabbit anti-thymocyte globulin (rATG) was associated with higher freedom from treated acute rejection grade 3A or more compared to basiliximab (83% vs. 65%) in heart transplant patients receiving cyclosporine, mycophenolate mofetil, and prednisone [100].

A multicenter study including 380 patients undergoing de novo cardiac transplants showed lower incidence of severe rejections (6.9% vs. 17.7%) but similar allograft and recipient survivals comparing CsA microemulsion and oil-based formulation of CsA after 24 months of followup [101].

To further explore the ideal combination of immunosuppressive agents for cardiac transplant recipients, 343 de novo cardiac transplant recipients were randomized to receive steroids and either TAC and SRL, TAC and MMF, or CsA and MMF, with antilymphocyte induction therapy. There was no difference in the incidence of ≥3A rejection or hemodynamic compromise rejection requiring treatment at 6 months (TAC/MMF 22.4%, TAC/SRL 24.3%, CsA/MMF 31.6%). Compared to CsA, patients receiving TAC showed lower incidence of any treated rejection (TAC/SRL 35%, TAC/MMF 42%, CsA/MMF 59%). Altogether, the data suggested that the TAC/MMF combination appears to offer more advantages than TAC/SRL or CsA/MMF in cardiac transplant patients, showing higher efficacy for the prevention of acute rejection and improved side effect profile [102].

A large prospective study involving 634 recipients of heart transplants receiving cyclosporine, corticosteroids, and statins showed lower efficacy failure (27% vs. 36.4% vs. 46.7%), smaller increase in maximal coronary intimal thickness, lower incidence of vasculopathy (35.7% vs. 30.4% vs. 52.8%), and CMV infections (7.7%

vs. 7.6% vs. 21.5%), but higher incidence of bacterial infections and inferior renal function comparing patients receiving everolimus 3.0 mg, everolimus 1.5 mg or azathioprine [103].

In a subsequent study, cardiac transplant patients receiving induction therapy (as per center practice) and corticosteroids were randomized to initiate everolimus, with doses adjusted to maintain whole blood through concentrations between 3 and 8 ng/mL, in combination with reduced CsA or MMF (3 g/day) with standard CsA. The 12-month incidence of biopsy-proven acute rejection ≥3A was 22.8% with everolimus and 29.8% with MMF, with a 3.9 ml/min mean lower glomerular filtration rate in the everolimus group at 12 months [104].

In a follow-up study, 282 maintenance thoracic transplant patients >1-year post-transplant were randomized to continue their current CNI-based immunosuppression or start everolimus with predefined CNI exposure reduction. From baseline to month 12, mean cyclosporine and tacrolimus through concentrations in the everolimus cohort decreased by 57% and 56%, respectively. Mean change in measured glomerular filtration rate from baseline to month 12, was 4.6 mL/min with everolimus and −0.5 mL/min in controls. While there was no difference in the incidence of biopsy-proven treated acute rejection, the incidence of adverse event and serious adverse events was higher after conversion to everolimus [105].

In an open-label, 24-month trial, 721 de novo heart transplant recipients receiving induction therapy (as per center practice) and were randomized to everolimus 1.5 or 3.0 mg with reduced-dose cyclosporine, or mycophenolate mofetil (MMF) 3 g/day with standard-dose cyclosporine. Everolimus 3.0 mg was terminated prematurely due to higher mortality. There was no difference in the incidence of efficacy failure (biopsy-proven acute rejection, acute rejection associated with hemodynamic compromise, graft loss/retransplant, death or loss to follow-up) comparing everolimus 1.5 mg and MMF (35.1% vs. 33.6%) and month 24. The mean increase in maximal intimal thickness was lower with everolimus 1.5 mg versus MMF. Everolimus 1.5 mg still showed inferior renal function and higher incidence of serious adverse events. Everolimus 1.5 mg with reduced-dose cyclosporine offers similar efficacy to MMF with standard-dose cyclosporine and reduces intimal proliferation at 12 months in de novo heart transplant recipients [106].

In a randomized, open-label trial, de novo heart transplant recipients receiving MMF and steroids were randomized to everolimus with reduced-exposure calcineurin inhibitor followed by cyclosporine withdrawal or standard-exposure cyclosporine. Patients in the EVR/MMF group showed superior renal function (77.4 mL/min vs. 59.2 mL/min), reduced progression of allograft vasculopathy at 36 months but higher biopsy-proven acute rejection (10.2% vs. 5.9%), serious adverse events (37.3% vs. 19.6%), suggesting that early CNI withdrawal after heart transplantation supported by everolimus, mycophenolic acid and steroids with lymphocyte-depleting induction is feasible for selected patients [107].

In de novo heart transplant recipients receiving reduced-dose cyclosporine and corticosteroids, higher incidence of a composite safety endpoint (wound healing delays, pericardial effusion, pleural effusion needing drainage, and renal insufficiency events) was observed comparing immediate (EVR-I) or delayed everolimus

(EVR-D) (44.9% vs. 32.6%), without difference in efficacy failure, defined as the cumulative incidence of biopsy-proven rejection ≥2R, rejection with hemodynamic compromise, graft loss, or death (37.1% vs. 28.3%) [108].

In summary, the traditional combination of a calcineurin inhibitor, CSA or TAC, an anti-metabolite drug, AZA or MMF, and corticosteroids are used in the majority of patients. There is no definitive conclusion on the risk and benefit assessment of the clinical utility of induction therapy. Novel immunosuppressive drugs, such as mTORi, and strategies to minimize the use of CNIs and corticosteroids are under investigation, aiming to reduce several short- and long-term complications including nephrotoxicity, vasculopathy, viral infections and malignancies [109].

4.4 Lung

Transplantation became a successful treatment option for patients with chronic lung disease after the introduction of cyclosporine, in combination with azathioprine, and prednisone, with or without the use of anti-thymocyte globulin, despite the relatively high incidence of acute rejection [110].

After the demonstrations of the efficacy of MMF for the prevention of acute rejection after kidney transplantation, several clinical trials were conducted in lung transplant recipients. In one of the first studies, including 81 consecutive lung transplant recipients receiving cyclosporine and corticosteroids, there was no difference in the incidence of acute rejection (58% vs. 63%) and patient survival (86% vs. 82%) at 6 months comparing patients receiving AZA or MMF [111]. Another study compared the effects of MMF with AZA in combination with induction therapy, cyclosporine and corticosteroids in patients receiving their first lung transplant. The incidence of acute rejection did not differ between groups (56.6% vs. 60.3%), and there was no difference in survival or in the incidence, severity or time to acquisition of bronchiolitis obliterans syndrome (BOS) between the two groups [112].

There were no differences in the freedom from acute rejection and in 1-year patient survival (73.1% vs. 79.2%) among 50 lung transplant recipients received induction therapy with rabbit anti-thymocyte globulin (ATG), MMF, and steroids and were randomized to TAC or CsA [113]. In another trial including 249 recipients of lung transplant receiving MMF and prednisone without induction therapy, the incidence of BOS was lower among patients receiving tacrolimus compared to cyclosporine (11.6% vs. 21.3%) with no difference in the incidence of acute rejection (67.4% vs. 74.9%) and patient survival (78.7% vs. 88.6%) at 3 years [114]. In a prospective, two-center, open randomized trial, 74 lung transplant recipients receiving induction therapy with rabbit anti-thymocyte globulin, mycophenolate, and corticosteroids were randomized to receive either cyclosporine A (n = 37) or tacrolimus (n = 37). There was no difference in freedom from acute rejection (35% vs. 46%) and patient survival (82% vs. 71%) at 12 months. The incidence of new-onset diabetes mellitus was higher (11% vs. 0%) but the incidence of hypertension (60% vs. 11%) was lower among patients receiving tacrolimus [115].

This multicenter trial in 181 patients receiving tacrolimus-based immunosuppressive regimen showed no difference in the incidence of acute and chronic rejection and in graft survival comparing patients receiving sirolimus (SRL) or azathioprine (AZA). The incidence of cytomegalovirus was lower, but the incidence of adverse events was higher (64% vs. 49%) in patients receiving SRL study [116]. In another study, the use of everolimus was associated with reduced progression of BOS in recipients of lung transplantation compared to AZA. Yet, treatment discontinuations, serious adverse events and high serum creatinine values were more common with everolimus [117]. In another trial, the use of enteric-coated mycophenolate sodium was compared to delayed-onset of everolimus, in combination with cyclosporine monitored and corticosteroids without induction therapy. There was no difference in 3 years freedom from BOS Grade 1 (70% vs. 71%), patient survival (84% vs. 76%). The incidence of biopsy-proven acute rejection, leucopenia, diarrhea, and cytomegalovirus infection was higher in the MPS group, whereas venous thromboembolism was more frequent in the everolimus group. There was no difference in mean creatinine values at 3 years (160 ± 112 μmol/L vs 152 ± 98 μmol/L [118].

In a prospective multicenter trial, patients 3–18 months after lung transplantation were randomized to receive quadruple low CNI regimen ($n = 67$, everolimus, tacrolimus or cyclosporine, AZA/MMF/MPS, and prednisone) or the standard triple CNI regimen ($n = 63$, tacrolimus or cyclosporine, AZA/MMF/MPS, and prednisone). The eGFR after 12 months was superior in the quadruple low CNI regimen (64.5 mL/min vs. 54.6 mL/min). Biopsy-proven acute rejection, chronic lung allograft dysfunction, death and safety endpoints were similar between both groups [119].

In summary, immunosuppression in lung transplant is evolving with the development of newer drugs, such as costimulation blockers and mTOR inhibitors, and promising strategies to optimize immunosuppression, attempting to mitigate the long-term nephrotoxic effects of calcineurin inhibitors. Further studies with multicenter randomized trials are required to increase the strength of the evidence [120].

4.5 Pancreas

Similar to liver, heart, and lung, simultaneous pancreas-kidney transplantation has become an accepted therapy for type 1 diabetic patients with end-stage renal disease, after the introduction of cyclosporine. After a few single-center studies, an open-label, multicenter trial compared the efficacy and safety of tacrolimus ($n = 103$) with the microemulsion (ME) formulation of cyclosporine ($n = 102$). All patients received concomitant rabbit anti-T-cell globulin induction therapy, mycophenolate mofetil (MMF), and short-term corticosteroids. The 1-year incidence of biopsy-proven kidney or pancreas acute rejection was lower with tacrolimus (27.2% vs. 38.2%). Pancreas graft survival was higher with tacrolimus (91.3% vs. 74.5%) but no difference was observed in kidney graft survival [121].

The role of induction therapy with anti-IL-2 blocker was investigated in a subsequent multicenter, prospective, open-label study, where simultaneous kidney-pancreas transplant (SKPT) recipients receiving TAC, MMF, and steroids were randomized to receive daclizumab 1 mg/kg/dose every 14 days for five doses (Group I, $n = 107$), daclizumab 2 mg/kg/dose every 14 days for two doses (Group II, $n = 112$), and no antibody induction (Group III, $n = 78$). At 6 months, there were no differences in patient, kidney, and pancreas graft survival rates among the three groups. The probability of either kidney or pancreas allograft rejection at 6 months was 21%, 17%, and 32%. The actuarial event-free survival (no acute rejection, allograft loss, or death) rates were 66%, 77%, and 56%. Daclizumab is safe and effective in reducing the incidence of acute rejection in SKPT recipients compared with no antibody induction. Moreover, the two-dose regimen of daclizumab (2 mg/kg on days 0 and 14) compares favorably with the standard five-dose regimen [122]. A subsequent study compared clinical outcomes of SPKT recipients ($n = 174$) receiving tacrolimus, mycophenolate mofetil, and corticosteroids without or with any type of induction therapy. There were no differences between treatment groups for treated of biopsy-confirmed or presumptive rejection episodes, patient, kidney, and pancreas graft survival at 1 year. Decisions regarding the routine use of induction therapy in SPKT must take into consideration its differential effects on risk of rejection and infection [123].

mTORis are generally considered second-line immunosuppressive agents because of associations with increased rejection rates and impaired wound healing. Yet, because its association with decreased inflammatory response in pancreatitis, and antiproliferative and antiangiogenic activity, it has been used after SPKT in some centers. Despite the lack of large multicenter trials, a registry data analysis including 25,837 patients suggested that the use of mTORi group was associated with higher patient survival rate 1, 3, 5, and 10 years post-transplant compared to non-mTORi-based immunosuppression [124].

4.6 Multivisceral

There is a paucity of data on long-term outcomes following visceral transplantation. Types of visceral transplants include isolated intestinal transplant, combined liver-intestinal transplant, multivisceral transplant, and modified multivisceral transplant. These types remain a good option for treatment of end-stage intestinal failure with parenteral nutritional complications. Proper graft selection, shorter cold ischemia time, and improvement of immunosuppression regimens could significantly improve the long-term survival. These patients receive typically induction therapy with rATG and triple therapy with tacrolimus, mycophenolate, and prednisone [125]. Current guidelines restrict intestinal transplantation to patients who have had significant complications from parenteral nutrition including liver failure and repeated infections. Future research should focus on detecting biomarkers of early rejection, enhanced immunosuppression protocols, improved postoperative care, and early referral to transplant centers [126].

4.7 Vascularized Composite Allotransplant

Vascularized composite allotransplantation (VCA) has become a viable reconstructive option for individuals with amputations and severe facial disfigurements. VCA is not a life-saving procedure, raising concerns on the long-term adverse effects of standard maintenance triple therapy with corticosteroids, tacrolimus, and mycophenolate mofetil. Furthermore, it is uncertain whether VCA recipients may require greater maintenance immunosuppression than solid organ transplant recipients (SOTRs) due to the higher antigenicity of skin. A recent systematic literature review suggests VCA and kidney recipients receive comparable MMF/prednisone doses, including tacrolimus target through concentrations [127].

5 Risks and Benefits of the Immunosuppressive Drug Regimens

The historical development of immunosuppressive regimens started with the first kidney transplant performed in 1950. Interestingly, there was no mechanistic rational for the development of the drugs and the drug combinations to prevent and treat rejection of the transplanted organ. In fact, the in vitro and in vivo experimental use of several compounds was the tool to further understand the cellular and molecular mechanisms of the alloimmune response.

The key systems affected by the immunosuppressive regimens are infection, cardiovascular, malignancies, and bone marrow and metabolic disturbances.

Induction with depleting agents has been associated with increased incidence of bone marrow toxicity and infections, particularly viral infections such as herpes simples, herpes zoster, cytomegalovirus, and polyomavirus. Historically, high doses of depleting agents were also associated with an increase incidence of malignancies [10, 128, 129].

CNIs have been associated with worsening of preexisting cardiovascular diseases, increased incidence of new cardiovascular disease, acute and chronic nephrotoxicity, increased incidence of metabolic disturbances such as post-transplant diabetes mellitus and dyslipidemia, and malignancies [130, 131].

Anti-metabolites have been associated with bone marrow toxicity and infections, particularly viral infections such as herpes simples, herpes zoster, cytomegalovirus and polyomavirus, and malignancies.

mTORi have been associated with worsening of preexisting cardiovascular diseases, increased incidence of new cardiovascular disease, acute and chronic nephrotoxicity, increased incidence of metabolic disturbances such as post-transplant diabetes mellitus and dyslipidemia, and malignancies [32].

Corticosteroids have been associated with worsening of preexisting cardiovascular diseases, increased incidence of new cardiovascular disease, increased incidence of metabolic disturbances such as post-transplant diabetes mellitus and dyslipidemia, growth retard in children, bone diseases [40].

While each drug has a particular safety profile, and many have been associated with distinct and typical adverse events, the safety profile is routinely attributed to the drug combination. Currently, the majority of SOTRs receive a combination of three drugs as maintenance therapy, with or without an induction agent depending upon the perceived risk. Typically, this drug combination is constituted of a CNI in association with mycophenolate and corticosteroids [70].

An alternative regimen includes the association of a CNI with an mTORi and corticosteroids [72]. One relevant aspect is the data that suggests that the use of mTORi is associated with lower incidence of malignancies after transplantation, primarily malignancies associated with oncoviruses [69, 132].

Skin cancers account for 40–50% of all post-transplant malignancies and tend to be more aggressive than in the general population. The most commonly reported skin cancers are cutaneous squamous cell carcinoma (SCC) and basal cell carcinoma (BCC), together accounting for 90–95% of skin cancers, followed by Kaposi sarcoma (KS), Merkel cell carcinoma (MCC), and malignant melanoma (MM). Skin cancers are associated with higher morbidity and mortality in SOTRs and therefore screening and early diagnosis are critical to institute timely and effective treatments [133]. A meta-analysis of randomized clinical trials indicated that the use of sirolimus-based immunosuppression was associated with a reduced risk of non-melanoma skin cancer among kidney transplant recipients [134]. Yet, a recent meta-analysis did not show a significant risk reduction against primary or secondary non-melanoma skin cancer (NMSC) in non-kidney transplant recipients receiving mTOR inhibitors [135].

Recipients of solid organ transplants are at higher risk for other virus-associated cutaneous lesions [136], including human papillomavirus (HPV) infections, with clinical presentation ranging from premalignant lesions, warts, or cancer of the cervix, penis, vulva, scrotum, and anal canal adverse events [137]. There are mechanistic evidences suggesting that mTOR inhibition protects HPV-E6/E7 expressing tissues form SCC development upon carcinogen exposure, supporting the clinical use of mTOR inhibitors for the prevention of HPV-associated malignancies [138, 139]. In fact, conversion to mTORi-based immunosuppressive regimen has been associated with clinical improvement in transplant recipients with recalcitrant warts [140–142].

Despite the mechanistic rationale for mTOR inhibitors in cancer therapy [143], success rates in clinical trials with advanced malignancies are not consistent, except for Kaposi sarcoma [144] and mantle cell lymphoma [145]. Because mTOR inhibitors are primarily cytostatic, not cytotoxic, the observed clinical efficacy is a reflection of disease stabilization rather than tumor regression, and is influenced by timing of initiation, use of concomitant immunosuppressive drugs, and type of cancer. Non-melanoma skin cancers, in particular cutaneous SCCs, have the highest standardized incidence ratios in transplant recipients. Recent meta-analyses and randomized trials on secondary prevention of SCC observed a reduction in cumulative tumor load, suggesting most benefit to be gained by early conversion to an mTOR inhibitor-based maintenance regime. There is ongoing debate on the mechanisms involved including withdrawal of the carcinogenic effects of calcineurin inhibitors and/or their impact on chronic (oncogenic) viral infections [146].

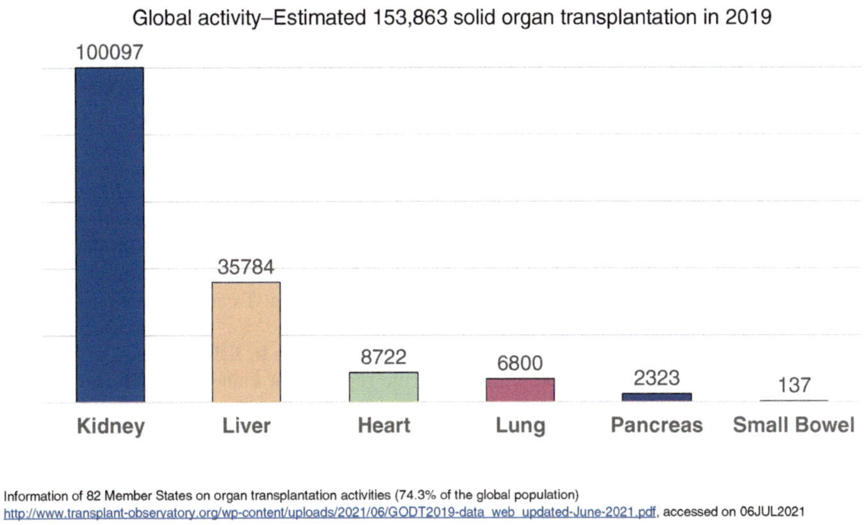

Fig. 9 Global activity in 2019—solid organ transplantation

More recently, belatacept has been approved for the prevention of acute rejection after kidney transplantation. Yet, higher earlier and more severe rejection episodes, the increased risk of opportunist infections, the need for monthly infusions and the associated cost, and the limited production are limiting their widespread use, including among recipients of other solid organ transplants [34].

It is estimated that in 2019 more than 153,000 solid organ transplants were performed worldwide (Fig. 9). Intuitively, millions of patients are living with a solid organ transplant. While we somehow have standard of care regimens for each organ transplants, many transplant recipients are discontinued from one of these drugs or require a switch from one drug to another due to an adverse event. The frequency of discontinuation or conversion varies among the organs and according to the demographic characteristics of the recipients, as increasing age and the number of comorbidities are associated with higher incidence of adverse events. Novel agents such as costimulatory blockers are under development and may allow a more personalized strategy for each recipient of solid organ transplant in the future, producing improved efficacy with reduced long-term toxicities. Ultimately, the goal is not only increasing long-term patient survival but also quality of life of solid organ transplant recipients.

References

1. He H, Stone JR, Perkins DL. Analysis of differential immune responses induced by innate and adaptive immunity following transplantation. Immunology. 2003;109(2):185–96.
2. Halloran PF. Immunosuppressive drugs for kidney transplantation. N Engl J Med. 2004;351(26):2715–29.

3. Kwun J, Manook M, Page E, Burghuber C, Hong J, Knechtle SJ. Crosstalk between T and B cells in the germinal center after transplantation. Transplantation. 2017;101(4):704–12.
4. Zeiser R, Negrin RS. Interleukin-2 receptor downstream events in regulatory T cells: implications for the choice of immunosuppressive drug therapy. Cell Cycle. 2008;7(4):458–62.
5. Wiland AM, Philosophe B. Daclizumab induction in solid organ transplantation. Expert Opin Biol Ther. 2004;4(5):729–40.
6. Ponticelli C. Basiliximab: efficacy and safety evaluation in kidney transplantation. Expert Opin Drug Saf. 2014;13(3):373–81.
7. van der Zwan M, Baan CC, van Gelder T, Hesselink DA. Review of the clinical pharmacokinetics and pharmacodynamics of alemtuzumab and its use in kidney transplantation. Clin Pharmacokinet. 2018;57(2):191–207.
8. Mohty M. Mechanisms of action of antithymocyte globulin: T-cell depletion and beyond. Leukemia. 2007;21(7):1387–94.
9. Alloway RR, Woodle ES, Abramowicz D, Segev DL, Castan R, Ilsley JN, et al. Rabbit antithymocyte globulin for the prevention of acute rejection in kidney transplantation. Am J Transplant. 2019;19(8):2252–61.
10. Gaber AO, Monaco AP, Russell JA, Lebranchu Y, Mohty M. Rabbit antithymocyte globulin (thymoglobulin): 25 years and new frontiers in solid organ transplantation and haematology. Drugs. 2010;70(6):691–732.
11. Shibasaki F, Hallin U, Uchino H. Calcineurin as a multifunctional regulator. J Biochem. 2002;131(1):1–15.
12. Dunn CJ, Wagstaff AJ, Perry CM, Plosker GL, Goa KL. Cyclosporin: an updated review of the pharmacokinetic properties, clinical efficacy and tolerability of a microemulsion-based formulation (neoral)1 in organ transplantation. Drugs. 2001;61(13):1957–2016.
13. Garnock-Jones KP. Tacrolimus prolonged release (Envarsus®): a review of its use in kidney and liver transplant recipients. Drugs. 2015;75(3):309–20.
14. Staatz CE, Tett SE. Clinical pharmacokinetics of once-daily tacrolimus in solid-organ transplant patients. Clin Pharmacokinet. 2015;54(10):993–1025.
15. Bowman LJ, Brennan DC. The role of tacrolimus in renal transplantation. Expert Opin Pharmacother. 2008;9(4):635–43.
16. Farouk SS, Rein JL. The many faces of calcineurin inhibitor toxicity-what the FK? Adv Chronic Kidney Dis. 2020;27(1):56–66.
17. Van Scoik KG, Johnson CA, Porter WR. The pharmacology and metabolism of the thiopurine drugs 6-mercaptopurine and azathioprine. Drug Metab Rev. 1985;16(1–2):157–74.
18. van Gelder T, van Schaik RH, Hesselink DA. Pharmacogenetics and immunosuppressive drugs in solid organ transplantation. Nat Rev Nephrol. 2014;10(12):725–31.
19. Mohammadi O, Kassim TA. Azathioprine. In: StatPearls. Treasure Island, FL: StatPearls Publishing; 2021.
20. Ransom JT. Mechanism of action of mycophenolate mofetil. Ther Drug Monit. 1995;17(6):681–4.
21. Ferreira PCL, Thiesen FV, Pereira AG, Zimmer AR, Fröehlich PE. A short overview on mycophenolic acid pharmacology and pharmacokinetics. Clin Transplant. 2020;34(8):e13997.
22. Bergan S, Brunet M, Hesselink DA, Johnson-Davis KL, Kunicki PK, Lemaitre F, et al. Personalized therapy for mycophenolate: consensus report by the International Association of Therapeutic Drug Monitoring and Clinical Toxicology. Ther Drug Monit. 2021;43(2):150–200.
23. Le HL, Francke MI, Andrews LM, de Winter BCM, van Gelder T, Hesselink DA. Usage of tacrolimus and mycophenolic acid during conception, pregnancy, and lactation, and its implications for therapeutic drug monitoring: a systematic critical review. Ther Drug Monit. 2020;42(4):518–31.
24. Kajiwara M, Masuda S. Role of mTOR inhibitors in kidney disease. Int J Mol Sci. 2016;17(6):975.
25. Boutouja F, Stiehm CM, Platta HW. mTOR: a cellular regulator interface in health and disease. Cell. 2019;8(1):18.

26. Buhaescu I, Izzedine H, Covic A. Sirolimus—challenging current perspectives. Ther Drug Monit. 2006;28(5):577–84.
27. van Gelder T, Fischer L, Shihab F, Shipkova M. Optimizing everolimus exposure when combined with calcineurin inhibitors in solid organ transplantation. Transplant Rev (Orlando). 2017;31(3):151–7.
28. Moes DJ, Guchelaar HJ, de Fijter JW. Sirolimus and everolimus in kidney transplantation. Drug Discov Today. 2015;20(10):1243–9.
29. Ventura-Aguiar P, Campistol JM, Diekmann F. Safety of mTOR inhibitors in adult solid organ transplantation. Expert Opin Drug Saf. 2016;15(3):303–19.
30. Jara-Palomares L, Solier-López A, Russo M, Suñer M, González-Roncero F, Peters-Sengers H, et al. Thromboprophylaxis after renal transplantation and patient risk stratification: the case of mTOR inhibitors. Thromb Res. 2020;195:100–2.
31. Baas MC, Gerdes VE, Ten Berge IJ, Heutinck KM, Florquin S, Meijers JC, et al. Treatment with everolimus is associated with a procoagulant state. Thromb Res. 2013;132(2):307–11.
32. Kaplan B, Qazi Y, Wellen JR. Strategies for the management of adverse events associated with mTOR inhibitors. Transplant Rev (Orlando). 2014;28(3):126–33.
33. Snanoudj R, Zuber J, Legendre C. Co-stimulation blockade as a new strategy in kidney transplantation: benefits and limits. Drugs. 2010;70(16):2121–31.
34. Schroder PM, Fitch ZW, Schmitz R, Choi AY, Kwun J, Knechtle SJ. The past, present, and future of costimulation blockade in organ transplantation. Curr Opin Organ Transplant. 2019;24(4):391–401.
35. Vincenti F. Belatacept and long-term outcomes in kidney transplantation. N Engl J Med. 2016;374(26):2600–1.
36. Garcia VD, Meinerz G, Keitel E. A safety evaluation of belatacept for the treatment of kidney transplant. Expert Opin Drug Saf. 2016;15(8):1125–32.
37. Del Bello A, Marion O, Milongo D, Rostaing L, Kamar N. Belatacept prophylaxis against organ rejection in adult kidney-transplant recipients. Expert Rev Clin Pharmacol. 2016;9(2):215–27.
38. Viana LA, Cristelli MP, Santos DW, Tavares MG, Dantas MTC, Felipe CR, et al. Influence of epidemiology, immunosuppressive regimens, clinical presentation, and treatment on kidney transplant outcomes of patients diagnosed with tuberculosis: a retrospective cohort analysis. Am J Transplant. 2019;19(5):1421–31.
39. Almawi WY, Hess DA, Rieder MJ. Multiplicity of glucocorticoid action in inhibiting allograft rejection. Cell Transplant. 1998;7(6):511–23.
40. De Lucena DD, Rangel ÉB. Glucocorticoids use in kidney transplant setting. Expert Opin Drug Metab Toxicol. 2018;14(10):1023–41.
41. Murray JE, Merrill JP, Harrison JH, Wilson RE, Dammin GJ. Prolonged survival of human-kidney homografts by immunosuppressive drug therapy. N Engl J Med. 1963;268:1315–23.
42. Calne RY. The present position and future prospects of organ transplantation. Ann R Coll Surg Engl. 1968;42(5):283–306.
43. Tomlinson SA, Joslin MP, Evans DB, Joysey VC, Calne RY. Kidney transplantation: analysis of 200 cases. Br Med J. 1974;4(5944):553–7.
44. Starzl TE, Marchioro TL, Hutchinson DE, Porter KA, Cerilli GJ, Brettschneider L. The clinical use of antilymphocyte globulin in renal homotransplantation. Transplantation. 1967;5(4 Suppl):1100–5.
45. Calne RY, White DJ, Thiru S, Evans DB, McMaster P, Dunn DC, et al. Cyclosporin A in patients receiving renal allografts from cadaver donors. Lancet. 1978;2(8104–5):1323–7.
46. Cyclosporin a as sole immunosuppressive agent in recipients of kidney allografts from cadaver donors. Preliminary results of a European multicentre trial. Lancet. 1982;2(8289):57–60.
47. Ferguson RM, Rynasiewicz JJ, Sutherland DE, Simmons RL, Najarian JS. Cyclosporin A in renal transplantation: a prospective randomized trial. Surgery. 1982;92(2):175–82.
48. A randomized clinical trial of cyclosporine in cadaveric renal transplantation. N Engl J Med. 1983;309(14):809–15.

49. Hall BM, Tiller DJ, Hardie I, Mahony J, Mathew T, Thatcher G, et al. Comparison of three immunosuppressive regimens in cadaver renal transplantation: long-term cyclosporine, short-term cyclosporine followed by azathioprine and prednisolone, and azathioprine and prednisolone without cyclosporine. N Engl J Med. 1988;318(23):1499–507.
50. Lindholm A, Albrechtsen D, Tufveson G, Karlberg I, Persson NH, Groth CG. A randomized trial of cyclosporine and prednisolone versus cyclosporine, azathioprine, and prednisolone in primary cadaveric renal transplantation. Transplantation. 1992;54(4):624–31.
51. Kasiske BL, Heim-Duthoy K, Ma JZ. Elective cyclosporine withdrawal after renal transplantation. A meta-analysis. JAMA. 1993;269(3):395–400.
52. Fung JJ, Abu-Elmagd K, Todo S, Shapiro R, Tzakis A, Jordan M, Armitage J, Jain A, Alessiani M, Martin M, et al. Overview of FK506 in transplantation. Clin Transpl. 1990:115–21. PMID: 1715740; PMCID: PMC3079459.
53. Shapiro R, Jordan M, Scantlebury V, Vivas C, Fung J, McCauley J, et al. A prospective, randomized trial of FK-506 in renal transplantation—a comparison between double- and triple-drug therapy. Clin Transplant. 1994;8(6):508–15.
54. Sollinger HW. Mycophenolate mofetil for the prevention of acute rejection in primary cadaveric renal allograft recipients. U.S. Renal Transplant Mycophenolate Mofetil Study Group. Transplantation. 1995;60(3):225–32.
55. A blinded, randomized clinical trial of mycophenolate mofetil for the prevention of acute rejection in cadaveric renal transplantation. The Tricontinental Mycophenolate Mofetil Renal Transplantation Study Group. Transplantation. 1996;61(7):1029–37.
56. Placebo-controlled study of mycophenolate mofetil combined with cyclosporin and corticosteroids for prevention of acute rejection. European Mycophenolate Mofetil Cooperative Study Group. Lancet. 1995;345(8961):1321–5.
57. Pirsch JD, Miller J, Deierhoi MH, Vincenti F, Filo RS. A comparison of tacrolimus (FK506) and cyclosporine for immunosuppression after cadaveric renal transplantation. FK506 Kidney Transplant Study Group. Transplantation. 1997;63(7):977–83.
58. Mayer AD, Dmitrewski J, Squifflet JP, Besse T, Grabensee B, Klein B, et al. Multicenter randomized trial comparing tacrolimus (FK506) and cyclosporine in the prevention of renal allograft rejection: a report of the European Tacrolimus Multicenter Renal Study Group. Transplantation. 1997;64(3):436–43.
59. Nashan B, Moore R, Amlot P, Schmidt AG, Abeywickrama K, Soulillou JP. Randomised trial of basiliximab versus placebo for control of acute cellular rejection in renal allograft recipients. CHIB 201 International Study Group. Lancet. 1997;350(9086):1193–8.
60. Kahan BD, Rajagopalan PR, Hall M. Reduction of the occurrence of acute cellular rejection among renal allograft recipients treated with basiliximab, a chimeric anti-interleukin-2-receptor monoclonal antibody. United States Simulect Renal Study Group. Transplantation. 1999;67(2):276–84.
61. Ponticelli C, Yussim A, Cambi V, Legendre C, Rizzo G, Salvadori M, et al. A randomized, double-blind trial of basiliximab immunoprophylaxis plus triple therapy in kidney transplant recipients. Transplantation. 2001;72(7):1261–7.
62. Vincenti F, Kirkman R, Light S, Bumgardner G, Pescovitz M, Halloran P, et al. Interleukin-2-receptor blockade with daclizumab to prevent acute rejection in renal transplantation. Daclizumab Triple Therapy Study Group. N Engl J Med. 1998;338(3):161–5.
63. Nashan B, Light S, Hardie IR, Lin A, Johnson JR. Reduction of acute renal allograft rejection by daclizumab. Daclizumab Double Therapy Study Group. Transplantation. 1999;67(1):110–5.
64. Kahan BD. Efficacy of sirolimus compared with azathioprine for reduction of acute renal allograft rejection: a randomised multicentre study. The Rapamune US Study Group. Lancet. 2000;356:194–202.
65. MacDonald AS. A worldwide, phase III, randomized, controlled, safety and efficacy study of a sirolimus/cyclosporine regimen for prevention of acute rejection in recipients of primary mismatched renal allografts. Transplantation. 2001;71(2):271–80.

66. Johnson RW, Kreis H, Oberbauer R, Brattström C, Claesson K, Eris J. Sirolimus allows early cyclosporine withdrawal in renal transplantation resulting in improved renal function and lower blood pressure. Transplantation. 2001;72(5):777–86.
67. Yan HL, Zong HT, Cui YS, Li N, Zhang Y. Calcineurin inhibitor avoidance and withdrawal for kidney transplantation: a systematic review and meta-analysis of randomized controlled trials. Transplant Proc. 2014;46(5):1302–13.
68. Webster AC, Lee VW, Chapman JR, Craig JC. Target of rapamycin inhibitors (sirolimus and everolimus) for primary immunosuppression of kidney transplant recipients: a systematic review and meta-analysis of randomized trials. Transplantation. 2006;81(9):1234–48.
69. Montero N, Quero M, Melilli E, Pérez-Sáez MJ, Redondo-Pachón D, Bestard O, et al. Mammalian target of rapamycin inhibitors combined with calcineurin inhibitors as initial immunosuppression in renal transplantation: a meta-analysis. Transplantation. 2019;103(10):2031–56.
70. Ekberg H, Tedesco-Silva H, Demirbas A, Vitko S, Nashan B, Gurkan A, et al. Reduced exposure to calcineurin inhibitors in renal transplantation. N Engl J Med. 2007;357:2562–75.
71. Tedesco Silva H Jr, Cibrik D, Johnston T, Lackova E, Mange K, Panis C, et al. Everolimus plus reduced-exposure CsA versus mycophenolic acid plus standard-exposure CsA in renal-transplant recipients. Am J Transplant. 2010;10:1401–13.
72. Pascual J, Berger SP, Witzke O, Tedesco H, Mulgaonkar S, Qazi Y, et al. Everolimus with reduced calcineurin inhibitor exposure in renal transplantation. J Am Soc Nephrol. 2018;29(7):1979–91.
73. Flechner SM, Gurkan A, Hartmann A, Legendre CM, Russ GR, Campistol JM, et al. A randomized, open-label study of sirolimus versus cyclosporine in primary de novo renal allograft recipients. Transplantation. 2013;95(10):1233–41.
74. Glotz D, Charpentier B, Abramovicz D, Lang P, Rostaing L, Rifle G, et al. Thymoglobulin induction and sirolimus versus tacrolimus in kidney transplant recipients receiving mycophenolate mofetil and steroids. Transplantation. 2010;89(12):1511–7.
75. Weir MR, Mulgaonkar S, Chan L, Shidban H, Waid TH, Preston D, et al. Mycophenolate mofetil-based immunosuppression with sirolimus in renal transplantation: a randomized, controlled Spare-the-Nephron trial. Kidney Int. 2011;79:897–907.
76. Budde K, Becker T, Arns W, Sommerer C, Reinke P, Eisenberger U, et al. Everolimus-based, calcineurin-inhibitor-free regimen in recipients of de-novo kidney transplants: an open-label, randomised, controlled trial. Lancet. 2011;377:837–47.
77. Bemelman FJ, de Fijter JW, Kers J, Meyer C, Peters-Sengers H, de Maar EF, et al. Early conversion to prednisolone/everolimus as an alternative weaning regimen associates with beneficial renal transplant histology and function: the randomized-controlled MECANO trial. Am J Transplant. 2017;17(4):1020–30.
78. Budde K, Zeier M, Witzke O, Arns W, Lehner F, Guba M, et al. Everolimus with cyclosporine withdrawal or low-exposure cyclosporine in kidney transplantation from month 3: a multicentre, randomized trial. Nephrol Dial Transplant. 2017;32(6):1060–70.
79. Schena FP, Pascoe MD, Alberu J, del Carmen RM, Oberbauer R, Brennan DC, et al. Conversion from calcineurin inhibitors to sirolimus maintenance therapy in renal allograft recipients: 24-month efficacy and safety results from the CONVERT trial. Transplantation. 2009;87:233–42.
80. Holdaas H, Rostaing L, Serón D, Cole E, Chapman J, Fellstrøm B, et al. Conversion of long-term kidney transplant recipients from calcineurin inhibitor therapy to everolimus: a randomized, multicenter, 24-month study. Transplantation. 2011;92(4):410–8.
81. Vincenti F, Larsen C, Durrbach A, Wekerle T, Nashan B, Blancho G, et al. Costimulation blockade with belatacept in renal transplantation. N Engl J Med. 2005;353(8):770–81.
82. Vincenti F, Charpentier B, Vanrenterghem Y, Rostaing L, Bresnahan B, Darji P, et al. A phase III study of belatacept-based immunosuppression regimens versus cyclosporine in renal transplant recipients (BENEFIT study). Am J Transplant. 2010;10(3):535–46.

83. Durrbach A, Pestana JM, Pearson T, Vincenti F, Garcia VD, Campistol J, et al. A phase III study of belatacept versus cyclosporine in kidney transplants from extended criteria donors (BENEFIT-EXT study). Am J Transplant. 2010;10(3):547–57.
84. Masson P, Henderson L, Chapman JR, Craig JC, Webster AC. Belatacept for kidney transplant recipients. Cochrane Database Syst Rev. 2014;(11):CD010699.
85. Woodle ES, Kaufman DB, Shields AR, Leone J, Matas A, Wiseman A, et al. Belatacept-based immunosuppression with simultaneous calcineurin inhibitor avoidance and early corticosteroid withdrawal: a prospective, randomized multicenter trial. Am J Transplant. 2020;20(4):1039–55.
86. Randomised trial comparing tacrolimus (FK506) and cyclosporin in prevention of liver allograft rejection. European FK506 Multicentre Liver Study Group. Lancet. 1994;344(8920):423–8.
87. U.S. Multicenter FK506 Liver Study Group. A comparison of tacrolimus (FK 506) and cyclosporine for immunosuppression in liver transplantation. N Engl J Med. 1994;331(17):1110–5.
88. O'Grady JG, Burroughs A, Hardy P, Elbourne D, Truesdale A. Tacrolimus versus microemulsified ciclosporin in liver transplantation: the TMC randomised controlled trial. Lancet. 2002;360(9340):1119–25.
89. Levy G, Villamil F, Samuel D, Sanjuan F, Grazi GL, Wu Y, et al. Results of lis2t, a multicenter, randomized study comparing cyclosporine microemulsion with C2 monitoring and tacrolimus with C0 monitoring in de novo liver transplantation. Transplantation. 2004;77(11):1632–8.
90. Neuhaus P, Clavien PA, Kittur D, Salizzoni M, Rimola A, Abeywickrama K, et al. Improved treatment response with basiliximab immunoprophylaxis after liver transplantation: results from a double-blind randomized placebo-controlled trial. Liver Transplant. 2002;8(2):132–42.
91. Wiesner R, Rabkin J, Klintmalm G, McDiarmid S, Langnas A, Punch J, et al. A randomized double-blind comparative study of mycophenolate mofetil and azathioprine in combination with cyclosporine and corticosteroids in primary liver transplant recipients. Liver Transplant. 2001;7(5):442–50.
92. Boudjema K, Camus C, Saliba F, Calmus Y, Salamé E, Pageaux G, et al. Reduced-dose tacrolimus with mycophenolate mofetil vs. standard-dose tacrolimus in liver transplantation: a randomized study. Am J Transplant. 2011;11(5):965–76.
93. Teperman L, Moonka D, Sebastian A, Sher L, Marotta P, Marsh C, et al. Calcineurin inhibitor-free mycophenolate mofetil/sirolimus maintenance in liver transplantation: the randomized spare-the-nephron trial. Liver Transplant. 2013;19(7):675–89.
94. Saliba F, Duvoux C, Gugenheim J, Kamar N, Dharancy S, Salamé E, et al. Efficacy and safety of everolimus and mycophenolic acid with early tacrolimus withdrawal after liver transplantation: a multicenter randomized trial. Am J Transplant. 2017;17(7):1843–52.
95. De Simone P, Nevens F, De Carlis L, Metselaar HJ, Beckebaum S, Saliba F, et al. Everolimus with reduced tacrolimus improves renal function in de novo liver transplant recipients: a randomized controlled trial. Am J Transplant. 2012;12(11):3008–20.
96. Barnhart GR, Goldman MH, Hastillo A, Szentpetery S, Wolfgang T, Thompson J, et al. Comparison of immunosuppression therapy following heart transplantation: pretransfusion/azathioprine/ATG/prednisone versus cyclosporine/prednisone. J Heart Transplant. 1985;4(4):381–4.
97. Reichart B, Meiser B, Viganò M, Rinaldi M, Martinelli L, Yacoub M, et al. European Multicenter Tacrolimus (FK506) Heart Pilot Study: one-year results—European Tacrolimus Multicenter Heart Study Group. J Heart Lung Transplant. 1998;17(8):775–81.
98. Kobashigawa J, Miller L, Renlund D, Mentzer R, Alderman E, Bourge R, et al. A randomized active-controlled trial of mycophenolate mofetil in heart transplant recipients. Mycophenolate Mofetil Investigators. Transplantation. 1998;66(4):507–15.
99. Kobashigawa JA, Renlund DG, Gerosa G, Almenar L, Eisen HJ, Keogh AM, et al. Similar efficacy and safety of enteric-coated mycophenolate sodium (EC-MPS, myfortic) compared with mycophenolate mofetil (MMF) in de novo heart transplant recipients: results of a 12-month, single-blind, randomized, parallel-group, multicenter study. J Heart Lung Transplant. 2006;25(8):935–41.

100. Carrier M, Leblanc MH, Perrault LP, White M, Doyle D, Beaudoin D, et al. Basiliximab and rabbit anti-thymocyte globulin for prophylaxis of acute rejection after heart transplantation: a non-inferiority trial. J Heart Lung Transplant. 2007;26(3):258–63.
101. Eisen HJ, Hobbs RE, Davis SF, Carrier M, Mancini DM, Smith A, et al. Safety, tolerability, and efficacy of cyclosporine microemulsion in heart transplant recipients: a randomized, multicenter, double-blind comparison with the oil-based formulation of cyclosporine—results at 24 months after transplantation. Transplantation. 2001;71(1):70–8.
102. Kobashigawa JA, Miller LW, Russell SD, Ewald GA, Zucker MJ, Goldberg LR, et al. Tacrolimus with mycophenolate mofetil (MMF) or sirolimus vs. cyclosporine with MMF in cardiac transplant patients: 1-year report. Am J Transplant. 2006;6(6):1377–86.
103. Eisen HJ, Tuzcu EM, Dorent R, Kobashigawa J, Mancini D, Valantine-von Kaeppler HA, et al. Everolimus for the prevention of allograft rejection and vasculopathy in cardiac-transplant recipients. N Engl J Med. 2003;349(9):847–58.
104. Lehmkuhl HB, Arizon J, Viganò M, Almenar L, Gerosa G, Maccherini M, et al. Everolimus with reduced cyclosporine versus MMF with standard cyclosporine in de novo heart transplant recipients. Transplantation. 2009;88(1):115–22.
105. Gullestad L, Iversen M, Mortensen SA, Eiskjaer H, Riise GC, Mared L, et al. Everolimus with reduced calcineurin inhibitor in thoracic transplant recipients with renal dysfunction: a multicenter, randomized trial. Transplantation. 2010;89(7):864–72.
106. Eisen HJ, Kobashigawa J, Starling RC, Pauly DF, Kfoury A, Ross H, et al. Everolimus versus mycophenolate mofetil in heart transplantation: a randomized, multicenter trial. Am J Transplant. 2013;13(5):1203–16.
107. Andreassen AK, Andersson B, Gustafsson F, Eiskjaer H, Rådegran G, Gude E, et al. Everolimus initiation with early calcineurin inhibitor withdrawal in de novo heart transplant recipients: three-year results from the randomized SCHEDULE study. Am J Transplant. 2016;16(4):1238–47.
108. Potena L, Pellegrini C, Grigioni F, Amarelli C, Livi U, Maccherini M, et al. Optimizing the safety profile of everolimus by delayed initiation in de novo heart transplant recipients: results of the prospective randomized study EVERHEART. Transplantation. 2018;102(3):493–501.
109. Söderlund C, Rådegran G. Immunosuppressive therapies after heart transplantation—the balance between under- and over-immunosuppression. Transplant Rev (Orlando). 2015;29(3):181–9.
110. Griffith BP, Hardesty RL, Armitage JM, Kormos RL, Marrone GC, Duncan S, et al. Acute rejection of lung allografts with various immunosuppressive protocols. Ann Thorac Surg. 1992;54(5):846–51.
111. Palmer SM, Baz MA, Sanders L, Miralles AP, Lawrence CM, Rea JB, et al. Results of a randomized, prospective, multicenter trial of mycophenolate mofetil versus azathioprine in the prevention of acute lung allograft rejection. Transplantation. 2001;71(12):1772–6.
112. McNeil K, Glanville AR, Wahlers T, Knoop C, Speich R, Mamelok RD, et al. Comparison of mycophenolate mofetil and azathioprine for prevention of bronchiolitis obliterans syndrome in de novo lung transplant recipients. Transplantation. 2006;81(7):998–1003.
113. Treede H, Klepetko W, Reichenspurner H, Zuckermann A, Meiser B, Birsan T, et al. Tacrolimus versus cyclosporine after lung transplantation: a prospective, open, randomized two-center trial comparing two different immunosuppressive protocols. J Heart Lung Transplant. 2001;20(5):511–7.
114. Treede H, Glanville AR, Klepetko W, Aboyoun C, Vettorazzi E, Lama R, et al. Tacrolimus and cyclosporine have differential effects on the risk of development of bronchiolitis obliterans syndrome: results of a prospective, randomized international trial in lung transplantation. J Heart Lung Transplant. 2012;31(8):797–804.
115. Zuckermann A, Reichenspurner H, Birsan T, Treede H, Deviatko E, Reichart B, et al. Cyclosporine A versus tacrolimus in combination with mycophenolate mofetil and steroids as primary immunosuppression after lung transplantation: one-year results of a 2-center prospective randomized trial. J Thorac Cardiovasc Surg. 2003;125(4):891–900.

116. Bhorade S, Ahya VN, Baz MA, Valentine VG, Arcasoy SM, Love RB, et al. Comparison of sirolimus with azathioprine in a tacrolimus-based immunosuppressive regimen in lung transplantation. Am J Respir Crit Care Med. 2011;183(3):379–87.
117. Snell GI, Valentine VG, Vitulo P, Glanville AR, McGiffin DC, Loyd JE, et al. Everolimus versus azathioprine in maintenance lung transplant recipients: an international, randomized, double-blind clinical trial. Am J Transplant. 2006;6(1):169–77.
118. Glanville AR, Aboyoun C, Klepetko W, Reichenspurner H, Treede H, Verschuuren EA, et al. Three-year results of an investigator-driven multicenter, international, randomized open-label de novo trial to prevent BOS after lung transplantation. J Heart Lung Transplant. 2015;34(1):16–25.
119. Gottlieb J, Neurohr C, Müller-Quernheim J, Wirtz H, Sill B, Wilkens H, et al. A randomized trial of everolimus-based quadruple therapy vs standard triple therapy early after lung transplantation. Am J Transplant. 2019;19(6):1759–69.
120. Chandrashekaran S, Crow Pharm SA, Shah SZ, Arendt Pharm CJ, Kennedy CC. Immunosuppression for lung transplantation: current and future. Curr Transplant Rep. 2018;5(3):212–9.
121. Bechstein WO, Malaise J, Saudek F, Land W, Fernandez-Cruz L, Margreiter R, et al. Efficacy and safety of tacrolimus compared with cyclosporine microemulsion in primary simultaneous pancreas-kidney transplantation: 1-year results of a large multicenter trial. Transplantation. 2004;77(8):1221–8.
122. Stratta RJ, Alloway RR, Lo A, Hodge E. Two-dose daclizumab regimen in simultaneous kidney-pancreas transplant recipients: primary endpoint analysis of a multicenter, randomized study. Transplantation. 2003;75(8):1260–6.
123. Kaufman DB, Burke GW III, Bruce DS, Johnson CP, Gaber AO, Sutherland DE, et al. Prospective, randomized, multi-center trial of antibody induction therapy in simultaneous pancreas-kidney transplantation. Am J Transplant. 2003;3(7):855–64.
124. Siskind EJ, Liu C, Collins DT, Emery E, Steen E, Tran E, et al. Use of mammalian target of rapamycin inhibitors for pancreas transplant immunosuppression is associated with improved allograft survival and improved early patient survival. Pancreas. 2019;48(5):644–51.
125. Elsabbagh AM, Hawksworth J, Khan KM, Kaufman SS, Yazigi NA, Kroemer A, et al. Long-term survival in visceral transplant recipients in the new era: a single-center experience. Am J Transplant. 2019;19(7):2077–91.
126. Bharadwaj S, Tandon P, Gohel TD, Brown J, Steiger E, Kirby DF, et al. Current status of intestinal and multivisceral transplantation. Gastroenterol Rep (Oxf). 2017;5(1):20–8.
127. Rifkin WJ, Manjunath AK, Kantar RS, Jacoby A, Kimberly LL, Gelb BE, et al. A comparison of immunosuppression regimens in hand, face, and kidney transplantation. J Surg Res. 2021;258:17–22.
128. Bamoulid J, Staeck O, Crépin T, Halleck F, Saas P, Brakemeier S, et al. Anti-thymocyte globulins in kidney transplantation: focus on current indications and long-term immunological side effects. Nephrol Dial Transplant. 2017;32(10):1601–8.
129. Ballen K. New trends in transplantation: the use of thymoglobulin. Expert Opin Drug Metab Toxicol. 2009;5(3):351–5.
130. Naesens M, Kuypers DR, Sarwal M. Calcineurin inhibitor nephrotoxicity. Clin J Am Soc Nephrol. 2009;4:481–508.
131. Karolin A, Genitsch V, Sidler D. Calcineurin inhibitor toxicity in solid organ transplantation. Pharmacology. 2021;106:1–9.
132. Wolf S, Hoffmann VS, Habicht A, Kauke T, Bucher J, Schoenberg M, et al. Effects of mTOR-Is on malignancy and survival following renal transplantation: a systematic review and meta-analysis of randomized trials with a minimum follow-up of 24 months. PLoS One. 2018;13(4):e0194975.
133. Mittal A, Colegio OR. Skin cancers in organ transplant recipients. Am J Transplant. 2017;17(10):2509–30.
134. Gu YH, Du JX, Ma ML. Sirolimus and non-melanoma skin cancer prevention after kidney transplantation: a meta-analysis. Asian Pac J Cancer Prev. 2012;13(9):4335–9.

135. Phan K, Moloney FJ, Hogarty DT, Lenane P, McColl D, Yazdabadi A. Mammalian target of rapamycin (mTOR) inhibitors and skin cancer risk in nonrenal solid organ transplant recipients: systematic review and meta-analysis. Int J Dermatol. 2019; https://doi.org/10.1111/ijd.14549.
136. Naldi L, Venturuzzo A, Invernizzi P. Dermatological complications after solid organ transplantation. Clin Rev Allergy Immunol. 2018;54(1):185–212.
137. Chin-Hong PV, Reid GE. Human papillomavirus infection in solid organ transplant recipients: guidelines from the American Society of Transplantation Infectious Diseases Community of Practice. Clin Transplant. 2019;33(9):e13590.
138. Callejas-Valera JL, Iglesias-Bartolome R, Amornphimoltham P, Palacios-Garcia J, Martin D, Califano JA, et al. mTOR inhibition prevents rapid-onset of carcinogen-induced malignancies in a novel inducible HPV-16 E6/E7 mouse model. Carcinogenesis. 2016;37(10):1014–25.
139. Molinolo AA, Marsh C, El Dinali M, Gangane N, Jennison K, Hewitt S, et al. mTOR as a molecular target in HPV-associated oral and cervical squamous carcinomas. Clin Cancer Res. 2012;18(9):2558–68.
140. Vance KK, Krunic AL, Fishman PM, Kadkol SS, Nuovo GJ. Dramatic regression of recalcitrant human papillomavirus type 1-related palmar verrucae and squamous cell carcinoma in situ following R-CHOP chemotherapy and transition to sirolimus in a renal transplant patient with diffuse large B cell lymphoma. Int J Dermatol. 2015;54(5):e119–21.
141. Shahidi S, Moeinzadeh F, Mohammadi M, Gholamrezaei A. Sirolimus-based immunosuppression for treatment of cutaneous warts in kidney transplant recipients. Iran J Kidney Dis. 2011;5(5):351–3.
142. Dharancy S, Catteau B, Mortier L, Boleslawski E, Declerck N, Canva V, et al. Conversion to sirolimus: a useful strategy for recalcitrant cutaneous viral warts in liver transplant recipient. Liver Transplant. 2006;12(12):1883–7.
143. Fania L, Didona D, Di Pietro FR, Verkhovskaia S, Morese R, Paolino G, et al. Cutaneous squamous cell carcinoma: from pathophysiology to novel therapeutic approaches. Biomedicines. 2021;9(2):171.
144. Hosseini-Moghaddam SM, Soleimanirahbar A, Mazzulli T, Rotstein C, Husain S. Post renal transplantation Kaposi's sarcoma: a review of its epidemiology, pathogenesis, diagnosis, clinical aspects, and therapy. Transpl Infect Dis. 2012;14(4):338–45.
145. Camara-Clayette V, Hermine O, Ribrag V. Emerging agents for the treatment of mantle cell lymphoma. Expert Rev Anticancer Ther. 2012;12(9):1205–15.
146. de Fijter JW. Cancer and mTOR inhibitors in transplant recipients. Transplantation. 2017;101(1):45–55.

Overview of Dermatological Diseases After Transplantation

Sarah Tuttleton Arron

1 Overview

Survival after organ transplantation has improved dramatically since the procedure was developed in the 1950s. The immunosuppressive agents required to maintain the transplanted graft put the patient at risk for two major categories of complication: infections and malignancies. Dermatologists are frequently called upon to evaluate inflammatory skin eruptions or concerning lesions, and understanding the frequency and timing of these opportunistic events can assist in diagnosis.

The association between solid organ transplantation and skin cancer was first reported by Walter et al. in 1971 [1], and the field of transplant dermatology developed rapidly to meet the growing need. In 2000 and 2001, the Skin Care in Organ Transplant Patients, Europe (SCOPE) and International Transplant Skin Cancer Collaborative (ITSCC) were formed, and the first of many joint meetings was held in Berlin in 2002. Members of these organizations have led the field in clinical and basic science research on the topic, expanding our understanding and informing multidisciplinary guidelines for the dermatologic care of transplant recipients. Over time, this expertise was expanded to include patients immunosuppressed for other reasons such as hematologic malignancy and iatrogenic immunosuppression; in 2016, ITSCC formally updated their name to International Immunosuppression and Transplant Skin Cancer Collaborative to reflect the growing field.

Clinical signs and symptoms of cutaneous infection may vary in solid organ transplant recipients (SOTR); immunosuppression may reduce the inflammatory response and attenuate fever and rashes. Empiric antimicrobial treatment may be complicated by drug interactions with immunosuppressive agents, but fortunately the new era of rapid molecular testing for microbes and antimicrobial resistance has enabled physicians to optimize therapy in a rapid time frame.

S. T. Arron (✉)
Peninsula Dermatology, Burlingame, CA, USA

J. Tomimori et al. (eds.), *Atlas of Dermatologic Diseases in Solid Organ Transplant Recipients*, https://doi.org/10.1007/978-3-031-13335-0_2

In contrast, skin cancers typically occur with the usual morphology in SOTR, but the increased frequency and aggressive nature of many skin cancers create a high burden of disease and management challenges.

Balancing the level and type of immunosuppression to maintain graft function while reducing the risks of infection and malignancy requires clear communication between the transplant team and dermatologist. Understanding the local immunosuppressive regimens used, local infection rates, and patient-specific risk factors can contribute to optimal screening and care.

2 Timeline of Skin Disease

The epidemiology of skin disease after transplantation reflects changing risks over time (Fig. 1). Risk is typically broken down into three phases: phase 1, the 1st month posttransplantation; phase 2, the end of the 1st month posttransplantation—12th month; and phase 3, beyond 12th month. In the immediate posttransplant period, the transplant team is typically focused on postoperative care and induction immunosuppression. As the patient and graft function stabilize, dermatologic issues may become more important. Close communication between the dermatologist and transplant team can assist in understanding the skin condition in the overall context of care.

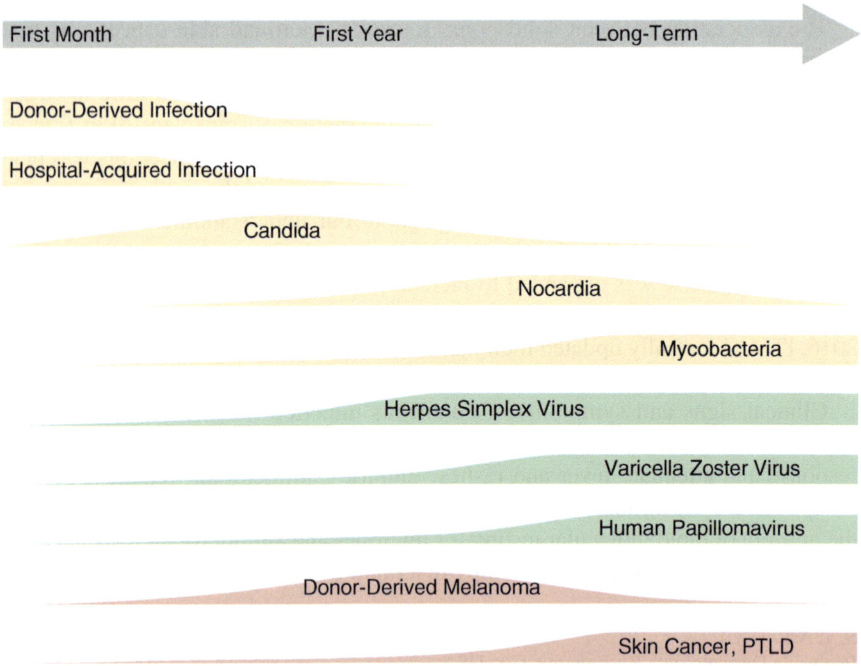

Fig. 1 Timeline of common dermatologic conditions after transplantation. *PTLD* posttransplant lymphoproliferative disorder

3 Pretransplant Evaluation

Transplant candidates should be formally reviewed by the transplant center selection committee. The pretransplant evaluation typically includes an assessment of organ function in the context of regional or national eligibility guidelines and a review of potential contraindications to transplantation. The dermatologist may be asked to review a patient with a prior history of melanoma or invasive nonmelanoma skin cancer. While there are dermatologic recommendations for patients with pretransplant skin cancer [2], the committee must view these in the context of patient prognosis, individual patient advocacy, and population organ stewardship [3].

While it would be ideal for every transplant candidate to receive a full body skin examination and skin cancer prevention counseling by a dermatologist, in practice this is simply not feasible. Candidates may be too physically ill for an additional outpatient visit among the many required for evaluation. Patients may be overwhelmed by the amount of information they are receiving and unable to focus on sun protection teaching. Access to dermatology may also be limited due to the small workforce; and as many transplant candidates may not go on to receive transplant, or may be at low risk for skin cancer due to demographics, screening these patients would burden the healthcare system unnecessarily. Therefore, the recommendation in the USA is to rely on the transplant team to triage patients to dermatology for pretransplant evaluation and counseling based on sun damage or skin cancer history, or suspicious lesions [4].

The protocols for organ donor harvesting should include a skin examination of the donor; any suspicious pigmented lesions should be biopsied if time permits. In the case of a remote organ harvest, a photograph can be sent to the transplant dermatologist for evaluation [5]. Educating the transplant team on evaluation of pigmented lesions is a key contribution, as donor-derived melanoma is invariably lethal.

In the immediate preoperative period, the dermatologist may be asked to consult on acute skin infections or allergic skin reactions. In most cases, these can be quickly identified and addressed. Figure 2 depicts a liver transplant candidate with jaundice

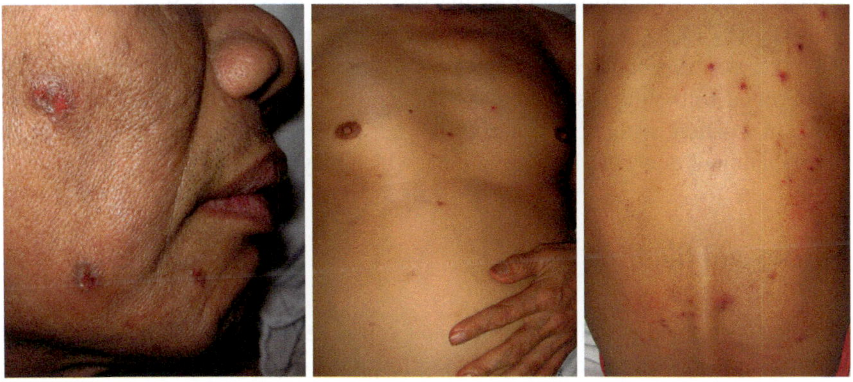

Fig. 2 Liver transplant candidate with jaundice and ascites. Diagnosis of prurigo nodularis after dermatological evaluation. His itch was significantly improved after transplantation

and ascites; the dermatologist was called to see him in the preoperative evaluation to rule out bacterial infection. The diagnosis of prurigo nodularis was made and the patient received his transplant. His itch was significantly improved the next day.

4 Immediate Postoperative Period

In the first month after transplantation, the organ transplant team prioritizes the immediate postoperative care and organ function. The initiation of high-level immunosuppression can predispose the patient to acute bacterial or fungal infection. Patients are at risk from procedures- and hospital-acquired infections which may include surgical wound infection, nosocomial infections (such as aspiration pneumonia or *C. difficile* colitis), or environmental mold infections from hospital ventilation systems or construction. For the consulting dermatologist, awareness of the surgical procedure and current hospital infection control guidelines can assist in identifying these risks. Corticosteroid-related acne can also arise in this period though this is commonly recognized by the transplant team and does not require consultation.

5 First Year After Transplant

The first year after transplantation is a fragile time during which the transplant team is optimizing immunosuppression and the patient is adjusting to a new lifestyle. During this phase, patients are prone to reactivation of latent infections such as herpes simplex virus (HSV) or varicella zoster virus (VZV). Opportunistic infections may also arise, such as *Pneumocystis jirovecii* pneumonia (PCP). Most medication regimens include prophylaxis against common infections in this period.

Patients with extensive sun damage and a history of pretransplant UV-associated skin cancer such as squamous cell carcinoma (SCC) may also develop explosive growth of new skin lesions during the first year. The SUNTRAC algorithm and SUNTRAC 4TXP smartphone app utilizes prediction modeling data to guide providers on skin cancer screening after transplantation; the highest risk group should be screened within the first 6 months [6]. Rapid development of a metastatic melanoma in a patient without a history of pretransplant skin cancer should prompt an investigation of donor-derived melanoma, which is typically lethal.

6 Beyond the First Year

Patients with stable graft function beyond the first year remain at increased risk for community-acquired infections including respiratory and gastrointestinal disease. However, those with unstable allografts may require higher levels of immunosuppression and become prone to recurrent infections. In this phase, skin cancer may overtake infection as the predominant dermatologic concern.

7 Posttransplant Infections

7.1 *Viral Infection*

Evaluation for transplant candidacy and organ donation typically include serologic screening for human immunodeficiency virus (HIV), hepatitis B and C virus, and herpes simplex virus (HSV).

Viral infections in the first 2–12 months after transplantation include newly acquired virus, reactivation of latent virus, or donor-derived viral disease (particularly in seronegative recipients) (see Chap. Viral Diseases). The herpesviruses are particularly concerning, including cytomegalovirus (CMV), herpes simplex virus (HSV), varicella zoster virus (VZV), human herpesvirus 6 and 7 (HHV-6, HHV-7), and Epstein-Barr virus (EBV). CMV prophylaxis with valganciclovir or ganciclovir can reduce other herpesvirus infections as well. The incidence of herpes zoster is up to 12% in SOTR and 10–100-fold higher than the general population [7]. Heart and lung transplant recipients are at highest risk, and previous history of graft rejection also confers additional risk [8]. Herpes simplex carries less risk for disseminated or fatal disease but may cause symptomatic lesions in up to 10% of SOTR [9].

Viral warts are the most common skin infection in SOTR, and these lesions can be widespread and refractory to treatment [7, 10]. The majority of viral warts are caused by human papillomavirus (HPV), a ubiquitous virus that can infect cutaneous and mucosal epithelium. Initiation of transplant immunosuppression dramatically increases the cutaneous manifestations of sexually transmitted and non-sexually transmitted types of HPV. These include flat warts, common warts, genital warts, and anogenital carcinoma [11]. The common and flat warts associated with human papillomavirus (HPV) are the most frequently seen in SOTR, followed by molluscum warts caused by the molluscum contagiosum virus (MCV).

7.2 *Bacterial Infection*

Bacterial infection after transplantation includes hospital/community-acquired infection as well as opportunistic infections (see Chap. Bacterial Diseases). In the immediate posttransplant period, wound or line infections may be seen. Prolonged hospitalization may result in colonization with multi-drug-resistant organisms such as *Klebsiella* spp. or methicillin-resistant *Staphylococcus* spp. [12].

SOTR are typically placed on trimethoprim-sulfamethoxazole prophylaxis to prevent *Pneumocystis jirovecii* pneumonia (PCP); this reduces the risk for other bacterial infections as well. Later in the transplant course, opportunistic bacterial infections include Nocardia, *Toxoplasma gondii*, and *Listeria monocytogenes*. Nocardia should be in the differential for a draining abscess, ulcer, or deeper mycetoma.

7.3 Mycobacterial Infection

SOTR are susceptible to mycobacterial tuberculosis and Hansen's disease, in areas where these are endemic (see Chap. Mycobacterial Diseases). Community-acquired disease typically appears after the first year, but reactivation of latent disease after transplantation is possible. The incidence of tuberculosis is 20–74 times higher in SOTR compared to the general population, with risk factors including prior exposure to *M. tuberculosis* and intensity of immunosuppression [13]. Treatment for latent tuberculosis infection is effective in SOTR, with only 2% of SOTR going on to develop TB after treatment [14]. Tuberculosis appearing within the first few months after transplant should raise a concern for donor-derived tuberculosis [15]. *M. leprae* is primarily observed in endemic regions such as Brazil, India, and Indonesia.

The non-tuberculous mycobacteria may also present after transplantation, particularly impacting lung transplant recipients through aerosolized infection. Cutaneous manifestations are typically found when these mycobacteria infect through skin trauma.

7.4 Fungal Infection

Invasive fungal infection is a significant source of morbidity after transplantation, with invasive candidiasis representing approximately half of cases, followed by invasive mold infections such as aspergillosis or mucormycosis [16]. The most common fungal skin infection in transplant recipients is *Candida albicans*, which typically arises in the first year after transplantation. Deep fungal infections are less frequent, and typically arise after the first year. Of these, phaeohyphomycosis is the most common and typically presents as nodules [17]. In contrast, community-acquired cutaneous dermatophytosis and pityriasis versicolor become more common after the first year (see Chaps. Superficial Fungal Diseases and Deep Fungal Diseases). Prompt treatment of superficial dermatomycoses may prevent invasive or extensive disease [18].

Additional diagnostic clues may come from the patterns of prophylactic antifungal use after transplantation. Liver, pancreas, and small bowel recipients are frequently placed on prophylactic fluconazole in the first month posttransplant, while lung transplant recipients are typically placed on voriconazole or a newer azole antifungal to prevent pulmonary aspergillosis [16]. Dermatologists may observe antifungal-resistant cutaneous infections, or new disease presenting arising upon cessation of prophylaxis. Management of fungal infection is best undertaken in partnership with the transplant team, as many antifungals interact with transplant immunosuppression and alter drug levels.

8 Posttransplant Skin Cancer

Many of the risk factors for skin cancer after organ transplantation mirror those in the general population. The UV-associated keratinocyte carcinomas and melanoma are increased in patient with fair skin, light hair and eyes, older age, male sex, a tendency to burn in the sun, and an extensive history of sun exposure [19]. Additional risk after transplantation is associated with age at transplant, level and duration of immunosuppression, and specific medications such as voriconazole and azathioprine [20].

It is difficult to capture patient-specific levels of immunosuppression in large epidemiologic studies, and no specific biomarker of immunosuppression has yet proven to be indicative of skin cancer risk. In general, the lung and the heart are the most immunogenic organs and require the highest levels of immunosuppression, followed by small bowel, pancreas, kidney, and then liver. These categories, or the rough split into thoracic vs. abdominal transplant, have been used as high-level proxies for level of immunosuppression in multiple studies of skin cancer risk after transplant. However, patient-specific care entails a detailed review of demographic risk factors, sun exposure and sun protection behaviors, and pre- and posttransplant immunosuppression regimens.

While UV-induced skin cancers, and particularly SCC, are the most common malignancies after transplantation, the viral-associated skin cancers are also increased in SOTR. Reactivation of human herpesvirus 8 (HHV-8) can lead to posttransplant Kaposi sarcoma (KS), which arises from endothelial cells (see Chap. Kaposi Sarcoma). KS is most common among SOTR of color and those in geographic areas where HHV-8 is endemic, such as the Mediterranean and sub-Saharan Africa [21]. HPV-associated anogenital carcinoma is another oncoviral cancer that is increased in SOTR. A thorough skin examination is crucial, as occult HPV-associated genital lesions have been reported in over 40% of SOTR, frequently unrecognized by the patient [22]. Merkel cell carcinoma (MCC), which may be UV-associated or driven by the MCC polyomavirus (MCPyV) is extremely rare but aggressive (see Chap. Other Rare Cancers) [23]. Posttransplant lymphoproliferative disorder (PTLD) is frequently associated with Epstein-Barr virus (EBD), particularly in those PTLD that develop within the first-year posttransplant (see Chap. Lymphoproliferative Diseases) [24].

References

1. Walder BK, Robertson MR, Jeremy D. Skin cancer and immunosuppression. Lancet. 1971;2(7737):1282–3. https://doi.org/10.1016/s0140-6736(71)90602-7.
2. Zwald F, Leitenberger J, Zeitouni N, et al. Recommendations for solid organ transplantation for transplant candidates with a pretransplant diagnosis of cutaneous squamous cell carcinoma, Merkel cell carcinoma and melanoma: a consensus opinion from the International

Transplant Skin Cancer Collaborative (ITSCC). Am J Transplant. 2016;16(2):407–13. https://doi.org/10.1111/ajt.13593.
3. Volk ML, Biggins SW, Huang MA, Argo CK, Fontana RJ, Anspach RR. Decision making in liver transplant selection committees: a multicenter study. Ann Intern Med. 2011;155(8):503–8. https://doi.org/10.7326/0003-4819-155-8-201110180-00006.
4. Crow LD, Jambusaria-Pahlajani A, Chung CL, et al. Initial skin cancer screening for solid organ transplant recipients in the United States: Delphi method development of expert consensus guidelines. Transpl Int. 2019;32(12):1268–76. https://doi.org/10.1111/tri.13520.
5. Juszczak H, Lowenstein SE, Crow L, Roll GR, McCalmont TH, Arron ST. Potential for overlooked melanoma in solid organ donors with a severely dysplastic nevus. JAAD Case Rep. 2018;4(7):682–3. Published 2018 Aug 11. https://doi.org/10.1016/j.jdcr.2018.04.018.
6. Jambusaria-Pahlajani A, Crow LD, Lowenstein S, et al. Predicting skin cancer in organ transplant recipients: development of the SUNTRAC screening tool using data from a multicenter cohort study. Transpl Int. 2019;32(12):1259–67. https://doi.org/10.1111/tri.13493.
7. Piaserico S, Sandini E, Peserico A, Alaibac M. Cutaneous viral infections in organ transplant patients. G Ital Dermatol Venereol. 2014;149(4):409–15.
8. Kwon DE, Lee HS, Lee KH, La Y, Han SH, Song YG. Incidence of herpes zoster in adult solid organ transplant recipients: a meta-analysis and comprehensive review. Transpl Infect Dis. 2021;23(4):e13674. https://doi.org/10.1111/tid.13674.
9. Lee DH, Zuckerman RA, AST Infectious Diseases Community of Practice. Herpes simplex virus infections in solid organ transplantation: guidelines from the American Society of Transplantation Infectious Diseases Community of Practice. Clin Transpl. 2019;33(9):e13526.
10. Tan HH, Goh CL. Viral infections affecting the skin in organ transplant recipients: epidemiology and current management strategies. Am J Clin Dermatol. 2006;7(1):13–29. https://doi.org/10.2165/00128071-200607010-00003.
11. Chin-Hong PV, Reid GE, AST Infectious Diseases Community of Practice. Human papillomavirus infection in solid organ transplant recipients: guidelines from the American Society of Transplantation Infectious Diseases Community of Practice. Clin Transpl. 2019;33(9):e13590.
12. Fishman JA. Infection in organ transplantation. Am J Transplant. 2017;17(4):856–79. https://doi.org/10.1111/ajt.14208.
13. Aguado JM, Silva JT, Samanta P, Singh N. Tuberculosis and transplantation. Microbiol Spectr. 2016;4:6. https://doi.org/10.1128/microbiolspec.TNMI7-0005-2016.
14. Abad CLR, Deziel PJ, Razonable RR. Treatment of latent TB infection and the risk of tuberculosis after solid organ transplantation: comprehensive review. Transpl Infect Dis. 2019;21(6):e13178. https://doi.org/10.1111/tid.13178.
15. Abad CLR, Razonable RR. Donor derived Mycobacterium tuberculosis infection after solid-organ transplantation: a comprehensive review. Transpl Infect Dis. 2018;20(5):e12971. https://doi.org/10.1111/tid.12971.
16. Garcia-Vidal CG, Carratala J, Lortholary O. Defining standards of CARE for invasive fungal diseases in solid organ transplant patients. J Antimicrob Chemother. 2019;74(Suppl 2):ii16–20.
17. Galezowski A, Delyon J, Le Cleach L, et al. Deep cutaneous fungal infections in solid-organ transplant recipients. J Am Acad Dermatol. 2020;83(2):455–62. https://doi.org/10.1016/j.jaad.2019.12.064.
18. Rouzaud C, Chosidow O, Brocard A, et al. Severe dermatophytosis in solid organ transplant recipients: a French retrospective series and literature review. Transpl Infect Dis. 2018;20(1) https://doi.org/10.1111/tid.12799.
19. Lowenstein SE, Garrett G, Toland AE, et al. Risk prediction tools for keratinocyte carcinoma after solid organ transplantation: a review of the literature. Br J Dermatol. 2017;177(5):1202–7. https://doi.org/10.1111/bjd.15889.
20. Madeleine MM, Patel NS, Plasmeijer EI, et al. Epidemiology of keratinocyte carcinomas after organ transplantation. Br J Dermatol. 2017;177(5):1208–16. https://doi.org/10.1111/bjd.15931.

21. Andreoni M, Goletti D, Pezzotti P, et al. Prevalence, incidence and correlates of HHV-8/KSHV infection and Kaposi's sarcoma in renal and liver transplant recipients. J Infect. 2001;43(3):195–9. https://doi.org/10.1053/jinf.2001.0899.
22. Nadhan KS, Larijani M, Abbott J, Doyle AM, Linfante AW, Chung CL. Prevalence and types of genital lesions in organ transplant recipients. JAMA Dermatol. 2018;154(3):323–9. https://doi.org/10.1001/jamadermatol.2017.5801.
23. Arron ST, Canavan T, Yu SS. Organ transplant recipients with Merkel cell carcinoma have reduced progression-free, overall, and disease-specific survival independent of stage at presentation. J Am Acad Dermatol. 2014;71(4):684–90. https://doi.org/10.1016/j.jaad.2014.05.054.
24. King RL, Khurana A, Mwangi R, et al. Clinicopathologic characteristics, treatment, and outcomes of post-transplant lymphoproliferative disorders: a single-institution experience using 2017 WHO diagnostic criteria. Hemasphere. 2021;5(10):e640. Published 2021 Sept 6. https://doi.org/10.1097/HS9.0000000000000640.

Cutaneous Side Effects of Immunosuppressive Drugs Other Than Neoplasms

Isadora Zago Miotto and Walmar Roncalli Pereira de Oliveira

1 Introduction

Solid organ transplant recipients (SOTRs) may present with a wide spectrum of cutaneous findings related to the immunosuppressant regimens. Although cutaneous malignancies associated with SOTRs are well described, there is less information regarding nonmalignant skin changes that may occur after transplantation. There are numerous dermatological toxicities secondary to the immunosuppressive drugs, which can vary in presentation and severity in this population. Cutaneous side effects related to the following drugs will be discussed: systemic steroids, azathioprine, mycophenolate mofetil, cyclosporine, tacrolimus, mTOR inhibitors (sirolimus and everolimus), and newer agents, such as monoclonal antibodies and biologic drugs. It may be difficult to attribute some dermatological finding to a specific immunosuppressant or to a combination of drugs, as well as it may be challenging to define if an event is directly imputed to the drug's mechanism of action or if it is due to immunosuppression. Transplant care providers must be able to recognize and properly manage these cutaneous side effects in order to limit associated morbidity and mortality.

I. Z. Miotto (✉) · W. R. P. de Oliveira
Department of Dermatology, Hospital of Clinics, University of São Paulo Medical School, São Paulo, SP, Brazil
e-mail: isadora.miotto@usp.br; walmar.roncalli@hc.fm.usp.br

J. Tomimori et al. (eds.), *Atlas of Dermatologic Diseases in Solid Organ Transplant Recipients*, https://doi.org/10.1007/978-3-031-13335-0_3

2 Systemic Steroids

2.1 Epidemiology

Systemic steroids are used in most of the immunosuppressant regimens, often prescribed at higher doses earlier in the posttransplantation period before being progressively tapered down to lower doses or suspended in the following months or years. Skin changes related to steroids occur in up to 50% of patients treated with prednisone >20 mg/day for at least 3 months [1, 2].

2.2 Pathogenesis

Steroids are nonspecific immunosuppressants that inhibit B- and T-cell lymphocytes and cytokines. Dosing regimens vary based on organ transplant and patient needs, and adverse effects related to its chronic administration contribute to significant morbidity [3].

Steroids reduce the collagen and elastin synthesis and decrease fibroblastic proliferation leading to skin fragility. Through inhibiting fibroblastic function, angiogenesis and the production of ground substance, steroids also limit reepithelization of wounds [1]. Acneiform eruption is associated with the induction of Toll-like receptor 2 (TLR2) and *Cutibacterium acnes* proliferation [4].

2.3 Clinical Presentation

Cutaneous manifestations related to steroids include: acneiform eruption, striae distensae, impaired wound healing, hirsutism, skin fragility, and purpura [5]. The occurrence of exogenous Cushing syndrome, characterized by redistribution of body fat, is dependent on steroid dose and therapy length [1].

Striae distensae usually occur on the abdomen, thighs, and buttocks. The early stage (striae rubra) presents as symmetrical linear red or violaceus lesions following the lines of cleavage. As lesions mature, they become white, atrophic, and wrinkled (striae alba) [1] (Fig. 1a–d).

Steroid acne is characterized by the abrupt onset of monomorphic erythematous papules and pustules on the face and upper trunk (Fig. 2a–f). In contrast to acne vulgaris, steroid acne rarely presents with comedones, cysts, nodules, and scarring [1, 4, 6].

Predisposing factors for acneiform eruption include higher doses of steroids and age below 30 years old. The severity depends on the dose, treatment length, and medical history of acne vulgaris [4, 6].

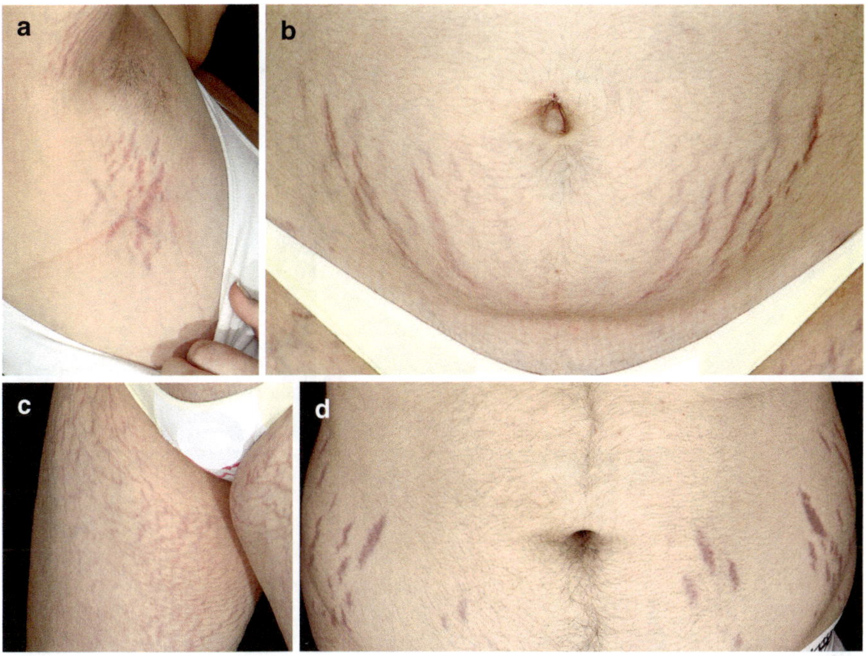

Fig. 1 (**a–d**) Striae distensae. Multiple erythematous, linear, atrophic lesions on the trunk, abdomen, and thighs. (Images collection, Department of Dermatology, Hospital of Clinics, University of São Paulo Medical School (HC-FMUSP))

2.4 *Histopathology*

Steroid acne affects the hair follicles, sebaceous glands, and epidermal structures. The major histopathologic pattern includes superficial perifolliculitis, characterized by neutrophilic infiltrate surrounding the hyperkeratotic follicular infundibula with rupture of the epithelial lining [6].

Regarding striae distensae, its early stages are characterized by mast cell degranulation, elastolysis and, elastophagocytosis by activated macrophages. In stablished striae, the epidermis appears atrophic, the thickness of the dermis is reduced, and the collagen bundles are oriented in a horizontal plane [7].

2.5 *Treatment*

Steroid acne can be managed with conventional treatments for acne vulgaris, including topical and systemic retinoids, benzoyl peroxide, and topical and/or systemic antibiotics. Persistent cases may need steroid dose reduction or cessation, when possible [1, 4].

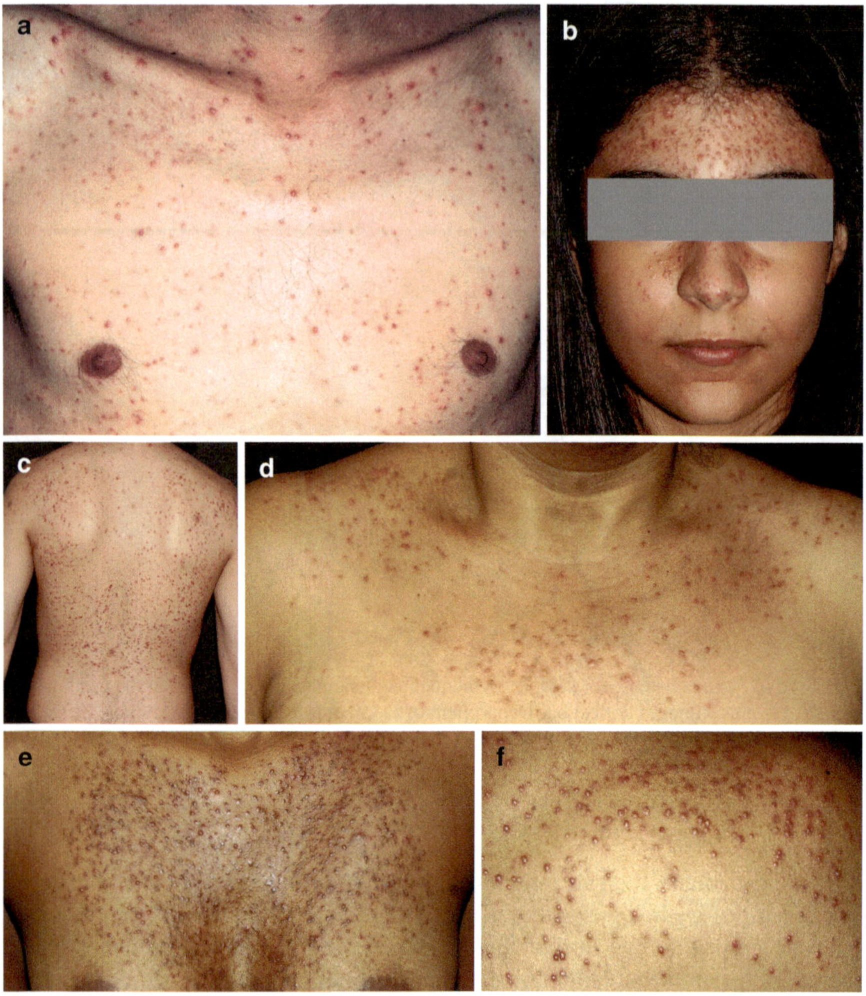

Fig. 2 (**a–f**) Acneiform eruption. Monomorphic erythematous papules and pustules on the face and upper trunk. (Images collection, Department of Dermatology, Hospital of Clinics, University of São Paulo Medical School (HC-FMUSP))

Mild atrophy induced by steroids can be resolved by reduction or suspension of the drug. Significant atrophy and striae distensae are difficult to treat. Topical retinoids and ammonium lactate may be useful in minimizing atrophy, striae, and related purpura [1].

3 Azathioprine

3.1 Epidemiology

Azathioprine was one of the first drugs approved for use in transplantation and a hallmark of the immunosuppressive therapy until the development of other drugs, such as calcineurin inhibitors [3]. The overall incidence of side effects leading to drug withdrawal ranges from 10% to 15%. Around 2% of the patients taking azathioprine develop some cutaneous toxicity [1, 8].

3.2 Pathogenesis

Azathioprine is a synthetic purine analog derived from 6-mercaptopurine. The drug is a nonspecific antimetabolite that interrupts the DNA synthesis phase of lymphocyte proliferation and leads to myelosuppression [3, 9].

Cutaneous reactions associated with azathioprine are mostly related to type IV hypersensitivity reactions and usually occur in the first 4 weeks after initiation of the drug [1, 9, 10].

3.3 Clinical Presentation

The hypersensitivity syndrome related to azathioprine is characterized by fever, cutaneous manifestations, and inflammation of internal organs such as liver, kidneys, lungs, and/or heart [11]. It is a rare yet life-threatening clinical phenomenon [12].

Azathioprine-induced hypersensitivity might be confused with infections or exacerbation of an underlying condition [8]. Skin manifestations may include maculopapular exanthema, acute generalized exanthematous pustulosis, urticaria, erythema nodosum (Fig. 3), neutrophilic dermatosis (mostly Sweet's syndrome) (Fig. 4), purpura, and leukocytoclastic vasculitis. Additional cutaneous findings include mild alopecia and photosensitivity [1, 8, 9, 11].

Diagnostic criteria for azathioprine-induced Sweet's syndrome include abrupt onset of painful erythematous plaques or nodules, fever, temporal relation of drug ingestion, and onset of symptoms or recurrence of symptoms with drug rechallenge [13].

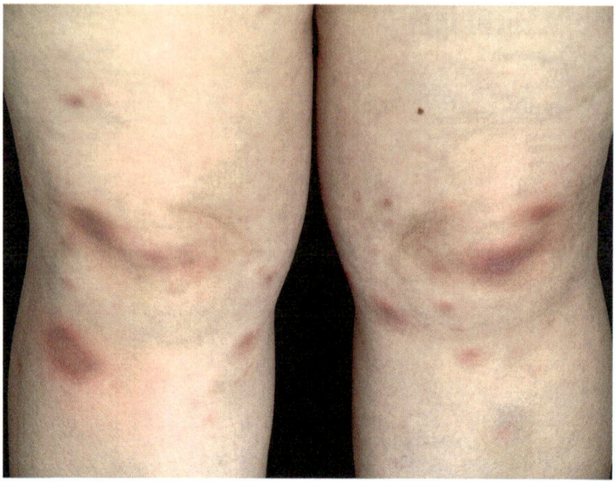

Fig. 3 Erythema nodosum. Multiple tender erythematous nodules on the lower legs. (Images collection, Department of Dermatology, Hospital of Clinics, University of São Paulo Medical School (HC-FMUSP))

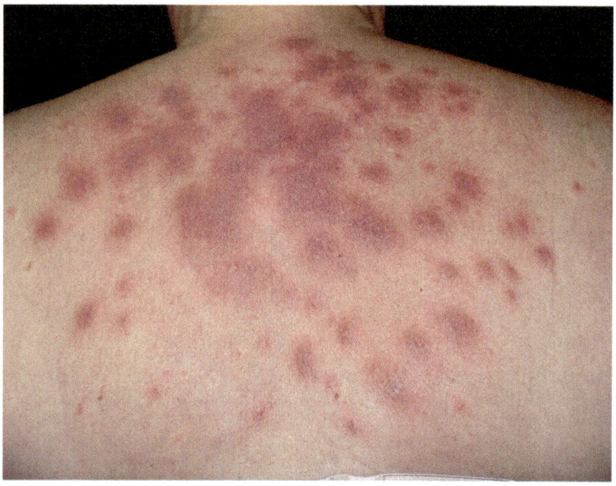

Fig. 4 Sweet's syndrome. Multiple erythematous edematous nodules and plaques on the upper back. (Images collection, Department of Dermatology, Hospital of Clinics, University of São Paulo Medical School (HC-FMUSP))

3.4 Histopathology

Erythema nodosum is characterized by septal inflammation, hemorrhage, vascular damage, and a variable degree of acute or chronic panniculitis. The overlying dermis typically shows a perivascular and periadnexal chronic inflammatory cell infiltrate [7].

Neutrophilic dermatoses, such as Sweet's syndrome, are characterized by a dense neutrophilic infiltrate within the reticular dermis, that may be diffuse or have a perivascular distribution pattern, without evidence of vasculitis [7, 13].

3.5 Treatment

Cutaneous side effects related to azathioprine can be managed with the discontinuation of the drug and/or replacement by other immunosuppressant. Hypersensitivity symptoms typically resolve in a few days after drug withdrawal, and it should not be reintroduced afterwards, as clinical manifestations may recur [9, 11].

4 Mycophenolate Mofetil

4.1 Epidemiology

Mycophenolate mofetil (MMF) has limited cutaneous toxicities and is preferred over azathioprine due to its increased efficacy with fewer side effects [3]. In contrast to other immunosuppressants, the drug has not been found to be nephrotoxic or neurotoxic. Systemic side effects may include mild myelodepression and gastrointestinal disturbances such as vomiting and diarrhea. Oral ulcers can also be found in SOTRs taking mycophenolate mofetil [14].

4.2 Pathogenesis

MMF and mycophenolate sodium are prodrugs of mycophenolic acid, which inhibits the enzyme dehydrogenase monophosphate [3]. This enzyme is required in purine synthesis pathway, obligatory for the proliferation and function of T and B lymphocytes [14].

The exact mechanism of oral ulcers induced by MMF is not completely understood although theories regarding direct toxic damage to the mucosa associated with bacterial or viral proliferation induced by immunosuppression have been proposed [14, 15].

4.3 Clinical Presentation

Aphthous stomatitis presents on the oral mucosa as ulcers with a greyish pseudomembrane surrounded by erythema and edema (Fig. 5a–c). Some cases may be severe, multiple, confluent, and large. These lesions are usually not accompanied by other side effects and time between starting the drug and the onset of ulcers varies greatly, ranging from 1 week to 3 years. Other rare side effects include acne, dyshidrotic eczema, and peripheral edema [1, 14].

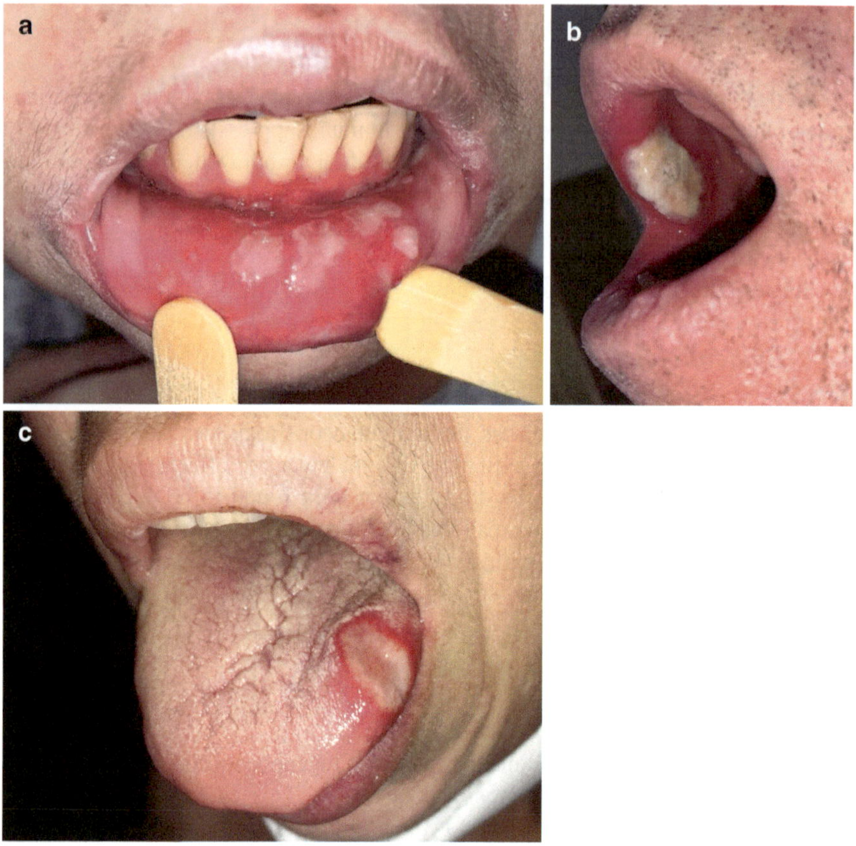

Fig. 5 (**a**–**c**) Aphthous stomatitis. Multiple oral ulcers with a greyish pseudo-membrane on the jugal mucosa and tongue. (**a**, **b**: Images collection, Department of Dermatology, Hospital of Clinics, University of São Paulo Medical School (HC-FMUSP), **c**: Courtesy of Carla Ferrándiz-Pulido, MD, PhD)

4.4 Histopathology

Aphthous ulcers show nonspecific inflammatory changes on hematoxylin-eosin (H&E) staining. The ulcer bed is characterized by the presence of granulation tissue with inflammatory cells [7].

4.5 Treatment

Other causes of aphthous ulcers, such as infections and hematologic disorders, need to be ruled out through physical examination, laboratory tests, and histopathological analysis. Drug discontinuation should be considered and leads to regression of lesions [1, 14].

5 Cyclosporine

5.1 Epidemiology

Cyclosporine is a potent immunosuppressant drug that has been used since early 1980s to prevent organ rejection after transplantation. The great majority of cutaneous side effects due to cyclosporine found in SOTRs are caused by its harmful effects in the follicular units [1].

Sebaceous hyperplasia and hypertrichosis occur in up to 30% and 70% of SOTRs taking cyclosporine, respectively. The prevalence of sebaceous hyperplasia is around 16% in heart transplant recipients and 10% in renal transplant recipients [16]. Gingival overgrowth has been observed in about one-third of patients after 3 months of therapy [1, 17].

5.2 Pathogenesis

Cyclosporine blocks IL-2 production and T lymphocytes function through the formation of a complex with cyclophilin, thus inhibiting calcineurin activation. It is metabolized via the CYP450 3A4 enzymes. Its therapeutic levels can vary due to other drugs that are metabolized via the same enzyme pathway [2, 3].

Cyclosporine releases the inhibition of a nuclear factor on hair follicle stem cells, leading to an increase in the anagen phase of hair growth on the face and body [1]. It has been suggested that cyclosporine might cause morphological changes in the follicular units [18, 19].

The pathogenesis of gingival overgrowth is not fully understood, but some studies suggest that dental plaque and gingivitis are important contributing factors. Chronic gingivitis promotes a decrease in matrix metalloproteinases and an increase in collagen and extracellular matrix production [1, 7, 20].

5.3 Clinical Presentation

The gingival overgrowth is usually characterized by a growth beginning in the anterior labial gingiva [1]. Multiple gingival areas can be affected, initially by nodular hyperplasia in the interdental areas, which become coalescent to form diffuse masses and may lead to alveolar bone loss [20]. Such gingival overgrowth is rare in edentulous patients and if the teeth are extracted, lesions tend not to recur, reinforcing the theory of dental bacteria as playing an important role in its pathogenesis [7] (Fig. 6a, b).

Most of the cutaneous side effects related to cyclosporine involve the pilosebaceous units: hypertrichosis (Fig. 7a, b), sebaceous hyperplasia, folliculitis, acne, keratosis pilaris, and epidermoid cysts [1, 18, 21].

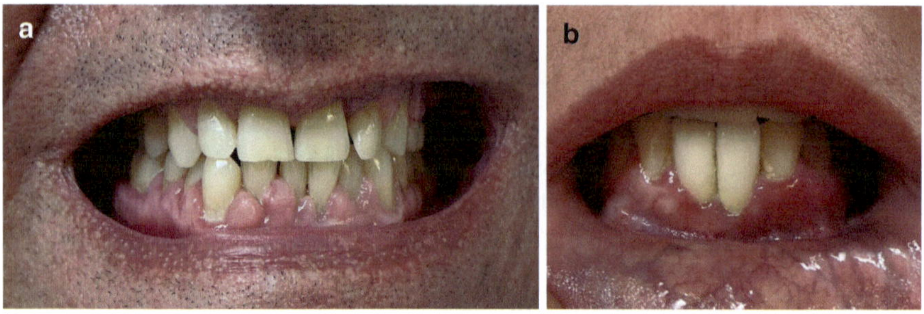

Fig. 6 (**a**, **b**) Gingival hyperplasia. Gingival overgrowth in the interdental areas. (Images collection, Department of Dermatology, Hospital of Clinics, University of São Paulo Medical School (HC-FMUSP))

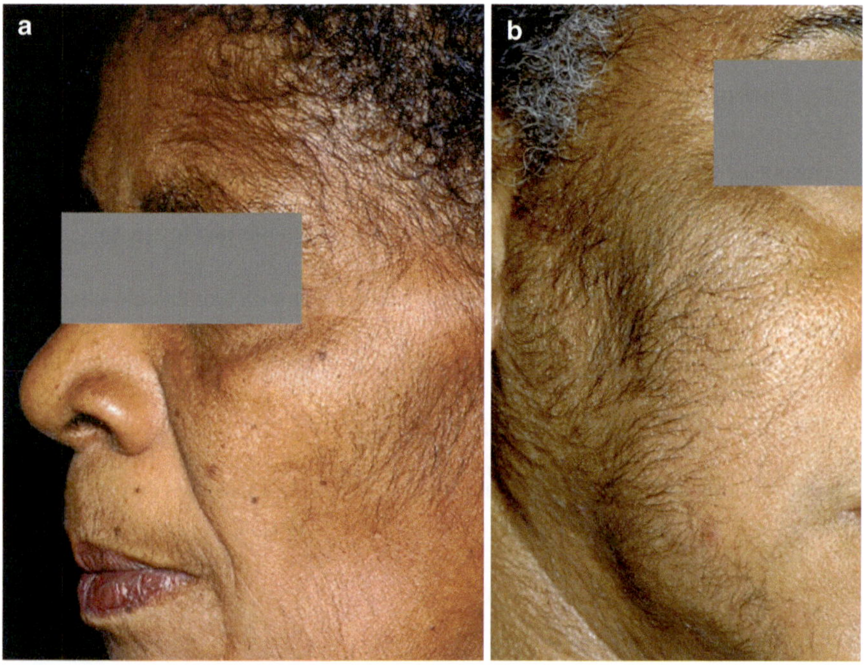

Fig. 7 (**a**, **b**) Hypertrichosis. Abnormal hair growth on the forehead, temporal, malar, and mandibular area. (Images collection, Department of Dermatology, Hospital of Clinics, University of São Paulo Medical School (HC-FMUSP))

Sebaceous hyperplasia presents as multiple, isolated, or grouped, yellowish asymptomatic umbilicated papules predominantly on the forehead and cheeks. In SOTRs, these lesions are large and may involve atypical locations, such as the upper trunk and genital area [1, 7, 16, 21] (Fig. 8a–d).

Acne due to cyclosporine is typically nodulocystic, contrasting to the acneiform eruption induced by steroids. Another possible side effect is the occurrence of

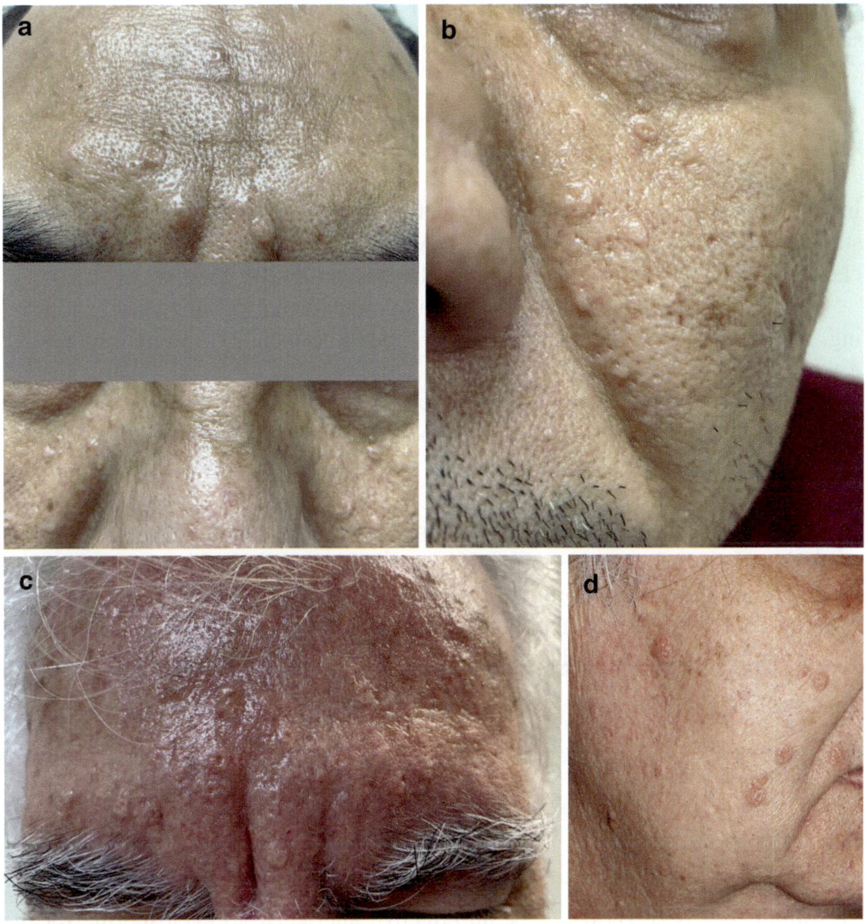

Fig. 8 (**a**–**d**) Sebaceous hyperplasia. Multiple yellowish umbilicated papules on the forehead and cheeks. (Images collection, Department of Dermatology, Hospital of Clinics, University of São Paulo Medical School (HC-FMUSP))

pseudofolliculitis barbae, a chronic inflammatory disorder of facial hair-bearing areas characterized by folliculocentric papules and pustules [1, 21].

5.4 Histopathology

Gingival hyperplasia presents histologically as a proliferation of collagen fibers with variable fibroblasts hyperplasia. The epithelium is parakeratinized. Lymphoplasmacytic infiltrate and vascular ectasia can be found [7, 20].

Sebaceous hyperplasia is characterized by hyperplastic sebaceous glands. Individual sebaceous lobules are increased in number, and lobules drain to a central duct, which is often associated with a hair follicle. In confluent lesions, multiple sebaceous glands are similarly affected [7, 16].

5.5 Treatment

Improvement of dental hygiene and reduction of cyclosporine dosage are the main strategies for reducing gingival growth. Antibiotic therapy, such as azithromycin, clarithromycin, and metronidazole, may also be useful [20].

Hypertrichosis can be managed with epilation methods, including laser and waxing. An alternative is the switch from cyclosporine to other immunosuppressive drug like tacrolimus, when possible [1].

Treatment of sebaceous hyperplasia consists in destructive methods such as electrodessication and cryotherapy. Carbon dioxide-laser and pulsed dyed-laser may be viable options [1]. Isotretinoin can also be prescribed in a low dosage [16].

Systemic antibiotics and isotretinoin are the most effective therapy for nodulocystic acne induced by cyclosporine. If isotretinoin is prescribed in association with cyclosporine, a close monitoring of serum lipid levels is recommended [1].

Drug-induced pseudofolliculitis barbae is usually resistant to topical treatment options and may require cyclosporine dose reduction [1].

6 Tacrolimus

6.1 Epidemiology

Tacrolimus has been shown to be an effective alternative to cyclosporine for the prevention of organ rejection with fewer cutaneous side effects. Alopecia and telogen effluvium are the most common and affect up to 30% of SOTRs. Shapiro et al. first described tacrolimus-related alopecia in 1990 and only a few cases have been reported so far [22].

6.2 Pathogenesis

Tacrolimus binds to an immunophilin, FK506-binding protein (FKBP), and inhibits calcineurin phosphatase. The drug inhibits calcium-dependent events, such as interleukin-2 expression by T-lymphocytes. Its properties are similar to cyclosporine [3]. The mechanism of alopecia related to calcineurin inhibitors have not yet been elucidated, but it might be related to tacrolimus-induced vasoconstriction and apoptosis [1].

Telogen effluvium is caused by an impairment of the hair cycle that results in shifting of a large proportion of hair follicles from anagen to telogen phase, leading to widespread shedding and thinning of hair [1, 23]. It can occur as a result of five different functional changes in the hair follicle: immediate anagen release, delayed anagen release, short anagen syndrome, immediate telogen release, and a delayed telogen release [7].

6.3 Clinical Presentation

Telogen effluvium is characterized by diffuse hair shedding. There are two main presentations: an acute self-limiting presentation that last less than 6 months and is generally precipitated by a recognizable event, and a chronic presentation of an unknown etiology [1].

An extensive range of events and diseases, such as thyroid dysfunction, infectious diseases, surgery, iron-deficiency anemia, eating disorders, neoplasms, psychological distress, severe systemic illness, and drugs may precipitate acute telogen effluvium. When related to tacrolimus, telogen effluvium usually occurs around 3 months after the initiation of the drug and resolves after its withdrawal [1, 7].

Telogen effluvium presents as a diffuse noninflammatory hair loss involving the entire scalp although baldness is never observed (Fig. 9a–c). The hair pull-test is positive and trichogram shows increase of the telogen hair follicles [1, 7].

6.4 Histopathology

The histological findings in telogen effluvium are subtle and include an increase in the number of telogen germinal units, telogen hair follicles, and follicular stelae in the deep scalp layers with a normal number of hair follicles. There is no significant inflammatory infiltrate or follicular miniaturization [7].

6.5 Treatment

Due to the great number of diseases and clinical scenarios that may be related to telogen effluvium, a detailed medical history is necessary to establish the role of tacrolimus in the hair loss, as well as laboratory tests in order to exclude illnesses that might provoke alopecia [1].

Tacrolimus may be discontinued and/or replaced by another immunosuppressant drug, if possible. Patients may also be treated with topical minoxidil 5% [23]. The vasodilatory effect of minoxidil is believed to improve local vasoconstriction that occurs in the scalp of these patients [24].

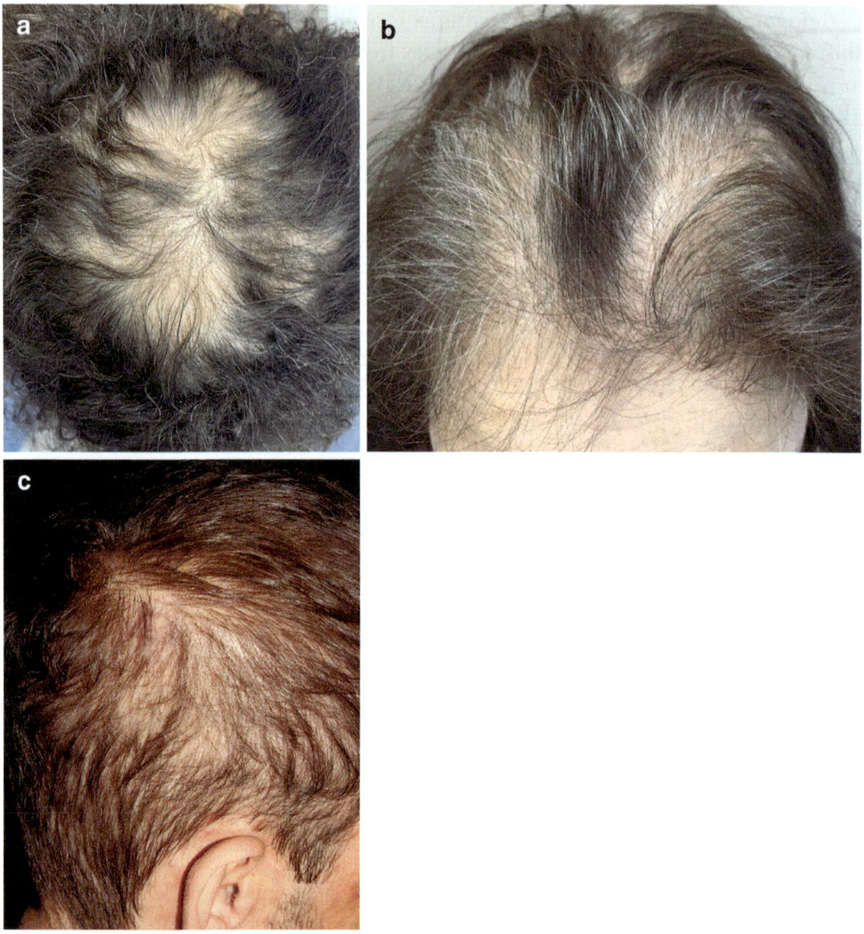

Fig. 9 (**a–c**) Tacrolimus-related alopecia. Diffuse noninflammatory hair loss. (Images collection, Department of Dermatology, Hospital of Clinics, University of São Paulo Medical School (HC-FMUSP))

7 mTOR Inhibitors: Sirolimus and Everolimus

7.1 Epidemiology

The mammalian target of rapamycin (mTOR) inhibitor class is well established as part of the immunosuppressive regimen used in SOTRs. Sirolimus and everolimus can be prescribed in association with steroids, azathioprine, or MMF [25]. These drugs can also be used to replace calcineurin inhibitors, in case of important side effects related to the latter [26].

Although generally well-tolerated, aphthous ulcers may occur in 10–20% of patients taking mTOR inhibitors and are dose dependent. Acneiform eruption can be seen in 15–45% of patients, with a higher prevalence in men [26–29]. Nail abnormalities may occur in more than half of patients, such as fragility and slow growth [30].

An important and common side effect of mTOR inhibitors is the development of peripheral edema, predominantly on the lower limbs. It can be painful and may limit daily activities. The use of mTOR inhibitors-based immunosuppressive regimens can also lead to a higher prevalence of wound-healing complications [30, 31].

7.2 Pathogenesis

Sirolimus is a macrocyclic lactone produced by *Streptomyces hygroscopicus*, and everolimus is the 40-*O*-(2-hydroxyethyl) derivative of sirolimus [25]. Everolimus has higher oral biodisponibility and better metabolic stability in comparison to sirolimus. However, their side effect profile is quite similar and seem to be dose related [2].

These drugs inhibit T lymphocyte activation and proliferation. They bind to FK-binding protein-12 (FKBP-12) to generate an immunosuppressive complex that inhibits the activation of mTOR and cause suppression of cytokine-driven T-cell proliferation [25, 27–30].

The inhibition of vascular endothelial growth factor (VEGF) is related to most of the reported side effects, such as impaired wound healing, acneiform eruption, and peripheral edema [1]. This drug class is also believed to have a direct toxic effect on hair follicles and mucous membranes, as well as impairing fibroblasts function and inhibiting angiogenesis [26–29, 31].

7.3 Clinical Presentation

Sirolimus and everolimus may cause multiple dermatological side effects, including aphthous ulcers, impaired wound healing and dermatoses affecting the pilosebaceous units [1].

Aphthous ulcers affect non-keratinized mucosae, like the labial and buccal mucosa, the floor of the mouth, or the ventral surface of the tongue [26]. Lesions appear as oval ulcers with a central grey area surrounded by an erythematous band and usually develop in the first month of therapy [1, 32]. They can present as small or larger and confluent lesions, the latter defined as the major type of aphthous stomatitis (Fig. 10). Patients may complain of severe pain and anorexia. Diagnosis is

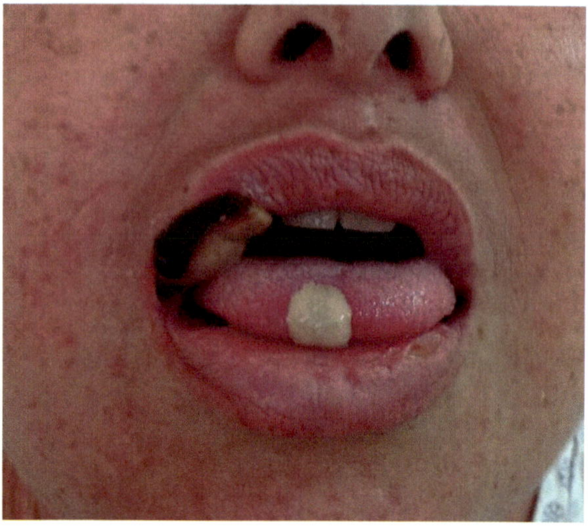

Fig. 10 Oral ulcer related to everolimus. Large oral ulcer with a yellowish pseudo-membrane on the tongue (Reproduced from Pasin et al. 2015; Images collection, Department of Dermatology, EPM/Unifesp)

made clinically and biopsy should be reserved for persistent cases, in order to exclude cytomegalovirus infection [33, 34].

The most common form of pilosebaceous inflammation related to mTOR inhibitors is acneiform eruption. It usually occurs in the first month of therapy and presents as erythematous lesions on sebaceous areas, such as the head and upper trunk, but may also extend to the arms and cervical area [26–28]. Folliculitis, hidradenitis suppurativa, furuncles, and chalazion can also be found [1, 27].

Transplant recipients taking mTOR inhibitors have a higher rate of wound-healing complications due to their anti-proliferative effects, including wound dehiscence, seromas, hematomas, abscesses, ulcers, and lymphoceles [22, 28, 31, 35].

Palmoplantar peeling is characterized by tenderness, dry vesicles, and skin desquamation, and may occur in the first weeks of sirolimus therapy. It can resolve spontaneously or after drug discontinuation [1, 36].

Peripheral edema is another common side effect. It is not dose related, and there is no clear relationship between time since starting the drug or time since transplantation and the occurrence of edema. Most cases are located in the lower limbs, tend to be asymmetrical and painful [1, 27] (Fig. 11a–e). Lymphedema is less frequent and is related to lymphatic drainage impairment [37].

Other toxicities related to sirolimus include leukocytoclastic vasculitis and nail changes, such as onycholysis, splinter hemorrhages, brittle nails, leukonychia, and pyogenic granulomas [26]. The nail fragility increases the risk of periungual traumatisms, which leads to perionyxis and infections [27].

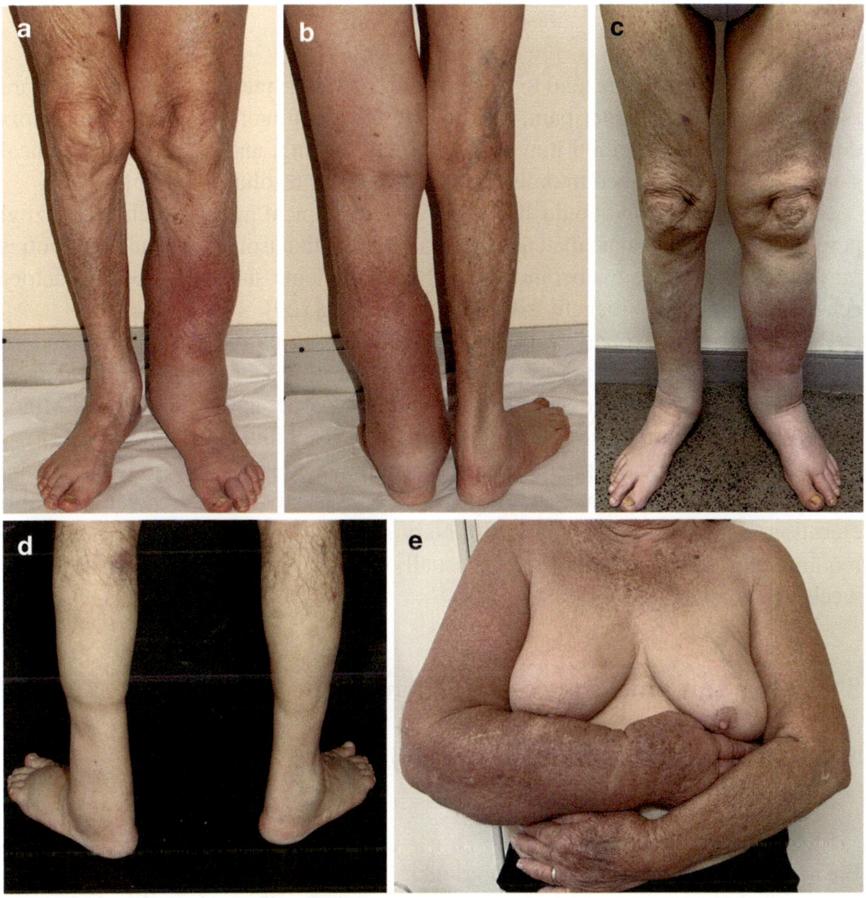

Fig. 11 (**a–e**) Peripheral edema related to mTOR inhibitors. Asymmetrical peripheral edema on the lower and upper limbs. (Images collection, Department of Dermatology, Hospital of Clinics, University of São Paulo Medical School (HC-FMUSP))

7.4 Histopathology

Histological findings of acneiform eruption related to mTOR inhibitors are similar to those related to other drugs, including follicular plugging, perifolliculitis, and neutrophilic suppurative folliculitis [7].

Palmoplantar peeling is histologically characterized by orthokeratosis, parakeratosis, and may present with some degree of interface damage. Periodic acid-Schiff (PAS) stain is usually negative for fungal organisms [36].

The histological appearance of aphthous ulcers is not specific. There is ulceration of the mucosa with a thick fibrin clot enmeshed with neutrophils [7].

7.5 Treatment

Although aphthous ulcers tend to be self-limited, lesions may last for weeks and are associated with significant pain, resulting in transient anorexia. mTOR inhibitors dose reduction or cessation may lead to ulcers healing, and high potency topical steroids can be prescribed in order to provide a faster resolution [1, 26].

Acneiform eruption should be managed with topical agents, such as benzoyl peroxide, tretinoin, and adapalene. Systemic agents like isotretinoin and antibiotics may be used in more exuberant cases [1, 28]. Patients suffering from refractory acneiform lesions may benefit from drug withdrawal [29].

The majority of wound-healing complications can be managed with standard clinical care. Wound dehiscence may demand surgical debridement. Fluid collections may require drainage and infections require proper antibiotic therapy. Minor wound-healing complications do not require mTOR inhibitors cessation [1, 31].

Regarding chronic peripheral edema, if left untreated it may lead to lymphedema and stasis dermatitis. Management includes conservative measures such as limb elevation, compression therapy, and dietary salt restriction [1]. Severe cases may require drug discontinuation, which usually leads to a slow resolution in a few weeks or months [30].

8 Other Immunosuppressive Agents

8.1 Monoclonal Antibodies (mAbs): Basiliximab and Daclizumab

Basiliximab and daclizumab are interleukin-2 receptor-directed monoclonal antibodies used to prevent acute organ rejection in SOTRs. These drugs block the proliferation of activated T lymphocytes and are considered effective in preventing acute cellular rejection, especially in recipients with renal disfunction, which would benefit from the delay in the introduction of calcineurin inhibitors [38].

Monoclonal antibodies have selective immunosuppressive activity and a narrower side effect profile. Some cases of severe acute hypersensitivity reactions have been reported, which presents as urticaria and angioedema within the first hours of drug administration. Besides that, 3–10% of SOTRs taking basiliximab may develop cysts, hypertrichosis, herpes simplex, herpes zoster, and pruritus [38].

8.2 Belatacept

Belatacept is a B7 ligand antagonist and is an emerging biologic for immunosuppression maintenance in SOTRs. The drug is a potent antagonist of B7-1 (CD80) and B7-2 (CD86) ligands present in antigen-presenting cells that are responsible for

2 Herpes Simplex Virus (HSV)

2.1 Epidemiology

HSV is one of the most common infections of humans throughout the world [5]. We distinguish two types of herpes simplex viruses: type-1 (HSV-1), which usually causes orolabial HSV and type-2 (HSV-2) historically connected with genital lesions. However, in the last few years, HSV-1 is an increasing cause of genital lesions although is characterized by less frequent reactivation than HSV-2. HSV-1 is acquired from early childhood through adulthood [4]. The infection is usually minimal and often subclinical [5]. HSV-2 is strongly connected with sexual debut [4]. The primary HSV-2 infection is more commonly symptomatic [5].

HSV-1 seroprevalence ranges from 27% in 14- to 19 years old and 59.7% in 40- to 49 years old. HSV-2 has a seroprevalence of 0.8% of persons aged 14–19 years and 21.2% of persons aged 40–49 years. Many SOTR adults are infected with HSV with a prevalence similar to the distribution by age in the general population. Infection may be acquired from contact with infected mucocutaneous surface lesions or infected donor's tissue. Most of the HSV is acquired from asymptomatic carriers, as viral shedding is also often asymptomatic. After primary inflammation, HSV persists latent in sensory ganglia lifelong with recurrent reactivation [4].

2.2 Histopathology

Histopathology of the cutaneous lesions of HSV is characterized by the cytoplasm of infected epithelial cells becoming edematous, and swollen causing ballooning degeneration. Thick-walled vesicles are formed by the combination of intra- and intercellular oedema. The dermis and the epidermis are infiltrated with polymorphonuclear leukocytes. Intranuclear inclusions can usually be seen in a single section. Moreover, giant cells containing 2–15 or more nuclei are almost always present in the cutaneous and corneal epithelium [5].

2.3 Clinical Manifestation

The clinical manifestation of HSV is associated with localized multiple painful lesions in the orolabial, genital, and perianal area. Lesions may be vesicular (Fig. 1) or ulcerative with local extensions [4, 6]. When primary lesions develop, the severity is usually greater than in recurrences [5].

Herpes gingivostomatitis is the most common clinical manifestation of a primary infection of HSV1. After the incubation period of nearly 5 days, the gums become swollen, inflamed, and bleed easily. Vesicles looking like white plaques are present in the oral cavity and can develop into ulcers with a yellowish pseudomembrane [5] (Fig. 2).

Viral Diseases

Karolina Cekala, Alicja Debska-Slizien, and Beata Imko-Walczuk

1 Introduction

Solid organ transplant recipients (SOTR) are a population at high risk for cutaneous adverse events [1]. Infections are an important cause of morbidity and mortality among this group [2]. Viral and fungal diseases including cutaneous manifestations are far more common than bacterial ones. Their quick recognition and suitable treatment are an important element of the clinical management of SOTR and should be dealt with by dermatologists cooperating with transplantologists [1]. Skin examination should be a standard procedure before performing organ transplantation, and the dermatological care should also be maintained after transplantation since some important skin complications may occur several years after the transplant. However, about 70% of severe skin infections appear during the first 3 months after organ transplantation. Viral skin infections are the most frequent complications which decrease the quality of life in SOTR, and they usually result from reactivation of a previous infection such as the varicella-zoster virus (VZV) or cytomegalovirus (CMV) [3, 4]. Other frequent viral diseases that are found among this population are the human papilloma virus (HPV), herpes simplex virus (HSV), molluscum contagiosum (MC), trichodysplasia spinulosa (TS), and acquired epidermodysplasia verruciformis (EDV).

K. Cekala (✉)
Medicine, University Clinical Centre in Gdansk, Gdansk, Pomeranian, Poland

A. Debska-Slizien
Department of Nephrology, Transplantology and Internal Medicine, University Hospital in Gdansk, Gdansk Medical University, Gdansk, Pomeranian, Poland
e-mail: adeb@gumed.edu.pl

B. Imko-Walczuk
Dermatology Outpatient Clinic, Copernicus Hospital, Gdansk, Pomeranian, Poland

J. Tomimori et al. (eds.), *Atlas of Dermatologic Diseases in Solid Organ Transplant Recipients*, https://doi.org/10.1007/978-3-031-13335-0_4

activation of CD28 [39]. The transmembrane immunoglobulin CD28 of naïve T cells is stimulated by CD80 and CD86 and is well known as an essential component of co-stimulation in T-cell activation. Belatacept can be used as maintenance immunosuppression to replace other traditional drugs, such as calcineurin inhibitors [3, 39].

Belatacept has shown an increased risk of posttransplant lymphoproliferative disorder. However, aside from an increased risk of malignancy, the drug's side effect profile is narrow and may be an attractive option for immunosuppressive maintenance therapy [39].

Infusion-related reactions, including flushing, infusion site pain, and swelling are infrequent and usually are well tolerated [39]. Peripheral edema may occur in up to 35% of patients and hirsutism has been reported to occur in 1% of cases [40].

References

1. Ilyas M, Colegio OR, Kaplan B. Cutaneous toxicities from transplantation-related medications. Am J Transplant. 2017;17:2782–9.
2. Miotto IZ, Souza BDCE, Tyring SK, de Oliveira WRP. Immunosuppressant-induced cutaneous drug reactions in solid organ transplant recipients. Transpl Immunol. 2021;64:101355. https://doi.org/10.1016/j.trim.2020.101355.
3. Allison TL. Immunosuppressive therapy in transplantation. Nurs Clin North Am. 2016;51(1):107–20. https://doi.org/10.1016/j.cnur.2015.10.008.
4. Kazandjieva J, Tsankov N. Drug-induced acne. Clin Dermatol. 2017;35(2):156–62. https://doi.org/10.1016/j.clindermatol.2016.10.007.
5. Fardet L, Flahault A, Kettaneh A, Tiev KP, Généreau T, Tolédano C, et al. Corticosteroid-induced clinical adverse events: frequency, risk factors and patient's opinion. Br J Dermatol. 2007;157(1):142–8.
6. Dessinioti C, Antoniou C, Katsambas A. Acneiform eruptions. Clin Dermatol. 2014;32(1):24–34. https://doi.org/10.1016/j.clindermatol.2013.05.023.
7. Kee M. Pathology of the skin, vol. 51. London: Elsevier; 1999. p. 348–53.
8. Bidinger JJ, Sky K, Battafarano DF, Henning JS. The cutaneous and systemic manifestations of azathioprine hypersensitivity syndrome. J Am Acad Dermatol. 2011;65(1):184–91. https://doi.org/10.1016/j.jaad.2010.04.041.
9. Patel AA, Swerlick RA, McCall CO. Azathioprine in dermatology: the past, the present, and the future. J Am Acad Dermatol. 2006;55(3):369–89.
10. Calbo Mayo JM, Blasco Colmenarejo M, Rivera Vaquerizo PJ, Vicente Gutierrez M. Hypersensitivity reaction to azathioprine in a patient with ulcerative colitis. Inflamm Bowel Dis. 2004;10(5):700.
11. Yiasemides E, Thom G. Azathioprine hypersensitivity presenting as a neutrophilic dermatosis in a man with ulcerative colitis. Australas J Dermatol. 2009;50(1):48–51.
12. Frank J, Fett N. Azathioprine hypersensitivity syndrome. J Rheumatol. 2017;44(12):1876–7.
13. Choonhakarn C, Chaowattanapanit S. Azathioprine-induced Sweet's syndrome and published work review. J Dermatol. 2013;40(4):267–71.
14. Weng RR, Foster CE, Hsieh LL, Patel PR. Oral ulcers associated with mycophenolate mofetil use in a renal transplant recipient. Am J Health Syst Pharm. 2011;68(7):585–8.
15. Van Gelder T, Ter Meulen CG, Hené R, Weimar W, Hoitsma A. Oral ulcers in kidney transplant recipients treated with sirolimus and mycophenolate mofetil. Transplantation. 2003;75(6):788–91.

16. McDonald SK, Goh MS, Chong AH. Successful treatment of cyclosporine-induced sebaceous hyperplasia with oral isotretinoin in two renal transplant recipients. Australas J Dermatol. 2011;52(3):227–30.
17. Oliveira WRP, Tirico MCCP, Souza AAV, Codarin FR, Silva LLC, Festa NC. Skin lesions in organ transplant recipients: a study of 177 consecutive Brazilian patients. Int J Dermatol. 2019;58(4):440–8.
18. Heaphy MR, Shamma HN, Hickmann M. Cyclosporine-induced folliculodystrophy. J Am Acad Dermatol. 2004;50:310–5.
19. Salim A, Reece SM, Smith AG, Harrison D, Ramsay HM, Harden PN, et al. Sebaceous hyperplasia and skin cancer in patients undergoing renal transplant. J Am Acad Dermatol. 2006;55(5):878–81.
20. Tokgöz B, Sari HI, Yildiz O, Aslan S, Sipahioğlu M, Okten T, et al. Effects of azithromycin on cyclosporine-induced gingival hyperplasia in renal transplant patients. Transplant Proc. 2004;36(9):2699–702.
21. Dromer C, Doutre M, Beylot C. Cyclosporine-induced follicular eruption. Ann Dermatol Vénéréol. 2008;135:58–62.
22. Shapiro R, Fung JJ, Jain AB, Parks P, Todo S, Starzl TE. The side effects of FK 506 in humans. Transplant Proc. 1990;22(1):35–6.
23. Tricot L, Lebbé C, Pillebout E, Martinez F, Legendre C, Thervet E. Tacrolimus-induced alopecia in female kidney-pancreas transplant recipients. Transplantation. 2005;80(11):1546–9.
24. Iorizzo M, Tosti A. Treatments options for alopecia. Expert Opin Pharmacother. 2015;16(15):2343–54.
25. Klawitter J, Nashan B, Christians U. Everolimus and sirolimus in transplantation-related but different. Expert Opin Drug Saf. 2015;14(7):1055–70.
26. Campistol JM, de Fijter JW, Flechner SM, Langone A, Morelon E, Stockfleth E. MTOR inhibitor-associated dermatologic and mucosal problems. Clin Transpl. 2010;24(2):149–56.
27. Mahe E. Cutaneous adverse events in renal transplant recipients receiving sirolimus-based therapy 1. Transplantation. 2005;79(4):476–82.
28. Mahé E, Morelon E, Lechaton S, Drappier JC, de Prost Y, Kreis H, et al. Acne in recipients of renal transplantation treated with sirolimus: clinical, microbiologic, histologic, therapeutic, and pathogenic aspects. J Am Acad Dermatol. 2006;55(1):139–42.
29. Kunzle N, Venetz J, Pascual M, Panizzon RG, Laffi E. Sirolimus-induced acneiform eruption. Dermatology. 2005;211:366–9.
30. Montalbano M, Neff GW, Yamashiki N, Meyer D, Bettiol M, Slapak-Green G, et al. A retrospective review of liver transplant patients treated with sirolimus from a single center: an analysis of sirolimus-related complications. Transplantation. 2004;78(2):264–8.
31. Valente JF, Hricik D, Weigel K, Seaman D, Knauss T, Siegel CT, et al. Comparison of sirolimus vs. mycophenolate mofetil on surgical complications and wound healing in adult kidney transplantation. Am J Transplant. 2003;3(9):1128–34.
32. Sonis S, Treister N, Chawla S, Demetri G, Haluska F. Preliminary characterization of oral lesions associated with inhibitors of mammalian target of rapamycin in cancer patients. Cancer. 2010;116(1):210–5.
33. Dioguardi M, Troiano G, Lo Russo L, Giannatempo G, Rubini C, Bertossi D, et al. Occult co-infection in the oral cavity with cytomegalovirus during immunosuppression. J Transl Sci. 2015;1(2):26–30.
34. Pasin VP, Pereira AR, de Carvalho KA, de Paiva JMG, Enokihara MMSS, Porro AM. New drugs, new challenges for dermatologists: mucocutaneous ulcers secondary to everolimus. An Bras Dermatol. 2015;90(3):S165–7.
35. Totonchy MB, Colegio OR, Christensen SR. Sirolimus-associated rapid progression of leg ulcers in a renal transplant recipient. JAMA Dermatol. 2017;153(1):105–6.
36. Liu LS, McNiff JM, Colegio OR. Palmoplantar peeling secondary to sirolimus therapy. Am J Transplant. 2014;14(1):221–5.

37. Moro JA, Almenar L, Martínez-Dolz L, Sánchez-Lázaro I, Agüero J, Salvador A. Tolerance profile of the proliferation signal inhibitors everolimus and sirolimus in heart transplantation. Transplant Proc. 2008;40(9):3034–6. https://doi.org/10.1016/j.transproceed.2008.09.049.
38. de Ataide EC, Perales SR, Bortoto JB, Peres MAO, Filho FC, Stucchi RSB, et al. Immunomodulation, acute renal failure, and complications of basiliximab use after liver transplantation: analysis of 114 patients and literature review. Transplant Proc. 2017;49(4):852–7. https://doi.org/10.1016/j.transproceed.2017.01.047.
39. Martin ST, Tichy EM, Gabardi S. Belatacept: a novel biologic for maintenance immunosuppression after renal transplantation. Pharmacotherapy. 2011;31(4):394–407.
40. Grinyó J, Charpentier B, Pestana JM, Vanrenterghem Y, Vincenti F, Reyes-Acevedo R, et al. An integrated safety profile analysis of belatacept in kidney transplant recipients. Transplantation. 2010;90(12):1521–7.

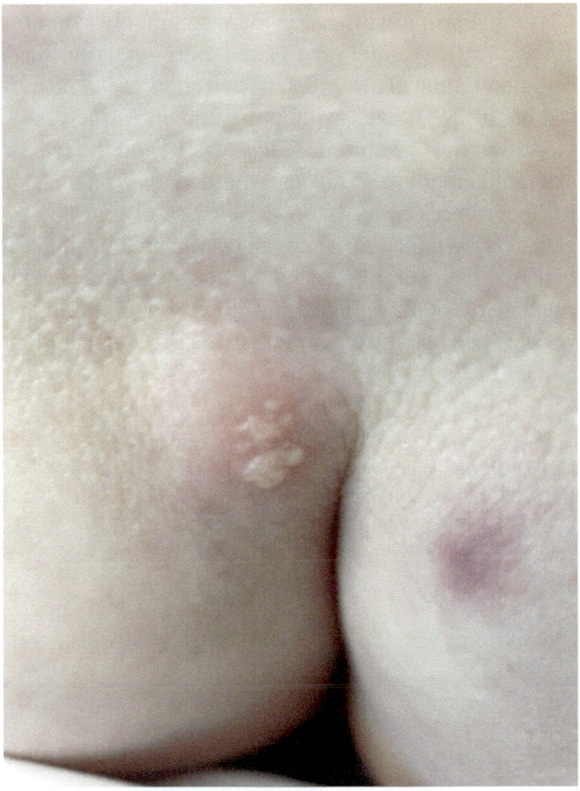

Fig. 1 Grouped vesicles on an erythematous base on the buttock after kidney transplantation

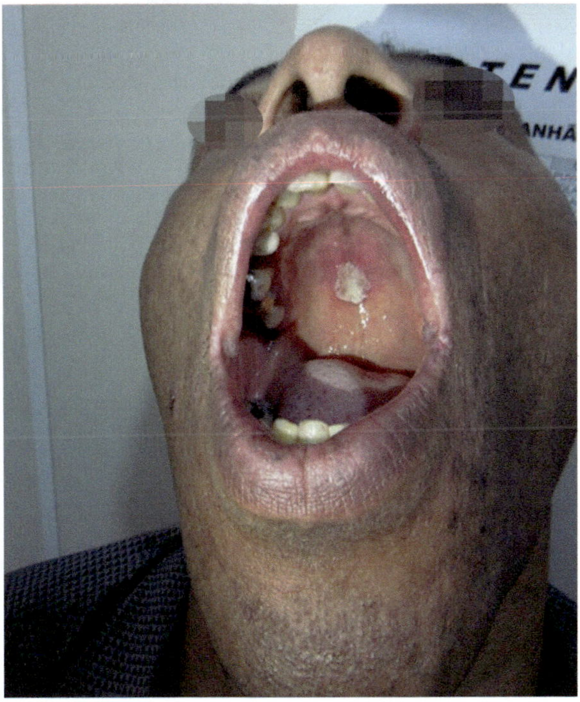

Fig. 2 Oral herpes simplex, ulcer covered by yellowish pseudomembrane on a hard palate in a 44-year-old man after kidney transplantation

Genital primary disease is more commonly symptomatic than oral infection. The disease in the genital area is generally sexually transmitted. The ulcers are most common on the glans, prepuce, and shaft of the penis. They are sore or painful and last about 2–3 weeks without treatment. In the case of the absence of immunity, ulceration may be chronic (Figs. 3 and 4). In the female, similar lesions arise on the external genitalia and mucosae of the vulva, vagina, and cervix [5].

Recurrences occur in 30–50% cases of oral herpes but are more frequent after genital HSV infection. They can be triggered by minor trauma, infections, ultraviolet radiation, an operation, or by the pre-menstrual period. Recurrent infections have a smaller size of the vesicles, and closer grouping, compared to primary infection. The vesicles become pustular and crusted before healing in 7–10 days without scarring.

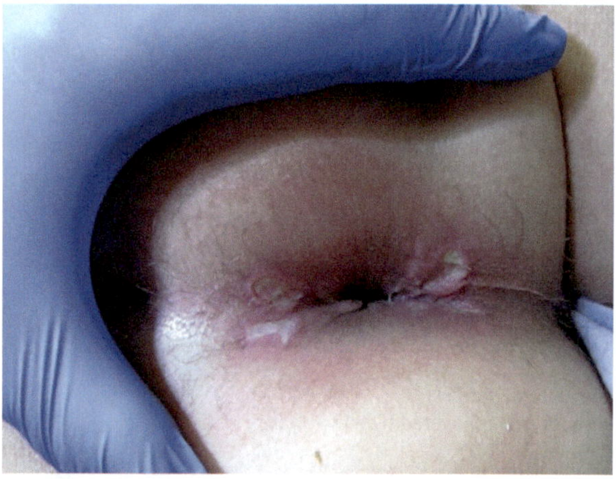

Fig. 3 Chronic mucocutaneous herpes simplex in a 67-year-old man after kidney transplantation

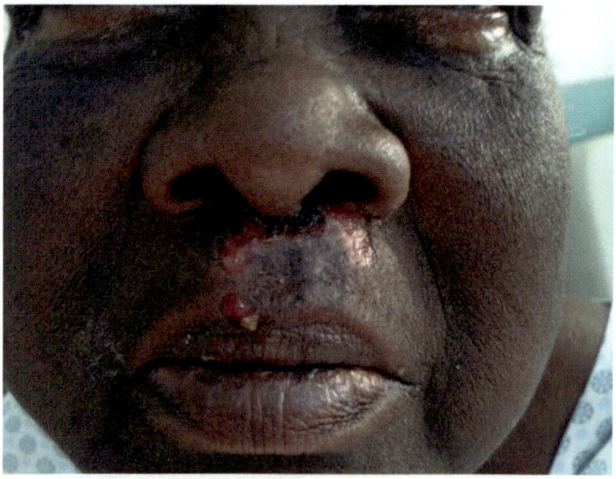

Fig. 4 Chronic mucocutaneous herpes simplex in a 70-year-old woman after kidney transplantation

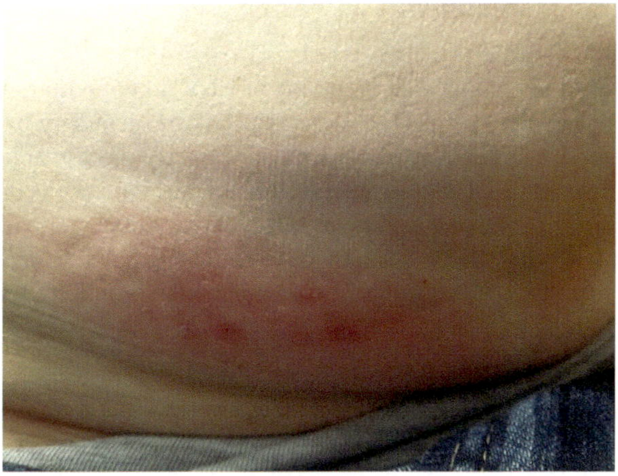

Fig. 5 HSV on the lower abdomen in a 48-year-old woman after kidney transplantation

They occur most frequently on the face, especially around the mouth. Recurrent herpetic lesions are most commonly vesicular and ulcerative, but they may be atypical with the appearance of folliculitis, candida fissures, or minor fractional ulcers [5].

Recurrences of genital herpes are more common and consist of small vesicles which produce non-indurated ulcers on the glans or shaft of the penis, or on the labia, vagina, or cervix. They have a shorter duration than the primary infection and are more likely in HSV-2 infections [5].

Among the population with immunodeficiency, both primary and recurrent herpetic infections can be increased in incidence and severity and may have a prolonged and atypical course [5]. HSV in SOTR occurs mainly as a reactivation of a latent infection, and rarely as de novo involving donor-derived infection. The most common of HSV infections in the post-transplant period are mucocutaneous lesions of which 85% are orolabial followed by anogenital manifestations [7]. HSV in SOTR can be more persistent than in immunocompetent patients, and in some cases may cause atypical lesions or localization not only in recurrence but also in a primary disease [4, 6] (Fig. 5).

2.4 *Diagnosis*

The diagnosis may be based on growing a viral culture or polymerase chain reaction (PCR), both of which can differentiate type-specific HSV [4].

2.5 Treatment

Mild uncomplicated eruptions of HSV do not require treatment. Topical antiseptic agents may be used to reduce the risk of secondary bacterial infection. In a severe primary infection or problematic recurrent disease antiviral therapy should be considered [5]. The treatment of limited mucocutaneous disease consists of nucleoside analogs like oral acyclovir, valacyclovir, or famciclovir. The therapy should be continued for a minimum 5–7 days until complete healing of the lesions. In the case of more extensive lesions in the immunocompromised host, intravenous acyclovir can also be used [4].

3 Trichodysplasia Spinulosa (TS)

3.1 Epidemiology

Trichodysplasia spinulosa (TS) is a distinctive infrequent dermatologic complication among immunosuppressed patients caused by a human polyomavirus, trichodysplasia spinulosa-associated polyomavirus (TSPyV). TS has been primarily observed in SOTR [8].

Unfortunately, the epidemiology of TS is poorly defined to date and is estimated based on the volume of cases reported in the literature. As of 2016, the assessed complete reported cases of TS were 32 [9]. The disease has been described in a wide range of ages, between 5 and 69 years, with no known gender prejudice, and a changeable duration of immunosuppression at the time of TS development.

3.2 Histopathology

Distinctive histological features of TS contain follicular dilation, absence of a papilla, proliferation of inner root sheath cells with enlarged trichohyalin granules, and infundibular keratin plugs.

3.3 Clinical Manifestation (Fig. 6)

TS is characterized by distinctive spiny folliculocentric papular eruptions on the face, ears, extremities, and trunk, and moreover this condition is also connected with alopecia with xerosis [8, 9].

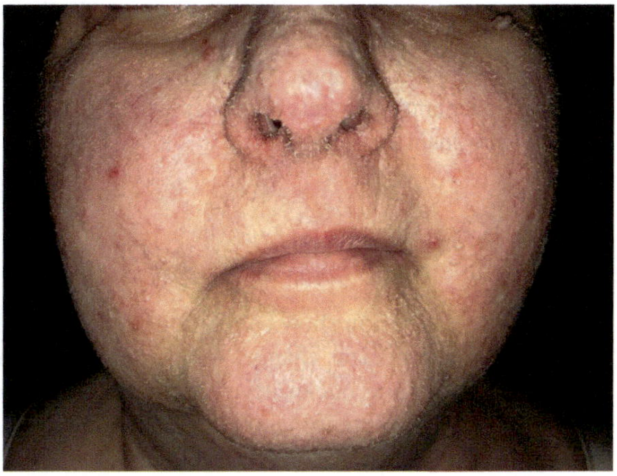

Fig. 6 Follicular spiny skin-colored papules on an erythematous base on face

3.4 Treatment

Unfortunately, there is no extensively accepted standard of treatment of TS. It is known that a reduction in immunosuppressive medications allows immune recovery and enables a reduction in viral load. Some authors estimate as effective alternatives intravenous cidofovir, topical cidofovir (1–3%) cream, oral valganciclovir, or leflunomide. A cost-effective and safe option for temporary improvement in appearance is also the physical extraction of keratin spicules. Regrettably, this technique has limited use when large body surface areas are involved, lesions can also return after removal due to ongoing immunosuppression [10].

4 Varicella-Zoster Virus (VZV)

4.1 Epidemiology

Shingles, also known as herpes zoster (HZ) is a disease characterized by neuralgia and a vesicular rash, which is due to reactivation of a latent varicella-zoster virus (VZV) infection [11]. The first manifestation of zoster is usually pain, which may be localized to the same area as the rash or be more diffuse [5].

Primary infection is acquired through direct contact with skin lesions or through airborne spread from respiratory droplets. It is known that the majority of SOTR are seropositive. After primary infection VZV stays lifelong latent in the cranial nerve and dorsal root ganglia and can reactivate years to decades later as HZ [12]. The lifetime risk of HZ in the general population ranges from 20% to 30% but the risk increases dramatically after 50 years of age, with the lifetime risk of HZ reaching 50% at the age of 85 years [13]. Longitudinal studies established that the older transplant recipients are at greater risk for the development of HZ. In addition, heart and lung transplant recipients have increased rates of HZ compared to patients after other organ transplantations [12].

4.2 Histopathology

In varicella, cells of skin show ballooning of their cytoplasm by intracellular edema and characteristic nuclear changes containing eosinophilic inclusions and marginated chromatin. Some nuclei develop other nuclear membranes which divide the nucleus into small compartments. Cell fusion produces multinucleated giant cells with up to 15 nuclei. Intra- and intercellular edema forms the vesicle. Moreover, in zoster there are inflammatory changes in the posterior nerve roots, ganglia, and sometimes in the anterior horn [5].

4.3 Clinical Manifestation

The reactivation of VZV presents as a unilateral dermatomal rash, which does not cross the midline and is primarily maculopapular on an erythematous base (Figs. 7, 8, and 9a, b). The skin lesions evolve into a vesicular-pustular appearance which after 7–10 days begins to crust over and heals within 2–4 weeks. The onset of the rash is frequently preceded by neuropathic pain like aching, burning, or lancinating over the involved dermatome(s) [13].

The clinical manifestation of HZ among the population of SOTR is more likely to present multi-dermatomal or disseminated zoster compared to the immunocompetent population. The definition of disseminated zoster is having more than 20 vesicles outside the area of the primary and adjacent dermatomes or affecting three or more dermatomes. Some authors estimate that the level of immunosuppression may increase the risk of developing disseminated HZ [12] (Figs. 10a, b and 11). Among the population under immunosuppression, HZ can have unusual clinical presentations like persistent, crusted, verrucous lesions, or post-herpetic hyperhidrosis [14] (Fig. 12). Moreover, rates of HZ complications, such as post-herpetic

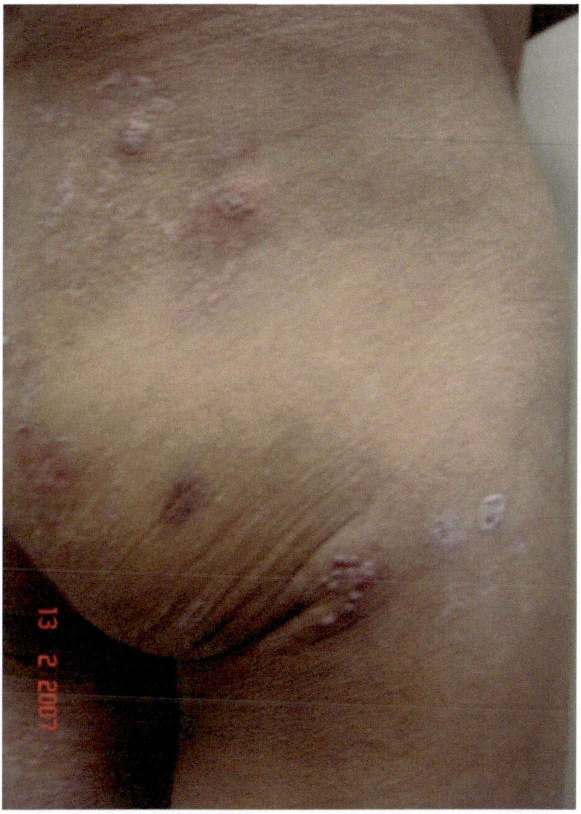

Fig. 7 Grouped vesicles on an erythematous base distributed along the dermatome of the lower back and right buttock

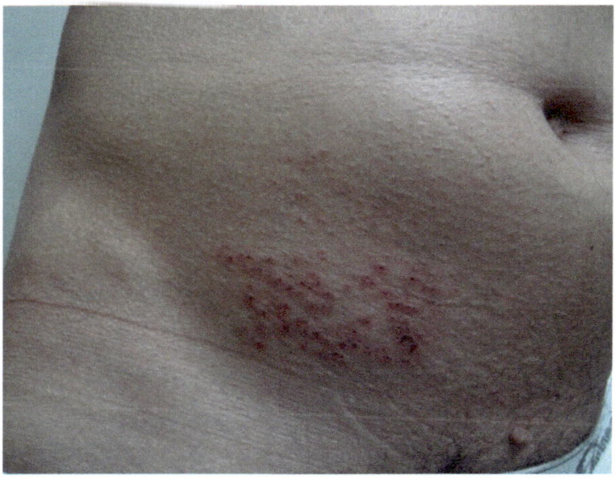

Fig. 8 VZV in a 62-year-old man after kidney transplantation

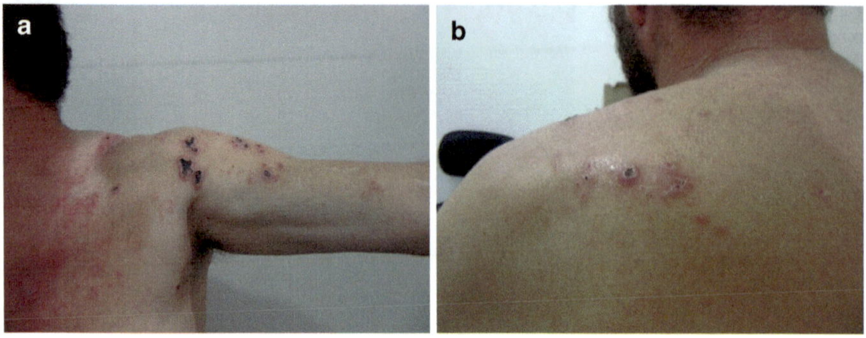

Fig. 9 (**a**, **b**) VZV affecting the region of cervical dermatome in a 57-year-old man after kidney transplantation

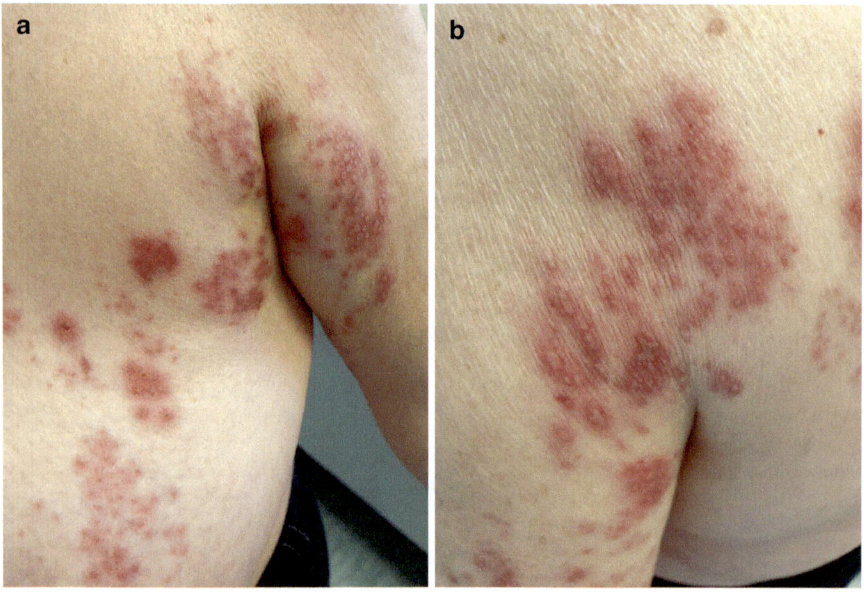

Fig. 10 (**a**, **b**) Disseminated shingles in a 37-year-old man after kidney transplantation

neuralgia are thought to be much higher in SOTR than in the general population [12]. In most patients, the history and classic dermatomal appearance of the rash allows for a clinical diagnosis of HZ.

Among patients with atypical clinical presentation of HZ, laboratory-based diagnostic tools can be used [13].

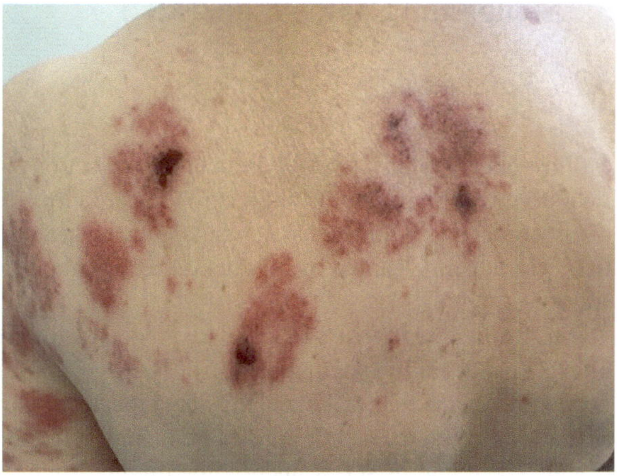

Fig. 11 Disseminated shingles in a woman after kidney transplantation. Deep erosions covered by crust in 65-year-old woman after kidney transplantation

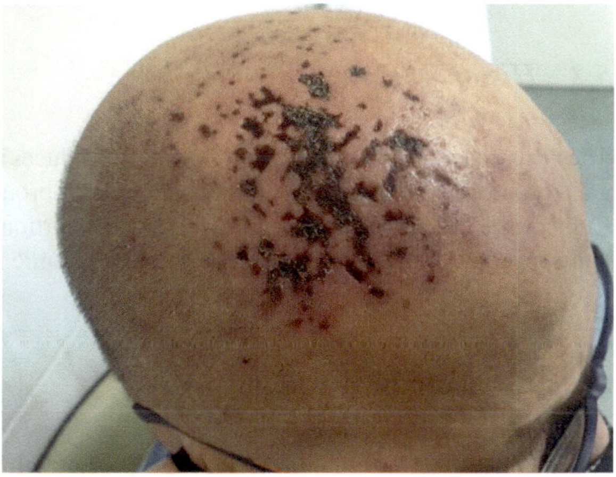

Fig. 12 Shingles on the skin of the scalp. Deep ulcers covered by crusts in a 60-year-old man after kidney transplantation

4.4 Treatment

The treatment of shingles depends on the extent of the disease. Non-severe and localized dermatomal HZ can usually be treated with oral acyclovir, valacyclovir, or famciclovir as an outpatient in most adult patients, with close follow-up. Antiviral therapy should be performed for at least 7 days, or until the lesions have crusted over. The time of treatment can be delayed in SOTR in connection to immunosuppression. Post-transplant patients with disseminated HZ should receive intravenous over the oral acyclovir as an initial therapy. In the case of allergies to acyclovir or similar drugs, or documented viral resistance, foscarnet, or cidofovir can be used [12].

5 Molluscum Contagiosum (MC)

5.1 Epidemiology

Molluscum contagiosum (MC) is an highly infectious benign dermatosis associated with an infection of double-stranded DNA poxvirus. MC is mainly transmitted by direct contact with infected skin, which may be sexual, non-sexual, or autoinoculation. Moreover, it can be transmitted by contaminated fomites like towels or bath sponges.

MC occurs worldwide and there are no gender differences. This infection mainly affects the pediatric population [15]. The age of peak incidence is reported as between 2 and 5 years. A later incidence peak in young adults is connected with sexual transmission, with lesions more common in the genital area [5]. Although it can also be found in SOTR undergoing immunosuppression [15].

5.2 Histopathology

The virus causes cellular proliferation, which produces lobulated epidermal growths and compresses the papillae until they appear as fibrous septa between the lobules. Cells of the core of the lesions show greater distortion, then are finally destroyed; and appear as large hyaline bodies having cytoplasmic masses of virus material [5].

5.3 Clinical Manifestation

The clinical manifestation of MC is multiple smooth pearly pink or skin-colored and umbilicated papules, usually 2–5 mm in size (Fig. 13). The lesions may be single, multiple, or clustered, and occasionally they may have an erythematous halo or be pediculated (Figs. 14 and 15). Moreover, pruritus could be present. The skin lesions have variable duration, however in most cases, they are self-limited to a period of 6–9 months; however, some cases could persist for more than 3 or 4 years. In adults, lesions are most commonly located in the lower abdomen,

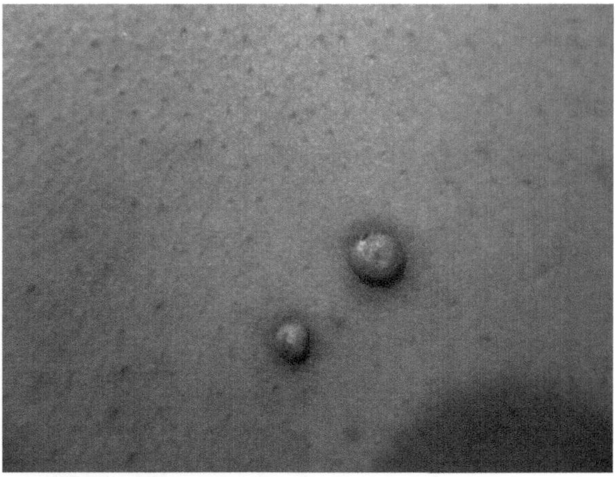

Fig. 13 Molluscum contagiosum—pink colored umbilicated papules

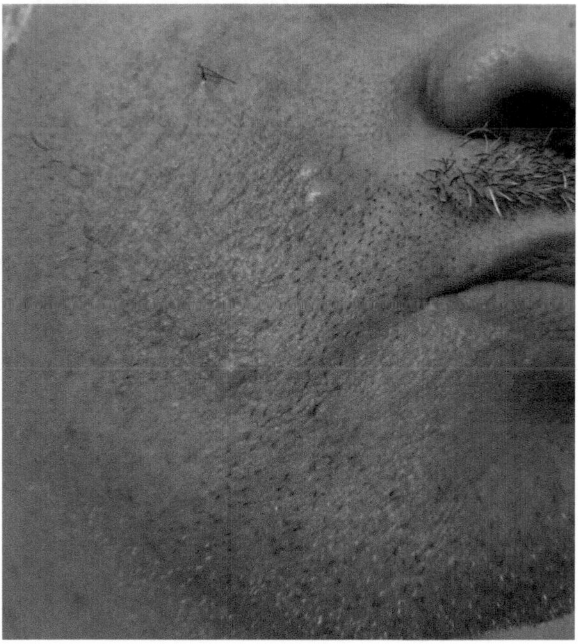

Fig. 14 Molluscum contagiosum on the face of a 65-year-old man after kidney transplantation

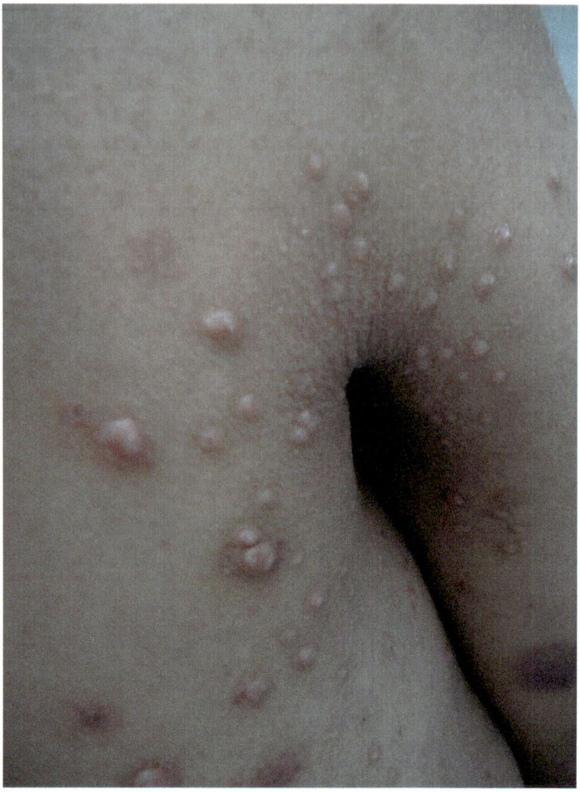

Fig. 15 Molluscum contagiosum, multiple skin colored umbilicated papules

thighs, genitals, and perianal area (Fig. 16). Most of these cases are transmitted by sexual contact. The viral infection among the population of immunosuppressed patients is connected with a recalcitrant and more extensive manifestation. The skin lesions may vary in size, shape, and location, or be refractory to treatment. SOTR are also at risk of presenting complications such as eczema and a bacterial superinfection.

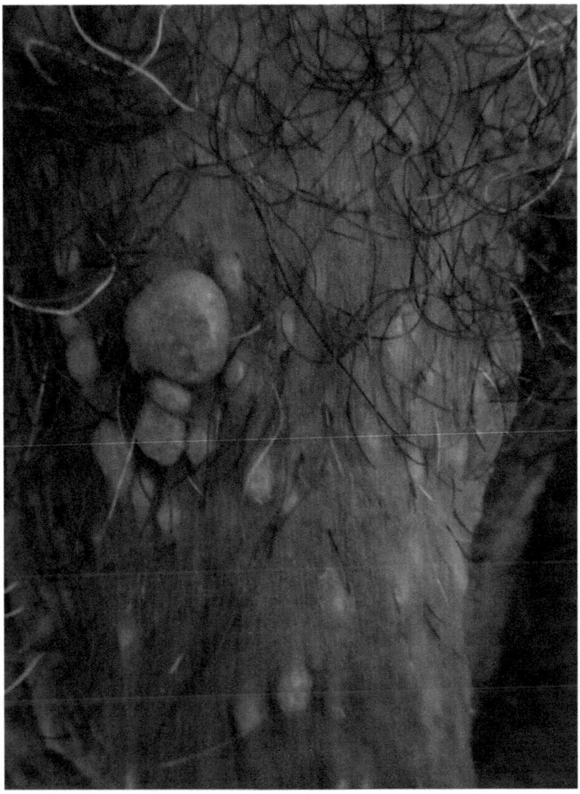

Fig. 16 Molluscum contagiosum in a 66-year-old man after kidney transplantation

5.4 Diagnosis

The diagnosis is based on clinical findings with the use of dermatoscopy. Moreover, we also distinguished giant MC, which is a specific variant of the condition with the presence of multiple or single lesions larger than 5 mm. The diagnosis of this variant of MC is usually connected with immunocompromised patients like SOTR. Giant MC could mimic other benign or malignant lesions, and the definitive diagnosis is typically based on histopathological examination [15].

5.5 *Treatment*

Actually, the necessity for active treatment of MC is controversial due to both the self-limited course of infection and the lack of evidence to define the best therapy. Many researchers agree that treatment should be indicated in cases with extensive disease, secondary complications like bacterial superinfection or molluscum dermatitis or esthetic complaints. There are multiple treatment alternatives which may be classified as mechanical, chemical, immunomodulatory, and antiviral. Some effective mechanical methods are cryotherapy, curettage, and a pulsed dye laser therapy. Chemical therapy destroys skin lesions through the inflammatory response they produce. The most popular chemical agents are cantharidin, a topical agent, which is an inhibitor of phosphodiesterase or potassium hydroxide—an alkaline compound that dissolves keratin. Immunomodulatory medications stimulate the individual's immune response against the infection. The most known method is imiquimod— an immunostimulatory agonist of the toll-like receptor 7. Other immunomodulatory agents are oral cimetidine, interferon alfa, candidin, and diphencyprone. Antiviral therapy, used in immunocompromised patients includes cidofovir, which could be used topically at a concentration of 1–3% or intravenously [16, 17].

6 Human Papillomavirus (HPV)

6.1 *Epidemiology*

Human papillomavirus (HPV) is a double-stranded circular DNA virus belonging to the papillomavirus family. HPVs include more than 150 types each identified by a number. It is a widespread disease, which can be transmitted by skin-to-skin or mucosa-to-mucosa contact and enters the body through cutaneous or mucosal damage. There is also the possibility of autoinoculation from scratching, eczema, shaving, or hyperhidrosis.

HPV disease is the most common sexually transmitted infection and the global risk of being infected at least once in a lifetime including both men and women is around 50%. The most frequent types worldwide are HPV 16 and 18, which are the major types connected with carcinogenesis. Fortunately, there are vaccines against both types: HPV 16 and HPV 18.

6.2 *Histopathology*

HPV warts histologically present acanthosis and hyperkeratosis, typically with the characteristic feature of koilocytosis of the upper keratinocytes. Moreover, in most warts there is papillomatosis. In koilocytes and other granular layer cells, basophilic nuclear inclusion bodies can be seen. These upper epidermal cells have eosinophilic inclusions representing irregular, clumped keratohyaline granules [5].

6.3 Clinical Manifestation

There is a wide range of clinical manifestations of HPV infection. The most common is the development of warts (verrucae), which are pleomorphic tumors and may affect generally the skin of extremities, genital skin and mucosa, larynx and oral mucosa. Verrucae on the skin can present many different morphological forms dependent on HPV type, body site, immunological status of the patient, and environmental influences. We can distinguish mainly: common warts, plantar warts, plane warts, and anogenital warts.

Common warts are firm papules with a rough, corneous surface, which range in size from less than 1 mm to over 1 cm in diameter and can also form large masses. They are most often placed on the back of the hands and fingers but can occur anywhere on the skin (Figs. 17, 18a, b, and 19).

Plantar warts have the typical appearance of a sharply rounded lesion, with a rough, keratotic surface surrounded by a smooth collar of thickened horn. Most commonly, they are placed under pressure points, the heel, or the metatarsal heads (Figs. 20 and 21a, b).

Plane warts are smooth, flat, or slightly elevated skin lesions which are most often skin-colored or grayish yellow but can be pigmented. They are round or polygonal in shape and vary in size from 1 to 5 mm or more in diameter (Fig. 22). They are most commonly found on the face and the back of the hands and the number present ranges from two or three to many hundreds.

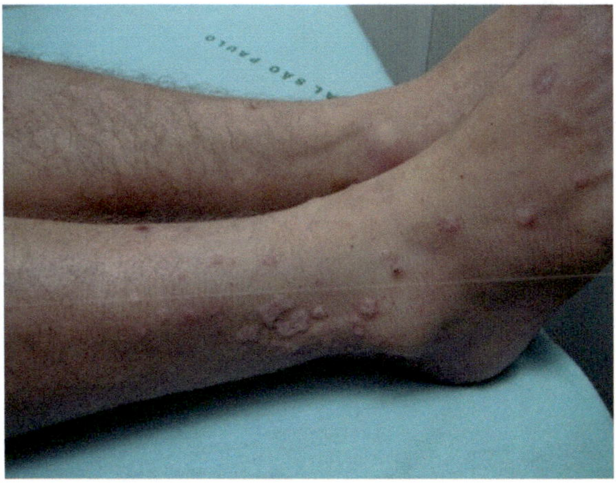

Fig. 17 Flat warts in a 38-year-old man after kidney transplantation

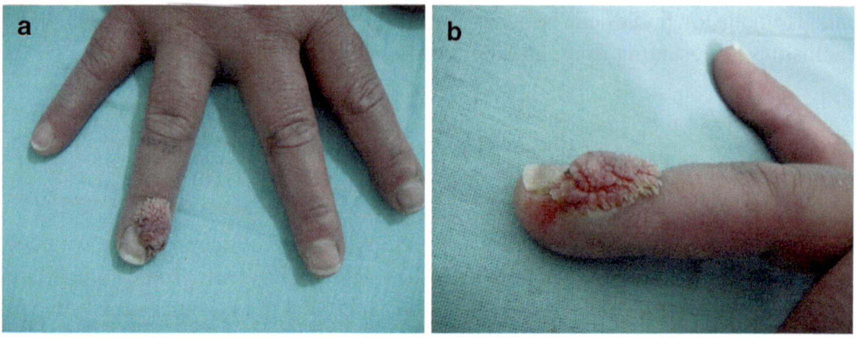

Fig. 18 (**a**) Common wart in a 50-year-old woman after kidney transplantation. (**b**) Close-up

Fig. 19 Multiple periungual warts

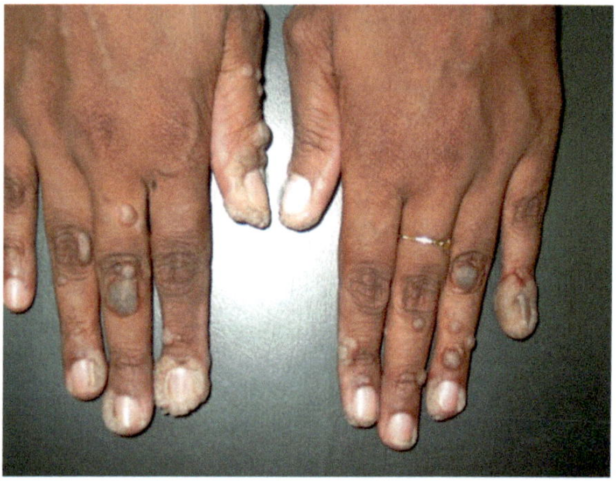

Fig. 20 Multiple plantar warts in a 52-year-old woman after kidney transplantation

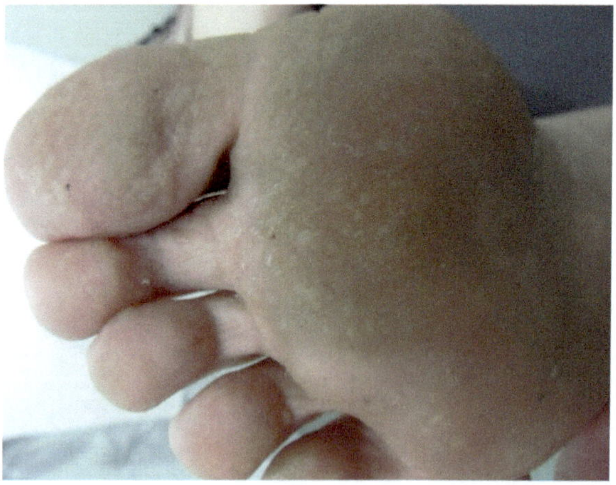

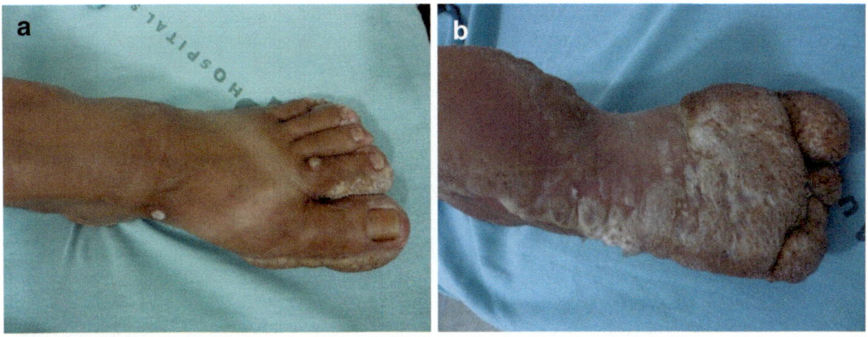

Fig. 21 (**a**, **b**) Extensive plantar wart in a 38-year-old woman after kidney transplantation

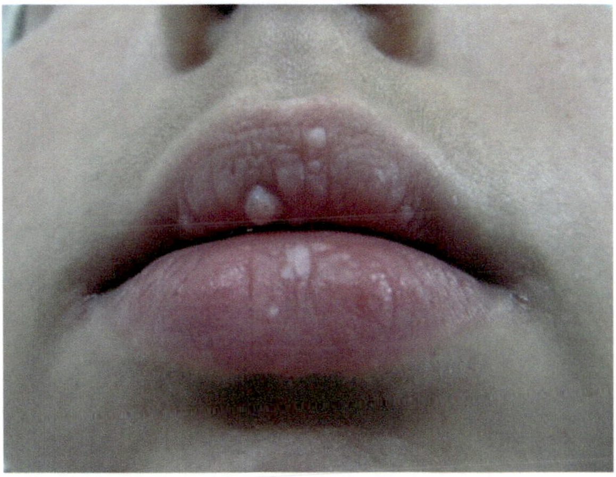

Fig. 22 Flat warts on lips in a 21-year-old woman after kidney transplantation

Anogenital warts are typically soft, pink, elongated, and occasionally filiform or pedunculated. They are most common and multiple, mainly on moist surfaces, such as on frenulum, corona, and glans in men, and the posterior fourchette in women [5].

Another less common manifestation of HPV, which is observed in immunosuppressed patients is the Buschke-Löwenstein tumor (BLT) or giant condylomata acuminata (GCA) (Fig. 23a, b), which is a pseudoepithelial proliferation belonging to the verrucous carcinomas. BLT is caused by HPV, especially by HPV-6 and HPV-11 [18]. Histologically, BLT is described as a well-differentiated malpighian proliferation with local aggressive behavior [19]. The condition is quite rare, and it is always preceded by condylomata acuminata. It is known that BLT's annual incidence seems to be 0.1% among the sexually active population. It may appear at any age after puberty, but it is mainly diagnosed in the population between 40 and 60 years. BLT most commonly appears in males and mainly affects the anogenital area. It can result in progressive degeneration and recur after therapy. Immunocompromised

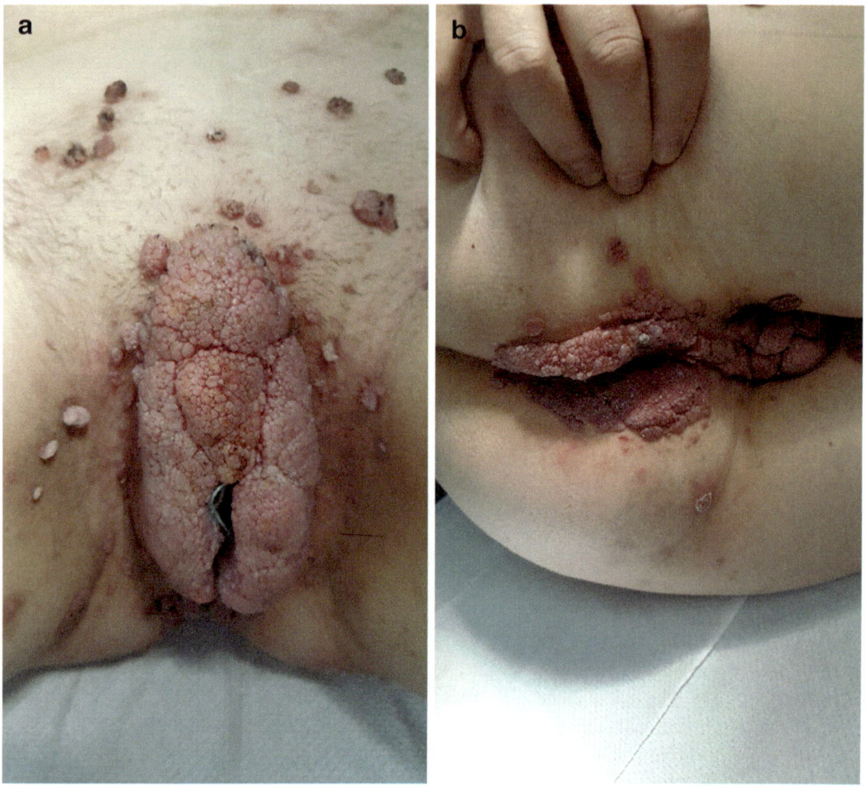

Fig. 23 (**a**, **b**) Giant condyloma acuminatum in a 45-year-old woman after kidney transplantation

patients are predisposed to this condition. Early treatment of condylomata acuminata is crucial for the prevention of BLT. It is recommended to perform a wide excision of the lesions [18].

We can also distinguish low- and high-risk oncogenic types of HPV. Infection of the low-risk oncogenic types is associated with anogenital warts, some types of cutaneous warts, and recurrent respiratory papillomatosis. While high-risk oncogenic types are connected with cervical, penile, anal, vaginal, vulvar, and oropharyngeal cancers. Low-risk group HPV types 6 and 11 cause 90% of external anogenital warts, known as a condylomata and also low-grade changes in cervical cells. High-risk HPVs, mainly HPV 16 and 18, are connected with high-grade cervical and anal dysplasia and invasive carcinoma. There are also HPV-related skin cancers. HPV has been implicated in several non-melanoma skin cancers (NMSC). The two most common subtypes of NMSC include basal cell carcinomas (BCCs) and squamous cell carcinomas (SCCs). Some authors estimate that HPV DNA is

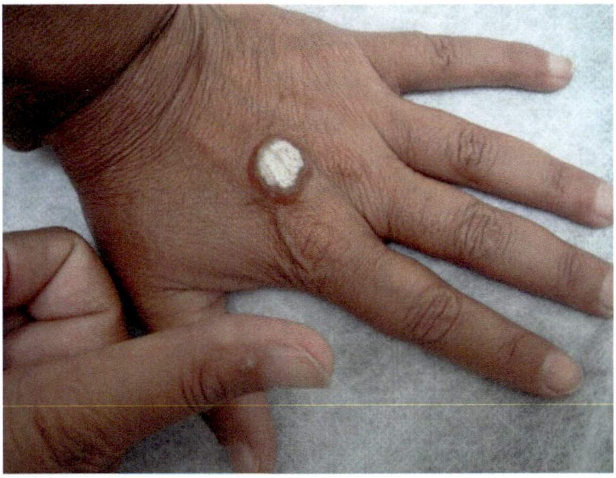

Fig. 24 Atypical common wart in a 43-year-old woman after kidney transplantation

found in 30–50% of NMSCs from immunocompetent patients, while this number goes up to 90% in lesions from immunocompromised patients. Moreover, HPV viruses may also be found in premalignant lesions like actinic keratosis, where the virus is transcriptionally active, or even in normal skin. Curiously, there seems to be an inverse correlation between viral load and the malignancy of the lesion [20, 21].

Among SOTR warts and HPV-related genital lesions are most commonly observed, reaching about 85% at 5 years, regardless of the immunosuppressive drug used. Warts in immunocompromised patients appear more often on the hands, feet, and face but mostly are more warty (Fig. 24), grayish, larger in size, and turning into large plaques. Furthermore, among this population widespread and diffuse HPV-related verruciformis lesions are also frequent.

6.4 *Treatment*

Given the widespread range of clinical manifestations of HPV infections, study data about the treatment of warts is very inhomogeneous. Moreover, the therapy of HPV infections is not easy because the infection is frequently recurrent, and therapy is not very successful. The success of the therapy depends on several clinical factors including disease duration, thickness, and location of the warts. The majority of patients need multiple treatments over a course of months. It is recommended to start the therapy at an early stage, which may prevent the infection from becoming chronic or disseminated in at least 50% of affected patients. First-line therapy includes medical treatments like salicylic acid or silver nitrate and are mainly useful to treat common warts of short duration-less than 1 year. If the first-line therapy is not effective, cryotherapy may be considered. In the case of recurrent or difficult to treat lesions, it is possible to use a diversity of alternative therapeutic options, such as local treatment with tretinoin, imiquimod, ablative or nonablative laser, or photodynamic therapy. On the assumption of disseminated lesions the acitretin may be used to reduce the number of warts, but lesions frequently recur. Vaccination as a preventive measure is recommended to reduce the risk of acquiring mucosal HPV infection in young candidates for transplant procedures [1, 21].

7 Cytomegalovirus (CMV)

7.1 Epidemiology

Cytomegalovirus (CMV), which is common in SOTR, is a highly prevalent double-stranded DNA virus in the Herpesviridae family. It is known that over 60% of the population in the Western world have been exposed to CMV. Based on some studies, CMV infection is significantly connected with an increased risk of graft rejection [1, 22].

CMV is mainly transmitted through saliva or the placenta, breastfeeding, sexual contact, blood transfusions, and hematopoietic stem cell transplant or organ transplant. CMV persists lifelong latent without causing symptoms unless reactivated, most frequently during periods of immunosuppression. Most CMV infections are related to the reactivation of a latent virus. The primary reservoir for CMV latency is myeloid progenitor cells and monocytes [1, 22].

7.2 Histopathology

A characteristic histological feature of CMV is the presence of cytomegalic cells in vascular endothelium, which can progress in some cases to vasculitis [5] (Fig. 25).

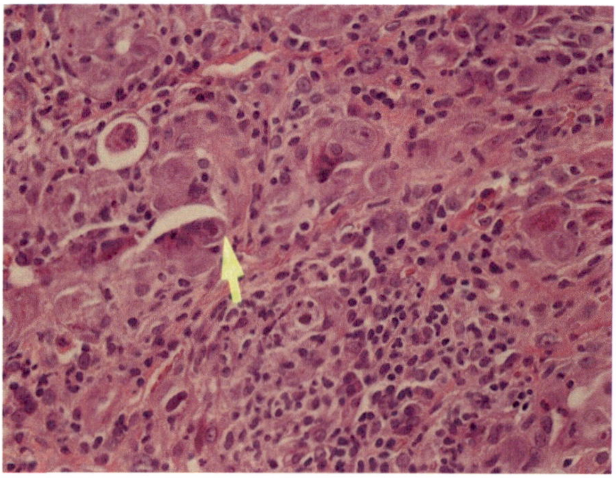

Fig. 25 Histopathology: cytomegalovirus, owl eye (arrow)

7.3 *Clinical Manifestation*

Cutaneous manifestations of CMV infection in SOTR are less common than systemic effects of infection although it may be the first sign of a disadvantageous prognosis. In the case of CMV, it manifests as a visible lesion and the infection is early diagnosed; there is the potential to significantly reduce the morbidity and mortality of infected patients. CMV may have many dermatological manifestations like morbilliform rash, petechiae, purpura, plaques, vesicles, bullae, erosions, erythema, nodules, papules, edema, vasculitis, and pustules. As researchers say, the most prevalent lesions are ulcers. The most common areas where ulcers are found are the genital, perianal, gluteal, or oral regions (Fig. 26). However, ulcers can be located in various locations [1, 16]. Among the population under immunosuppression, keratotic skin lesions, severe oral and skin ulceration have been found [5].

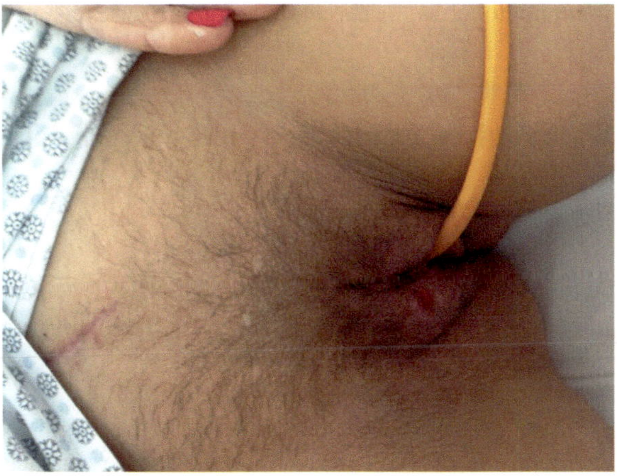

Fig. 26 Cytomegalovirus infection in a 39-year-old woman after kidney transplantation

7.4 Diagnosis

The clinical diagnosis of a CMV infection based on skin lesions is problematic. The main methods used for diagnosis of CMV are skin biopsy followed by histopathological identification of intranuclear inclusion, as well as PCR, IHC, and blood antigen testing [1, 22].

7.5 Treatment

The basis of treatment of CMV includes intravenous or oral antiviral medications: ganciclovir or valganciclovir. With this therapy, the symptoms are resolved in 1 week to several months. In the population of patients under immunosuppression, using antivirals for prophylaxis may be concerned. In addition, during the antiviral therapy immunosuppressive medication should be reduced, if possible, this concerns mainly mycophenolate. Other useful methods of treatment are intravenous immunoglobulins, foscarnet, leflunomide, or excision of the skin lesion [1, 22].

8 Acquired Epidermodysplasia Verruciformis (EDV)

8.1 Epidemiology

Acquired epidermodysplasia verruciformis (EDV) is an infrequent complication of immunosuppression among SOTR [22]. Although the predisposition to the virus is inherited, it is generally autosomal recessive; however, autosomal dominant and X-linked dominant patterns are reported [5].

There is a positive correlation between the length of immunosuppression and the development of HPV lesions. This disease characteristically manifests within 5 years of starting the immunosuppression therapy.

8.2 Histopathology

Distinguishing histopathologic features are enlarged keratinocytes with perinuclear halos and blue-gray cytoplasm with hypergranulosis.

8.3 *Clinical Manifestation*

Clinical manifestation of acquired EDV may present as multiple hypopigmented to red macules that can connect into patches with a fine scale, clinically they look like the lesions of pityriasis versicolor. The condition may also present as multiple flesh-colored flat-topped verrucous papules that clinically resemble the lesions of verruca plana on sun-exposed areas [23]. The warts are most numerous on the face and neck and backs on the hands and feet, but may be generalized over the entire body surface [5] (Figs. 27a, b, 28, 29a, b, 30a, b, and 31).

The most commonly isolated EDV-HPV subtypes as well as the most oncogenic are HPV types 5 and 8. These subtypes are associated with the highest risk for malignant transformation into squamous cell carcinoma (SCC). A diagnosis of acquired HPV is based on the clinical and histopathologic features.

Infection of EDV-HPV among immunosuppressed patients is associated with more severe dysplasia than in the general population. It is known that UV light increases the risk for malignant transformation of EDV lesions. In order to reduce the risk for malignant transformation, patients with EDV should be recommended to avoid UV radiation and examine skin lesions every year.

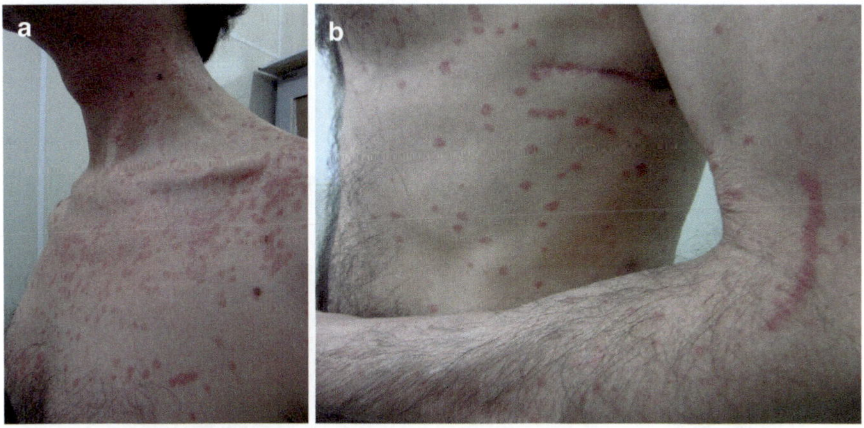

Fig. 27 (**a**, **b**) Epidermodysplasia verruciformis in a 44-year-old man after kidney transplantation

Fig. 28 Epidermodysplasia verruciformis in a 50-year-old woman after kidney transplantation

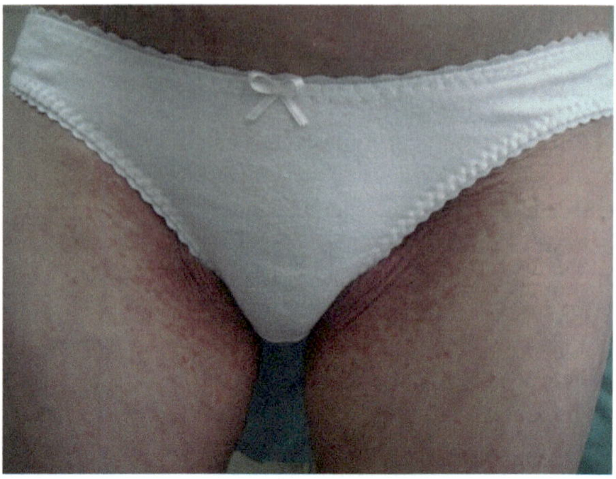

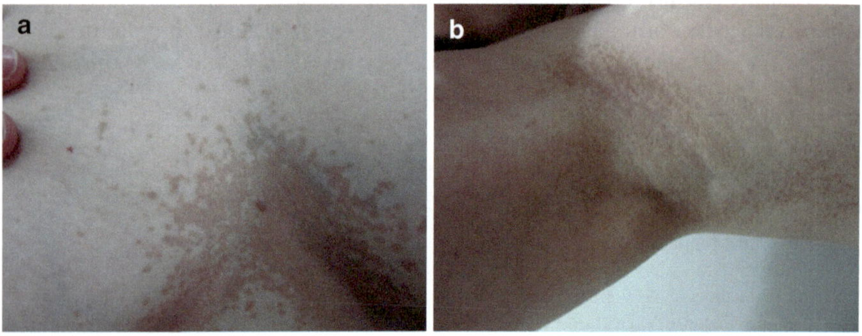

Fig. 29 (**a**, **b**) Epidermodysplasia verruciformis in a 52-year-old woman after kidney transplantation

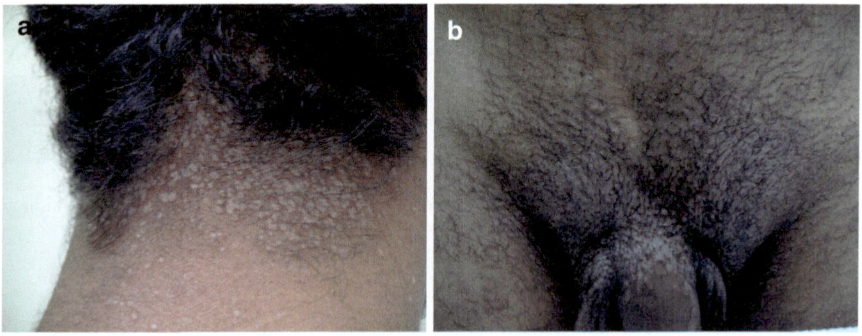

Fig. 30 (**a**, **b**) Epidermodysplasia verruciformis in a patient with dark skin

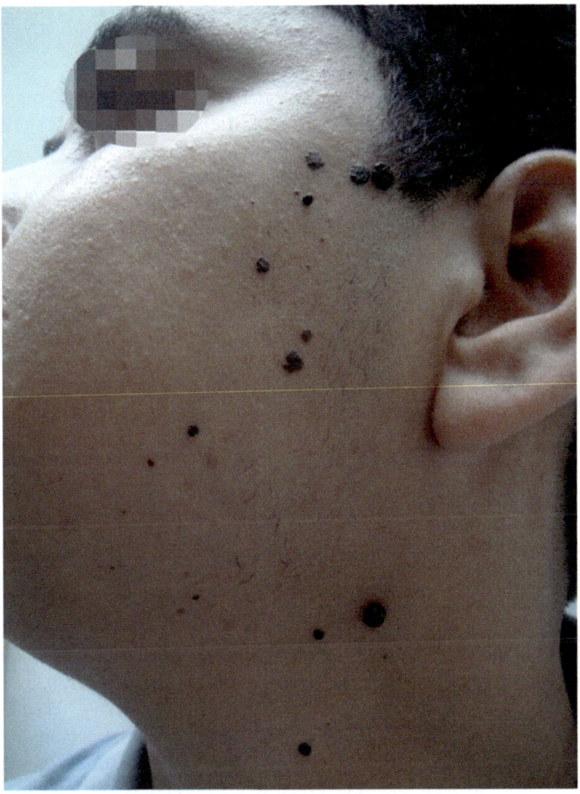

Fig. 31 Pigmented epidermodysplasia verruciformis in a 31-year-old man after kidney transplantation

8.4 Treatment

The treatment of EDV is based on topical imiquimod, 5-fluorouracil, tretinoin, and tazarotene with variable success. Some therapies are carried out with acitretin alone, or in combination with interferon alfa-2a. Highly active antiretroviral therapy in patients with immunodeficiencies has successfully decreased the number of lesions in this population. Some authors also have had success using photodynamic therapy. SCC among patients with EDV may be managed by excision or by Mohs micrographic surgery [23].

References

1. Naldi L, Venturuzzo A, Invernizzi P. Dermatological complications after solid organ transplantation. Clin Rev Allergy Immunol. 2018;54(1):185–212. https://doi.org/10.1007/s12016-017-8657-9.
2. Arze S, Arze L, Abecia C. Post-transplantation infections in Bolivia. Transplant Proc. 2016;48(2):646–53. https://doi.org/10.1016/j.transproceed.2016.02.049.
3. Sulowicz J, Wojas-Pelc A, Kuzniewski M, Ignacak E, Janda K, Sulowicz W. Cutaneous viral infections in patients after kidney transplantation: risk factors. Pol Arch Med Wewn. 2013;123(12):686–92. https://doi.org/10.20452/pamw.2013. Epub 2013 Nov 15
4. Lee DH, R. A. Zuckerman RA. Herpes simplex virus infections in solid organ transplantation: guidelines from the American Society of Transplantation Infectious Diseases Community of Practice. Clin Transpl. 2019;33(9):e13526–36. https://doi.org/10.1111/ctr.13526.
5. Sterling JC. Virus infections. In: Burns T, Breathnach S, editors. Rook's textbook of dermatology. Hoboken, NJ: Wiley Blackwell; 2010. p. 33.
6. Martin-Gandul C, Stampf S, Héquet D, Mueller NJ, Cusini A, van Delden C, et al. Preventive strategies against cytomegalovirus and incidence of α-herpesvirus infections in solid organ transplant recipients: a nationwide cohort study. Am J Transplant. 2017;17(7):1813–22. https://doi.org/10.1111/ajt.14192.
7. Jothimani D, Venugopal R, Vij M, Rela M. Post liver transplant recurrent and de novo viral infections. Best Pract Res Clin Gastroenterol. 2020;46:101689–707. https://doi.org/10.1016/j.bpg.2020.101689.
8. Kassar R, Chang J, Chan AW, Lilly LB, Al Habeeb A, Rotstein C. Leflunomide for the treatment of trichodysplasia spinulosa in a liver transplant recipient. Transpl Infect Dis. 2017;19(4):e12702–18. https://doi.org/10.1111/tid.12702.
9. Barone H, Brockman R, Johnson L, Al-Uzri A, Wright M, Mengden-Koon S, et al. Trichodysplasia spinulosa mimicking lichen nitidus in a renal transplant patient. Pediatr Transplant. 2019;23(4):e13394. https://doi.org/10.1111/petr.13394.
10. Narayanan D, Rady PL, Tyring SK. Recent developments in trichodysplasia spinulosa disease. Transpl Infect Dis. 2020;22(6):e13434. https://doi.org/10.1111/tid.13434.
11. Rondaan C, de Joode AEA, Wang L, Siderius M, Raveling-Eelsing R, van Leer-Buter C, et al. Immune response to varicella-zoster virus before and after renal transplantation. Antivir Res. 2020;183:104938–45. https://doi.org/10.1016/j.antiviral.2020.104938.
12. Pergam SA, Limaye AP. Varicella zoster virus in solid organ transplantation: guidelines from the American Society of Transplantation Infectious Diseases Community of Practice. Clin Transpl. 2019;33(9):e13622–34. https://doi.org/10.1111/ctr.13622.
13. John AR, D. H. Canaday DH. Herpes zoster in the older adult. Infect Dis Clin N Am. 2017;31(4):811–26. https://doi.org/10.1016/j.idc.2017.07.016.
14. Madkan V, Sra K, Brantley J. Human herpesviruses. In: Bolognia JL, Jorizzo JL, Rapini RP, editors. Dermatology. 2nd ed. Madrid: Elsevier; 2008. p. 1199–217.
15. Sławińska M, Hlebowicz M, Iżycka-Świeszewska E, Sikorska M, Sokołowska-Wojdyło M, Smiatacz T. Dermoscopic features of giant molluscum contagiosum in a patient with acquired immunodeficiency syndrome. Acta Dermatovenerol Croat. 2020;28(7):233–5.
16. Fisher C, McLawhorn JM, Adotama P, Stasko T, Collins L, Levin J. Pulsed dye laser repurposed: treatment of refractory molluscum contagiosum in renal transplant patient. Transpl Infect Dis. 2019;21(2):e13036–43. https://doi.org/10.1111/tid.13036.
17. Meza-Romero R, Navarrete-Dechent C, Downey C. Molluscum contagiosum: an update and review of new perspectives in etiology, diagnosis, and treatment. Clin Cosmet Investig Dermatol. 2019;12:373–81. https://doi.org/10.2147/CCID.S187224.
18. Kadouri Y, Nouini Y. La tumeur de Buschke-Löwenstein [Buschke-Löwenstein' tumor]. Pan Afr Med J. 2020;36:359–62. https://doi.org/10.11604/pamj.2020.36.359.1329.

19. Ben Kridis W, Werda I, Charfi S, Toumi N, Boudawara T, Mzali R, et al. Buschke-Lowenstein anal tumor: an ambiguous entity. Exp Oncol. 2019;41(2):182–4. https://doi.org/10.32471/exp-oncology.2312-8852.
20. Brianti P, De Flammineis E, Mercuri SR. Review of HPV-related diseases and cancers. New Microbiol. 2017;40(2):80–5.
21. Ockenfels HM. Therapeutic management of cutaneous and genital warts. J Dtsch Dermatol Ges. 2016;14(9):892–9. https://doi.org/10.1111/ddg.12838.
22. Drozd B, Andriescu E, Suárez A, De la Garza Bravo MM. Cutaneous cytomegalovirus manifestations, diagnosis, and treatment: a review. Dermatol Online J. 2019;25(1):2–11. https://doi.org/10.5070/D3251042608.
23. Henley JK, Hossler EW. Acquired epidermodysplasia verruciformis occurring in a renal transplant recipient. Cutis. 2017;99(5):E9–E12.

Bacterial Diseases

Daniel Wagner de Castro Lima Santos and Marilia Marufuji Ogawa

1 Introduction

The infectious disease complications that occur in patients with impaired host defenses represents a formidable challenge to the clinicians, especially for assuming an opportunistic character and sometimes with atypical clinical manifestation. Dermatological evaluation should start before transplantation when possible. Some dermatological features and morbid conditions may help in predicting complications in the posttransplant phase. Despite the frequent publication in the literature on cutaneous malignancies in SOTRs and other opportunistic diseases caused by viruses, fungi, and mycobacteria, information on the diagnosis and management of bacterial skin infections is scarce [1–3]. Bacterial infections can present with a variety of symptoms and can cause significant morbidity. In general, skin bacterial infections may represent hematogenous dissemination with systemic involvement or only a local process, similarly to other immunosuppressive conditions, such as all solid organ transplantation, neutropenia, chemotherapy, HIV/aids, and corticotherapy [4–6]. In case of hematogenous dissemination with systemic involvement, one of the principal risk factors for cutaneous and systemic bacterial infections in the SOTRs is granulocytopenia that predispose to potentially severe infectious complications. In addition, frequently performed procedures bypassing the skin or mucous membrane barriers (intravenous catheters, urinary catheters, surgical interventions,

D. W. de Castro Lima Santos
Instituto D'Or de Pesquisa e Ensino, Rio de Janeiro, Brazil

Department of Infectious Diseases, Hospital Universitário Presidente Dutra da Universidade Federal do Maranhão (HUUFMA), São Luis, Maranhão, Brazil

M. M. Ogawa (✉)
Department of Dermatology, Escola Paulista de Medicina, Universidad de Federal de São Paulo, São Paulo, SP, Brazil

J. Tomimori et al. (eds.), *Atlas of Dermatologic Diseases in Solid Organ Transplant Recipients*, https://doi.org/10.1007/978-3-031-13335-0_5

inhalation therapy) facilitate microbial invasion. Likewise, patients who have undergone major transplant surgery, especially heart and liver recipients, may develop wound infections and secondary septicemia during the early posttransplant period. In cases of localized disease, represented by local invasion of the skin after trauma, cellulitis, impetigo, and folliculitis are the most common bacterial skin infections seen by the transplant team, mostly occurring after 6 months [5–7].

2 Epidemiology

The different bacterial genera can cause different clinical syndromes in the organ transplant scenario:

Staphylococcus aureus: Folliculitis, furunculosis, impetigo contagiosa, bullous impetigo, ecthyma, necrotizing fasciitis, and staphylococcal scalded skin syndrome. Prior to transplantation, *Staphylococcus aureus* colonizes the anterior nares of transplant candidates (heart and liver), and a majority of nasal carriers of *S. aureus* have methicillin-resistant *S. aureus* (MRSA) or risk for develop bacteremia after transplantation compared to immunocompetent individuals. The most common cutaneous manifestation of *S. aureus* in the transplant patient is cellulitis [5, 8]. Wolfson et al. reported three interesting cases of a condition they termed "*transplant elbow*" due to the combination of steroid-induced myopathy of the legs and steroid-induced thinning of the skin. Due to the myopathy, the patients had to push their elbows against the arms of a chair to rise up, causing trauma to the elbows and recurrent cellulitis [9].

***Streptococcus* spp.**: Impetigo contagiosa, ecthyma, cellulitis; *Streptococcus pyogenes* is the most common pathogen to cause monomicrobial necrotizing fasciitis [10].

***Pseudomonas aeruginosa* and other Gram-negative rods (*Stenotrophomonas maltophilia, E. coli*)**: Necrotizing fasciitis, ecthyma gangrenosum; *P. aeruginosa* is a Gram-negative rod present in soil and water. It especially has an affinity for man-made bodies of water such as pools and hot tubs. Cutaneous infections include malignant otitis externa, necrotizing fasciitis, and ecthyma gangrenosum, which is pathognomonic for pseudomonal sepsis [11].

3 Pathogenesis and Clinical Presentation

Impetigo is a common type of superficial pyoderma that is characterized by inflammation and infection localized in the epidermis, caused by *Staphylococcus aureus* or β-hemolytic streptococcus. It consists of yellowish, eroded plaques appearing on the skin of face and limbs, that may be painful or itchy. The bullous is usually caused by exfoliating toxins produced by *Staphylococcus aureus* and is characterized by large blisters. Nonbullous impetigo is more frequent and caused by

Streptococcus sp., characterized by an erythematous macule or papule, which can progress to pustules and erosions. Serous and purulent drainage forms a characteristic honey-colored crust. Impetigo usually is transmitted through direct contact. In many cases, there is antecedent of cutaneous trauma, such as an insect bite or minor scratch. Bacterial colonization of the nares, axilla, or perineum may serve as a reservoir for infection. Impetigo is more common in tropical climates and in crowded living conditions and can be associated with poor hygiene. Impetigo is a bacterial condition that frequently occurs in SOTRs during the first posttransplant year and has an excellent prognosis. The infection may be self-limited, but it can spread and persist on the skin, becoming it contagious to others [2, 12–14] (Fig. 1a, b).

Folliculitis refers to the inflammation of the hair follicles mostly caused by *Staphylococcus aureus* and represents the most frequent bacterial infection occurring during the early phase after transplantation. The most common form is superficial folliculitis that manifests as a tender or painless pustule that heals without scarring. The clinical lesions of folliculitis begin as small pustules in follicular orifices, often accompanied by a halo of perifollicular erythema. Pustules may rupture followed by crust formation at the follicular opening. The papulo-pustular eruption is often regionalized, and lesions are typically located on the trunk, buttocks, and extremities. Pruritus is the most common symptom of folliculitis. Although prominent excoriations are usually not seen, children may excoriate each pustule leaving behind only papules and crusts. Systemic signs and symptoms are rare. Superficial staphylococcal folliculitis is very common and is also known as *Bockhart impetigo*. The hair shaft will frequently be seen in the center of the pustule. Multiple or single lesions can appear on any skin bearing hair including the head, neck, trunk, buttocks, and extremities. Similar to impetigo, folliculitis is more common in tropical climates and in settings characterized by crowded living conditions and poor hygiene [1, 15]. Gram-negative folliculitis usually involves the face and affects patients with a history of long-term antibiotic therapy for acne. Pathogens include *Klebsiella*, *Enterobacter*, and *Proteus* species. "Hot tub" folliculitis is caused by *Pseudomonas aeruginosa* contamination of under-treated water in a hot tub or

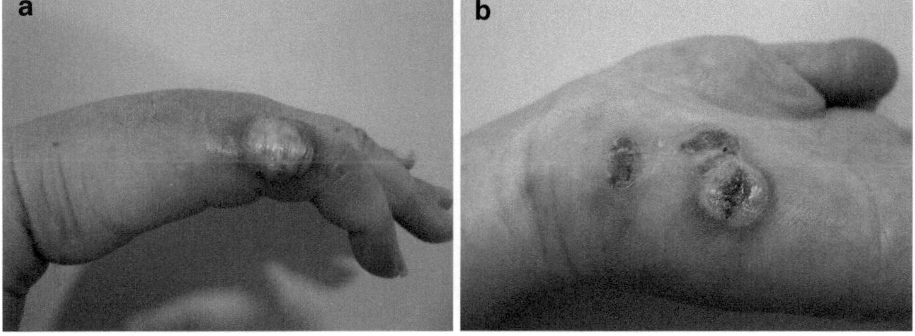

Fig. 1 (**a**, **b**) Impetigo. Pustular lesions on the dorsal hand and meliceric crust with a pustular lesion on the palm of the hand of a heart transplanted recipient

whirlpool. Multiple pustular or papular perifollicular lesions appear on the trunk and sometimes extremities within 6–72 h after exposure, and mild fever and malaise may occur [16] (Figs. 2, 3a, b, and 4).

Furunculosis are inflammatory nodules associated with a hair follicle that extend into the dermis and the subcutaneous tissue. They usually affect moist, hairy, friction-prone areas of the body, such as the face, axilla, neck, and buttocks. These lesions are firm and tender. Typically, the furuncle will develop into a fluctuant mass and eventually open to the skin surface, allowing the purulent contents to drain, either spontaneously or following incision of the furuncle. Fever and other constitutional symptoms are rarely present. The most common causative microorganism is *S. aureus.* Carbuncles are an aggregate of infected hair follicles that form broad, swollen, erythematous, deep, and painful masses that usually open and drain through multiple tracts [5, 17, 18].

Erysipelas and cellulitis are common infections of the skin. Erysipelas is a superficial infection, affecting the upper layers of the skin (the dermis and the

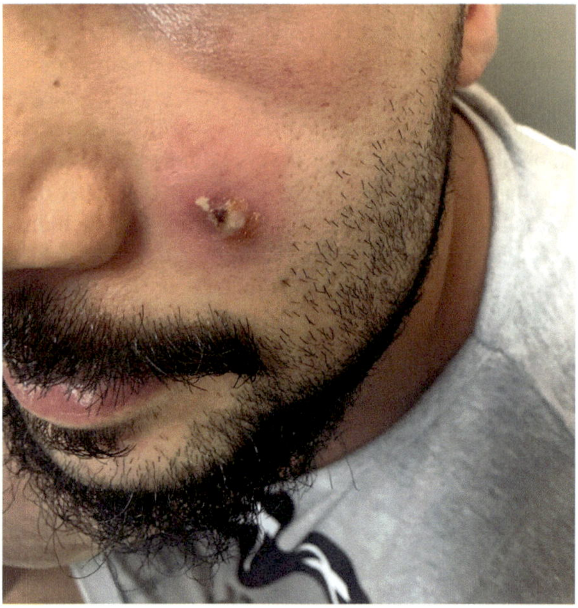

Fig. 2 Impetigo on a malar region in a kidney transplant recipient after razor injury

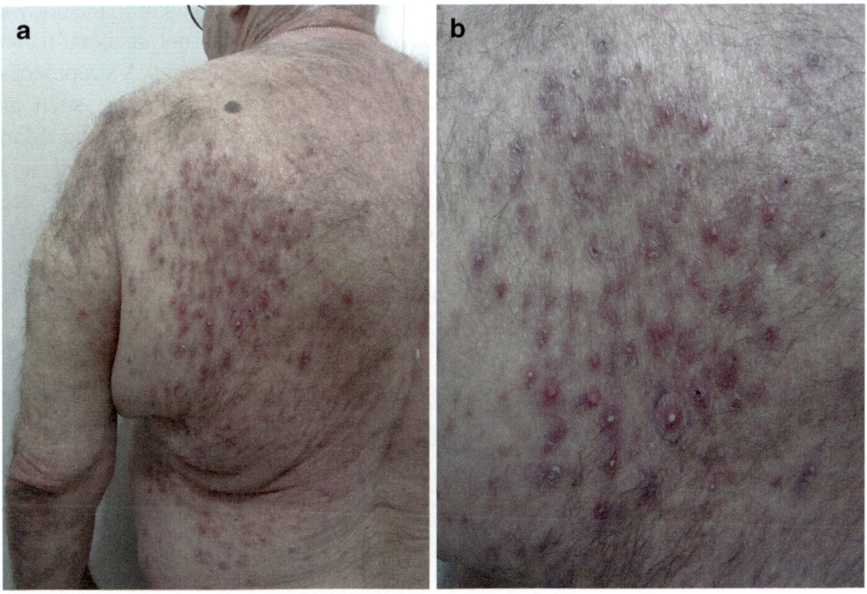

Fig. 3 (**a**) Kidney transplant recipient with folliculitis. Multiple pustules with perifollicular erythema on his back. (**b**) Close-up of the lesions

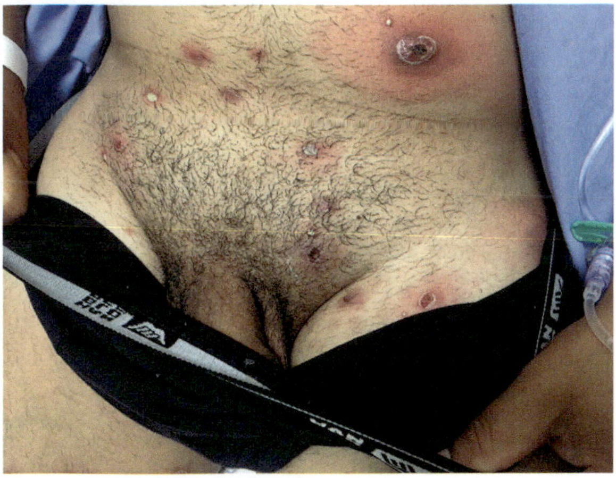

Fig. 4 Folliculitis on the pubic and lower abdomen after hair removal in a kidney transplant recipient (*S. pyogenes* was isolated from the purulent drainage)

superficial lymphatic vessels), while cellulitis affects the deeper tissues (involving the dermis and subcutis). They can overlap, so it is not always possible to make a definite diagnosis between the two. Bacteria (germs) get through a break in the skin. This break can be very small, such as from a scratch, insect bite or injection, or from another skin disease such as athlete's foot, eczema, or a leg ulcer. The body's immune system tries to stop the bacteria spreading. If this is not successful, an infection will develop. The more commonly causative agent is group A streptococcus. If bullous, hemorrhagic, or necrotic lesions occur, other germs, such as *Staphylococcus aureus* or Gram-negative bacteria, are more likely involved. Skin lesions may be accompanied by systemic symptoms such as fever, fatigue, and headache. The main risk factors for erysipelas in immunocompetent patients are venous stasis, obesity, and the presence of fissures in interdigital spaces; in SOT, immunosuppression is an additional contributing factor. Patients should be aware of the importance of an adequate feet hygiene, in order to prevent the infection [15, 16, 18–20] (Figs. 5, 6, 7, 8, 9, 10, and 11).

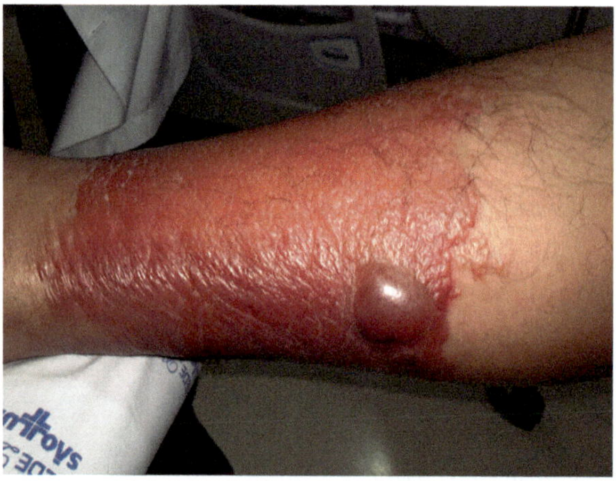

Fig. 5 Bullous erysipelas on the leg of a heart transplant recipient with a very well-defined border

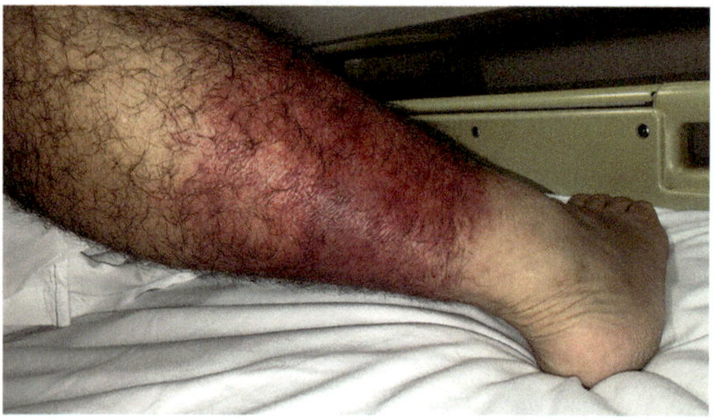

Fig. 6 Erysipelas on the leg of a 33-year-old kidney transplant recipient. Shiny erythema with well-circumscribed margins, warm and pain to the touch

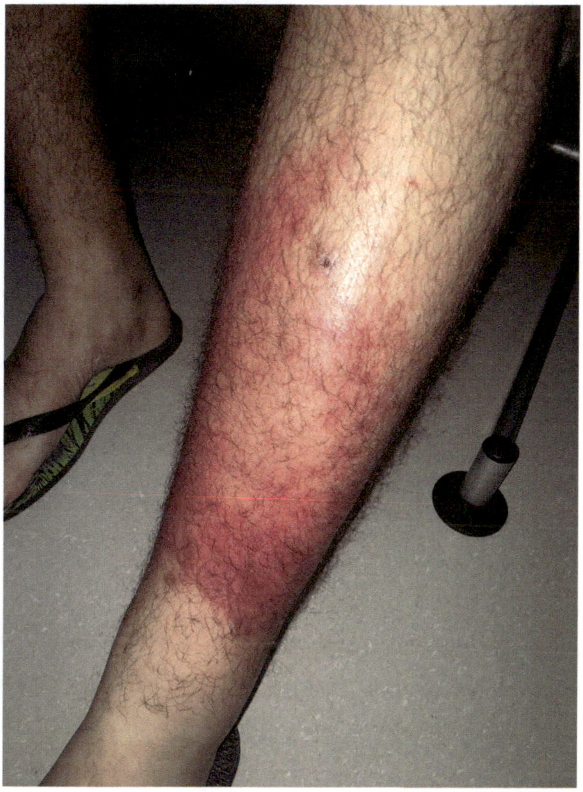

Fig. 7 Erysipelas on the leg of a 23-year-old kidney transplant recipient, insulin-dependent, with fever and pain

Necrotizing fasciitis (NF) is a severe infection resulting in life-threatening soft tissue destruction and necrosis and is caused by toxin-secreting bacteria. Extensive, rapid, and widespread progression of the infection and necrosis along soft tissue planes is the essential characteristics of the disease, a devastating cutaneous infection, especially so in the transplant population. NF spreads through the superficial fascia, subcutaneous fat, and deep fascia. It is most commonly seen in the extremities and abdominal wall, and it is associated with a mortality rate between 25% and 30%. Along with immunosuppression, other

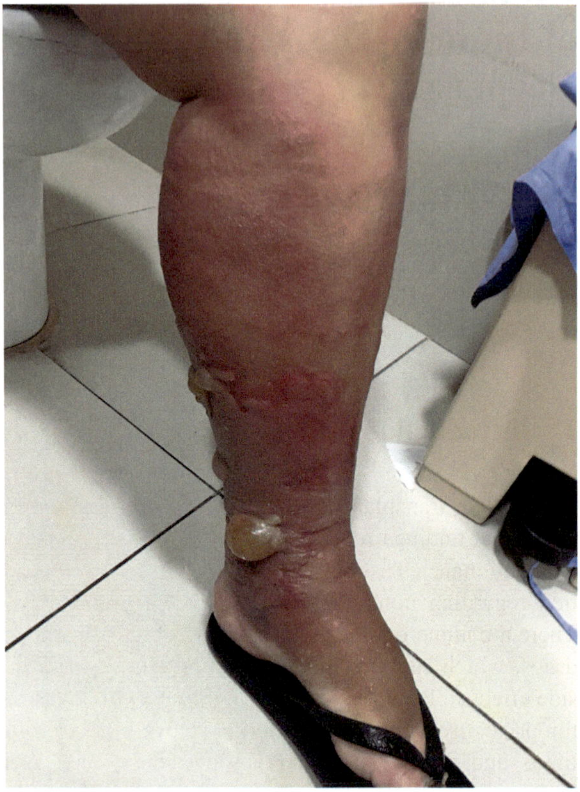

Fig. 8 Bullous erysipelas with well-defined erythema, with blisters and ascending lymphatic spread on the left leg of a female, 43 years old, kidney-pancreas transplant patient. *S. aureus* was isolated from the peripheral blood culture

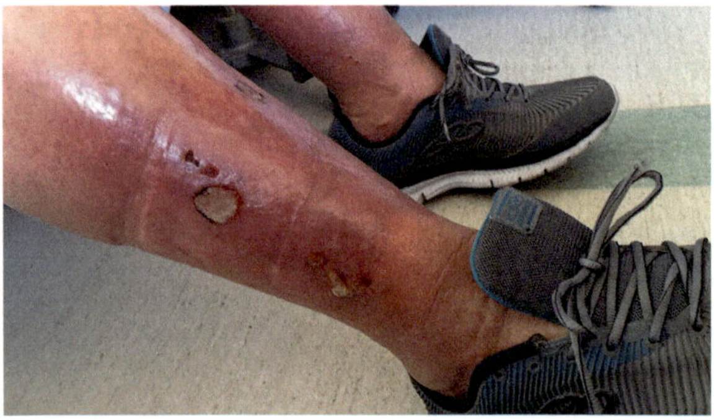

Fig. 9 Cellulitis. Erythema, with irregular margin and was warm and painful to the touch with an ulcer draining pus on the right leg in a 37-year-old kidney transplant recipient (*S. aureus* was isolated)

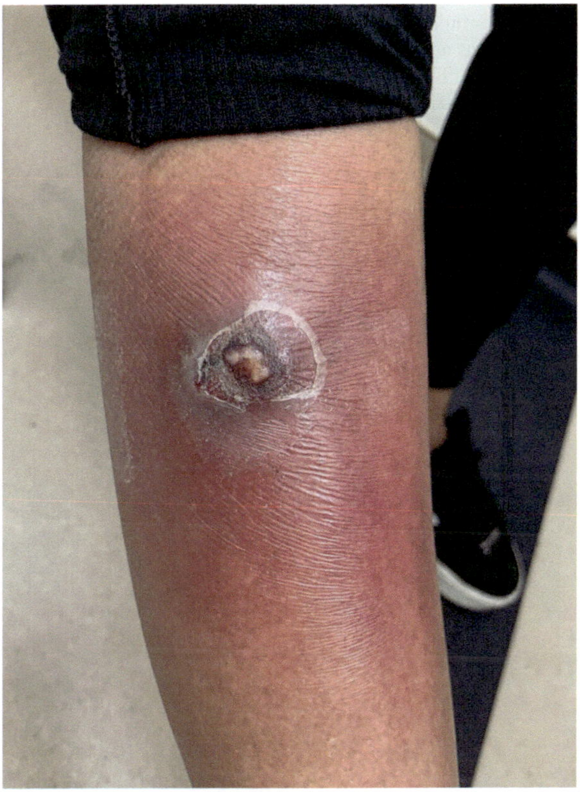

Fig. 10 Cellulitis on a leg in consequence of chronic ulcers caused by arterial disease in a 65-year-old kidney transplant patient

risk factors for NF include older age, diabetes, atherosclerosis, and drug or alcohol addiction. Although, commonly due to polymicrobial infection, staphylococcal species may be implicated. SOTRs with NF are also much more likely to present with shock (50%) when compared to a control group (20.2%) [10, 21, 22] (Figs. 12 and 13).

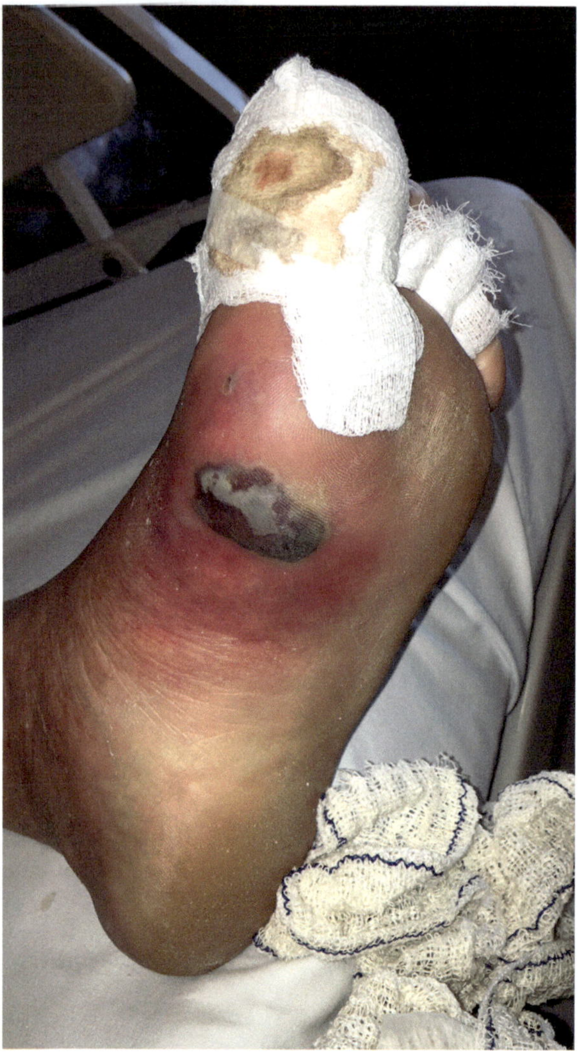

Fig. 11 Cellulitis with subcutaneous necrosis and hemorrhagic blister on left foot of a 64-year-old kidney transplant recipient. Methicillin-resistant *S. aureus* was isolated from peripheral blood culture

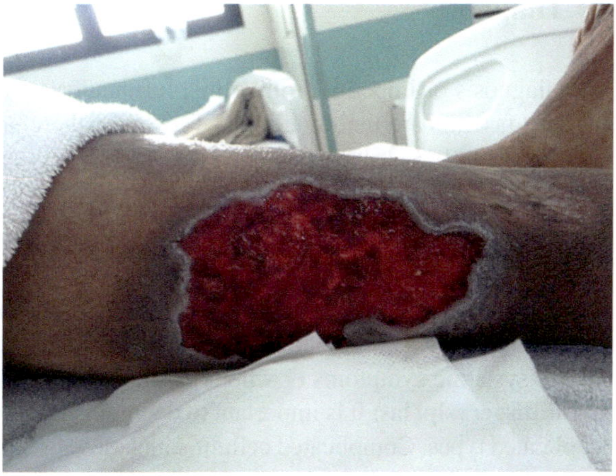

Fig. 12 Necrotizing fasciitis on the lateral face of the right leg in a 51-year-old kidney transplant recipient with diabetes and systemic arterial hypertension. Two peripheral blood cultures grew *Myroides odoratimimus*

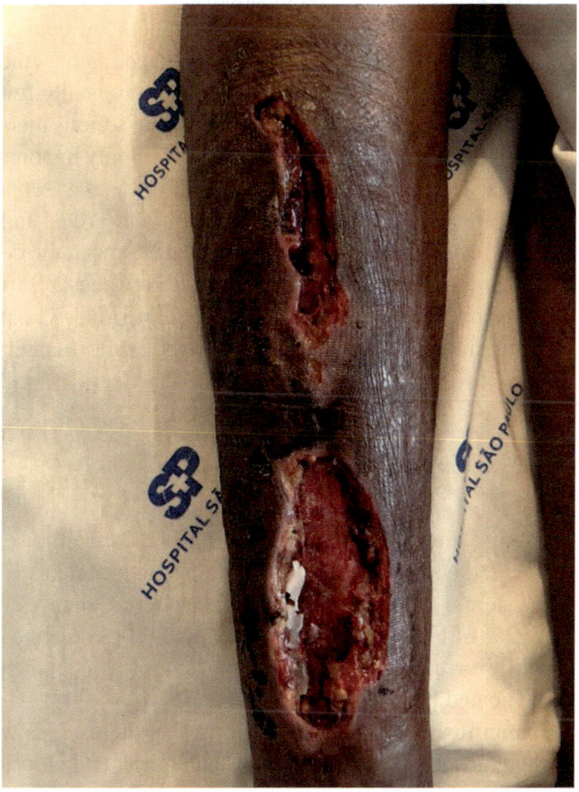

Fig. 13 Necrotizing fasciitis in a 41-year-old kidney-pancreas transplant patient with diabetes and systemic arterial hypertension. Massive ulcers with necrosis and purulent drainage on the right leg. There was isolation of *Pseudomonas aeruginosa* and *Streptococcus pyogenes* in purulent material after debridement

4 Diagnosis

The diagnosis of impetigo, folliculitis, furunculosis, cellulitis, erysipelas, and necrotizing fasciitis are mainly clinical. However, there are some remarks that should be considered [23–25]:

Impetigo and folliculitis: Bacterial culture and antimicrobial susceptibilities are important especially when the causative agent is the *S. aureus*, which can be resistant to various antibiotics.

Furunculosis: Gram stain and culture of purulent material are particularly useful in recurrent cases; blood culture can be requested for patients presenting with fever and systemic symptoms or who are immunocompromised.

Cellulitis, erysipelas: It is important to distinguish between complicated and uncomplicated types. Complicated cellulitis includes abscess requiring surgical drainage, lymphadenitis, underlying soft-tissue malformation, bite or penetrating injury, foreign body, fracture, lymphedema, medical comorbidities, and immunosuppression. Imaging (i.e., ultrasound, magnetic resonance imaging [MRI], computed tomography [CT] scan) can help in detecting the emergence of complications.

Necrotizing fasciitis: Laboratory workup typically reveals significant leukocytosis with marked left shift or even bandemia, serious metabolic disturbances, and multiple electrolyte imbalances, most commonly hyponatremia and acidosis. Creatine kinase levels are also often elevated. In cases of septic shock, creatinine clearance is compromised with early signs of acute renal failure. Computed tomography scan reveals soft tissue stranding and edema at the deeper fascial or muscular layers and occasionally will show gas between these tissue layers, even when the causative agent is not anaerobic or clostridial. The presence of gas on computed tomography scan is highly specific but, unfortunately, has a low sensitivity.

5 Treatment

Impetigo and folliculitis: Fusidic acid 2% cream or ointment: 2–3 times daily for 7–12 days; Mupirocin 2% cream* or ointment: 3 times daily for 7–10 days; Systemic treatment should be considered in cases of extensive/multiple lesions (>2% of total body surface area in child). First-line oral treatment with flucloxacillin or a first-generation cephalosporin (cephalexin) for 7–10 days could be indicated [23–25].

Furunculosis: Small lesions can resolve themselves without treatment, with spontaneous drainage. Treatment with oral trimetoprim-sulfamethoxazole (TMP-SMX) or clindamycin (if the local clindamycin resistance rate is <10%) for 7–10 days (or until complete resolution). Decolonization strategies based on chlorhexidine body wash or bleach baths and nasal mupirocin ointment, including for all household contacts, have been suggested [23–25].

Cellulitis and erysipelas: Mild cellulitis may be treated empirically with oral β-lactams, either alone or in association with TMP-SMX. The addition of an MRSA-active agent (i.e., TMP-SMX, clindamycin, linezolid) could be considered in areas where the MRSA incidence rate in the community is >10% or in cases of clinical suspicion. Severe cellulitis with rapid progression of erythema or clinical sepsis, treatment with parenteral antibiotics is indicated [23–25].

Necrotizing fasciitis: Surgical exploration is mandatory and are characterized by pale or necrotic soft tissue/muscle/fascia, absence of abrupt bleeding on sharp tissue surgical dissection, "dishwasher-like" gray discharge, and effortless separation and elevation of tissue planes with easy finger "sliding" between the muscle and fascia layers, as well as between subcutaneous tissue and fascia layers (the "finger test"). Hemodynamic support and fluid resuscitation are required. As soon as, a necrotizing fasciitis is suspected, broad-spectrum antibiotics should be instituted. The regimen should address Gram-positive, Gram-negative, and anaerobic bacteria. A combination of a β-lactam/β-lactamase inhibitor (e.g., piperacillin/tazobactam) or cephalosporin (e.g., cefepime) with an antimethicillin-resistant *Staphylococcus* [23–25].

References

1. Ponticelli C, Bencini PL. Nonneoplastic mucocutaneous lesions in organ transplant recipients. Transplant Int. 2011;24:1041–50.
2. Hogewoning AA, Goettsch W, van Loveren H, de Fijter JW, Vermeer BJ, Bouwes Bavinck JN. Skin infections in renal transplant recipients. Clin Transplant. 2001;15(1):32.
3. Bakr NI, El-Sawy E, Hamdy AF, Bakr MA. Skin infections in Egyptian renal transplant recipients. Transplant Infect Dis. 2011;13:131–5.
4. Euvrard S, Kanitakis J, Cochat P, Cambazard F, Claudy A. Skin diseases in children with organ transplants. J Am Acad Dermatol. 2001;44:932–9.
5. Lopez FA, Lartchenko S. Skin and soft tissue infections. Infect Dis Clin N Am. 2006;20(759–772):v–vi.
6. Florescu D, Qiu F, West S, et al. Staphylococcus aureus infections in kidney transplantation: a matched case controlled study. Scand J Infect Dis. 2012;44:427–32.
7. McNeil J, Munoz F, Hulten G, et al. Staphylococcus aureus infections among children receiving a solid organ transplant: clinical features, epidemiology, and antimicrobial susceptibility. Transplant Infect Dis. 2015;17:39–47.
8. Cohen PR. Community-acquired methicillin-resistant *Staphylococcus aureus* skin infections: a review of epidemiology, clinical features, management, and prevention. Int J Dermatol. 2007;46:1–11.
9. Wolfson JS, Sober AJ, Rubin RH. Dermatologic manifestations of infections in immunocompromised patients. Medicine (Baltimore). 1985;64(2):115–33.
10. Sarani B, Strong M, Pascual J, Schwab CW. Necrotizing fasciitis: current concepts and review of the literature. J Am Coll Surg. 2009;208:279–88.
11. Nakai N, Takenaka H, Kishimoto S. Ecthyma gangrenosum without pseudomonas septicemia in a kidney transplant recipient. J Dermatol. 2008;35:585–9.
12. Steer A, Danchin M, Carapetis J. Group A streptococcal infections in children. J Pediatr Child Health. 2007;43:209–13.
13. Cole C, Gazewood J. Diagnosis and treatment of impetigo. Am Fam Physician. 2007;75:859–64.

14. Euvrard S, Kanitakis J, Cochat P, Cambazard F, Claudy A. Skin diseases in children with organ transplants. J Am Acad Clin Rev Allergy Immunol Dermatol. 2001;44(6):932–9.
15. Sadick NS. Current aspects of bacterial infections of the skin. Dermatol Clin. 1997;15:341–9.
16. Jacob JS, Tschen J. Hot tub-associated pseudomonas folliculitis: a case report and review of host risk factors. Cureus. 2020;12(9):e10623. https://doi.org/10.7759/cureus.10623.
17. Lally A, Casabonne D, Imko-Walczuk B, Newton R, Wojnarowska F. Prevalence of benign cutaneous disease among Oxford renal transplant recipients. J Eur Acad Dermatol Venereol. 2011;25(4):462–70.
18. Salard D, Parriaux N, Derancourt C, Aubin F, Bresson-Hadni S, Miguet JP, Laurent R. Cutaneous complications following liver transplantation: epidemiologic and clinical study in 86 patients. Ann Dermatol Venereol. 2002;129(10 Pt 1):1134–8.
19. Galli L, Venturini E, Bassi A, Gattinara GC, Chiappini E, Defilippi C, Diociaiuti A, Esposito S, Garazzino S, Giannattasio A, Krzysztofiak A, Latorre S, Lo Vecchio A, Marchisio P, Montagnani C, Nicolini G, Novelli A, Rossolini GM, Tersigni C, Villani A, El Hachem M, Neri I, Italian Pediatric Infectious Diseases Society, Italian Pediatric Dermatology Society. Common community-acquired bacterial skin and soft-tissue infections in children: an intersociety consensus on impetigo, abscess, and cellulitis treatment. Clin Ther. 2019;41(3):532–551.e17.
20. Salard D, Parriaux N, Derancourt C, Aubin F, Bresson-Hadni S, Miguet JP, Laurent R. Manifestations dermatologiques chez les transplantés hépatiques [Cutaneous complications following liver transplantation: epidemiologic and clinical study in 86 patients]. Ann Dermatol Venereol. 2002;129(10 Pt 1):1134–8.
21. McHenry CR, Piotrowski JJ, Petrinic D, Malangoni MA. Determinants of mortality for necrotizing soft-tissue infections. Ann Surg. 1995;221:558–63.
22. Seal DV. Necrotizing fasciitis. Curr Opin Infect Dis. 2001;14:127–32.
23. Ruhe JJ, Smith N, Bradsher RW, Menon A. Community-onset methicillin-resistant Staphylococcus aureus skin and soft-tissue infections: impact of antimicrobial therapy on outcome. Clin Infect Dis. 2007;44(6):777–84.
24. Demos M, McLeod MP, Nouri K. Recurrent furunculosis: a review of the literature. Br J Dermatol. 2012;167(4):725–32.
25. Bruun T, Oppegaard O, Hufthammer KO, Langeland N, Skrede S. Early response in cellulitis: a prospective study of dynamics and predictors. Clin Infect Dis. 2016;63(8):1034–41.

Mycobacterial Diseases

Jane Tomimori and Marcos César Florian

1 Introduction

Mycobacteriosis is divided into three major groups: tuberculosis, leprosy, and non-tuberculous mycobacteriosis. They are caused by aerobic, acid fast, stick-shaped bacteria. Its wall is rich in lipids which leads to hydrophobia and mycolic acids. This waxy capsule impairs not only the supply of nutrients leading to slow growth, but also hinders the action of humoral immunity. Therefore, the main immunity involved in the pathogenesis of mycobacteriosis is cellular immunity. The mycobacteria identification is through staining with Fite-Faraco and Ziehl-Neelsen stains. These agents can be grown slowly in culture, except for *Mycobacterium leprae*.

Iatrogenic immunosuppression that is prescribed to solid organ transplant recipients (SOTRs) may facilitate mycobacterial infection or may change its natural course.

2 Tuberculosis

Tuberculosis is caused by *Mycobacterium tuberculosis* complex. It is the most common mycobacterial disease in the world. The genus *Mycobacterium* is part of the order *Actinomycetales* and the phylum *Actinobacteria*. *Mycobacterium tuberculosis* is part of the *M. tuberculosis* complex (MTBC), which includes other genetically related species that can also cause tuberculosis: *M. bovis*, *M. africanum*, *M. microti*, *M. pinnipedii*, *M. caprae*, *M. canettii*, *M. mungi*, and *M. orygis*. The association of tuberculosis and immunosuppression must be handled with special attention, with

J. Tomimori (✉) · M. C. Florian
Department of Dermatology, Escola Paulista de Medicina, Universidade Federal de São Paulo, São Paulo, SP, Brazil
e-mail: jane.tomimori@unifesp.br; mcflorian@unifesp.br

J. Tomimori et al. (eds.), *Atlas of Dermatologic Diseases in Solid Organ Transplant Recipients*, https://doi.org/10.1007/978-3-031-13335-0_6

the possibility of the emergence or reactivation of infection in immunosuppressed individuals. It most commonly affects the lungs. Other possible systems affected are the central nervous system, lymphatic, urinary, genital, cardiac, gastrointestinal, osteoarticular, ocular, and cutaneous systems. Tuberculosis is an ancient disease. The first report of cutaneous tuberculosis was made in 1826, a probable verrucous tuberculosis. Until March 1882, the disease remained without a known cause, when Dr. Roberto Koch discovered the etiologic agent [1].

2.1 *Epidemiology*

Tuberculosis is an endemic disease and one of the ten deadliest diseases in the world [1]. The main route of transmission is through inhalation of droplets expelled into the air by patients with pulmonary or laryngeal tuberculosis. In recent years, there are approximately 10 million new cases and about 1,400,000 deaths per year from the disease. Adults are the most affected (90% of cases), and it is more prevalent in men. It is a public health problem in many regions with a new potential for aggravation by global migration flows [2]. It is related to poverty and vulnerable populations. Patients also suffer from the stigmatization and prejudice surrounding the disease. It is estimated that about one-third of the world's population presents latent infection (ILTB) and 5–10% may develop active disease during their lifetime [3]. Extrapulmonary tuberculosis occurs in 6.4–13.7% of all tuberculosis cases. Cutaneous manifestations are uncommon and account for less than 2.0% of extrapulmonary manifestations. The World Health Organization has global goals for tuberculosis for reducing incidence rates by 80% and deaths by 90% by 2030 [1].

In SOTR, the prevalence of tuberculosis is about 3–4% and the median time between transplantation and tuberculosis is about 20 months [4–6]. Tuberculosis is more frequent in kidney and lung transplants recipients [7]. Cutaneous involvement is rare [6].

2.2 *Pathogenesis*

Tuberculous primoinfection usually occurs in the lung but can also occur in the skin. The interaction of the parasite with the host is important for the evolution of the disease and its clinical forms. A tuberculoid granuloma is composed of epithelioid cells, Langhans giant cells, caseous necrosis, and a lymphocytic halo. Cellular immunity response is crucial with the Th1 pathway, where macrophages and T lymphocytes are the main cells involved. Depending on this response and without interventions, the infection may evolve to spontaneous cure, remain latent, evolve to a disease with tissue damage, or spread.

Many cytokines participate in the recognition and immune response. Tumor necrosis factor alpha plays a central role in this process, since its production is essential for granulomas development, preventing the dissemination of the mycobacteria [8].

Overall, dependent on many factors, it is the agent-host-environment interaction that determines the natural history of tuberculosis (pulmonary, cutaneous, or other) in the individual who has acquired MTBC infection [8].

2.3 Clinical Presentation

The clinical manifestations of tuberculosis are varied, depending on factors related to host immunity, the environment, and type of inoculation of the etiologic agent. The same is true for the cutaneous tuberculosis [9], which has many clinical presentations that will be described below.

Attention should be paid to cutaneous tuberculosis in immunocompromised individuals (patients under immunosuppressive drugs and immunobiological drugs as well as HIV infected individuals). Diagnostic suspicion should always be made under these conditions.

- Primary inoculation tuberculosis
  It results from direct inoculation of the bacteria into the skin in individuals not previously infected by the bacillus. It is characterized by a slow growing, painless and difficult to heal papule, nodule, or ulcer.
- Tuberculosis verrucosa cutis
  It results from the inoculation of the tubercle bacillus in previously infected and sensitized individuals. It most commonly occurs on the hands and forearms. It begins as a papule that becomes keratotic. The lesion grows slowly with development of verrucous plaque with irregular outlines.
- Cutaneous tuberculosis after BCG vaccination
  BCG (bacillus Calmette-Guérin) is a preparation of attenuated *M. bovis* that has been used as a form of prevention of more severe forms of tuberculosis. It is applied by intradermal injection in many endemic countries in early childhood. Exceptionally, BCG vaccination can cause a specific tuberculous process (Fig. 1).
- Scrofuloderma
  Scrofuloderma results from an endogenous focus of tuberculosis with contiguous skin involvement. It may arise from lymph nodes (most common), bone, joint, or testicles. It begins as a firm, reddish or purple nodule adhering to the skin, which can evolve into fluctuation, suppuration, and fistulization. The lesions may be single or multiple, with a tendency to confluence, forming large infiltrated masses that intercommunicate through fistulous tracts (Fig. 2).
- Tuberculosis cutis orificialis
  It is rare and usually associated with severe forms of pulmonary, intestinal, or genitourinary tuberculosis. It may occur on oropharyngeal and anal mucosa or genital skin. It presents with erythematous papules or nodules that usually transform into painful ulcers with poorly delineated borders.

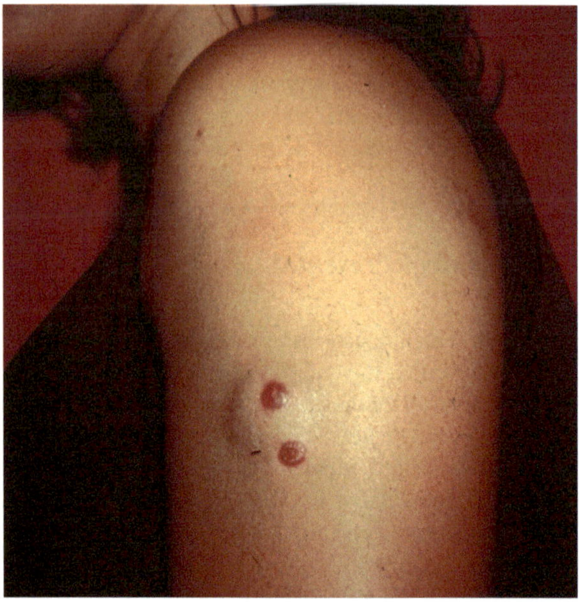

Fig. 1 Cutaneous tuberculosis after BCG vaccination on arm, in immunocompetent patient. (Tomimori J, Florian MC. Chapter 57 Cutaneous tuberculosis and atypical mycobacterioses. In: Belda Jr W, DiChiacchio N, Criado PR, eds. Treaty of Dermatology. 3rd edition. Sao Paulo, Editora Atheneu, 2018. ISBN: 978-85-388-0898-5)

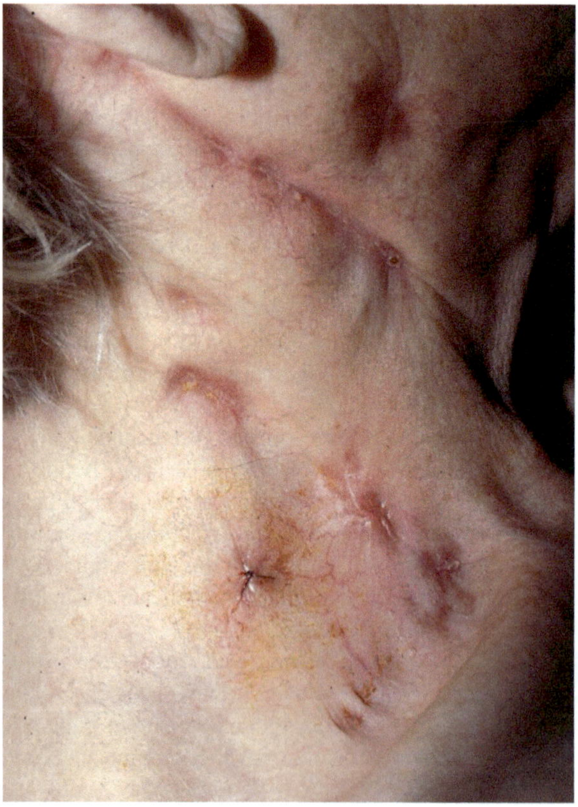

Fig. 2 Scrofuloderma on cervical region, in immunocompetent patient. (Tomimori J, Florian MC. Chapter 57 Cutaneous tuberculosis and atypical mycobacterioses. In: Belda Jr W, DiChiacchio N, Criado PR, eds. Treaty of Dermatology. 3rd edition. Sao Paulo, Editora Atheneu, 2018. ISBN: 978-85-388-0898-5)

- Lupus vulgaris
  It is a chronic and progressive form of cutaneous tuberculosis. The initial lesion is a slow growing, progressive, centrifugal papule or plaque, with a preference for the exposed areas: face (nose, malar regions, ears), hands, and forearms (Fig. 3). It can also have a nodule, tumor-like, ulcerated or vegetating clinical presentation.
- Acute miliary tuberculosis
  Miliary tuberculosis is a severe, acute, and rare form of TB. This form can be lethal in childhood, affecting children who are anergic to the bacillus. It also occurs in patients with compromised cellular immunity such as SOTRs [10]. The lesions are papules, nodules, or pustules spread all over the body. The manifestations may be accompanied by systemic signs and symptoms. It can be found in SOTR and is related to low immune response. The prevalence in immunosuppressed patients is higher compared to the general population [11].
- Tuberculous gumma
  The lesions are abscesses and nodules that liquefy in the center and drain material through fistulas or ulcers. Tuberculous gumma can occur in patients with acute miliary tuberculosis. This uncommon form of cutaneous tuberculosis has been described in immunocompromised individuals [12, 13]. Abscesses are also described in SOTRs [12, 13]. Figure 4 shows cutaneous tuberculosis manifestation as an abscess, with purulent secretion in a kidney transplant recipient.
- Tuberculids
  Tuberculids do not represent a local cutaneous infection. They are considered hypersensitivity reactions that occur in patients with moderate or high cellular immune response and are secondary to distant foci of tuberculosis. They disappear with the treatment of tuberculosis. Tuberculids comprise papulonecrotic tuberculids (Fig. 5), lichen scrofulosorum, and erythema induratum of Bazin.

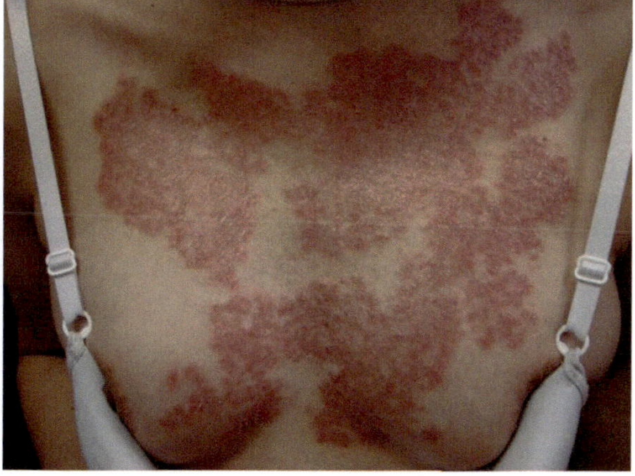

Fig. 3 Lupus vulgaris on chest, in immunocompetent patient. (Tomimori J, Florian MC. Chapter 57 Cutaneous tuberculosis and atypical mycobacterioses. In: Belda Jr W, DiChiacchio N, Criado PR, eds. Treaty of Dermatology. 3rd edition. Sao Paulo, Editora Atheneu, 2018. ISBN: 978-85-388-0898-5)

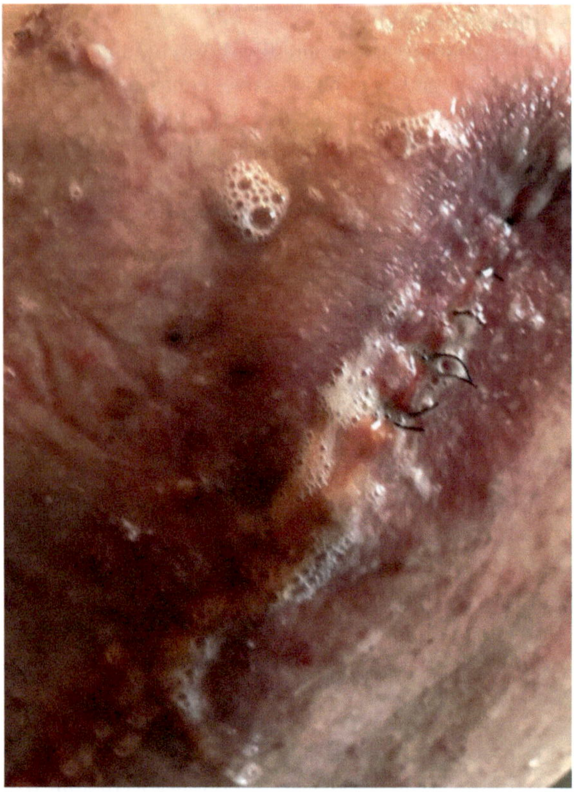

Fig. 4 Tuberculous abscess on upper trunk, lesion size of 10 cm with purulent secretion, in kidney transplant recipient

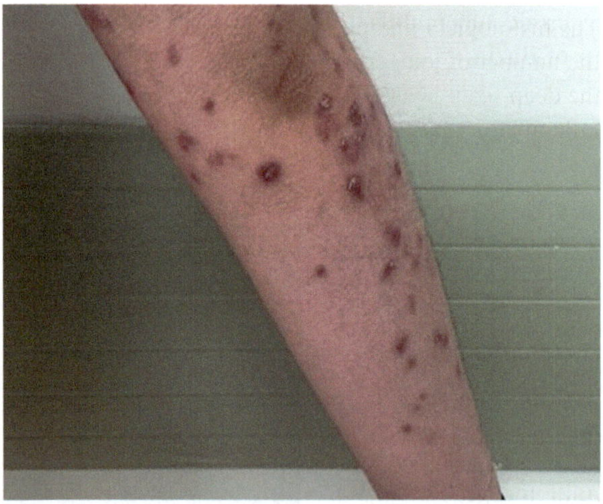

Fig. 5 Papulonecrotic tuberculid, multiple erythematous papules with crust on arm, in immunocompetent patient. (Tomimori J, Florian MC. Chapter 57 Cutaneous tuberculosis and atypical mycobacterioses. In: Belda Jr W, DiChiacchio N, Criado PR, eds. Treaty of Dermatology. 3rd edition. Sao Paulo, Editora Atheneu, 2018. ISBN: 978-85-388-0898-5)

2.4 Histopathology and Laboratorial Diagnosis

If there is a hypothesis of tuberculosis, the tuberculin skin test and chest radiograph should always be requested.

Skin biopsy for histopathological analysis, acid fast research, and culture for mycobacteria is crucial in suspected cases of cutaneous tuberculosis. PCR (polymerase chain reaction) should also be performed on the skin fragment and blood. It is very difficult finding the etiologic agent in the skin.

- Histopathology: It is a very important method in cases of cutaneous tuberculosis and tuberculids. There are differences in the histopathology of clinical presentations, but the common histological basis is the presence of tuberculoid granuloma and caseous necrosis. The absence of tuberculoid granuloma does not completely rule out the diagnosis of tuberculosis. Similarly, its presence alone is not definitive for the diagnosis. Tuberculids have other histopathological findings, but the granulomatous infiltrate is present.
- Bacilloscopy: Sputum is the most commonly requested test for suspected pulmonary tuberculosis and can also be obtained by bronchoscopy.
  If cutaneous tuberculosis is suspected, skin smear microscopy should be performed on the skin fragment obtained by biopsy. The Fite-Faraco or Ziehl-Neelsen stains can detect the presence of acid fast bacilli in infected tissue, but the negativity does not exclude the diagnosis. In the paucibacillary forms, the presence of bacillus is very rare. In tuberculids, the bacillus is not detected [1].
  The search for the bacillus by PCR techniques increases sensitivity in detecting the agent in tissue, without decreasing specificity. It can be performed on fresh tissue, blood, and paraffin-embedded tissue [14].
- Culture: It is the gold standard for diagnosing tuberculosis. The bacillus can be grown at 35–37 °C in an enriched aerobic medium. This test allows the isolation of the agent, characterizing the mycobacteria and determining its sensitivity to antibiotics. However, the growth of *M. tuberculosis* in culture media is slow (28 days or more) and treatment is often instituted even without identification of the agent. The sensitivity of culture in cutaneous forms of tuberculosis is low, around 23% [14, 15].
- Tuberculin skin test (TST): It measures the cellular immune response, indicating the sensitization of individuals to the bacillus. It shows the presence of infection but does not determine the presence of disease. It is indicated to identify cases of latent infection (ILTB) and diagnose active TB in children. It consists of the intradermal injection of 0.1 mL of antigen. The reading is after 48–72 h and may be extended to 96 h. Results from 0 to 4 mm indicate non-reactive: Individual not infected by *M. tuberculosis* or with reduced hypersensitivity; results ≥5 mm indicates individual infected by the tuberculosis bacillus.
- Interferon-gamma release assay (IGRA): It is based on the premise that cells previously sensitized with *M. tuberculosis* antigens produce high levels of interferon-gamma. It is a serological test for the detection of latent infection (ILTB), being more sensitive than the tuberculin skin test.

- Rapid molecular test for tuberculosis: It is a DNA amplification test by PCR for detection of tuberculosis and screening of rifampicin-resistant strains. It is mainly indicated for diagnosing pulmonary or laryngeal tuberculosis, performed on a sputum sample with result within 2 h. It is a diagnostic option in suspected cutaneous tuberculosis, such as scrofuloderma [16].
- Adenosine deaminase: Intracellular enzyme present in the active lymphocyte. Detection of its increased activity in pleural fluid indicates tuberculous pleuritis.

2.5 Treatment

The first drugs with anti-tuberculous effectiveness appeared in the 1940s. The first antimicrobial drug used was streptomycin in 1943. Subsequently, cases of resistant tuberculosis and multidrug-resistant tuberculosis appeared, requiring longer treatments and with a higher risk of toxicity.

This disease is curable. It is treated by a standard 6 months course of four antibiotics (rifampicin, isoniazid, pyrazinamide, and ethambutol). There are some cases of drug-resistant tuberculosis.

In the case of asymptomatic *M. tuberculosis* infection, the preconized treatment includes isoniazid or rifampicin.

The treatment of tuberculosis in transplant patients follows the usual regimens and should be instituted as soon as possible. However, interactions between anti-TB drugs and immunosuppressors can occur [17].

3 Leprosy

Leprosy is caused by *Mycobacterium leprae*. It is a chronic disease with cutaneous and peripheral neurological symptoms. Its incubation period is very long. Leprosy is considered a spectral granulomatous disease that can be classified as paucibacillary (tuberculoid-TT, borderline tuberculoid-BT) and multibacillary (mid-borderline-BB, borderline lepromatous-BL, and lepromatous-LL). In paucibacillary forms, Th1 response predominates, while in multibacillary forms Th2 response predominates. In 1973, Adu et al. described the first case of multibacillary leprosy in a kidney transplant recipient [18].

3.1 Epidemiology

The main endemic countries are Brazil, India, and Indonesia [19]. SOTRs susceptible to leprosy are those residing in endemic areas [20]. SOTRs have a similar chance to develop leprosy with respect to the risk of contamination when compared to immunocompetent individuals. Multibacillary leprosy can lead to renal changes that can determine organ failure and renal transplantation. There is no contraindication for solid organ transplantation in patients with leprosy [21].

3.2 Pathogenesis

The susceptible individuals are contaminated by Flügge's droplets, containing bacilli eliminated by multibacillary patients. The incubation period is around 5 years. The first cutaneous lesion is an anesthetic hypochromic macule. The infected individual can evolve to multibacillary forms, when the specific cellular immune response is not efficient or to paucibacillary forms, with few bacilli and limited lesion distribution.

Leprosy patients can develop two types of reactions: reversal reaction in which there is a greater cellular immune response and affects patients with borderline forms of disease and, erythema nodosum leprosum, which occurs in multibacillary forms with high levels of antibodies.

The reversal reaction could be considered an immune reconstitution inflammatory syndrome (IRIS). It occurs when the specific treatment is initiated in patients with unstable forms of disease (borderline form). Thus, when immunosuppression is reduced, this flare-up can also occur [22]. It is reported that the decreasing of iatrogenic immunosuppression in the leprosy patients can lead to the appearance of this reactive outbreak [18], or the reactions may evolve even in the course of immunosuppressive therapy [22, 23].

The association of leprosy and solid organ transplantation can result in a very complex clinical condition. The deficiency of cellular immunity of lepromatous leprosy could lead to a longer survival of the transplanted organ [18], while the use of immunosuppressants to avoid rejection could decrease the immune response against *M. leprae*, causing atypical forms of the disease or leading to relapses [21, 24].

3.3 Clinical Presentation

Multibacillary form is characterized by the presence of diffuse erythematous papules and nodules with symmetrical involvement of peripheral nerves. LL form presents brownish or erythematous disseminated papules and nodules (Fig. 6a, b). In BL form (Fig. 7), foveolar erythematous plaques, papules, and nodules are observed. The mid-borderline (BB) form (Fig. 8) is characterized by multiple foveolar plaques. Paucibacillary form presents a reduced number of erythematous plaques (less than 5 lesions), usually with local anesthesia and asymmetric neurological involvement. The BT form (Fig. 9) is observed the presence of erythematous annular plaques, less than 5 lesions. The TT form (Fig. 10) is characterized by a single erythematous

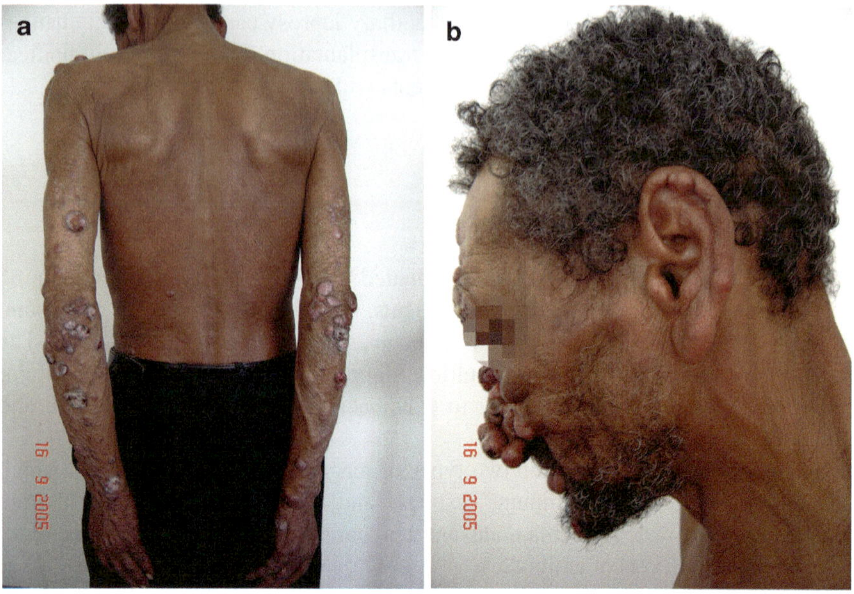

Fig. 6 Multibacillary form (LL: lepromatous-lepromatous) in immunocompetent patient, with disseminated multiple erythematous papules and nodules: (**a**) on arms, forearms, and elbows and (**b**) on face and ears

annular lesion. This is the spectral distribution of leprosy forms. The central nervous system is not affected in leprosy, except the peripheral portion of cranial nerves (for example, facial, trigeminal, glossopharyngeal nerves). Figure 11 shows right auricular nerve on sternocleidomastoid muscle and papules on ears in immunocompetent patient with LL form.

Leprosy can appear in the SOTRs during the transplant or afterwards [20]. Due to immunosuppressive therapy, clinical lesions can present with less signs of inflammation, as it can be observed in a kidney transplant recipient with LL form (Fig. 12a–c).

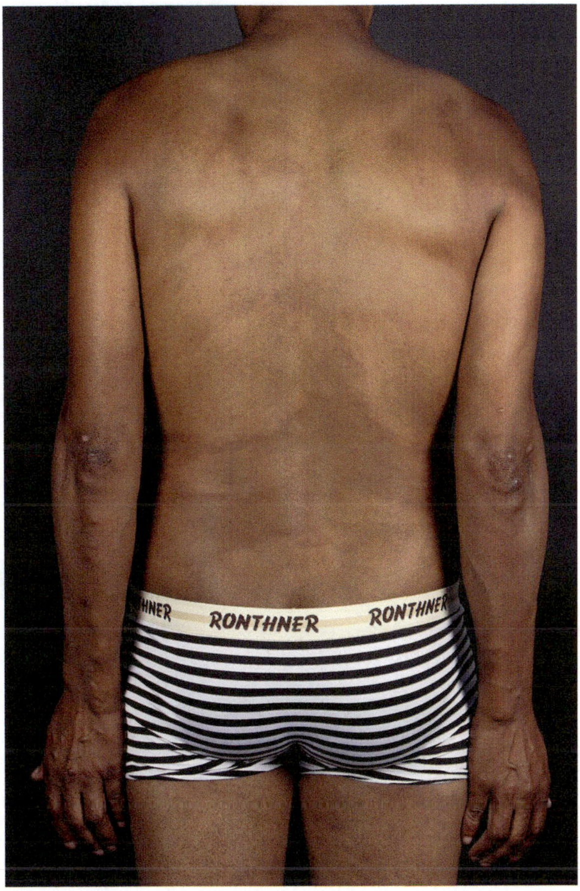

Fig. 7 Multibacillary form (BL: borderline-lepromatous), disseminated hypochromic plaques, and infiltrated papules on elbows and forearms, in immunocompetent patient

There are two complications that can occur during leprosy treatment. The reversal reaction (type 1 reaction) occurs in borderline patients. The primary lesions become edematous, infiltrated, and erythematous. Systemic symptoms can also be present such as fever, arthritis, and synovitis (Fig. 13a, b). Erythema nodosum

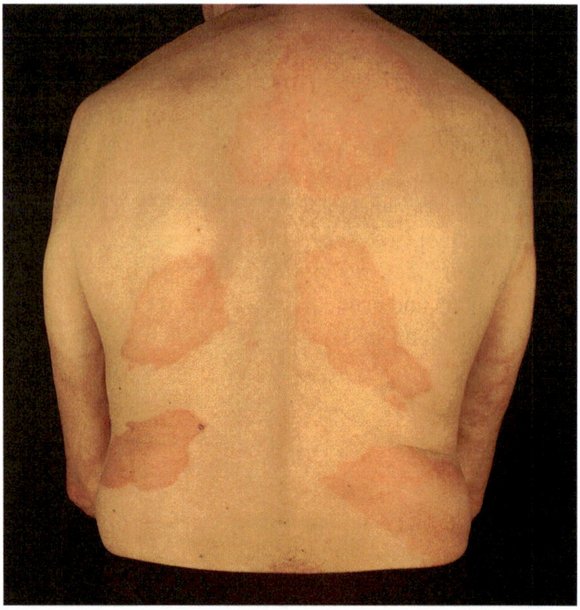

Fig. 8 Multibacillary form (BB: mid-borderline), multiples erythematous plaques on trunk and arms, in immunocompetent patient

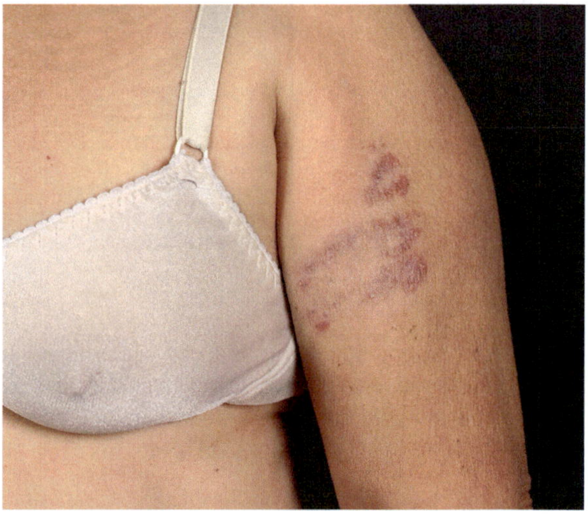

Fig. 9 Paucibacillary form (BT: borderline-tuberculoid), two erythematous plaques on left arm, in immunocompetent patient

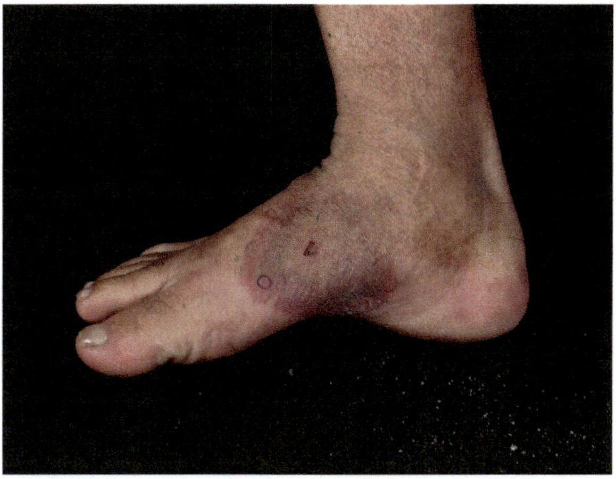

Fig. 10 Paucibacillary form (TT: tuberculoid-tuberculoid), single anesthetic cutaneous lesion on dorsal aspect of the right foot, in immunocompetent patient

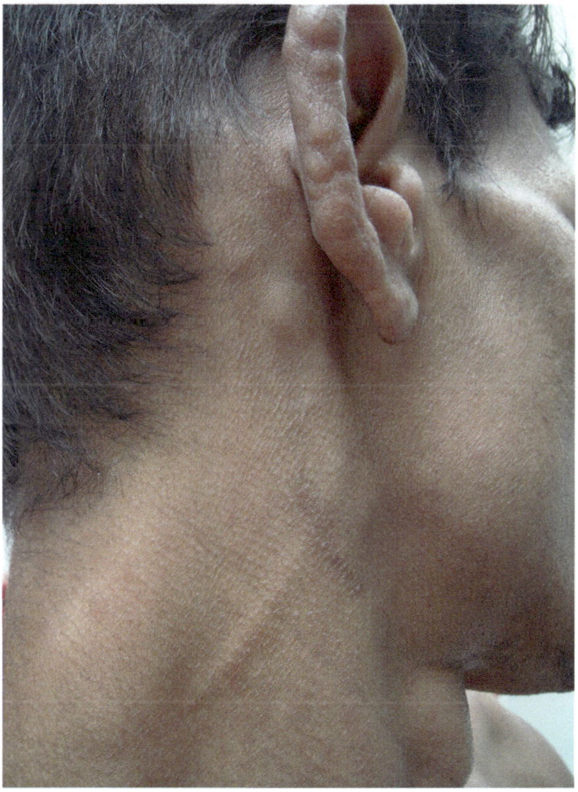

Fig. 11 Multibacillary form (LL), multiple papules on right ear and visible enlargement of auricular nerve (on sternocleidomastoid muscle), in immunocompetent patient

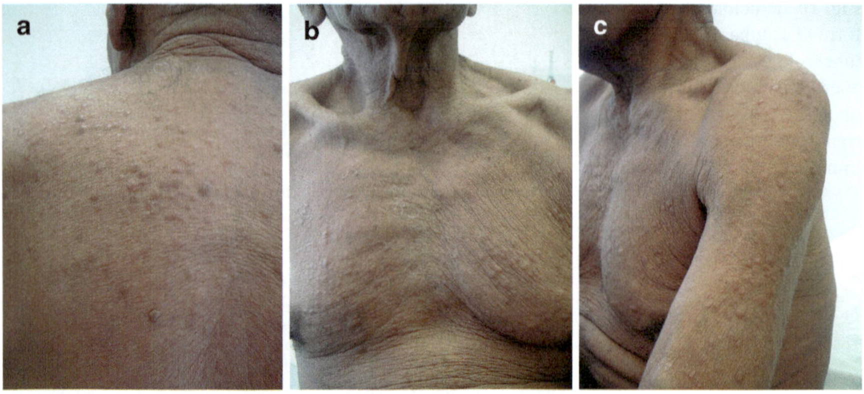

Fig. 12 Kidney transplant recipient with multibacillary leprosy (LL) with multiple and disseminated papules: (**a**) on upper back; (**b**) on chest; and (**c**) on arms

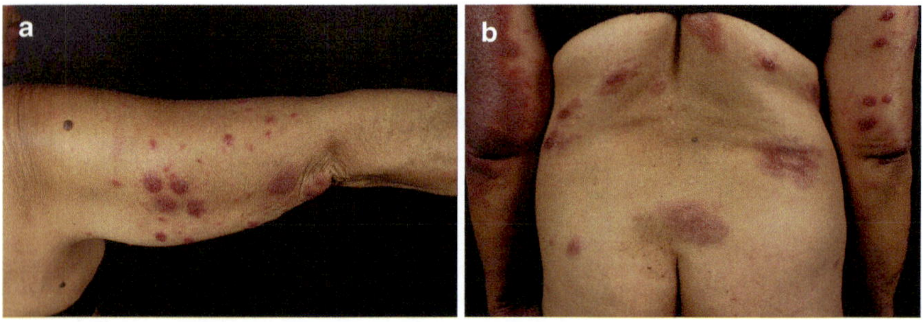

Fig. 13 Reversal reaction in immunocompetent patient with multiple erythematous and edematous plaques: (**a**) on arm and (**b**) on buttocks

leprosum (type 2 reaction) occurs in multibacillary form. It develops in patients with many bacilli and high levels of antibodies. The lesions are de novo and can be painful. Fever, orchitis, and arthritis can also be present (Fig. 14).

In SOTR, the reversal reaction can be observed when the immunosuppression is decreased or associated with other factors. These immunosuppressed patients do not develop an intense inflammatory reaction (Fig. 15a–c).

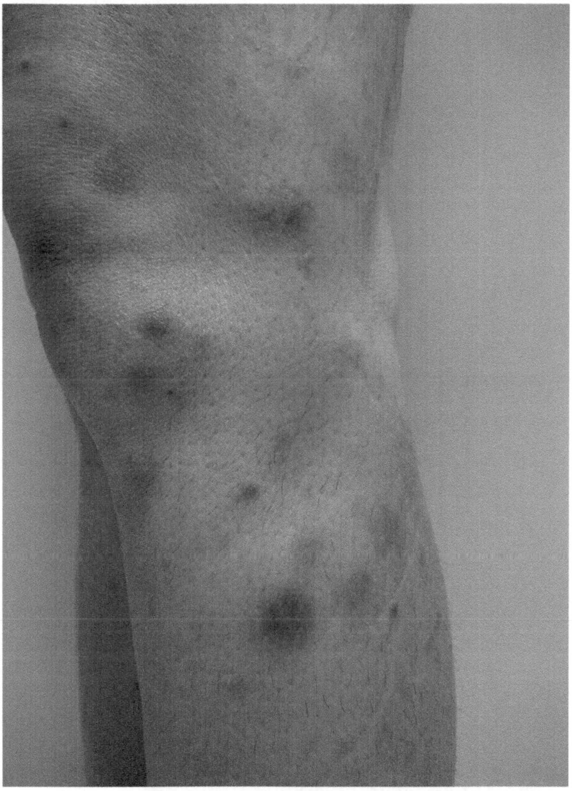

Fig. 14 Erythema nodosum leprosum, multiple erythematous papules and nodules on the leg, in immunocompetent patient

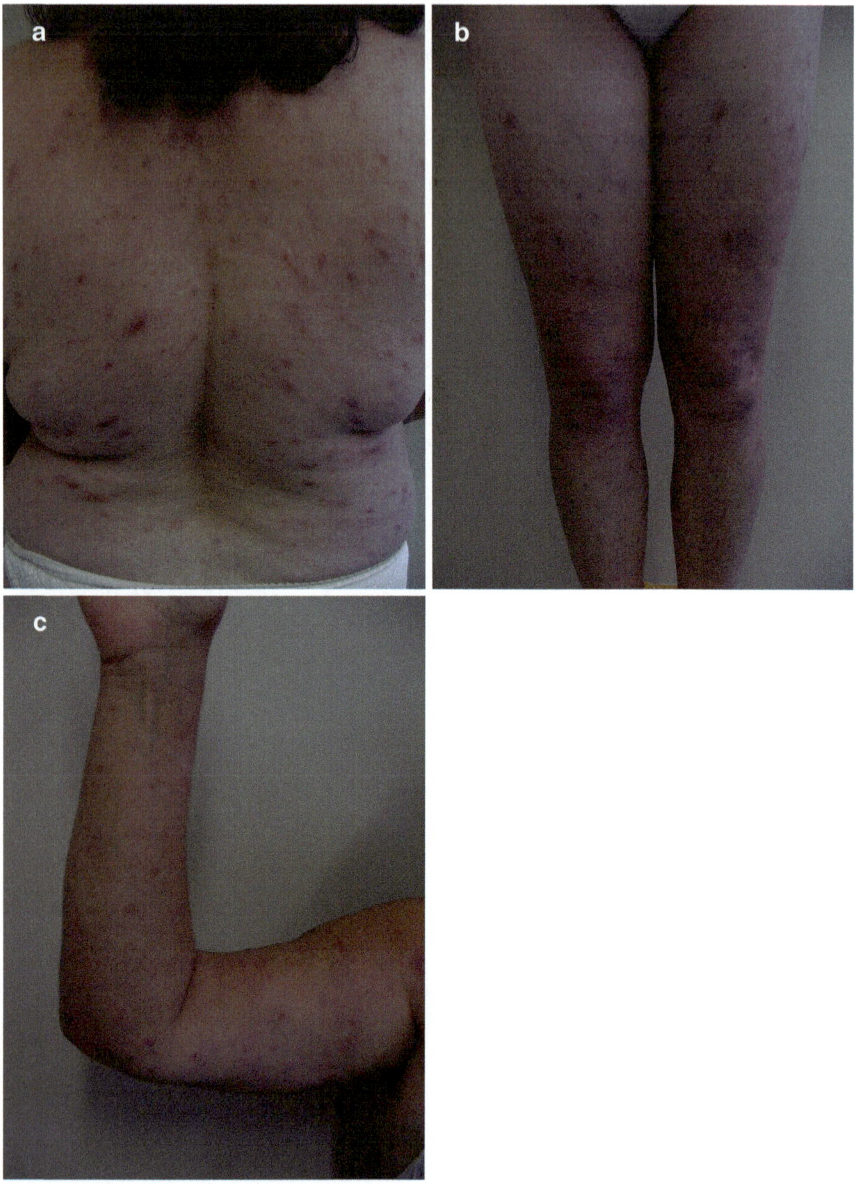

Fig. 15 Kidney transplant recipient with multibacillary leprosy (BL) and reversal reaction. Multiple erythematous papules and plaques: (**a**) on back; (**b**) on thighs; and (**c**) on arms

3.4 Histopathology and Laboratorial Diagnosis

In paucibacillary forms, the typical histopathology is the presence of tuberculoid granuloma with lymphocytic infiltrate, epithelioid cells, and Langhans giant cell. The infiltrate is localized around cutaneous nerves. There is also a scarcity of bacilli.

In multibacillary forms, there is a diffuse macrophagic granuloma, with an intense histiocytic infiltrate. There is a grenz zone, sparing the papillary dermis. The macrophages are vacuolated and the Fite-Faraco stain shows a large number of bacilli forming clusters (globi) (Fig. 16).

Serology anti-PGL-1 (phenolic glycolipid 1) or recombinant protein diagnoses multibacillary forms; however, it is not useful for diagnosing paucibacillary or indeterminate forms.

Mitsuda intradermal reaction employs the whole *M. leprae* bacilli. The reaction should be analyzed in 28 days. Paucibacillary patients develop tuberculous granuloma, showing papule bigger than 5 mm of diameter. Multibacillary patients do not react.

Bacilloscopy is performed collecting a slit skin smear from the cutaneous lesion, ears, elbows, and knees. Multibacillary patients present isolated bacilli and globi. In paucibacillary patients, bacilloscopy is negative.

Reports about the association of leprosy and solid organ transplantation do not show any difference in histopathological aspects [21, 23].

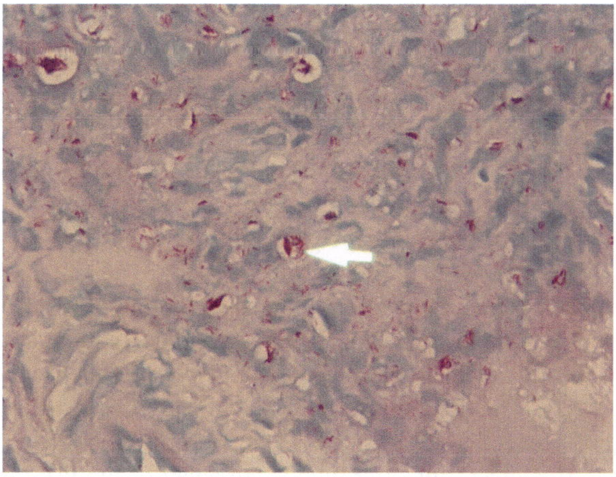

Fig. 16 Multibacillary leprosy, bacilli forming globi (Ziehl-Neelsen stain, 1000×)

3.5 Treatment

Treatment of leprosy in SOTRs is similar to the treatment recommended in immunocompetent leprosy patients. Greater care must be taken with rifampicin, which interacts with the calcineurin inhibitors. Rifampicin leads to a decrease of calcineurin inhibitors (cyclosporine and tacrolimus), so these immunosuppressive drug doses must be adjusted.

Leprosy reactions (reversal or erythema nodosum leprosum) in SOTRs should be treated with prednisone dosage increasing, without altering the other immunosuppressive drugs [22, 25]. Kidney transplantation is not contraindicated in patients with leprosy, as these patients often evolve with renal function damage [26].

Among liver transplant recipients, the use of rifampin should be well evaluated, due to its hepatotoxicity [27].

4 Non-tuberculous Mycobacteriosis

These infectious agents are non-tuberculous mycobacteria (NTM) and are also known as atypical mycobacteria and mycobacteria other than tuberculosis (MOTT). This group of bacilli can live as a saprophyte in soil, water, or vegetation.

4.1 Epidemiology

The incidence of NTM has been increased in the SOTRs, mainly within individuals with increased survival and greater environmental exposure [28]. The occurrence of NTM in SOTRs varies according to the geographic region. The highest incidence is among lung transplant recipients, followed by kidney and heart. NTM infection is rare in liver transplant recipients [29].

Infection with the *M. avium* complex (MAC) and *M. kansasii* can be transmitted by aerosol contamination, lodging in the lung [30]. Cutaneous lesions are uncommon and they can be due to hematogenous dissemination.

Buruli ulcer is caused by *Mycobacterium ulcerans* and occurs mainly in West Africa. This mycobacteriosis has already been reported in 27 countries [31]. Its occurrence in SOTRs has not been described so far.

Mycobacterium marinum is the agent of the fish tank granuloma. This agent is related to aquatic environments, involving fishmongers, pool, or aquarium caregivers. This infection is rare among SOTRs, as there are only 11 cases reported in the literature [32].

Among the SOTRs, the *M. fortuitum*, *M. chelonae*, and *M. abscessus* complex are usually related to local trauma [30]. In SOTRs, MAC infection represents the majority of NTM infections, followed by fast-growing mycobacteria (*M. fortuitum*,

M. chelonae, *M. abscessus* complex). The latter group is frequently related to catheter infection and bacteremia [33].

4.2 Pathogenesis

The majority of non-tuberculous mycobacterial infections result from minor traumas, as demonstrated in Buruli's ulcer and fish tank granuloma [31, 32].

Iatrogenic inoculations are an important cause, mainly involving *M. fortuitum*, *M. chelonae* and *M. abscessus* complex [30]. Disseminated infection by this complex is rare, but this possibility cannot be ruled out in immunosuppressed individuals [34].

Mycobacteria of MAC and *M. kansasii* complex are transmitted by aerosol and can be found in lung and heart transplant recipients [29]. Iatrogenic immunosuppression associated with invasive procedures increases the predisposition to NTM infection.

Mycobacterium haemophilum is a slow-growing mycobacteria with a genetic similarity with *M. marinum* [35]. There are descriptions of disseminated infection with *M. haemophilum* in SOTRs [36, 37].

4.3 Clinical Presentation

The predominant lesions are asymptomatic or slightly painful erythematous papules and nodules, which can progress to ulcers. Localized lesions can evolve following the lymphatic path, mimicking sporotrichosis. Disseminated lesions may indicate hematogenous spread [38, 39].

The most common sites are limbs, as most mycobacteria are inoculated through minor traumas of exposed skin. Buruli's ulcer can lead to intense edema of the affected limb with subsequent ulceration [31].

In SOTRs, the dermatologist can help the definitive diagnosis since systemic diseases such as those caused by *M. kansasii* or MAC complex, may present polymorphism of skin lesions as the result of hematogenous dissemination of the causative agent (Fig. 17a–c). There may be involvement of the pleuro-pulmonary, musculoskeletal, and lymph nodes with disseminated multi-organ disease [29, 40–42]. They are frequently caused by *M. fortuitum*, *M. chelonae,* and *M. abscessus* complex, as a single lesion (Fig. 18) or unilateral lymphangitic distribution papules and nodules (Fig. 19a, b).

The risk factors are male and aged around 50 years, who underwent lung transplantation with the diagnosis of NTM in the first year of transplantation. In the lung transplant recipients, mycobacteria affect mainly the transplanted organ, however disseminated skin lesions and involvement of the osteoarticular system may appear [43]. In SOTRs, cutaneous lesions may resemble multibacillary leprosy [44].

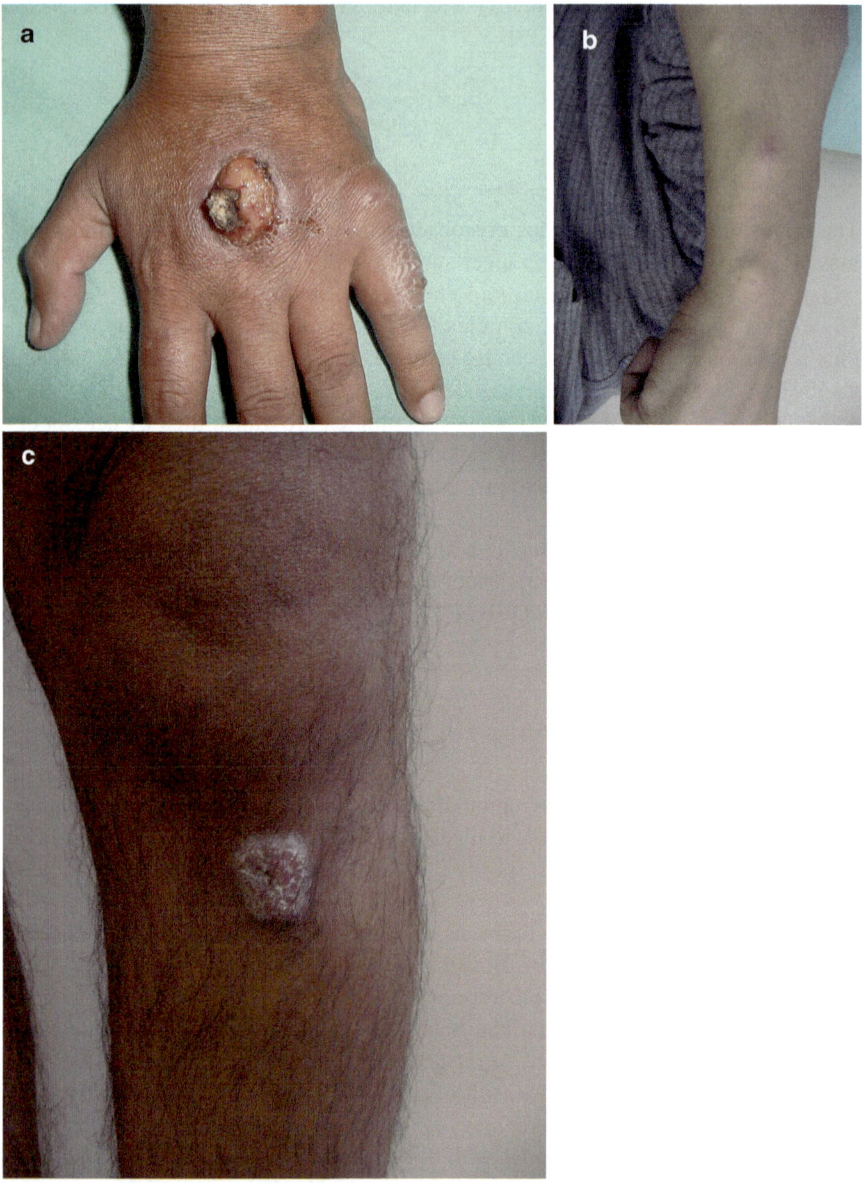

Fig. 17 *Mycobacterium avium* complex infection in kidney transplant recipient. Disseminated polymorphic lesions: (**a**) ulcer on the hand and abscess-like lesion on fifth finger; (**b**) subcutaneous nodular lesion with slight erythema; and (**c**) verrucous nodule on the knee

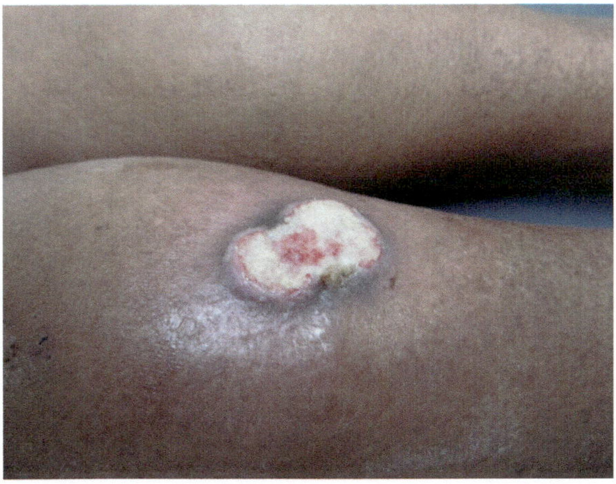

Fig. 18 *Mycobacterium chelonae* infection in kidney transplant recipient. Single ulcerated lesion on leg

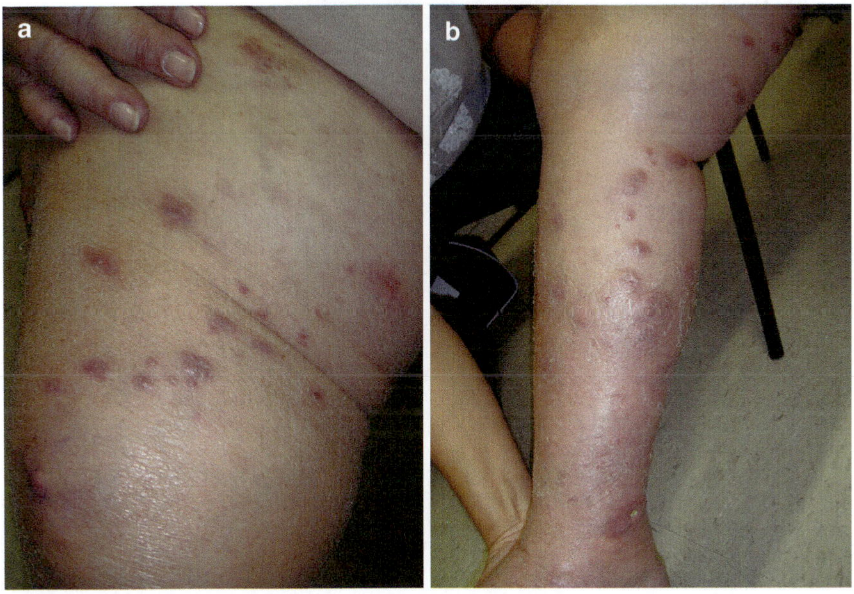

Fig. 19 *Mycobacterium chelonae* infection in kidney transplant recipient: (**a**) unilateral erythematous papules on medial region of right thigh and (**b**) unilateral lymphatic disposition of erythematous nodules on right leg

Figures 20 and 21 show different presentations of NTM in SOTRs. In Fig. 22, it is observed multiple lesions on abdomen, after serial use of the same syringe for subcutaneous injection of insulin.

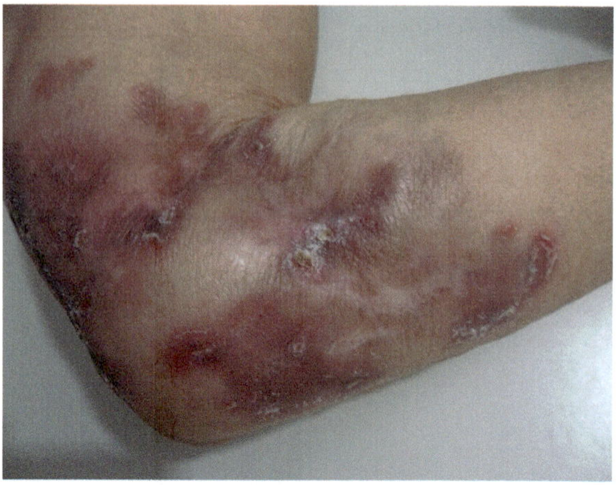

Fig. 20 Non-tuberculous mycobacteria infection in kidney transplant recipient. Infiltrated and inflammatory lesions with crust on elbow. Cicatricial atrophy is observed

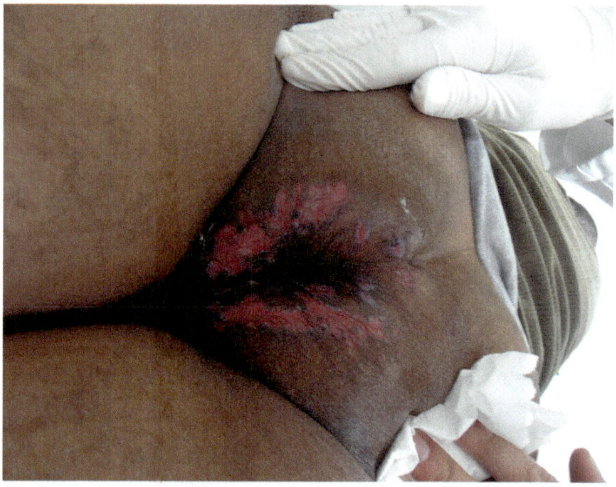

Fig. 21 Non-tuberculous mycobacteria infection in kidney transplant recipient. Perianal ulcers remarkably similar to tuberculosis cutis orificialis

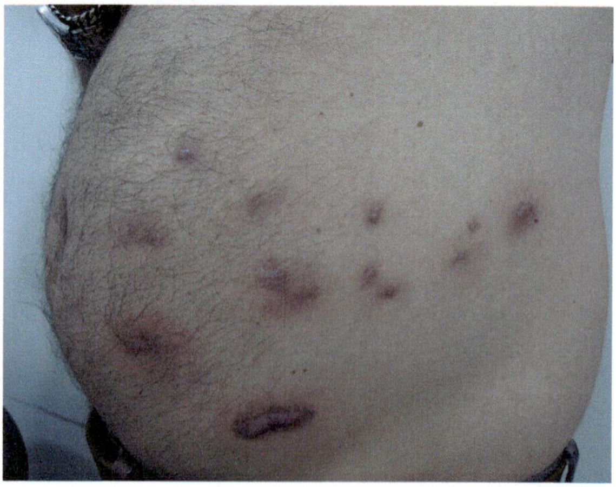

Fig. 22 Non-tuberculous mycobacteria infection in kidney transplant recipient with diabetes mellitus. Multiple erythematous papules and nodules on abdomen. The patient used the same syringe for serial subcutaneous injection of insulin

4.4 Histopathology and Laboratory Diagnosis

The histopathological characteristic findings is the tuberculoid granuloma with multinucleated giant cells, epithelioid cells, and lymphocytes (Fig. 23a–c). The presence of isolated and more elongated acid-fast bacilli compared to *M. leprae* and *M. tuberculosis* can help the diagnosis (Fig. 24a–c). Abscesses in the deep dermis with acid-fast bacilli clusters can also be found [38].

The material of secretion or skin biopsy can be sent for direct slit-smear microscopy and culture in Löwenstein-Jensen or Middlebrook medium. Interferon Gamma Rapid Assay (IGRA) used for the diagnosis of tuberculosis is not useful for the diagnosis of NTM, despite it can cross-react with *M. kansasii* and *M. marinum* [45].

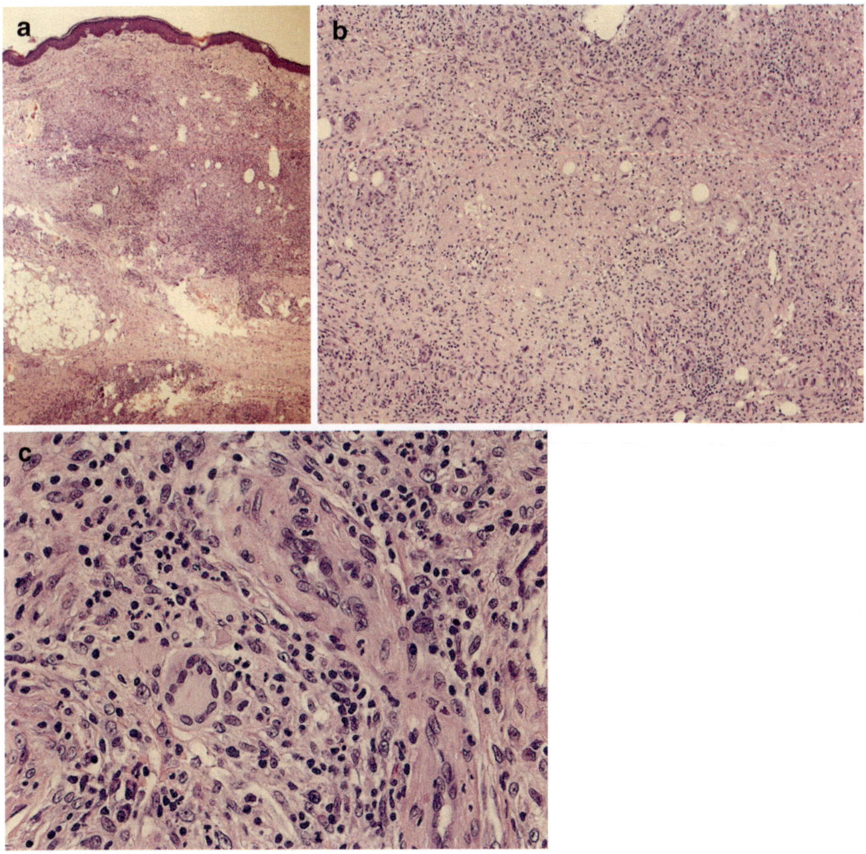

Fig. 23 Non-tuberculous mycobacteria infection histopathology: (**a**) inflammatory infiltrate in superficial and deep dermis (hematoxilin-eosin, 40×); (**b**) tuberculoid granulomatous infiltrate with multinucleated giant cells and necrosis areas (hematoxilin-eosin, 100×); and (**c**) tuberculoid granulomatous infiltrate with neutrophils and multinucleated giant Langhans cells (hematoxilin-eosin, 400×)

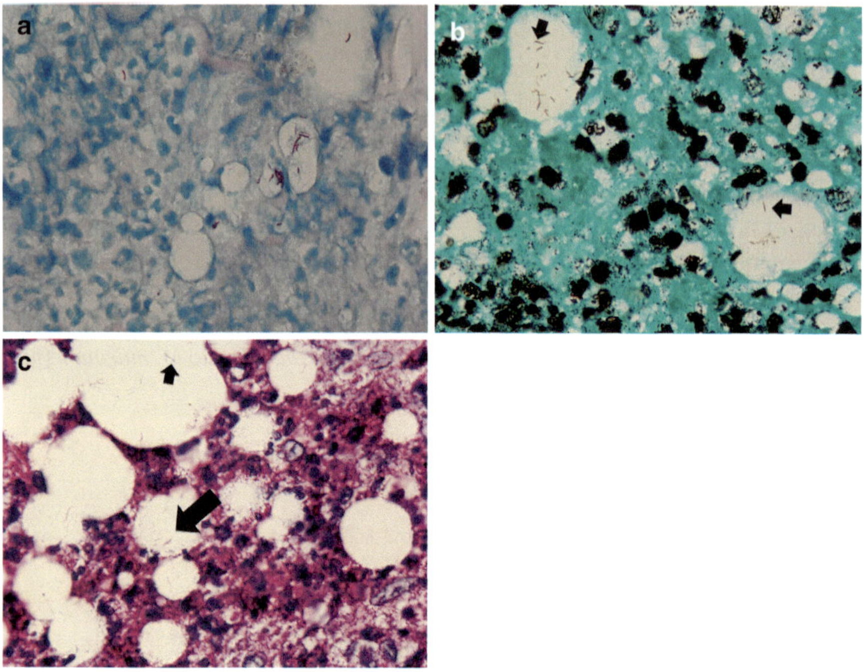

Fig. 24 Non-tuberculous mycobacteria infection histopathology. Presence of elongated acid-fast bacilli in vacuolated macrophages: (**a**) Ziehl-Neelsen stain, 1000×; (**b**) Grocott stain, 1000× (arrow); and (**c**) PAS stain, 1000× (arrow)

Skin lesions are often the primary sign of infection, so skin biopsies are important for early diagnosis of NTM [46].

4.5 *Treatment*

The NTM infection treatment in SOTRs is similar to that recommended for immunocompetent individuals. However, it needs special care for the possibility of drug interactions. Rifampicin reduces serum levels of calcineurin and mTOR inhibitors. Clarithromycin increases the levels of immunosuppressants. In this way, azithromycin seems to be more useful as it has minimal inhibitory effect on CYP450 [32, 47].

In severe disease, the combination of three active drugs is recommended. When the lesion is small, surgical excision is proposed. Surgical debridement, reduced immunosuppression, and use of anti-mycobacterial drug regimens are necessary for some SOTRs [48].

References

1. WHO. Global tuberculosis report 2020. Available: https://apps.who.int/iris/bitstream/handle/10665/336069/9789240013131-eng.pdf.
2. Chen Q, Chen W, Hao F. Cutaneous tuberculosis: a great imitator. Clin Dermatol. 2019;37:192–9.
3. Ahmad S. New approaches in the diagnosis and treatment of a latent tuberculosis infection. Respir Res. 2010;11(1):169.
4. Körner MM, Hirata N, Tenderich G, Minami K, Mannebach H, Kleesiek K, et al. Tuberculosis in heart transplant recipients. Chest. 1997;111(2):365–9.
5. Lattes R, Radisic M, Rial M, Argento J, Casadei D. Tuberculosis in renal transplant recipients. Transpl Infect Dis. 1999;1(2):98–104.
6. Ersan S, Celik A, Atila K, Sifil AA, Cavdar C, Soylu A, et al. Ren Fail. 2011;33(8):753–7.
7. Mamishi S, Pourakbari B, Moradzadeh M, van Leeuwen WB, Mahmoudi S. Prevalence of active tuberculosis infection in transplant recipients: a systematic review and meta-analysis. Microb Pathog. 2020;139:103894. https://doi.org/10.1016/j.micpath.2019.103894.
8. Dias MF, Bernardes Filho F, Quaresma MV, Nascimento LV, Nery JA, Azulay DR. Update on cutaneous tuberculosis. An Bras Dermatol. 2014;89(6):925–38.
9. Gunawan H, Achdiat PA, Hindritiani R, Essary ED, Ningtias LD, Siregar EP, et al. Various cutaneous tuberculosis with rare clinical manifestations: a case series. Int J Mycobacteriol. 2018;7(3):288–91.
10. Suraprasit P, Silpa-Archa N, Triwongwaranat D. Cutaneous miliary tuberculosis in a chronic kidney disease patient. Case Rep Dermatol. 2014;6(3):253–7.
11. Yodmalai S, Chiewchanvit S, Mahanupab P. Cutaneous military tuberculosis in a renal transplant patient: a case report and literature review. Southeast Asian J Trop Med Public Health. 2011;42(3):674–8.
12. Evans NS, Pritchett EN, Jones K, Doyle A, Chung CL, Allen HB, et al. Cutaneous gummatous tuberculosis in a kidney transplant patient. Cutis. 2019;103(2):E32–5.
13. Voigtländer T, Cornberg M, Gottlieb J, Welte T, Suerbaum S, Bange F-C. When a respiratory pathogen turns to the skin: cutaneous tuberculosis in a lung transplant patient. Ther Adv Respir Dis. 2015;9:260–2.
14. Agarwal P, Singh EM, Agarwal US, Meena R, Purohit S, Kumar S. The role of DNA polymerase chain reaction, culture and histopathology in the diagnosis of cutaneous tuberculosis. Int J Dermatol. 2017;56:1119–24.
15. Santos JB, Figueiredo AR, Ferraz CE, Oliveira MH, Silva PG, Medeiros VL. Cutaneous tuberculosis: diagnosis, histopathology and treatment—part II. An Bras Dermatol. 2014;89(4):545–55.
16. Costa LL, Veasey JV. Diagnosis of cutaneous tuberculosis (lymph node scrofuloderma) using the Xpert MTB/RIF method. An Bras Dermatol. 2021;96(1):82–4.
17. Epstein DJ, Subramanian AK. Prevention and management of tuberculosis in solid organ transplant recipients. Infect Dis Clin N Am. 2018;32(2):703–18.
18. Adu D, Evans DB, Millard PR, Calne RY, Shwe T, Jopling WH. Renal transplantation in leprosy. Br Med J. 1973;2:280–1.
19. WHO. Global leprosy (Hansen disease) update, 2019: time to step-up prevention initiatives. Wkly Epidemiol Rec. 2020;36(95):417–40.
20. Machado CM, Martins TC, Colturato I, et al. Epidemiology of neglected tropical diseases in transplant recipients. Review of the literature and experience of a Brazilian HSCT center. Rev Inst Med Trop S Paulo. 2009;51(6):309–24.
21. Aytekin S, Yasar S, Göktay F, et al. Lepromatous leprosy in a renal transplant recipient. Am J Transplant. 2017;17:2224–6.

22. Vieira AP, Trindade MAB, de Paula FJ, et al. Severe type 1 upgrading leprosy reaction in a renal transplant recipient: a paradoxical manifestation associated with deficiency of antigen-specific regulatory T-cells? BMC Infect Dis. 2017;17(1):305.
23. Trindade MAB, Palermo ML, Pagliari C, et al. Leprosy in transplant recipients: report of a case after liver transplantation and review of the literature. Transpl Infect Dis. 2011;13(1):63–9.
24. Teruel JL, Liaño F, del Hoyo M, et al. Successful kidney transplantation in leprosy and transitory recurrence of the disease. Int J Lepr Other Mycobact Dis. 1985;53(3):410–1.
25. Shih H-C, Hung T-W, Lian J-D, Tsao S-M, Hsieh N-K, Yang J-H. Leprosy in a renal transplant recipient: a case report and literature review. J Dermatol. 2005;32(8):661–6.
26. Roselino AM, de Almeida AM, Foss NT, Lima VJ, Raspanti EO, Ferraz AS. Renal transplantation in leprosy patients. Int J Lepr Other Mycobact Dis. 1993;61(1):102–5.
27. Date A, John GT, Thomas PP, Jacob CK. Leprosy and renal transplantation. Lepr Rev. 1998;69(1):40–5.
28. Ducette K, Fishman JÁ. Nontuberculous mycobacterial infection in hematopoietic stem cell and solid organ transplant recipients. Clin Infect Dis. 2004;38(10):1428–39.
29. Abad CL, Razonable RR. Non-tuberculous mycobacterial infections in solid organ transplant recipients: an update. J Clin Tuberc Other Mycobact Dis. 2016;4:1–8.
30. Morand J-J. Manifestations cutanéomuqueuses des mycobactéries environnementales (dont *Mycobacterium ulcerans*). In: Encyclopedie Médicale et Chirurgicale, vol. 1. Toulon: Elsevier; 2016. p. 1–10.
31. Asiedu K, Scherpbier R, Raviglione M, WHO. Buruli ulcer: *Mycobacterium ulcerans* infection. Paris, Tokyo: Association Française Raoul Follereau/The Nippon Foundation; 2000. p. 6. Available: https://apps.who.int/iris/bitstream/handle/10665/66164/WHO_CDS_CPE_GBUI_2000.1.pdf. Accessed 12/1/2021.
32. Assiri A, Euvrard S, Kanitakis J. Cutaneous Mycobacterium marinuma infection (fish tank granuloma) in renal transplant recipient: case report and literature review. Cureus. 2019;11(1):e6013. https://doi.org/10.7759/cureous.6013.
33. Henkle E, Winthrop K. Nontuberculous mycobacteria infections in immunosuppressed hosts. Clin Chest Med. 2015;36(1):91–9.
34. Ingram CW, Tanner DC, Durack DT, Kernodle GW Jr, Corey GR. Disseminated infection with rapidly growing mycobacteria. Clin Infect Dis. 1993;16(4):463–71.
35. Zappe CH, Barlow D, Zappe H, Bolton IJ, Roditi D, Steyn LM. 16S rRNA sequence analysis of an isolate of Mycobacterium haemophilum from a heart transplant patient. J Med Microbiol. 1995;43(3):189–91.
36. Brix SR, Iking-Konert C, Stahl RA, Wenzel U. Disseminated Mycobacterium haemophilum infection in a renal transplant recipient. BMJ Case Rep. 2016;2016:bcr2016216042.
37. Pacholec M, Sami F, Newell K, El Atrouni W. Fatal disseminated Mycobacterium haemophilum infection involving the central nervous system in a renal transplant recipient. J Clin Tuberc Other Mycobact Dis. 2020;21:100197.
38. Endzweig CH, Strauss E, Murphy F, Rao BK. A case of cutaneous Mycobacterium chelonae abscessus infection in a renal transplant patient. J Cutan Med Surg. 2001;5(1):28–32.
39. Lovric S, Becker JU, Kayser D, Wagner A, Haubitz M, Kielstein JT. Fish, flesh and a good red herring: a case of ascending upper limb infection in a renal transplant patient. Clin Nephrol. 2009;72(5):402–4.
40. Baisi A, Nosotti M, Chella B, Santambrogio L. Relapsing cutaneous Mycobacterium chelonae infection in a lung transplant patient. Transpl Int. 2005;18:1117–9.
41. Stelzmueller I, Dunst KM, Wiesmayr S, Zangerle R, Hengster P, Bonatti H. Emerg Infect Dis. 2005;11(2):352–3.
42. Malik S, Ghosh A, Husain S. Disseminated Mycobacteria chelonae infection in a kidney-pancreas transplant recipient: a case report and review of the literature. Saudi J Kidney Dis Transpl. 2016;27(6):1246–51.

43. Longworth SA, Vinnard C, Lee I, Sims KD, Barton TD, Blumberg EA. Risk factors for nontuberculous mycobacterial infections in solid organ transplant recipients: a case-control study. Transpl Infect Dis. 2014;16(1):76–83.
44. Copeland NK, Arora NS, Ferguson TM. Mycobacterium haemophilum masquerading as leprosy in a renal transplant recipient. Cas Rep Dermatol Med. 2013;2013:793127.
45. Kobashi Y, Mouri K, Yagi S, et al. Clinical evaluation of the QuantiFERON-TB Gold test in patients with non-tuberculous mycobacterial. Int J Tuberc Lung Dis. 2009;13:1422–6.
46. Morales P, Gil A, Santos M. Mycobacterium abscessus infection in transplant recipients. Transplant Proc. 2010;42(8):3058–60.
47. Torres F, Hodges T, Zamora MR. Mycobacterium marinum infection in a lung transplant recipient. J Heart Lung Transplant. 2001;20(4):486–9.
48. Piersimoni C. Nontuberculous mycobacteria infection in solid organ transplant recipients. Eur J Clin Microbiol Infect Dis. 2012;31(4):397–403.

Superficial Fungal Diseases

Carla Ferrándiz-Pulido

1 Introduction

Due to the long-term immunosuppressive therapy, solid organ transplant recipients (SOTR) are predisposed to a variety of cutaneous complications, being fungal infections one of them [1].

Fungi can cause infections in different structures of the human body including the skin by different mechanisms, among them through direct invasion of the skin causing various clinical pictures called dermatomycosis or cutaneous mycosis. According to their anatomical location, dermatomycoses are classified as: superficial mycoses, when they only affect the skin, hair or dermopapillary mucosa, and deep mycoses, when they penetrate more deeply and affect the deep dermis and subcutaneous cellular tissue. Some of the latter can spread, through lymphatic or hematologic vessels, and invade other organs of the economy (systemic mycoses) [2]. The skin may also be secondarily affected through the hematologic spread of a fungal infection originated in another organ [3]. In this chapter, we will focus on the

C. Ferrándiz-Pulido (✉)
Department of Dermatology, Hospital Universitari Vall d'Hebron, Universitat Autònoma de Barcelona, Barcelona, Spain
e-mail: Carla.ferrandiz@vallhebron.cat

J. Tomimori et al. (eds.), *Atlas of Dermatologic Diseases in Solid Organ Transplant Recipients*, https://doi.org/10.1007/978-3-031-13335-0_7

superficial fungal infection of the skin. The deep and systemic mycoses will be reviewed in the next chapter.

Fungal infections in SOTR tend to be more severe, show atypical clinical pictures, and are more resistant to standard treatments [4–7]. Moreover, it is worthy to know that drug interactions are common between antifungal systemic agents and calcineurin inhibitors frequently used by SOTR.

A higher-than-normal frequency of superficial fungal infection is expected among SOTR, mainly because of impaired cell-mediated immunity [6, 7]. The reduced numbers of epidermal antigen-presenting Langerhans' cells and the corticosteroid-induced atrophy of the skin and delay in desquamation of the stratum corneum due to treatment also have been suggested as contributing factors to the development of fungal infections in this group of patients [5].

2 Epidemiology

There are few studies evaluating the prevalence and clinical presentation of superficial fungal infections in SOTR [4–7]. A frequency of 15–64% has been reported, and most reports have described extensive lesions and mixed infections caused by different fungal species. A couple of studies comparing the prevalence in SOTR with an immunocompetent control group, identified a 1.5–2 fold increased prevalence [5, 6]. Depending on the study, *pityriasis versicolor* or dermatophytosis were the most common superficial fungal infections in SOTR. In one of the largest studies, *pityriasis versicolor* was the most frequent fungal infection, being identified in more than 35% of patients, followed by mucocutaneous candidiasis (about 25%), onychomycosis (about 13%), and *tinea pedis/ Candida* intertrigo (about 12%) [5]. Similarly, in a smaller study including 31 kidney transplant recipients, *pityriasis versicolor* was present in 27% of patients, followed by *tinea pedis* (14%) and onychomycosis (12%) [6]. Another study found *tinea cruris* and *tinea corporis* the more commonly clinical picture observed [4, 8, 9].

3 *Pityrosporum* Infections of the Skin

3.1 *Concept*

It is an infection of the most superficial layers of the epidermis caused by different species of *Malassezia*. The term *Pityrosporum* refers to the genus of the yeast form and the name *Malassezia* refers to the mycelial form. The infection by *Malassezia* causes a frequent, chronic, and asymptomatic infection of the skin, with a tendency to recur in predisposed people called *pityriasis versicolor* [2, 8, 9].

3.2 Etiology

The responsible agents, *Malassezia* spp. are lipophilic human saprophytes that are part of the normal flora of the skin, and colonization on the skin of the scalp, trunk, and flexural areas is particularly dense. Sometimes, it may switch from yeast to pathogenic mycelial form in circumstances that are not well determined, then adopting a filamentous form [9]. Its growth is favored in conditions of heat and humidity, sun tanning products containing oil, treatment with steroids and in states of immunosuppression, like SOTR [2, 8, 10].

3.3 Epidemiology

It is a mycosis of universal distribution, more frequent in countries with hot and humid climates, with an increasing incidence during the summer months. It affects all races and is somewhat more common in males than females. It has its maximum age incidence between 15 and 30 years and has been described to be the most frequent fungal infection (18–48%) in renal transplant recipients [5–7].

3.4 Pathogeny

The mechanism by which pigment alterations occur in this disease (hyperpigmentation in some lesions and hypopigmentation in others) is not clear. The fungus is capable of producing enzymes that oxidize some unsaturated fatty acids in skin lipids, giving rise to dicarboxylic acids that inhibit the action of tyrosinase, and possibly exert a cytotoxic effect on melanocytes, which would explain the hypochromic lesions, but not the hyperchromic ones.

3.5 Clinical Presentation

Cutaneous infections with *Malassezia* may take three forms: typical *pityriasis versicolor*, folliculitis, and inverse *tinea versicolor*.

Pityriasis versicolor is the most common presentation of *Malassezia* infection. It presents in the form of rounded, well-defined macules, with fine scales on their surface or dandruff, that when scraped with a fingernail, furfuraceous scaling is observed (scratch sign) (Fig. 1) [8–11]. Its color varies between hypo- and hyperpigmentation with a brownish color. When the patient is exposed to the sun, the hypopigmented macules become more evident (Fig. 2). Lesions are distributed throughout the chest, shoulders, back, abdomen, arms, and neck, and are very rare

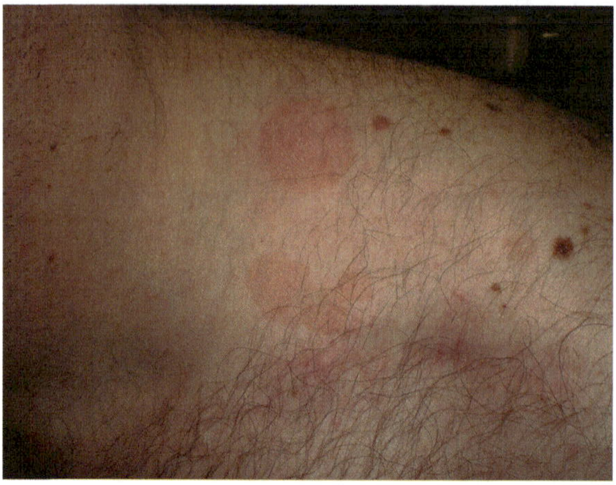

Fig. 1 A rounded, well-defined erythematous macule, with fine scales that appear more evident after scraping with a fingernail (scratch sign) in a patient with *pityriasis versicolor*

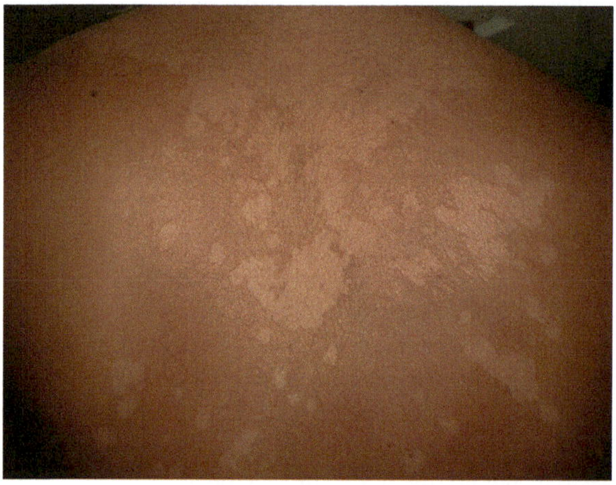

Fig. 2 Liver transplant recipient with hypopigmented *pityriasis versicolor* that becomes more evident with tanned skin

in the lower extremities, face, and genitalia. The lesions are usually asymptomatic; patients may complain of mild pruritus, but usually cosmetic concerns are the main problem for the patient. Sometimes, the macules coalesce into extensive patches (Fig. 3). When cured, the surface is smooth, without flakes, but hypopigmentation may retain for months or even years and sometimes until the patient is exposed to the sun again. It has a great tendency to relapse in predisposed individuals. Although superficial fungal infections have been described to be atypical, more severe, or widespread in SOTR in comparison to immunocompetent patients, other case-control studies did not find this [5]. The differential diagnosis should be established with seborrheic dermatitis, *pityriasis rosea*, secondary syphilis, vitiligo, post-inflammatory leukoderma, and *lichen scleroatrophicus* [12].

In *pityrosporum folliculitis*, lesions typically appear on the back, chest, and sometimes the extremities. It appears like an acneiform condition commonly misdiagnosed as *acne vulgaris*. Although often associated with common acne, this condition may persist for years without complete resolution with typical acne medication

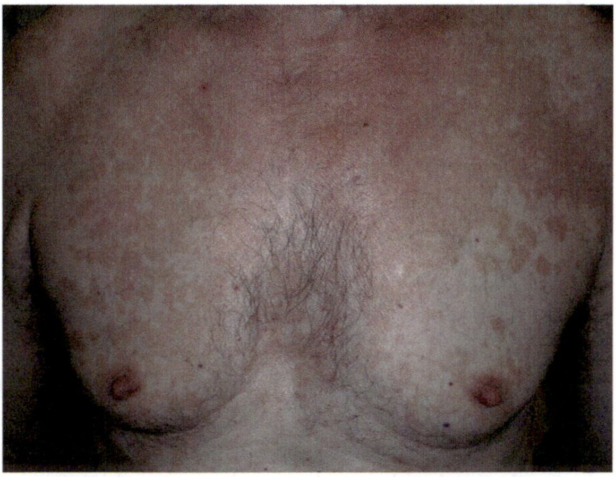

Fig. 3 A kidney transplant recipient with extensive erythematous *pityriasis versicolor* affecting the chest, coalescing in a large plaque

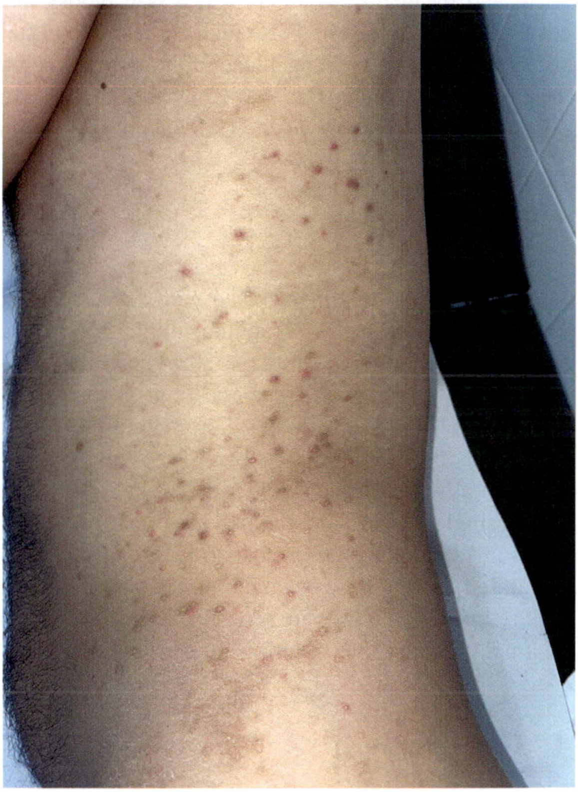

Fig. 4 *Pityrosporum* folliculitis, perifollicular erythematous 2–3 mm papules and pustules on the thorax

[13–15]. Clinically, the patient presents with a pruritic dermatosis characterized by the presence of perifollicular erythematous 2–3 mm papules or pustules (Fig. 4). In this case, a differential diagnosis with bacterial folliculitis is mandatory, and Potassium Hydroxide (KOH) examination as well as a biopsy with fungal stains may be necessary to distinguish both diseases.

Inverse tinea versicolor is similar to *tinea* versicolor but typically appears on flexural areas [16]. It may resemble a seborrheic dermatitis, psoriasis, erythrasma, candidiasis, or irritative dermatitis.

3.6 Diagnosis

The clinical diagnosis is easy in the presence of lesions such as those described, which show a pale yellow fluorescence when illuminated with Wood's light. It can be confirmed by direct microscopic examination of the scales, obtained by scratching the involved skin onto a glass or by the cellophane technique (a piece of cellophane is placed and adhered over the lesion, then it is pulled off and placed on a slide). The scales need to be treated with KOH and, under the microscope, short filaments can be observed mixed with round yeast elements, which form a characteristic image in "spaghetti and meatballs." Alternatively, a skin biopsy may show by hematoxylin and eosin (H&E) the yeast in the stratum corneum, PAS stain would confirm the diagnosis. In spite of a heavy fungal load of the lesions, there is no inflammation or even if there is, it is only minimal in the dermis [17]. In the case of *Malassezia* folliculitis, the organism may be seen in widened follicular ostia mixed with keratinous material [15].

3.7 Treatment

There are several treatments used with success. Most cases can be handled with topical treatments such as selenium sulfide 2.5% in a detergent base or an aqueous solution of sodium hyposulfite at 20%; however, nowadays, these treatments have been substituted by daily application of azole or allylamines derivatives or cyclopiroxolamine for 3 weeks. Terbinafine 1% in solution applied twice daily for 7 days has been reported to obtain 80% cure rates. In extensive cases, it can be treated orally with itraconazole at a dose of 200 or 400 mg daily for 5 days or fluconazole single dose of 400 mg. It is important to remark that oral azoles increase the levels of tacrolimus and cyclosporine; therefore, these patients need to be closely monitored and the dose of tacrolimus reduced. Despite the fact that the percentage of cures is high, relapses are frequent. Clinical improvement is seen 3–4 weeks after treatment because the epidermis must slough [8, 18].

4 Candidiasis

4.1 Concept

Cutaneo-mucosal candidiasis constitute a group of clinical pictures due to infection of the skin and/or mucous membranes by different species of the genus *Candida*.

4.2 *Ethiopathogenesis*

The genus *Candida* is made up of yeast fungi with more than 150 species. Of these, *C. albicans* is by far the most frequently implicated in skin and mucosal infections in the general population and also in the SOTR [11]. An important part of the individuals from the general population (30–50%) have *C. albicans*, in small numbers, in the oral and digestive mucosa taking part of their commensal flora, and in 20% of women taking part of the vaginal microflora. Therefore, the source of infection is usually endogenous. Some hosts characteristics, such as immunosuppression, facilitates infection by *Candida*.

4.3 *Epidemiology*

Oral candidiasis was significantly more frequent in renal transplant recipients than in controls despite the fact that there was no difference between the two groups regarding overall rate of cutaneous-oral colonization by *Candida* [5]. It has also been observed a greater susceptibility to this yeast in the early period after transplantation [7].

4.4 *Clinical Presentation*

Depending on the infected area, several pictures are distinguished [2]. In SOTR, the typical forms of *Candida* infection are the following:

4.4.1 Cutaneous Candidiasis

Intertrigo is the most common form of cutaneous candidiasis. The infection is located in large, macerated folds of the skin, such as the inguinal, intergluteal, axillary, and submammary folds, the abdominal folds in obese individuals, as well as in small cutaneous folds, such as the interdigital folds of the hands, mainly the third, and feet. In these areas, humidity and maceration due to the continuous rubbing of two surfaces favor the nesting of these yeasts. It starts with itching and vesiculo-pustules that converge and rupture, giving rise to erythematous, shiny, varnished-looking areas that spread centrifugally and symmetrically on both sides of the fold, the bottom of which tends to fissure (Fig. 5). On the periphery, an epidermal detachment collar is observed and the presence of some satellite vesiculo-pustules is characteristic.

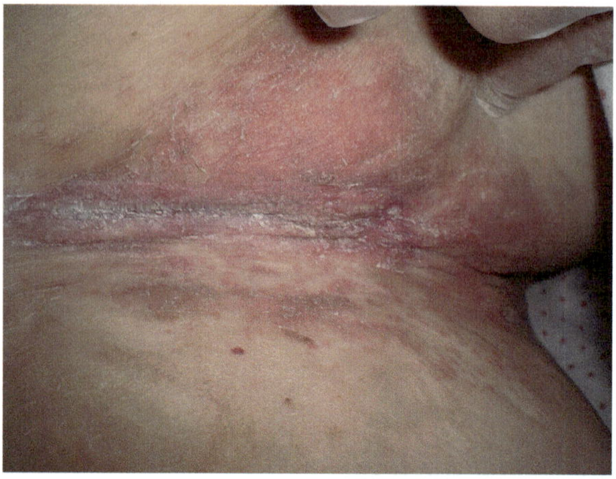

Fig. 5 A lung transplant recipient with cutaneous candidiasis on the submammary region

4.4.2 Vulvo-Vaginal Candidiasis

Infection of the female genital area is characterized by intense vulvar itching, with whitish, thick, creamy-looking leucorrhea. The vulvar and vaginal mucosa appears red and edematous, sometimes with whitish plaques on its walls. The infection frequently spreads to the neighboring cutaneous integument (Fig. 6). It is quite common, especially during pregnancy [2].

4.4.3 Balanitis or Balanoposthitis

It coexists most of the time with a vaginal yeast infection in the partner. It presents with itching and erythematous erosive lesions and superficial pustules on the glans and foreskin, covered by a whitish film and surrounded by a collarette of detached epithelium (Figs. 7 and 8). Lesions can extend to the scrotum and groin region [19].

4.4.4 Oral and Perioral Candidiasis

The most frequent form of oral candidiasis is mainly observed in infants and in immunosuppressed individuals. It is characterized by pseudomembranous whitish plaques that cover the entire oral mucosa as a creamy membrane that, when peeled off with the spoon, leaves a red, congestive, and bleeding surface (Figs. 9 and 10). It affects the jugal mucosa, tongue, palate, and gums, and in severe immunosuppressed patients, it can affect the pharyngeal and esophageal mucosa, with retrosternal pain and severe odynophagia [20].

Less frequently, oral infection by *Candida* may present as an atrophic oral candidiasis characterized by erythematous and atrophic plaques, more typically in elderly patients. Finally, hypertrophic oral candidiasis is an extremely rare form,

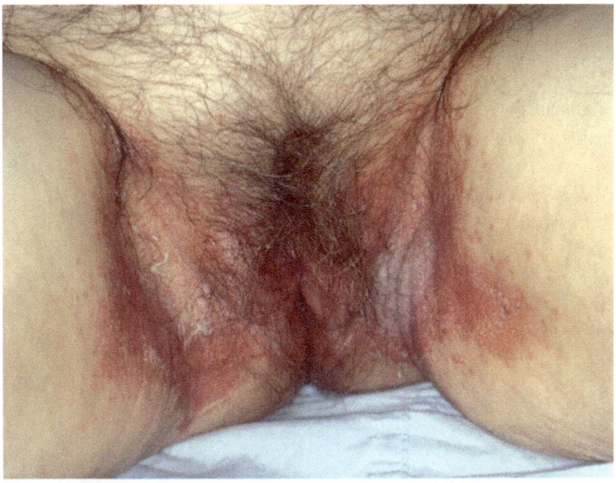

Fig. 6 Vulvar candidiasis spreading to the neighboring cutaneous integument. Note the characteristic peripheric pustules. (*Image courtesy of Prof. Vicente García-Patos, MD, PhD, Vall d'Hebron Hospital, Barcelona*)

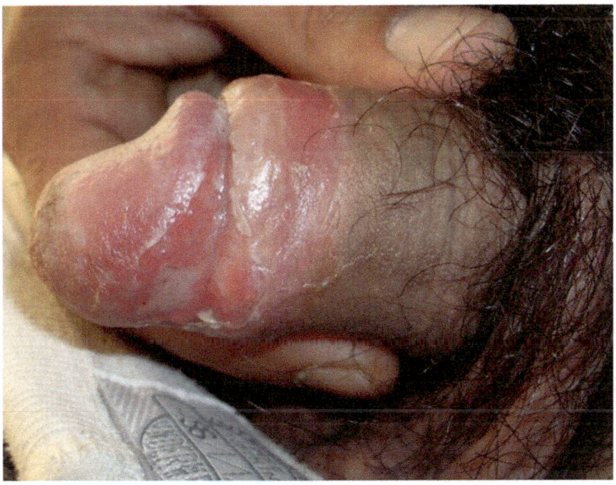

Fig. 7 Erythematous erosive lesions and superficial pustules on the glans caused by Candida infection

of chronic course, in which the whitish pseudomembrane, characteristic of oral candidiasis, is not removed by scraping (Fig. 11). When only the angles of the mouth are affected by erythema, fissuring and maceration is called angular cheilitis [20].

4.4.5 *Candida onixis* and *perionixis*

It is frequent in individuals who, due to their occupation, have frequently damp hands. Generally, it begins with swelling of the periungual soft tissues, with pain and erythema. By squeezing the area, a drop of pus can be seen coming out of the proximal nail fold (Fig. 12). Nail involvement is secondary and is manifested by discoloration and dystrophy of the nail plate that begins in the proximal or lateral part of the nail [21].

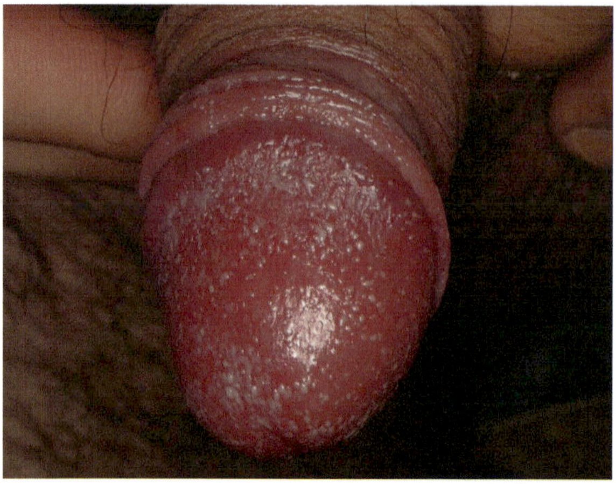

Fig. 8 Balanoposthitis by *Candida albicans*; superficial pustules on the glans and foreskin. (*Image courtesy of Prof. Vicente García-Patos, MD, PhD, Vall d'Hebron Hospital, Barcelona*)

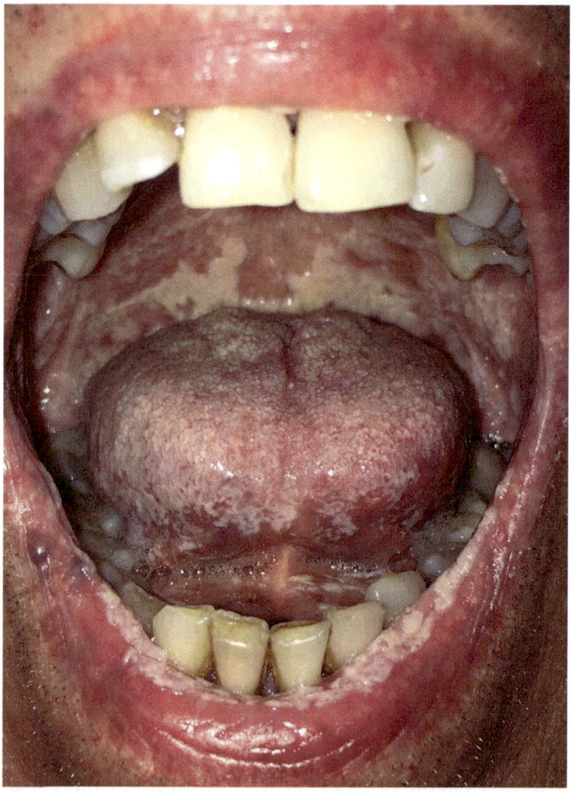

Fig. 9 Extensive oral candidiasis affecting all mucosal surfaces in a lung transplant recipient

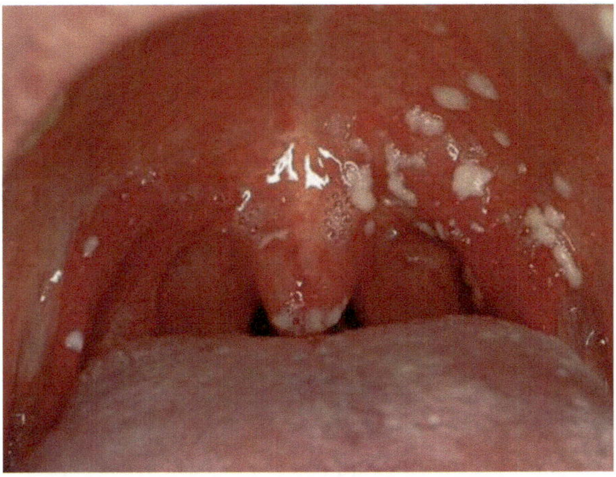

Fig. 10 Pseudomembranous whitish papules on the palate caused by *Candida* infection. (*Image courtesy of Prof. Vicente García-Patos, MD, PhD, Vall d'Hebron Hospital, Barcelona*)

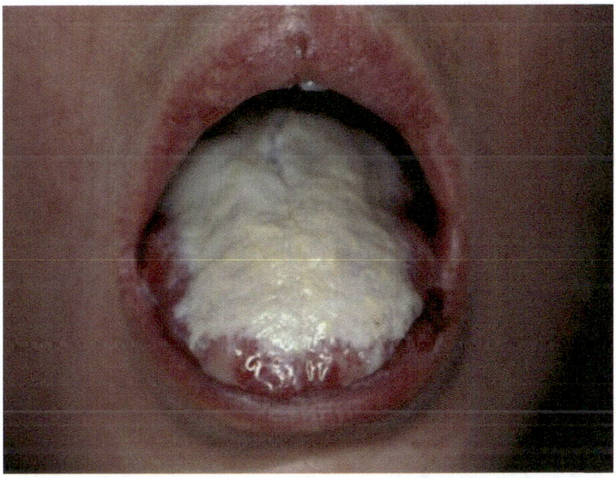

Fig. 11 Hypertrophic candidiasis in an immunosuppressed patient. (*Image courtesy of Prof. Vicente García-Patos, MD, PhD, Vall d'Hebron Hospital, Barcelona*)

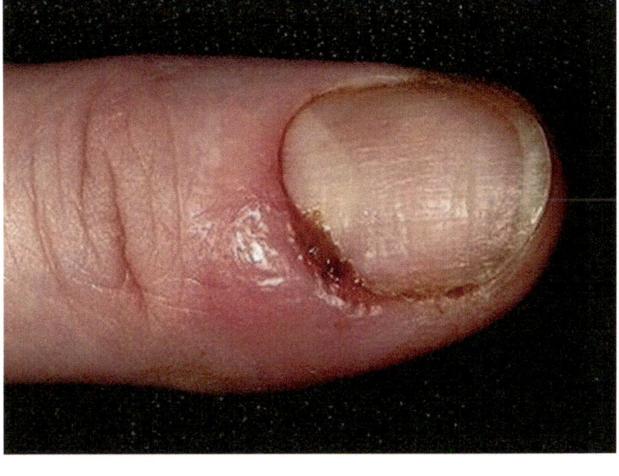

Fig. 12 Periungual erythematous swelling corresponding to a *Candida onixis*. (*Image courtesy of Prof. Vicente García-Patos, MD, PhD, Vall d'Hebron Hospital, Barcelona*)

4.5 *Diagnosis*

Although the symptoms are quite characteristic in all its forms, the diagnosis must be confirmed through direct examination (demonstration of blastospores or *pseudo-hyphae*) and culture of the material of the lesions (scales or content of pustules or secretions) in the middle of Sabouraud. *Candida* colonies have in cultures a whitish and creamy appearance and do not show carotenoid or melanic pigments [11].

4.6 *Treatment*

First, it is important to correct the predisposing factors, avoid humidity, and reduce the level of immunosuppression in case of extensive disease. Antifungal treatment can be topical or oral. Topically, either in the form of a cream, gel or vaginal ovules, clotrimazole, nystatin, and miconazole are the most studied topical drugs and all have demonstrated similar efficacy with complete cure rates of 73–100% [22]. Oral fluconazole is as effective as topical clotrimazole and is the only commercially available evidence-based option for systemic treatment of cutaneous candidiasis [22]. In most cutaneous candidiasis, topical treatment is sufficient. In oral candidiasis affecting immunosuppressed patients, oral treatment is convenient, as in onyxis and perionyxis and, sometimes, in vulvovaginitis due to its greater comfort in relation to topical treatment with vaginal ovules. Nail infections respond favorably to fluconazole treatment [2, 22].

5 Dermatophytosis or *Tineas*

5.1 *Concept*

Dermatophytosis defines the cutaneous and follicular infection by dermatophyte fungi [23, p. 1].

5.2 *Ethiopathogenesis*

Dermatophytes are primary filamentous pathogenic fungi with great keratinophilia, which is why they colonize the keratinized structures of animals and man, such as the epidermis, hair, and nails. These fungi possess keratinases that allow them to use the keratin in these structures as a source of nitrogen. There are three main genera of dermatophytes: *Microsporum*, *Epidermophyton*, and *Trichophyton*, each containing several species [24]. Several reports have identified *T. rubrum* to be the most common dermatophyte in SOTR [4, 5, 25], while others showed *T. mentagrophytes* to be a major isolate [6, 7].

5.3 Epidemiology

According to their natural reservoir, dermatophytes can be classified into three groups of epidemiological interest [2, 24]:

Anthropophilic: They only parasitize the human organism, produce little inflammatory reaction, and are transmitted with relative ease between sensitive individuals by direct contact or through fomites, producing epidemics in schools, gyms, swimming pools, etc.

Zoophilic: Their usual hosts are animals, and they are only occasionally transmitted to man. They produce family epidemics among members who are in contact with infected animals such as dogs, cats, or rabbits, among others. The clinical pictures they produce tend to have a greater inflammatory component than those produced by anthropophilic dermatophytes.

Geophilic: They have their reservoir in the ground, and feed with remains of keratin released by animals and humans. Although less frequently than the other groups of dermatophytes, they can parasitize man directly or through animals. It usually gives rise to sporadic cases with a very important inflammatory component.

In general, species of the genus *Trichophyton* can invade any skin structure, hair, and nails, *Microsporum* species rarely invade the folds or nails, and *Epidermophyton* mainly parasitize the feet, groins, and the *axillae*.

Even though, similar prevalence of dermatophyte infection have been found in SOTR and immunocompetent hosts, the length of the interval after transplantation seems to increase the appearance of dermatomycoses different from *pityriasis versicolor*, inducing several clinical forms of mycosis in the same patient and mixed infections with more than one species of fungi isolated from the same site [7].

5.4 Clinical Presentation

Many different species can invade the same structures, and with similar clinical expressiveness. Therefore, the resulting clinical pictures are described on a regional anatomical basis, rather than in relation to their etiology.

5.4.1 *Tinea Capitis*

The invasion of the scalp and associated hair by dermatophytes is called *tinea capitis* [26]. Three clinical types are distinguished:

Noninflammatory tinea capitis (tinea tonsurans)

It is the typical pattern observed by infection of anthropophilic dermatophytes, causing non-scarring alopecia with little inflammatory reaction. The lesion begins as a small erythematous papule surrounding a single hair shaft and spreads centrifugally, encompassing nearby hairs. Scaling is usually present and the hairs break off just above the level of the scalp (Fig. 13). They injure the hair without affecting the follicle, so that the alopecia they produce is reversible. There are two different forms depending on the etiology. In the trichophytic form, there are usually several small plaques, and in them healthy and parasitized hairs coexist, which are broken when emerging from the skin or very little above. The parasitization is usually endothrix. On the contrary, in microsporic ones there are usually few or a single plaque, larger in size, in which all the hairs are affected (perfect tonsure) and break a few millimeters from their emergence on the skin. In general, the parasitization of the hair is ectothrix (arrangement of spores and *hyphae* around the hair shaft).

Inflammatory tinea capitis (Kerion Celsi)

In general, they are produced by zoophilic or geophilic species that induce an important inflammatory reaction. It starts as a deep folliculitis or perifolliculitis. Within a few days, a very inflammatory plaque forms, usually single and painful, raised, bright red, and indurated covered with numerous follicular pustules (Fig. 14). When this plaque is pressed laterally, abundant suppuration appears through the follicular orifices [23, 27]. The inflammatory reaction itself removes hair, which is easily detached by traction. Occasionally, regional lymphadenopathy and fever develop and an episode of erythema nodosum can appear [28]. It can heal with more or less obvious scarring alopecia, depending on the number of affected follicles. This type of ringworm can also be seen in the beard and other hairy areas.

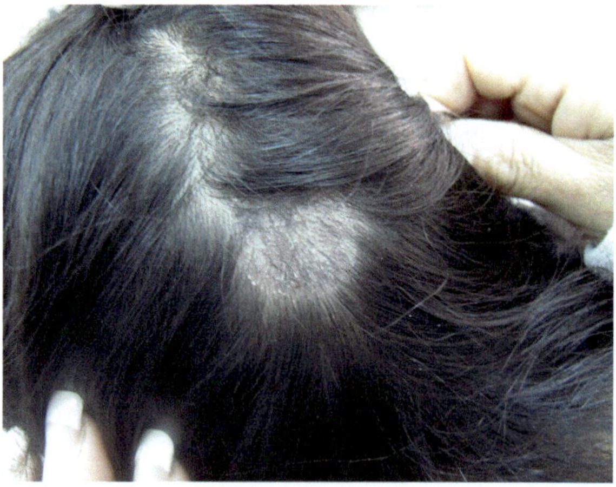

Fig. 13 Non-inflammatory *tinea capitis* caused by *Mychrosporum canis*, in a kidney transplanted child

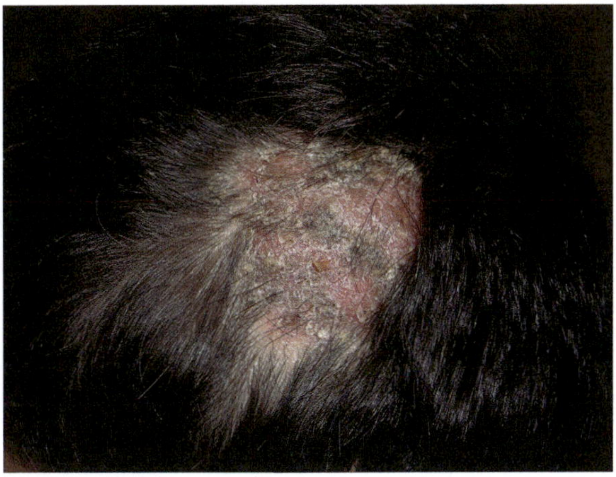

Fig. 14 Inflammatory *tinea capitis*: a single and painful, raised, erythematous and indurated plaque with pustules, crusts and alopecia

5.4.2 *Tinea Corporis (Tinea Circinata)*

It affects areas of glabrous skin on the face, trunk, or extremities, with the exception of the palms, soles, and flexural areas. It presents as one or more rounded erythematous-scaly plaque that grow centrifugally, with a well-defined and raised erythematous border, often scaly and with tiny pustules on its surface. The border of the plaque is always more active and inflammatory than the center of the lesion, giving it a very characteristic annular appearance (Figs. 15, 16, and 17) [23]. When the lesions are multiple, they sometimes converge to form plaques with polycyclic edges. In general, the lesions are itchy. There is a special form called Majocchi's granuloma, which is usually caused by *T. rubrum*, in which the lesions are deeper, often granulomatous and are manifested by violaceous papules (Fig. 18) [29].

5.4.3 *Tinea Cruris*

It is the parasitization of the crural area by dermatophytes, being *E. floccosum* and *T. rubrum* the most common dermatophytes isolated. It is seen more frequently during hot months of the year, especially in young males who play sports, sweat profusely, and wear tight clothing. The lesions consist of non-symmetrical, bilateral, erythematous-scaling plaques that extend downward and toward the inner thighs from both genitocrural folds, with a well-defined, progressing border, slightly raised, and more inflammatory than the rest of the thigh (Fig. 19). Occasionally, the lesions reach the scrotum and perineum as well as the gluteal crease. The infection is acquired through contaminated objects (clothing, towels, etc.) and by self-inoculation from interdigital lesions on the feet due to infections, sometimes asymptomatic, in this area [11].

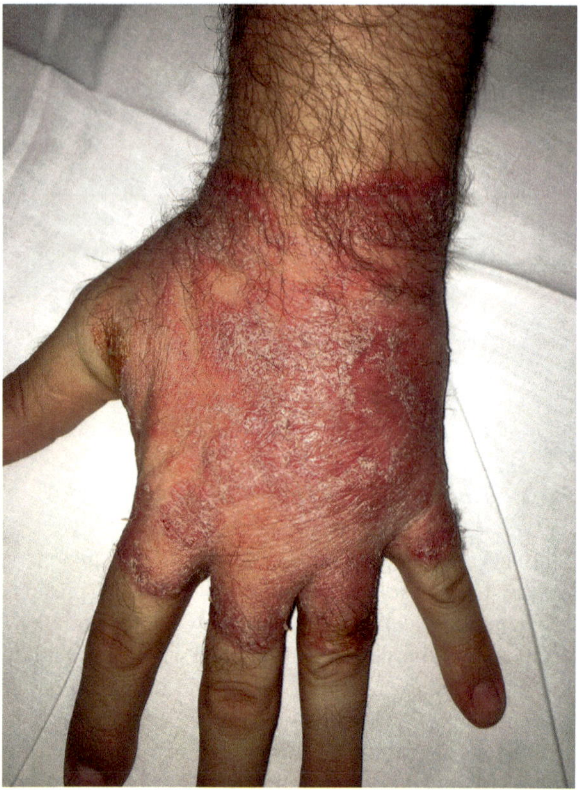

Fig. 15 *Tinea corporis*: a kidney transplant recipient with a plaque that grows centrifugally, with a well-defined erythematous and scaly border on the dorsum of the hand. A *Trychophytum interdigitale* was isolated

5.4.4 *Tinea Pedis*

It is the most common form of dermatophytosis [8]. It mainly affects young adults engaged in sports, mainly during summer, who wear occlusive footwear and often walk barefoot in public locker rooms [30, 31]. It is rare during childhood and in elderly people [32]. There are several clinical forms (Fig. 20).

Chronic Intertriginous Form

The causal species are usually anthropophilic, and the most frequent are *T. rubrum* and *T. mentagrophytes* var. *interdigital*. It is characterized by erythema and scaling of the interdigital folds, often with fissuring of the bottom of the fold. The fourth interdigital space is the one affected with the greatest intensity and frequency, to the point that the involvement of the other interdigital spaces, with preservation of the fourth, must make the diagnosis of *tinea pedis* doubtful (Fig. 21). Mild forms are often not given due attention, which is dangerous as they are excellent gateway

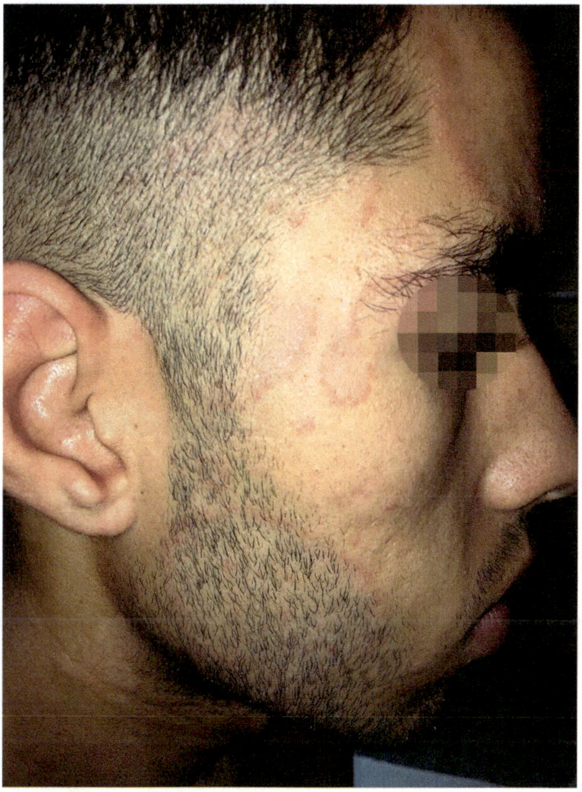

Fig. 16 *Tinea faciei* in a kidney transplant recipient

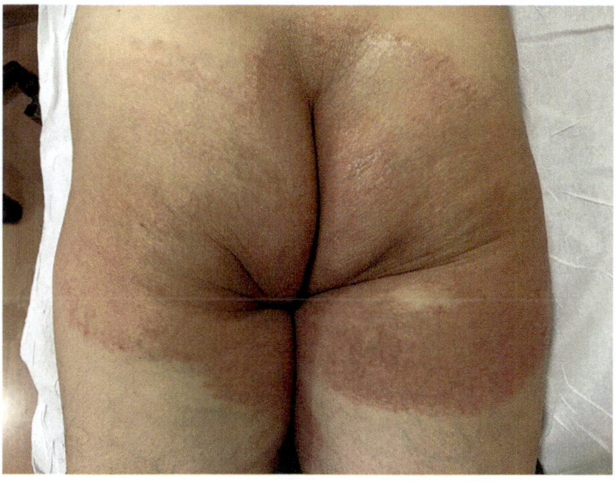

Fig. 17 *Tinea corporis*: extensive erythemato-brownish plaque affecting the lower part of the back and upper lower limbs with a scaly border in a lung transplant recipient. A *Trychophytum mentagrophytes* was isolated

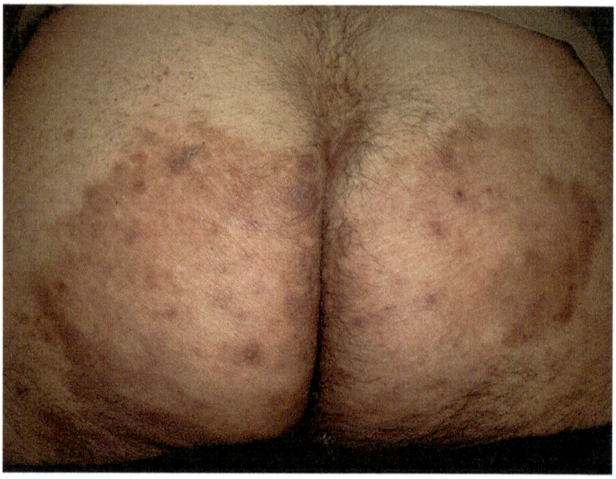

Fig. 18 Majocchi's granuloma: violaceous papules withing a brownish macule

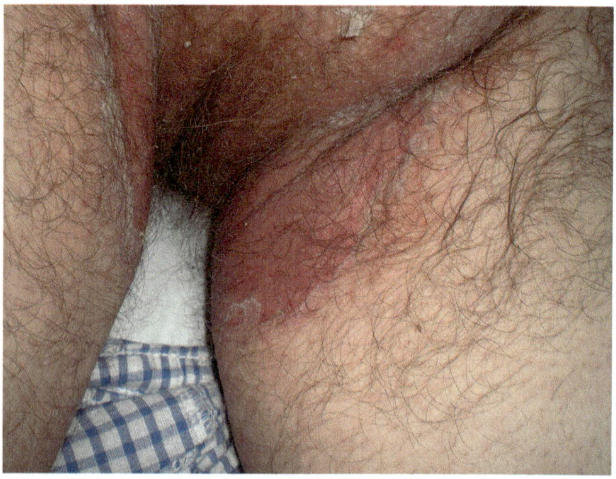

Fig. 19 *Tinea cruris*: a kidney transplant recipient with a bilateral erythematous-scaling plaque that extend downward and toward the inner thighs from both genitocrural folds

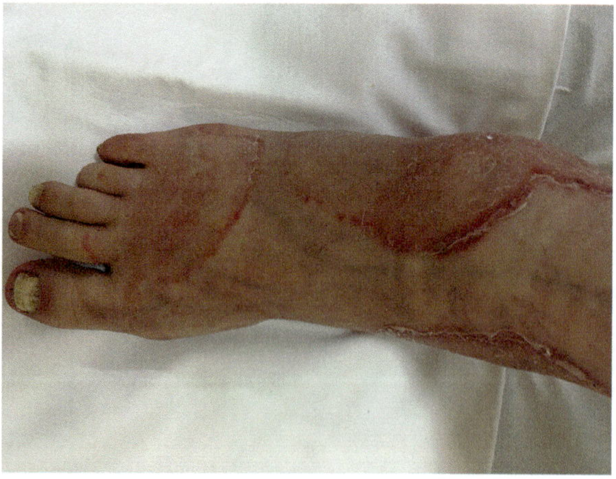

Fig. 20 *Tinea pedis*: an erythematous and scaly plaque affecting the lateral and dorsum of the foot associated with onychomycosis

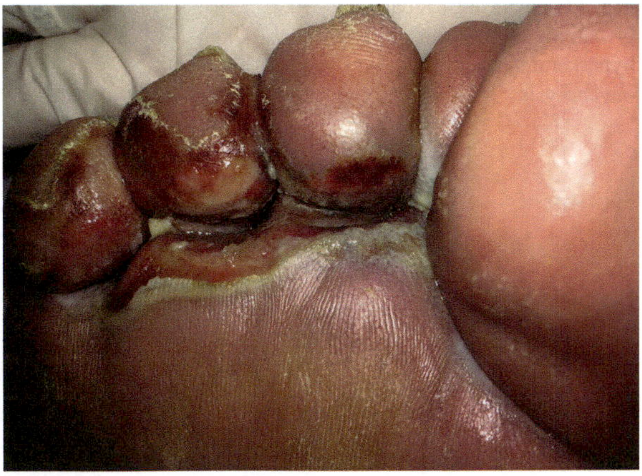

Fig. 21 Interdigital *tinea pedis* by *T. rubrum* with coinfection by *Pseudomonas aeruginosa* in a kidney transplant recipient

for streptococcal infections that cause repeated outbreaks of lymphangitis and cellulitis in the corresponding extremity. It must be differentiated from interdigital candidiasis, and from the Gram-negative infection with which it sometimes coexists [8, 11].

Chronic Hyperkeratotic Form

Characterized by a slight erythema and hyperkeratosis that symmetrically affects the soles, lateral margins, and heels and sometimes extends to the back of the feet, assuming a moccasin shape. It must be differentiated from eczema, psoriasis, and juvenile plantar dermatitis [23].

5.4.5 Onychomycosis

They are most frequently observed in adults and frequently associated with ringworms of the hands or feet. They are chronic infections affecting the nail bed and nail plate that may be chronic and difficult to treat [33]. There are various forms:

Distal Subungual

It is the most frequent form. It does not produce perionyxis, and the nail begins to be affected by its distal free end and by the lateral edges. Distal lateral yellowish or brownish discoloration appear that progress proximally or remain stationary for years. This is accompanied by abundant subungual hyperkeratosis that can lead to onycholysis (Figs. 22 and 23) [23]. The lamina becomes very thickened and brittle.

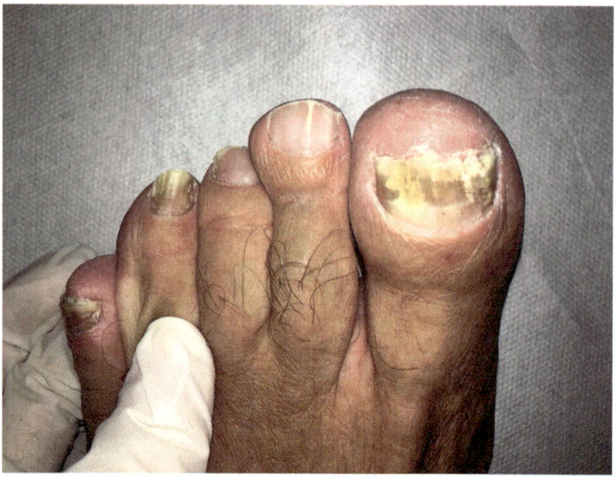

Fig. 22 Distal subungual onychomycosis; subungual hyperkeratosis and onycholysis

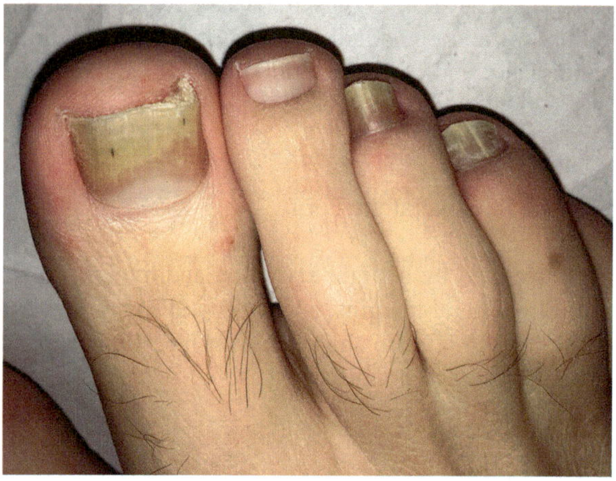

Fig. 23 Yellowish distal lateral nail fold corresponding to a distal subungueal onychomycosis

Proximal Subungual

This form is more frequent on immunosuppressed individuals, such as the SOTR. In it, the infection begins in the proximal fold and extends toward the distal fold. Its presence forces us to think of an associated immunodeficiency (Fig. 24) [23].

Dermatophytic Leukonychia or Superficial White Onychomycosis

Uncommon in fingernails. In it, the primary infection of the outer table of the lamina occurs, in general, by *T. mentagrophytes* var. *villous*, and leads to whitening of the nail (Fig. 25). Dermatophyte onychomycosis must be distinguished from those caused by *Candida*. In this sense, it is important to keep in mind that the latter are

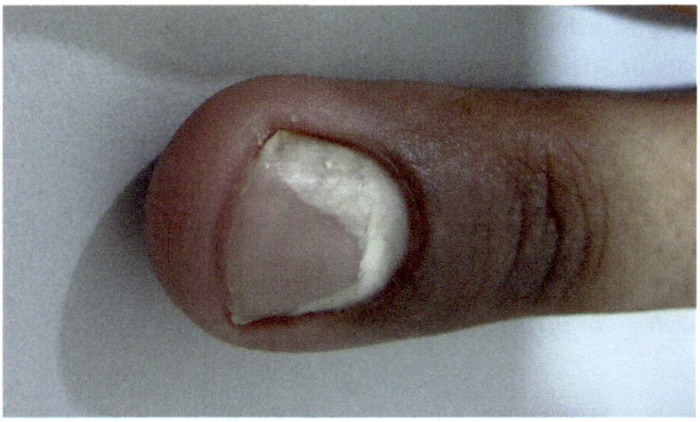

Fig. 24 Proximal subungueal onychomycosis. (*Image courtesy of Prof. Jane Tomimori, MD, Escola Paulista de Medicina, Sao Paulo, Brazil*)

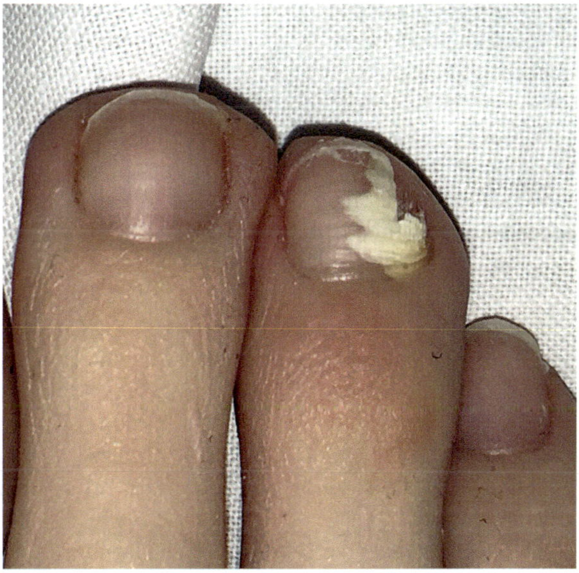

Fig. 25 Dermatophytic leukonychia

usually accompanied by intense perionyxis, which is rare in those produced by dermatophytes. On the other hand, when nail dermatophytosis is suspected, a meticulous mycological study must be carried out, the only way to confirm the diagnosis and exclude other similar-looking onychopathies, such as those caused by psoriasis, lichen planus, traumatic nail dystrophies or of circulatory origin [34].

5.5 Diagnosis

In general, the clinical diagnosis, at least of suspicion, does not present great difficulties. However, immediate diagnostic confirmation is always advisable by means of the microscopic search for fungal elements by direct examination (in parasitized scales or hair) that allows the diagnosis of dermatophytosis without specifying gender or species, and the isolation by culture and subsequent identification of the fungus. The sample must always be taken from the most active part of the lesion, generally the periphery in the skin lesions, the hair affected in the ringworm of the scalp, and the beard [2].

5.6 Treatment

There are excellent topical and oral antifungals. Topicals include imidazole derivatives, allylamine derivatives (terbinafine), and pyridone derivatives (cyclopyroxolamine). Amorolfine presented in the form of a 5% lacquer is useful in the treatment of distal onychomycosis, as are topical imidazoles formulated with 40% urea and occlusive treatment to favor the removal of the nail.

Among those for oral use, the following are available: griseofulvin, itraconazole, or terbinafine. Fluconazole is preferentially used in candidiasis rather than in dermatophytosis. Finally, ketoconazole, even though it is highly effective, it has a certain antiandrogen effect and is hepatotoxic, which is why it is reserved as a second-line treatment [11, 33].

In most cases, topical treatment for 3–4 weeks is sufficient to obtain a cure. However, there are some cases in which oral treatment is mandatory: ringworm of the scalp and nails, ringworm *incognito*, abnormally extensive ringworm of the glabrous skin and highly inflammatory acute ringworms. In these cases, the treatment duration is between 2 and 6 weeks depending on the drug and type of lesion. Onychomycosis usually requires a minimum of 3–6 months to be cured. Again, the oral antifungal agent interacts with tacrolimus and cyclosporine; therefore, SOTR need to be carefully monitored for drug levels and graft function during treatment.

In case of exudative lesions, before starting topical antifungal treatment, it is necessary to dry the lesions by using wet dressing with astringent solutions. On the contrary, when the lesions are very dry and with abundant hyperkeratosis, it is advisable to use topical keratolytics before antifungal medication in order to facilitate the subsequent penetration of the topical antifungal. In ringworms of the scalp, it is convenient to pluck the parasitized hairs [18].

Superficial mycotic infection in SOTR is facilitated not only by immunosuppressive treatments but also by environmental exposition. All our patients should be asked to reduce the risk of contamination, above all by avoiding contact with domestic animals. Moreover, we can offer a strict follow-up. Careful personal hygiene and the preventive measures adopted by our patients have been effective in limiting the onset of dermatomycoses with the result that prevalence no longer differs markedly from that of the immunocompetent population [7].

6 Other Superficial Fungal Infections

6.1 *Tinea Nigra*

It is a rare infection, usually of the palmar *stratum corneum*, caused by non-dermatophyte *Phaeoannellomyces werneckii* (*Exophiala*). It is typical from tropical or subtropical areas, including Central and South America. It presents as an asymptomatic, mottled brown to greenish-black macule with minimal to no scale (Fig. 26a, b). Usually found on the palmar or ventral surface of the fingers, plantar involvement is also possible. It is common to misdiagnose *tinea nigra* with a melanocytic nevus. It responds easily to topical therapy with a keratolytic field's ointment, an antifungal azole or terbinafine [9, 10].

6.2 *Piedra*

Piedra is an asymptomatic fungal infection of the hair shaft caused by *Piedraia hortae* and *Trichosporon beigelii*. Black piedra is characterized by firmly attached, hard brown-black nodules on the hair shaft that vary from microscopic to few millimeters in size and are gritty to palpation (Fig. 27). Black piedra weakens the hair shaft often resulting in broken hairs. White Piedra consists of softer and less adherent whitish to beige nodules that may be discrete or coalesce into sleeve-like structures (Fig. 28). Broken hairs are less common than with black piedra. The best treatment is to shave the infected hairs, but it may be accompanied by the use of topical azoles [9, 10].

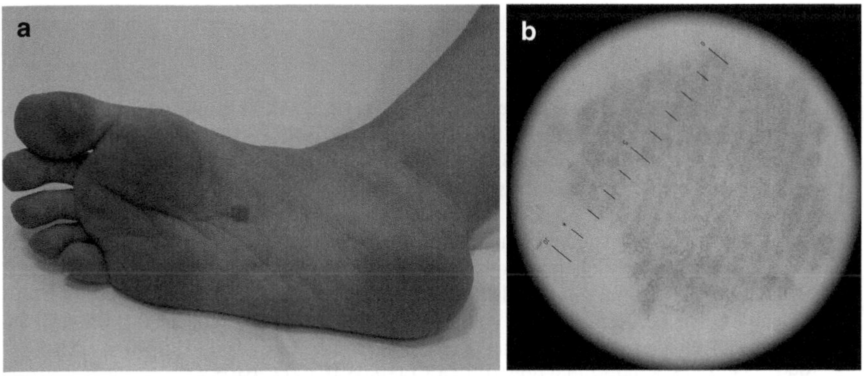

Fig. 26 (**a**) *Tinea nigra* affecting the sole of a child. (**b**) Dermatoscopy is very useful for distinguishing from a melanocytic lesion. (*Image courtesy Prof. Jane Tomimori, MD, Escola Paulista de Medicina, Sao Paulo, Brazil*)

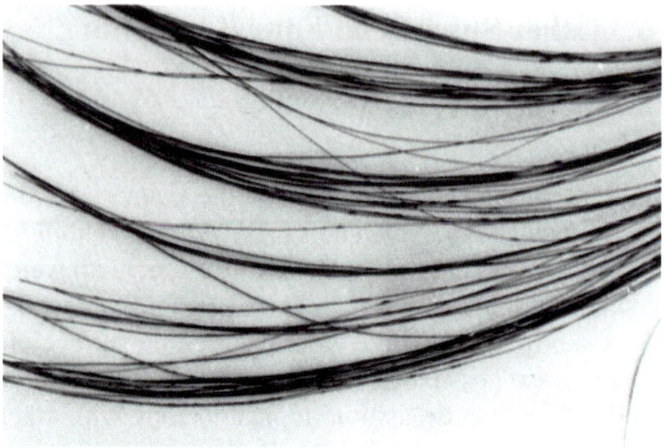

Fig. 27 Black Piedra: firmly attached, hard black nodules on the hair shaft. (*Image courtesy Prof. Jane Tomimori, MD, Escola Paulista de Medicina, Sao Paulo, Brazil*)

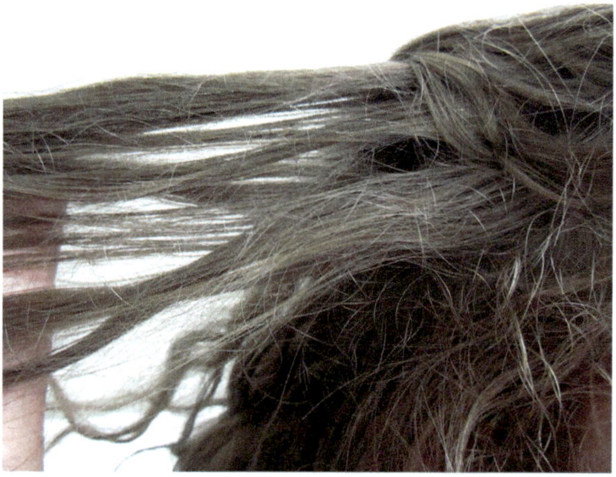

Fig. 28 White Piedra soft whitish to beige nodules along the hair shaft. (*Image courtesy Prof. Jane Tomimori, MD, Escola Paulista de Medicina, Sao Paulo, Brazil*)

References

1. Ulrich C, Hackethal M, Meyer T, Geusau A, Nindl I, Ulrich M. Skin infections in organ transplant recipients. JDDG. 2008;2:98–104. https://doi.org/10.1111/j.1610-0387.2008.06431.x.
2. Goldsmith LA, Katz SI, Gilchrest BA, Paller AS, Leffell DJ, Wolff K. Fitzpatrick's dermatology in general medicine. 8th ed. New York: McGraw-Hill Professional; 2012.
3. Shoham S, Dominguez EA, AST Infectious Diseases Community of Practice. Emerging fungal infections in solid organ transplant recipients: Guidelines of the American Society of Transplantation Infectious Diseases Community of Practice. Clin Transplant. 2019;33(9):e13525. https://doi.org/10.1111/ctr.13525.
4. Sentamil Selvi G, Kamalam A, Ajithados K, Janaki C, Thambiah AS. Clinical and mycological features of dermatophytosis in renal transplant recipients. Mycoses. 1999;42(1–2):75–8. https://doi.org/10.1046/j.1439-0507.1999.00405.x.
5. Güleç AT, Demirbilek M, Seçkin D, et al. Superficial fungal infections in 102 renal transplant recipients: a case-control study. J Am Acad Dermatol. 2003;49(2):187–92. https://doi.org/10.1067/s0190-9622(03)00861-2.
6. Shuttleworth D, Philpot CM, Salaman JR. Cutaneous fungal infection following renal transplantation: a case control study. Br J Dermatol. 1987;117(5):585–90. https://doi.org/10.1111/j.1365-2133.1987.tb07490.x.

7. Virgili A, Zampino MR, La Malfa V, Strumia R, Bedani PL. Prevalence of superficial dermatomycoses in 73 renal transplant recipients. Dermatology (Basel, Switzerland). 1999;199(1):31–4. https://doi.org/10.1159/000018174.
8. Gupta AK, Lyons DCA. Pityriasis versicolor: an update on pharmacological treatment options. Expert Opin Pharmacother. 2014;15(12):1707–13. https://doi.org/10.1517/14656566.2014.931373.
9. Schwartz RA. Superficial fungal infections. Lancet (London, England). 2004;364(9440):1173–82. https://doi.org/10.1016/S0140-6736(04)17107-9.
10. Bonifaz A, Gómez-Daza F, Paredes V, Ponce RM. Tinea versicolor, tinea nigra, white piedra, and black piedra. Clin Dermatol. 2010;28(2):140–5. https://doi.org/10.1016/j.clindermatol.2009.12.004.
11. Metin A, Dilek N, Demirseven DD. Fungal infections of the folds (intertriginous areas). Clin Dermatol. 2015;33(4):437–47. https://doi.org/10.1016/j.clindermatol.2015.04.005.
12. Gómez Moyanom E, Crespo Erchiga V, Martinez Pilar L. Dermatofitosis. Piel. 2016;31:546–59.
13. Rubenstein RM, Malerich SA. Malassezia (pityrosporum) folliculitis. J Clin Aesthet Dermatol. 2014;7(3):37–41.
14. Prindaville B, Belazarian L, Levin NA, Wiss K. Pityrosporum folliculitis: a retrospective review of 110 cases. J Am Acad Dermatol. 2018;78(3):511–4. https://doi.org/10.1016/j.jaad.2017.11.022.
15. Ferrándiz C, Ribera M, Barranco JC, Clotet B, Lorenzo JC. Eosinophilic pustular folliculitis in patients with acquired immunodeficiency syndrome. Int J Dermatol. 1992;31(3):193–5. https://doi.org/10.1111/j.1365-4362.1992.tb03934.x.
16. Ferry M, Shedlofsky L, Newman A, Mengesha Y, Blumetti B. Tinea InVersicolor: a rare distribution of a common eruption. Cureus. 2020;12(1):e6689. https://doi.org/10.7759/cureus.6689.
17. Crowson AN, Magro CM. Atrophying tinea versicolor: a clinical and histological study of 12 patients. Int J Dermatol. 2003;42(12):928–32. https://doi.org/10.1111/j.1365-4632.2003.02110.x.
18. Pereiro Ferreirós M, García-Martínez FJ, Alonso-González J. Update on the treatment of superficial mycoses. Actas Dermosifiliogr. 2012;103(9):778–83. https://doi.org/10.1016/j.ad.2012.01.009.
19. Lisboa C, Santos A, Dias C, Azevedo F, Pina-Vaz C, Rodrigues A. Candida balanitis: risk factors. J Eur Acad Dermatol Venereol (JEADV). 2010;24(7):820–6. https://doi.org/10.1111/j.1468-3083.2009.03533.x.
20. Scully C, el-Kabir M, Samaranayake LP. Candida and oral candidosis: a review. Crit Rev Oral Biol Med. 1994;5(2):125–57. https://doi.org/10.1177/10454411940050020101.
21. Hay RJ, Baran R, Moore MK, Wilkinson JD. Candida onychomycosis—an evaluation of the role of Candida species in nail disease. Br J Dermatol. 1988;118(1):47–58. https://doi.org/10.1111/j.1365-2133.1988.tb01749.x.
22. Taudorf EH, Jemec GBE, Hay RJ, Saunte DML. Cutaneous candidiasis—an evidence-based review of topical and systemic treatments to inform clinical practice. J Eur Acad Dermatol Venereol (JEADV). 2019;33(10):1863–73. https://doi.org/10.1111/jdv.15782.
23. Kovitwanichkanont T, Chong AH. Superficial fungal infections. Aust J Gen Pract. 2019;48(10):706–11. https://doi.org/10.31128/AJGP-05-19-4930.
24. Weitzman I, Summerbell RC. The dermatophytes. Clin Microbiol Rev. 1995;8(2):240–59. https://doi.org/10.1128/CMR.8.2.240.
25. McLelland J, Chu AC. Fungal infection in renal transplant patients. Br J Dermatol. 1988;118(5):734. https://doi.org/10.1111/j.1365-2133.1988.tb02587.x.
26. Moriarty B, Hay R, Morris-Jones R. The diagnosis and management of tinea. BMJ. 2012;345:e4380. https://doi.org/10.1136/bmj.e4380.
27. John AM, Schwartz RA, Janniger CK. The kerion: an angry tinea capitis. Int J Dermatol. 2018;57(1):3–9. https://doi.org/10.1111/ijd.13423.
28. Ferguson L, Fuller LC. Spectrum and burden of dermatophytes in children. J Infect. 2017;74(Suppl 1):S54–60. https://doi.org/10.1016/S0163-4453(17)30192-5.

29. Ilkit M, Durdu M, Karakaş M. Majocchi's granuloma: a symptom complex caused by fungal pathogens. Med Mycol. 2012;50(5):449–57. https://doi.org/10.3109/13693786.2012.669503.
30. Field LA, Adams BB. Tinea pedis in athletes. Int J Dermatol. 2008;47(5):485–92. https://doi.org/10.1111/j.1365-4632.2008.03443.x.
31. Szepietowski JC, Reich A, Garlowska E, Kulig M, Baran E, Onychomycosis Epidemiology Study Group. Factors influencing coexistence of toenail onychomycosis with tinea pedis and other dermatomycoses: a survey of 2761 patients. Arch Dermatol. 2006;142(10):1279–84. https://doi.org/10.1001/archderm.142.10.1279.
32. Andrews MD, Burns M. Common tinea infections in children. Am Fam Physician. 2008;77(10):1415–20.
33. Gupta AK, Cooper EA, Ryder JE, Nicol KA, Chow M, Chaudhry MM. Optimal management of fungal infections of the skin, hair, and nails. Am J Clin Dermatol. 2004;5(4):225–37. https://doi.org/10.2165/00128071-200405040-00003.
34. Bodman MA, Brlan MR. Superficial white onychomycosis. J Am Podiatr Med Assoc. 1995;85(4):205–8. https://doi.org/10.7547/87507315-85-4-205.

Deep Fungal Diseases

Carla Ferrándiz-Pulido, Marilia Marufuji Ogawa, and Daniel Wagner de Castro Lima Santos

1 Introduction

Deep cutaneous mycosis (DCM) are dermal and subcutaneous infections caused by fungi that have been introduced directly into the dermis or subcutaneous tissue through a penetrating injury. These infections are responsible for significant morbidity and mortality in solid organ transplant recipients (SOTR) [1]. Most of these infections occur in tropical or subtropical areas, where they are more prevalent although they may present anywhere as an imported disease. In SOTR, the most frequent DCM are phaeohyphomycosi*s* and zygomycosis [2]. All SOTR are at risk and infections can happen at any time along the posttransplant continuum. By sheer numbers, most emerging fungal infections occur in kidney transplant recipients [3]. Other risk factors include receiving a transplant after the age of 50 years, a prolonged and profound immunodeficiency, and breaks in skin integrity [4].

C. Ferrándiz-Pulido (✉)
Department of Dermatology, Hospital Universitari Vall d'Hebron, Universitat Autònoma de Barcelona, Barcelona, Spain
e-mail: Carla.ferrandiz@vallhebron.cat

M. M. Ogawa
Dermatology Department, Escola Paulista de Medicina, Universidade Federal de São Paulo, São Paulo, Brazil

D. W. de Castro Lima Santos
Infectious Diseases Department of Hospital Universitário Presidente Dutra, Universidade Federal do Maranhão (UFMA), São Luís, Brazil

Instituto D'or de Pesquisa e Ensino (IDOR, Rede D'or), Rio de Janeiro, Brazil

J. Tomimori et al. (eds.), *Atlas of Dermatologic Diseases in Solid Organ Transplant Recipients*, https://doi.org/10.1007/978-3-031-13335-0_8

2 Epidemiology

There are several series from Europe and America reviewing the frequency and etiology of opportunistic deep cutaneous fungal infections in SOTR. In Europe, Tessari et al. reported 22 opportunistic DCM in 3293 SOTR (0.7%) from Italy. The more commonly infections were phaeohyphomycoses (36%), mainly by *Alternaria* spp. but also *Scedosporium apiospermum* and *Cladosporium* spp. followed by other fungal infections such as *Aspergillus* spp. and *Histoplasma capsulatum* [5]. In Austria however, Stelzmueller et al. reported 11 opportunistic DCM in 2878 SOTR (0.38%), 8 due to a zygomycosis and one due to *Alternaria alternata* and one due to *Pseudallescheria boydii* [6]. Recently, Ferrándiz-Pulido et al. reported a series of 11 phaeohyphomycoses in SOTR from Spain, 8 of them due to *Alternaria* spp. [7]. Finally, Galezowski et al. reported a series of 46 SOTR from France with an opportunistic deep fungal infection, phaeohyphomycoses representing 46% of the cases, followed by hyalohyphomycoses and cryptococcoses/histoplasmoses [2].

In the USA, the Mayo Clinic reported 8 cases of DCM by *Alternaria* spp. from a population of 4668 SOTR in a 20-year period (0.17%) [8], and Schieffelin et al. reported 27 phaeohyphomycoses out of 3441 SOTR from New Orleans (0.8%), of which 11 were *Exophiala* spp. followed by *Ochroconis gallopava*, *Alternaria* spp., and *Phoma* spp., among others [9]. Finally, two papers from Brazil included a series of 17 phaeohyphomycoses out of 3885 kidney transplant recipients (0.4%), two of them due to *Exophiala* spp. and the others, to isolated cases of other dematiaceous fungi [10], and a larger series of 56 cases in which *Exophiala* spp. (34.2%) followed by *Alternaria* spp. (7.9%) that were the most frequent pathogens [11].

3 Pathogenesis

DCM may appear through two different routes. Mostly, in up to 90% of cases it is due to an exogenous inoculation through a trauma, reason for which has frequently been described in gardeners or farmers in whom slight inoculation with vegetable material may be the source of infection [2, 12]. The cutaneous fragility induced by the chronic use of corticosteroids may facilitate the cutaneous inoculation. However, in most cases, the patient does not refer a clear predisposing cause; in fact in some series, a previous local trauma could be identified in only 15–18% of cases [2, 7]. The second route results from the secondary cutaneous infection from a systemic spread.

4 Diagnosis

Diagnosis of these infections require a high degree of suspicion as they may show different clinical forms. There is usually a median delay of 4 months between onset of cutaneous lesions and DCM diagnosis [2]. Any unspecific cutaneous lesion in an SOTR should be biopsied and microscopically studied. Routine histopathologic examination of lesional skin tissue remains the primary method of confirming a DCM, but specimens should be thoroughly evaluated by both histopathology and

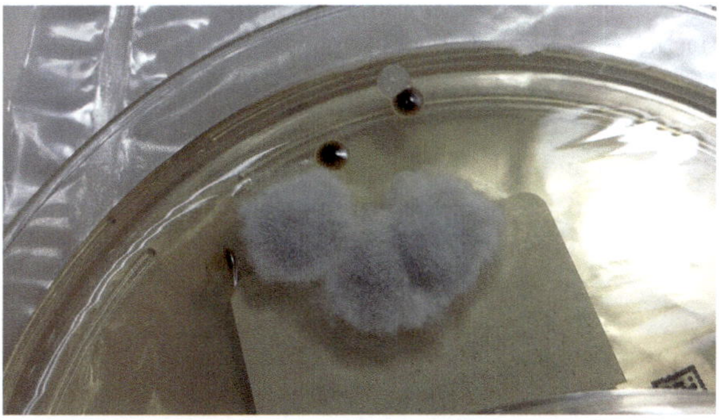

Fig. 1 Macroscopic appearance of colonies isolated of *Exophiala* spp. in Sabouraud's dextrose agar; the colony surface is white and velvety. The reverse side of the colony is black. (*Image courtesy of Mª Teresa Martín-Gómez, MD, PhD, Vall d'Hebron Hospital, Barcelona*)

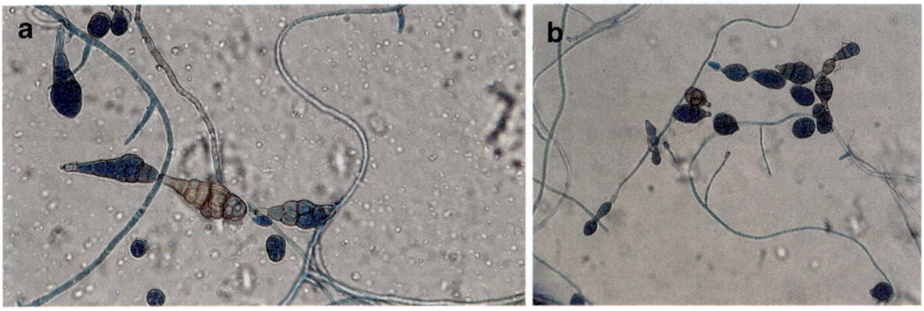

Fig. 2 (**a**, **b**) Septated ellipsoidal or cylindrical macroconidia corresponding to and *Alternaria* spp. Septated *hyphae* with poorly differentiated or sometimes tubular, short flask-shaped annellides are observed (lactophenol cotton blue stain). (*Image courtesy of Mª Teresa Martín-Gómez, MD, PhD, Vall d'Hebron Hospital, Barcelona*)

culture. Fungal elements are seen on hematoxylin-eosin (H&E)-stained samples [1], but Grocott methenamine silver and/or periodic acid–Schiff are useful stains to assist in histopathologic interpretation of most cases.

The fungus must also be isolated on a tissue sample obtained under sterile conditions by means of culture in Sabouraud media (Figs. 1 and 2a, b). The identification of the species usually requires molecular characterization by direct DNA sequencing by polymerase chain reaction. In order to confirm the involvement of the fungus in an infectious process and not just a colonization, it is also required to observe the fungal elements in smears or tissue samples (like a skin biopsy) with specific stains [7]. Discordant findings between histopathology and culture results are often seen and present a diagnostic and therapeutic challenge [13].

5 Specific Deep Cutaneous Mycosis

5.1 Phaeohyphomycosis

5.1.1 Concept

Phaeohyphomycoses are cutaneous or subcutaneous infections produced by a variety of dematiaceous fungi (filamentous molds characterized by their ability to form dark pigmented colonies as a result of the presence of melanin in their cell wall), that represent an emerging opportunistic infection in SOTR and the most frequent DCM in these group of patients [2, 9, 14]. Dematiaceous fungi are oligotrophic molds that can be found in man-made environments or heavily polluted habitats [15]. Most of these molds are recognized as plant pathogens and laboratory contaminant and only rarely produce disease in humans [16]. Usually, the combination of immunosuppression and a microtraumatic event as the entrance door is the pathogenic mechanism of this primary cutaneous mycoses [17–20].

5.1.2 Etiology

An heterogeneous group of more than 150 species of fungi can cause this infection. *Alternaria* spp., an ascomycete genus comprised in the *Pleosporaceae* family, are the most common cause of phaeohyphomycosis cutaneous infection in SOTR although differences in geographic locations and climate may be the reason for the differences in causative organisms [9]. Other common dematiaceous fungi causing phaeohyphomycosis in SOTR are *Exophiala* spp., *Cladosporium* spp., *Microsphaeropsis* spp., *Diaporthe* spp. or *Coelomycetous* spp., among others.

5.1.3 Pathogenesis

The pathogenicity of dematiaceous fungi causing phaeohyphomycosis is related to the presence of melanin in their wall. Melanin is an immunologically active compound, whose virulence is related to its ability to protect against the effect of reactive oxygen and nitrogen species, against proteolysis and to reduce phagocytosis, all of them defense mechanisms which are already altered in SOTR [21, 22].

5.1.4 Clinical Presentation (Figs. 3, 4a–f, 5, 6, 7a, b, 8, 9a, b, and 10)

SOTR are usually more susceptible to a phaeohyphomycosis in the first 2 years after transplantation [2, 4], but these infections have been described any time after transplantation [7, 11]. The clinical presentation is variable and dependent on host-related factors, the type of fungal organism, and the way the infection is acquired. Lesions may are usually unspecific and mostly asymptomatic and can present as nodules, that might ulcerate, cysts, ulcers, plaques, cellulitis or panniculitis, abscesses, blisters or erythematous-violaceous macules usually affecting the upper or lower limbs, and less frequently the trunk or the face [1, 2, 4, 7, 8, 11, 23]. Multiple sites of skin involvement is also a frequent event [1, 2, 7]. The lesions may progress and invade deeper structures as bones. Systemic dissemination needs to be always carefully ruled out, as it can be potentially mortal, although it is not a frequent event nowadays, probably due in part to the new high potency antifungal agents [2].

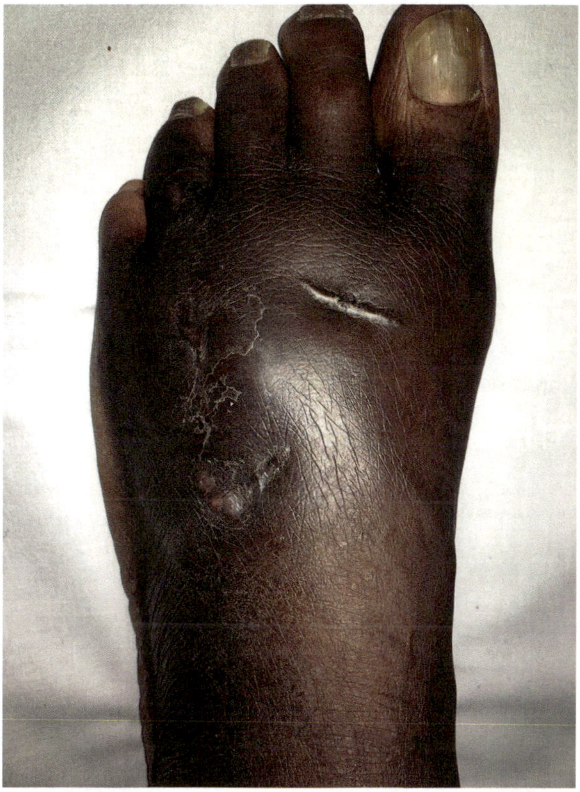

Fig. 3 Lung transplant recipient developing a deep subcutaneous infection with associated osteomyelitis on left foot by a filamentous fungus that required treatment with several surgeries and 2 years of oral isavuconazole

5.1.5 **Histopathology** (Fig. 11a, b)

The histological picture of a cutaneous infection by a dematiaceous fungi depends on the type of lesion and the days the lesion has been present. There is a variable degree of dermal granulomatous inflammation and/or abscess formation with filamentous *hyphae* with *septae* that can be distinguished by H&E stain and easily observed with special stains. The large, round to oval, thick walled refractile inclusion structures may be within histiocytes or disperse in the dermal infiltrate [23]. Even though these structures are unspecific from species, the fungal morphology can be easily distinguished from other cutaneous mycosis such as *Aspergillus*, *Fusarium,* or *Mucor* by the pigment production, the presence of *septae*, the diameter, and the absence of branching [7].

In the first 3 months, the lesions develop epidermal hyperplasia and acanthosis that may be eroded or ulcerated with mixed inflammatory infiltrates composed of histiocytes, neutrophils, and plasmocytic cells accompanied by microabscesses [23]. When the lesions evolve, it is characteristic the presence of inflammatory granulomas, either suppurative (more frequently), or sarcoid-like, accompanied by multinucleated giant cells. A granulomatous infiltrate can also be observed in earlier lesions [7]. As the lesions are treated, the inflammatory and granulomatous infiltrate is progressively substituted by fibrosis.

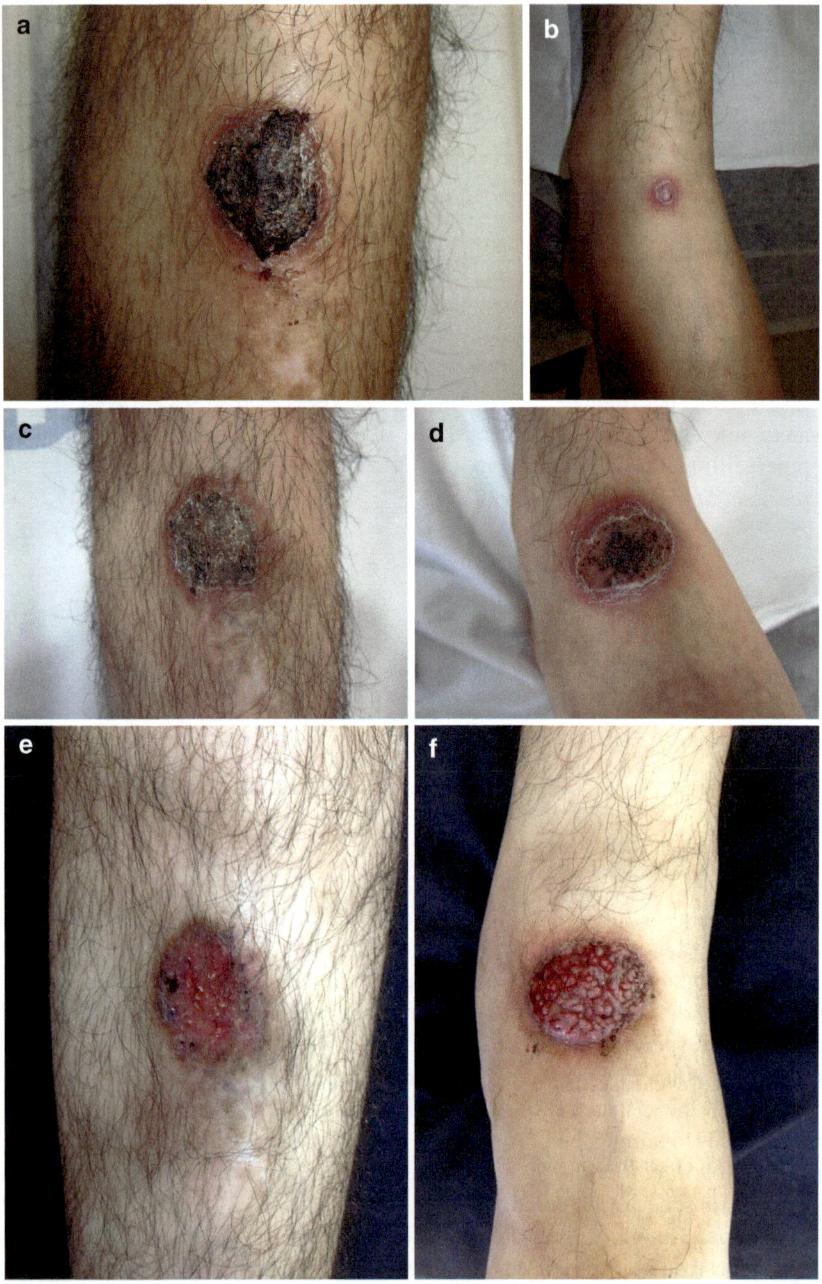

Fig. 4 A 32-year-old lung transplant recipient that developed multiple subcutaneous nodules with superficial ulceration and crust formation in both, lower and upper limbs. *Alternaria alternata* was isolated. The patient-initiated treatment with oral itraconazole 400 mg/day during 8 months, and the persistent lesions were surgically excised. (**a**) Initial lesion on the pretibial area. (**b**) Initial lesion in the instep. (**c**, **d**) Clinical evolution after 2 months of treatment. (**e**, **f**) Clinical evolution after 6 months of treatment. One of the lesions was almost healed, while the other continued to enlarge and was surgically removed

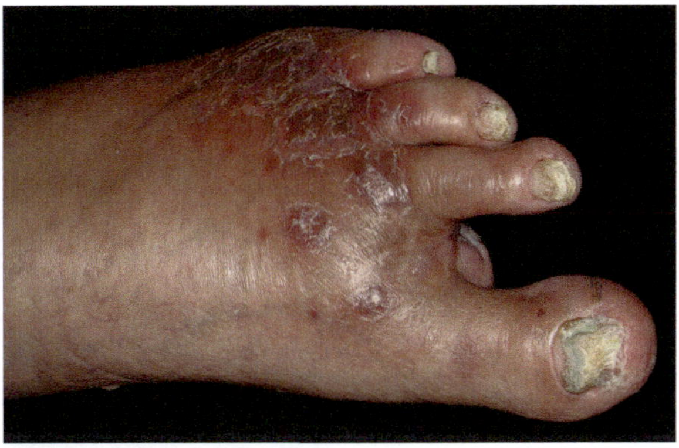

Fig. 5 A 58-year-old lung-transplanted male presented with an erythemato-violaceous plaque with nodules on his surface on the dorsum of his left foot. An *Alternaria alternata* was isolated and the patient received treatment with high-dose itraconazole for 2 months that needed to be switched to voriconazole that was maintained for 2 years

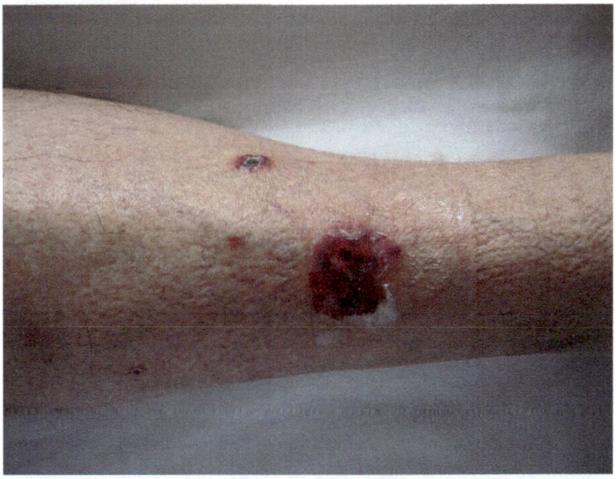

Fig. 6 A 64-year-old lung-transplanted male that presented with multiple slight ecchymotic lesions on his four limbs that rapidly progressed to suppurative ulcerated nodules. An *Alternaria infectoria* was isolated. The patient received oral antifungal agents for several months that needed to be modified because of the development of side effects

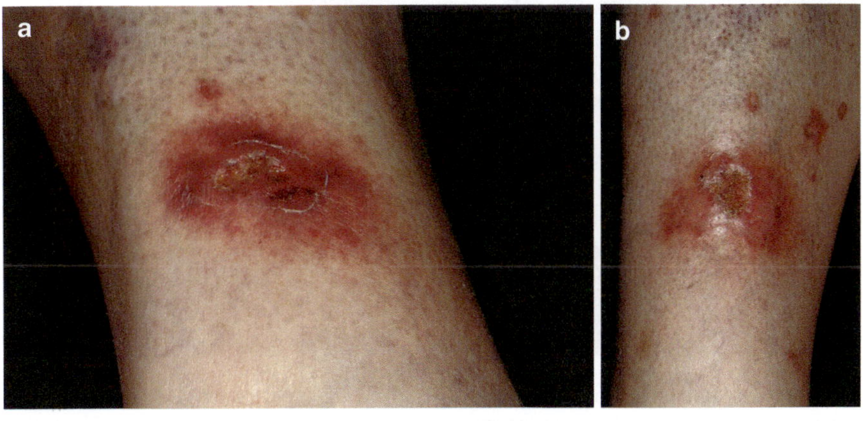

Fig. 7 A 53-year-old lung-transplanted patient that developed simultaneously several erythematous plaques on his legs that progressively ulcerated. An *Alternaria infectoria* was isolated and the patient received treatment with high-dose itraconazole for 7 months. (**a**) Left leg and (**b**) right leg

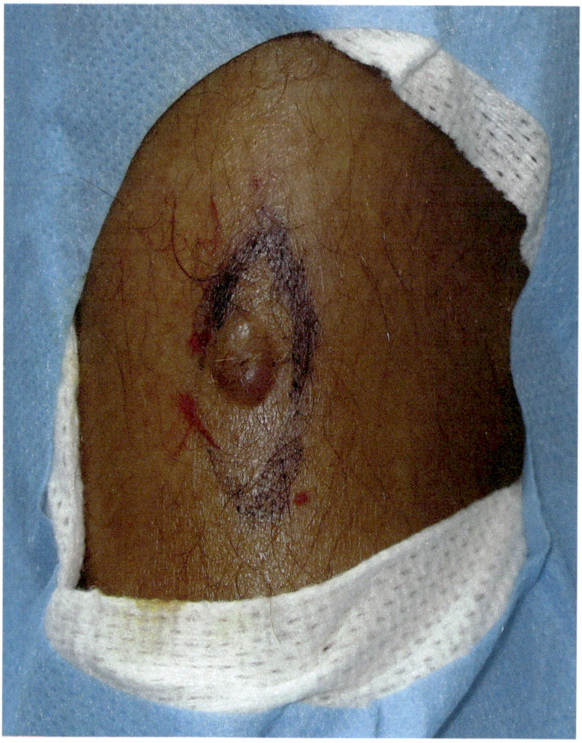

Fig. 8 A 53-year-old kidney-transplanted male with an isolated papular lesion on his leg. An *Alternaria infectoria* was isolated and the lesion surgically removed

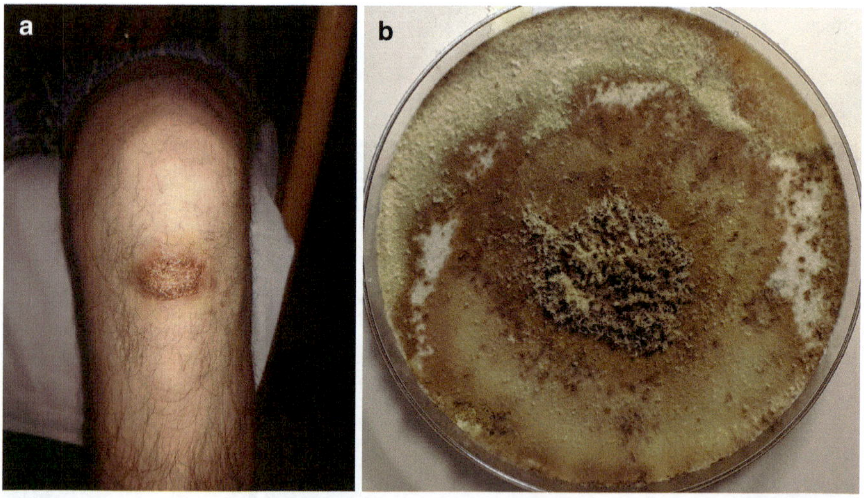

Fig. 9 A 62-year-old lung-transplanted male with a 3 cm infiltrated cutaneous plaque with superficial crusts on his knee. A *Diaporthe* spp., a dematiaceous fungus, was isolated. The patient received treatment with isavuconazole 200 mg/day for 4 months that was suppressed because of hepatotoxicity. The patient received additionally 3 MAL-photodynamic therapy sessions. (**a**) Initial clinical lesion. (**b**) Macroscopic appearance of colonies isolated of *Diaporthe* spp. in Sabouraud's dextrose agar; velvety and verrucose appearance with a deep brown pigmentation. (*Image courtesy of Mª Teresa Martín-Gómez, MD, PhD, Vall d'Hebron Hospital, Barcelona*)

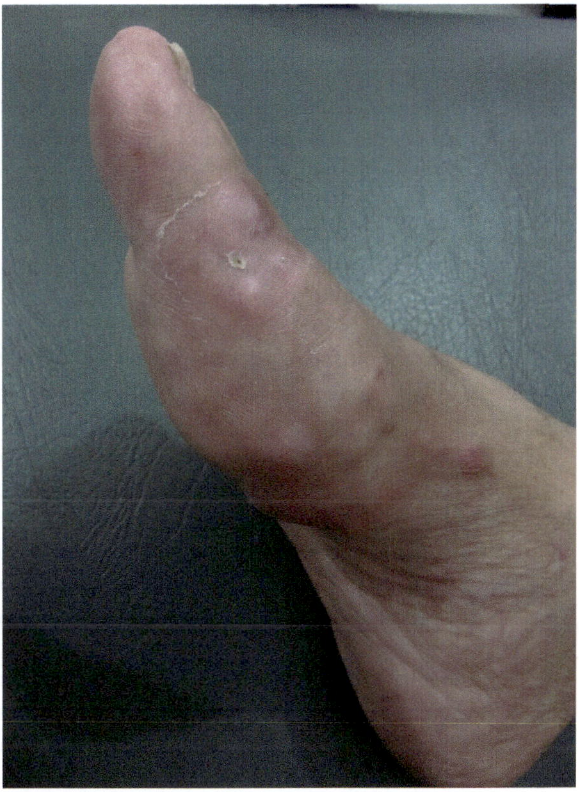

Fig. 10 Subcutaneous phaeohyphomycosis caused by *Exophiala* sp. in a male renal transplant recipient with multiple cystic lesions on his right foot

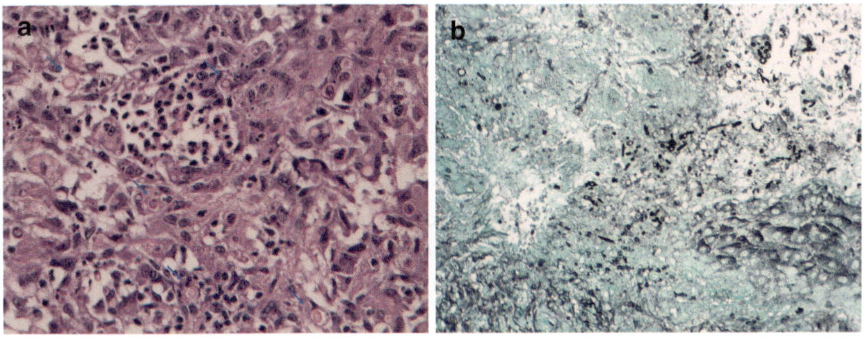

Fig. 11 (**a**) Microscopic findings in early lesions of phaeohyphomysosis: granulomatous infiltrate with microabscesses mixed with round-to-oval, thick refractile structures with *septae* (arrow) that correspond to a phaeohyphomycosis (Hematoxylin-eosin [H&E], magnification 40×). (**b**) Typical fungal structures corresponding to a cutaneous infection by *Alternaria alternata* (Grocott methenamine silver, magnification 20×)

5.1.6 Treatment

One of the main goals of treatment of phaeohyphomycosis in SOTR is preventing a life-threatening fungal dissemination [2]. The treatment of these infections in SOTR might be challenging and may require the combination of medical and surgical procedures as well as modulation of immunosuppressive therapy [7, 21].

Recently, the American Society of Transplantation Infectious Diseases Community of Practice published treatment guidelines for emerging fungal infections in SOTR [3]. Surgical excision would be the treatment of choice and may be sufficient for isolated cutaneous disease [7, 23]. If a complete excision is not possible, a debridement is recommended whenever feasible to decrease the fungal burden [3]. Large or multifocal lesions usually require combined antifungal and surgical treatment. Finally, reduction and/or modification of immunosuppression may help eliminate the fungal infection.

Since the late 90s, long-term and high doses of itraconazole (200–400 mg/day) maintained over several months have been empirically used to treat phaeohyphomycosis, as it is difficult to obtain molds susceptibility tests [7]. Other antifungal agents that have traditionally been used with success include terbinafine, intravenous caspofungin, or amphotericin B [8, 10]. Nowadays, most cases are treated with voriconazole 400 mg/day or isavuconazole although these drugs provoke more side effects, like myopathy, hepatopathy, phototoxicity, or the induction of squamous cell carcinoma [9]. Thermotherapy can also be used in combination with antifungals. When combining oral or intravenous antifungal agents with calcineurin inhibitor, the levels of the latter have to be closely followed and the dosage tapered to avoid increasing serum levels.

5.2 *Zygomycosis*

5.2.1 Concept and Etiology

Zygomycosis represents the second most frequent opportunistic DCM in SOTR [2]. Zygomycetes are ubiquitous fungi that can cause invasive disease associated with high mortality. Agents causing zygomycosis include *Mucor* spp., *Rhizopus* spp., *Rhizomucor* spp., *Absidia* spp., *Cunninghamella* spp., among others (note that the terms zygomycosis and mucormycosis are often used interchangeably).

5.2.2 Clinical Presentation (Figs. 12 and 13a, b)

Mucormycosis tends to be seen early after transplant. The most common clinical presentations are rhino-sino-orbital infection with or without cerebral involvement and pulmonary zygomycosis [24]. Cutaneous zygomycosis may be localized, may extend to deep underlying tissues, or may be disseminated. The exclusive cutaneous

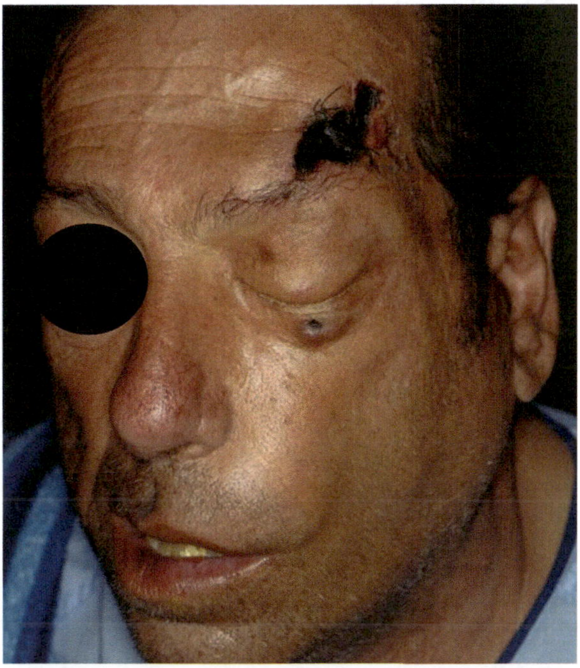

Fig. 12 A liver transplant recipient with diabetic cetoacidosis and rhino-ocular-cutaneous mucormycosis causing a facial paralysis. (*Image courtesy of Prof. Vicente García-Patos, MD, PhD, Vall d'Hebron Hospital, Barcelona*)

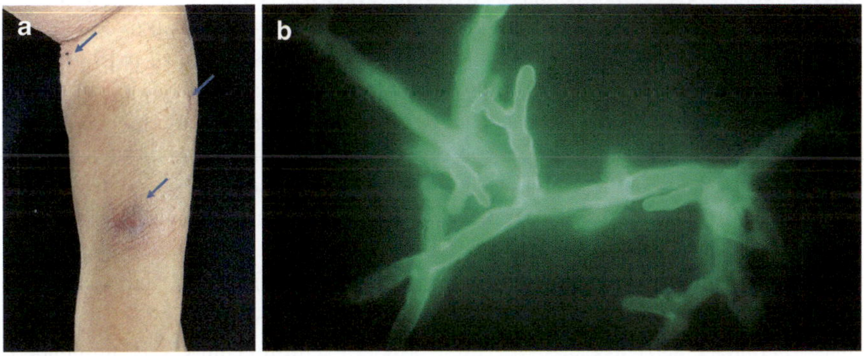

Fig. 13 (**a**) A 63-year-old lung-transplanted female that developed multiple subcutaneous nodules in a sporotrichoid pattern. A *Rhizopus oryzae* was isolated. Treatment with itraconazole was initiated and the patient developed myopathy, it was therefore switched to posaconazole. Finally, surgical excision was completed, but the patient died of medular aplasia. (**b**) Calcofluor-white dye showing wide and pauci septate hyphae with few branches corresponding to *Rhizopus* spp. (*Image courtesy of Mª Teresa Martín-Gómez, MD, PhD, Vall d'Hebron Hospital, Barcelona*)

form is less frequently seen because the infection may disseminate easily [1, 6]. The most common clinical presentation is induration of the skin with surrounding erythema, rapidly progressing to necrosis. When disseminated, mortality rates are approximately 30% [1].

5.2.3 Histopathology

Histological examination may reveal small, intravascular, hyaline, fungal hyphal forms in a granulomatous dermal infiltrate. Organisms of the Mucorales order should grow within 3 days on culture [1].

5.2.4 Treatment

Treatment consists of surgical debridement when possible, in order to decrease the fungal burden, that needs to be combined with administration of antifungal agents and, occasionally, hyperbaric oxygen [1]. Amphotericin B at higher doses or the lipid formulations have been the mainstay of medical treatment of zygomycosis. Posaconazole may also exhibit activity against zygomycetes. Finally, reduction in immunosuppression may also accompany a better survival [24].

5.3 Sporotrichosis

5.3.1 Concept and Etiology

Sporotrichosis is an endemic disease and considered a mycosis of implantation. The pathogenic agent is a dimorphic fungus, *Sporothrix schenckii* sensu *lato*. The disease is cosmopolitan but more prevalent in tropical and subtropical regions. New species have been described through molecular studies, and it is associated with geographical distribution. In the late 1990s, *S. brasiliensis* became the main etiological agent of human and animal sporotrichosis in Brazil, and it has been responsible for the largest outbreak reported worldwide for three decades in the State of Rio de Janeiro [25, 26]. In SOTR, like other endemic mycosis, the use of immunosuppressants increases the fungal burden, facilitates the fungal dissemination and increases the mortality rate. Sporotrichosis causes significant morbidity, but it is rarely associated with high mortality.

5.3.2 Epidemiology

S. schenckii is a species complex of six distinct cryptic species, three of them are clinically relevant (*S. brasiliensis*, *S. glob*osa, and *S. lurei*), two environmental fungi (*S. mexicana* and *S. albicans*) and *S. schenckii* sensu stricto. They are geographically distributed in distinct regions, such as *S. brasiliensis* is restricted to Brazil, *S. globosa* has a worldwide distribution, and finally *S. schenckii* sensu stricto has been isolated in the Americas, Europe, South Africa, and Asia [27].

The fungus is found in soil, tree bark, hay, rose shrubs, and decaying wood, so that human acquires the infection by traumatic implantation of contaminated plant or soil and it is usually related to *S. globosa* and *S. schenckii* [28]. So, the distribution of sporotrichosis across age and sex will depend on the exposure to the fungus [27], and it is also related to occupational and recreational habits. In Brazil, the contact with infected cats has been an important route of transmission of *S. brasiliensis* [25].

Sporotrichosis is rarely reported among SOTR and the kidney transplant recipients are the most common group associated with this infection since it is the most frequent solid organ transplantation performed worldwide [29, 30].

5.3.3 Pathogenesis

The dimorphic soil fungus *S. schenckii* is usually transmitted by the mold form from organic matter through cutaneous inoculation. Another route of inoculation is through scratch or bite of infected cats; in this case, *S. brasiliensis* is the fungus with the ability to transmit the disease between mammals in the yeast form. The third route of transmission is through inhalation, which is very rare [31]. Once the fungus is inoculated it takes from 1 to 10 weeks to develop the cutaneous lesion at the inoculation site. Later the fungus can disseminate through lymphatic channels (lymphocutaneous form) and less often by hematogenic dissemination. The most common extracutaneous infection sites are the bones, joints, tendon sheaths, and bursae.

5.3.4 Clinical Presentation (Figs. 14 and 15)

At the site of the fungal inoculation, a chancre appears that is characterized by a papulonodular lesion that may ulcerate and drain a purulent discharge. In the lymphocutaneous form, the most common presentation, new lesions may appear in the skin or subcutaneous tissue following the lymphatic pathway. These two clinical presentations comprise 95% of the cases [29]. There is a third skin presentation with multiple independent lesions without systemic invasion that occurs when the patient presents multiple traumas that give rise to multiple entry doors [31].

Sporotrichosis is rare in SOTR, and it may present as a cutaneous and lymphocutaneous form, as well as, the disseminated form, but it has also been reported extracutaneous manifestation without cutaneous or lymphocutaneous involvement [30, 31]. Fichman et al. reported the largest case series of sporotrichosis in renal transplant recipients [29]. Out of six patients, two presented disseminated forms involving skin, oral and nasal mucosa, and osteoarticular system. The oral and nasal mucosa involvement was also observed by Orofino-Costa et al. in immunosuppressed patients [31].

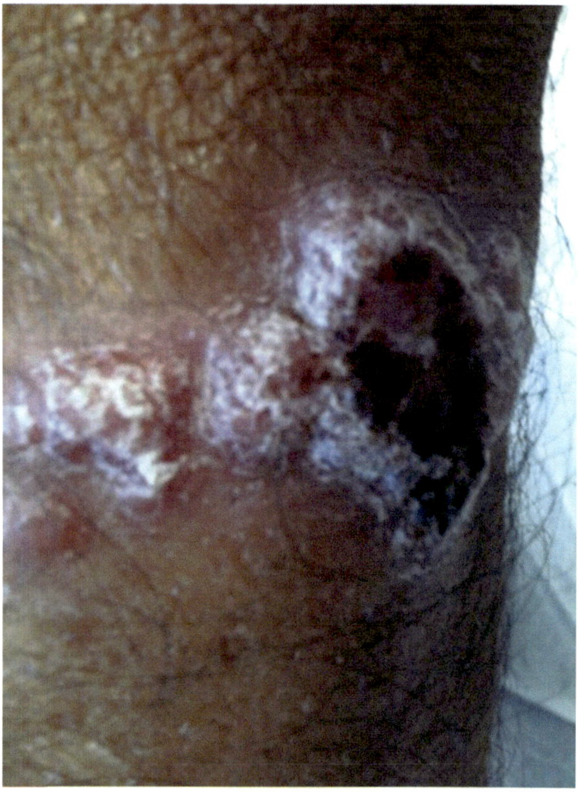

Fig. 14 Verrucous plaques on the leg caused by *S. schenckii*

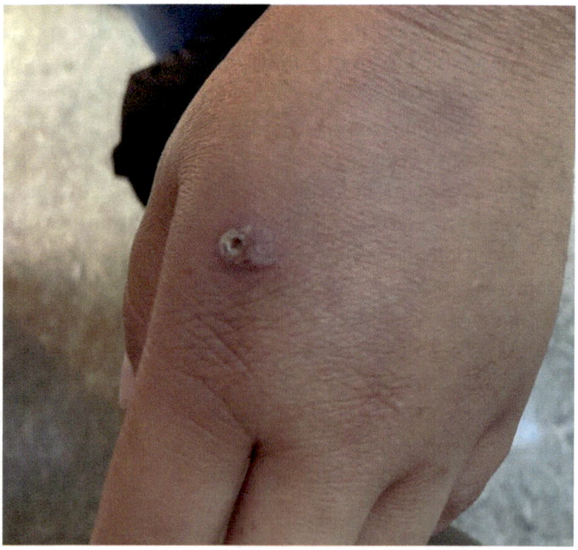

Fig. 15 Infection by *Sporothrix* spp.: verrucous plaque on the dorsum of the hand where a cat had bitten

5.3.5 **Histopathology** (Fig. 16a, b)

The histopathology reveals a granulomatous and pyogenic inflammatory process with oval or cigar-shaped yeast structures. However, due to the paucity of fungal elements, the histopathology has a low sensitivity.

5.3.6 **Diagnosis** (Fig. 17)

The golden standard is the isolation of *Sporothrix* species from cutaneous samples. The fungal culture is still a useful method since the *Sporothrix* species may be isolated in 4–6 days, from samples obtained from cutaneous lesions and in 10–19 days from extracutaneous lesions [31]. Molecular tools to identify the *Sporothrix* different species are still laborious, longstanding with variable results.

5.3.7 **Treatment**

Treatment of sporotrichosis in SOTR does not differ from the available drugs used in immunocompetent hosts. For patients with cutaneous or lymphocutaneous forms, itraconazole is the drug of choice and if it fails, terbinafine would be the second option [32, 33]. In the disseminated and visceral forms, amphotericin B deoxycholate or liposomal amphotericin B is recommended as an initial treatment until the patient presents a favorable response; subsequently amphotericin B is substituted by itraconazole. After the disease is controlled, itraconazole is maintained for a long

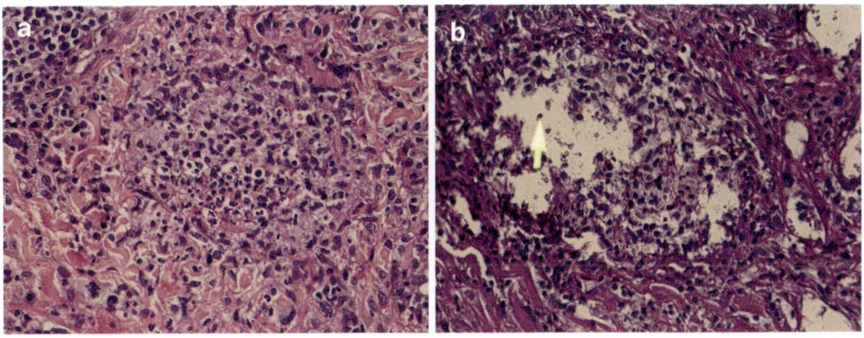

Fig. 16 Microscopic findings of Sporotrichosis infection. (**a**) Suppurative granulomatous inflammation (H&E, magnification 400×). (**b**) Presence of ovoid shape yeast structures (Periodic acid–Schiff (PAS) stain, 400×)

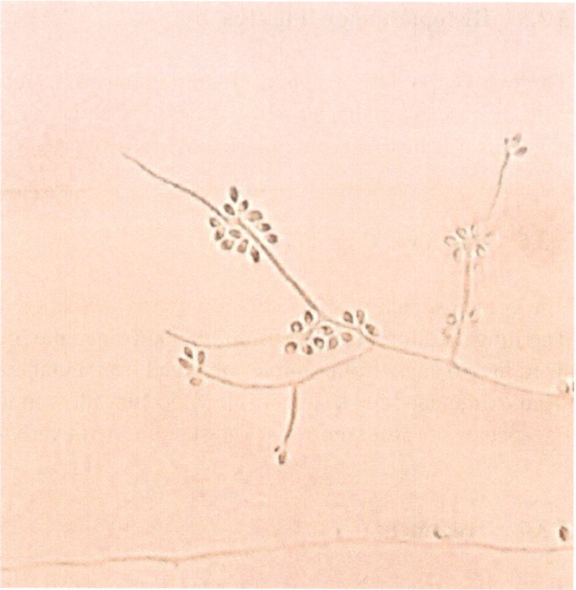

Fig. 17 Microscopy morphology of *Sporothrix* spp.: branched, hyaline septate *hyphae* with oval conidia arranged in a daisy-like pattern at the end of the conidiophore. (*Image courtesy of Patricio Christian Godoy Martinez, PhD, Universidad Austral de Chile*)

time as suppressive therapy at the dose of 200 mg daily [34, 35]. It has been reported strains of *Sporothrix* species resistant to antifungals [36–38], and it may be related to the presence of melanin, low genetic diversity, and mutation in cytochrome P-450 [37]. In this population, it is very important to emphasize the means of prevention by avoiding contact with soil, plant, and infected cats [29].

5.4 Other Emerging Deep Fungal Mycosis (*Figs. 18, 19a, b, 20a, b, and 21*)

Infections attributable to *Scedosporium* spp., a soil saprophyte commonly found in temperate climates are typical of lung transplant recipients appearing 3–4 months after transplantation [3]. Mycetoma, *Pseudallescheria boydii*, *Paraconiothyrium*

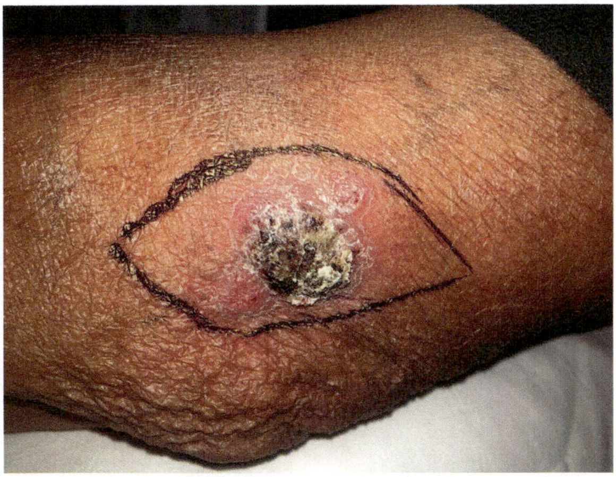

Fig. 18 A 66-year-old lung-transplanted male with a cutaneous single lesion on his elbow. A *Scedosporium apiospermum* was isolated and the patient was treated with surgical removal of the lesion. No relapse has been observed after 1-year follow-up

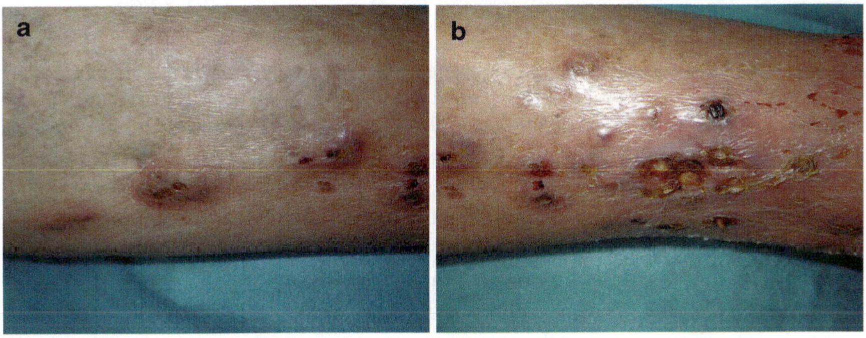

Fig. 19 A 75-year-old kidney transplant recipient that developed multiple nodules on both legs that evolved to ulcers. A *Scedosporium apiospermum* was isolated and the patient started treatment with voriconazole for 6 months associated with a large surgical debridement of the whole affected areas. Voriconazole was stopped 4 months after surgical removal because of the development of multiple cutaneous squamous cell carcinomas. (**a**) Nodular lesions on the upper part of his left leg. (**b**) Ulcerated lesions on the lower part of his left leg

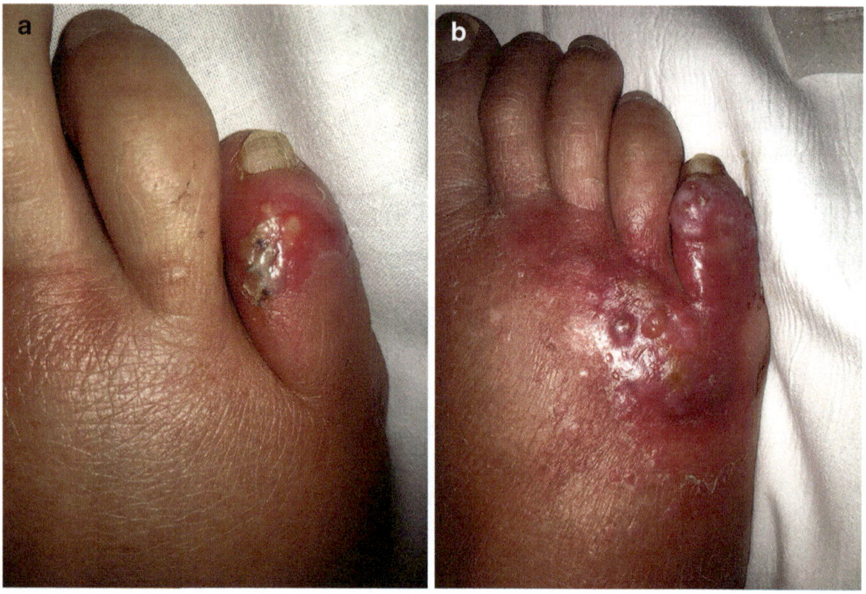

Fig. 20 A 44-year-old recently lung-transplanted male that developed a cutaneous infection by *Paraconiothyrium cyclothyrioides*. He received treatment with isavuconazole 200 mg/day for 8 months (**a**) Initial lesion as an erythematous plaque with a central pustule on the dorsum of his fifth toe. (**b**) Rapid progression after 2 weeks

spp., and others may also be responsible for opportunistic deep fungal infections in SOTR [11]. Their clinical presentation may be as varied as other etiological deep fungal infections and the treatment similar. Finally, although a deep cutaneous infection by *Candida* spp. is usually secondary to an hematogenous spread of a systemic infection, occasionally may also cause a single deep cutaneous lesion. In these cases, exclusion of a systemic infection is mandatory.

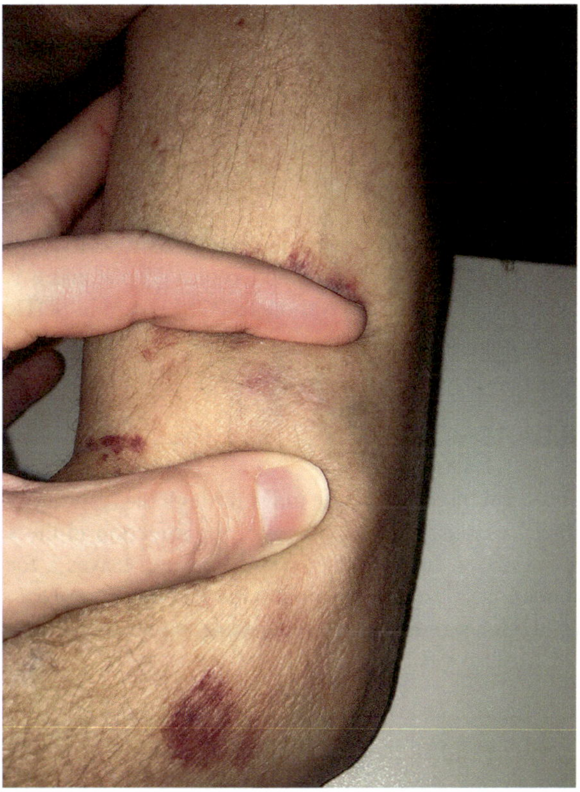

Fig. 21 A 60-year-old lung-transplanted male that developed a subcutaneous tumor on his elbow. A culture of a punch biopsy revealed infection by *Candida albicans*, a systemic spread was excluded. The patient initiated treatment with isavuconazole, that was stopped after 2 months because of asthenia and weakness. The lesion was surgically removed, and no clinical relapse has been observed after 1 year of follow-up

6 Systemic Mycosis

The frequency of invasive fungal disease in SOTR has decreased over the last decades [9], and non-*Aspergillus* species (hyalohyphomycetes, phaeohyphomycetes, zygomycetes) account for about 27% of invasive mycelial fungal infections [39].

6.1 Paracoccidioidomycosis

6.1.1 Introduction

Paracoccidioidomycosis (PCM) is a systemic fungal disease, endemic in some Latin American countries predominantly in South America. The infection is acquired by respiratory route and it is related to agricultural activities. The disease is characteristically chronic and requires long-term treatment. If not properly treated, the disease causes sequelae that may incapacitate the patient.

6.1.2 Epidemiology

PCM is caused by a dimorphic fungus called *Paracoccidioides brasiliensis* and *P. lutzii* that has been recently reported in Northwest and North of Brazil [40]. Brazil retains 80% of the reported cases of PCM followed by other Latin American countries. Infection by *P. brasiliensis* depends on the soil and air humidity, interaction between man and the environment that involves deforestation and agricultural activities [41, 42]. In non-endemic countries, the PCM reported were mostly imported [41]. It is rarely observed in children and young people, and it is more common in men aged 30 years or more [43]. Although, PCM is rare in SOTR, the morbidity and mortality have been increased in this population due to the difficulty in diagnosing and treating.

6.1.3 Pathogenesis

The conidia penetrate the lungs through the respiratory tract where the immune cellular response is able to control the infection in the vast majority of cases, but in some cases the immune system fails and leaves a focus of latent yeast cells. The infection is usually asymptomatic (98%) and only a small percentage of infected individuals progress to the disease, either the acute/juvenile form or the chronic PCM form [43].

6.1.4 Clinical Presentation (Fig. 22a, b)

PCM is a granulomatous disease that presents with two clinical forms: acute and chronic forms. The acute form occurs a few weeks to months after the contact with the fungal spores and approximately 5–10% of patients are symptomatic with generalized lymph node enlargement associated with hepatosplenomegaly, and involvement of other organs, such as the skin, gastrointestinal tract, and/or bones. The chronic form (74–90%) represents the reactivation of a fungal quiescent focus or exogenous reinfection. It may be focal, when only one organ is involved, usually the lungs, or multifocal when the lungs and other organs are also involved, such as the skin, oral mucosa, lymph nodes, adrenal glands, central nervous system, bones, genitals, and blood vessels [43]. The clinical manifestation depends on the host's immune response profile and characteristics inherent to the pathogen.

In SOTR, it is really hard to have a clinical suspicious of PMC as the clinical manifestation may be unspecific. The cutaneous manifestations are diverse as are the lungs' radiological findings, consequently there is usually a delay in the diagnosis [44, 45]. In this population, PCM presented as a disseminated disease in 60% of cases and had a faster evolution with lymphadenopathy, hepatosplenomegaly and manifestations of the digestive, cutaneo-mucosal and osteoarticular systems. It also presented with a higher mortality rate (33%) when compared to immunocompetent patients (5%) [46]. Clinical manifestation of endemic mycosis may occur

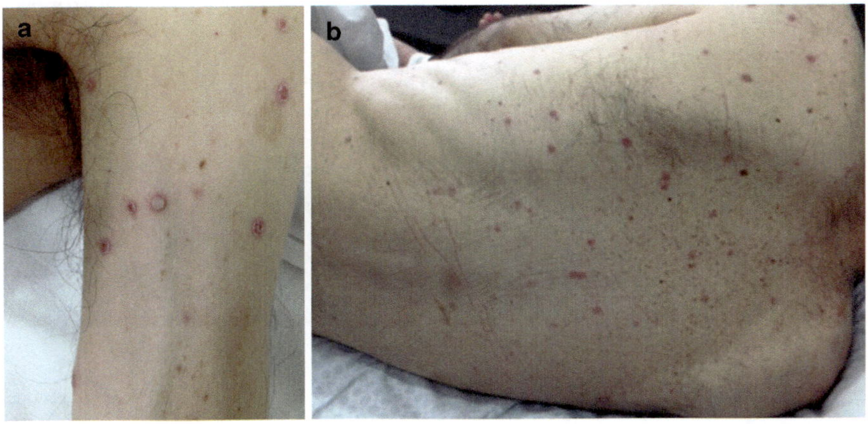

Fig. 22 Cutaneous spread of systemic paracoccidiomycosis in a renal-transplanted recipient. (**a**) Disseminated erythematous pustules and erosions covered with crusts on the leg. (**b**) Multiple erythematous papules on the back

many years after transplantation by the reactivation of the quiescent focus, new infection through a recent contact, or donor transmission in endemic areas [47]. Atypical clinical manifestation, late diagnosis, and an unsatisfactory management may impact negatively in their outcomes. Since PMC is considered not a common disease among SOTR, the screening for PMC in living donor and SOTR is not a routine recommendation; however, it has been strongly suggested in endemic areas [45].

6.1.5 **Histopathology** (Fig. 23a–c)

Microscopic findings of PCM are a granulomatous reaction pattern with numerous fungi within the giant cells. The characteristic feature of this organism is the multiple buds attached to the large and round fungal forms known as "captain wheel" or "pilot wheel" or Mickey Mouse head.

6.1.6 Diagnosis

The gold standard is the isolation of fungal elements on clinical specimen. Serology may be helpful for diagnosis when the fungal isolation is not possible, as well as, for the follow-up of response to treatment [43]. A double immunodiffusion is used and its titration correlates with disease severity [47]. However, in immunosuppressed patients the serology might be negative. Other diagnostic methods are molecular techniques and antigen detection although they are not available for the routine clinical use in most centers.

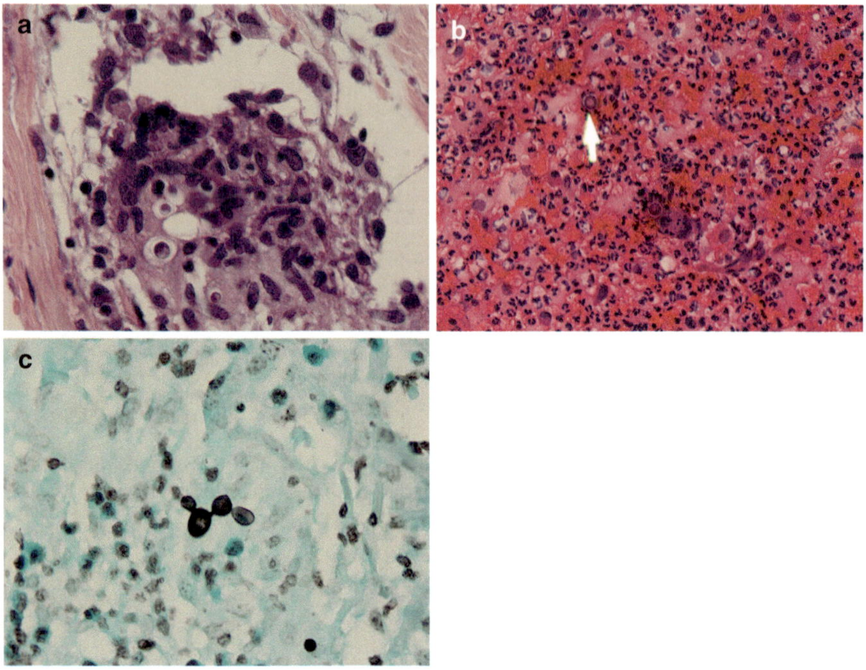

Fig. 23 Cutaneous paracoccidiomycosis. (**a**) Presence of double wall fungi with simple gemmulation within multinucleated giant cells (H&E, magnification 100×). (**b**) Double wall fungi (arrow) surrounded by numerous neutrophils (H&E, magnification 100×). (**c**) Grocott methenamine silver stain revealed yeast-like structures with multiple budding that resemble Mickey mouse ear (magnification 1000×)

6.1.7 Treatment

PMC is mainly treated with itraconazole 100–200 mg/day for 9–18 months in mild and moderate forms, or sulfamethoxazole/ trimethoprim as a second option. Amphotericin B deoxycholate (0.5–0.7 mg/kg/day) or its lipid formulation (3–5 mg/kg/day) are reserved for severe/disseminated forms, but they require a close monitoring due to adverse events mainly kidney toxicity [43, 48]. In SOTR, a close follow-up of the kidney function as well as calcineurin inhibitors levels need to be monitored.

6.2 *Fusariosis*

6.2.1 Introduction

Fusariosis is an emergent fungal disease caused by at least 10 complexes of human pathogenic *Fusarium* spp. [49]. The challenge of this infection is the treatment since *Fusarium* spp. presents an intrinsic resistance to most antifungal agents that makes the infection highly severe.

6.2.2 Epidemiology

More than 300 species of *Fusarium* have been identified, out of which 70 species are considered pathogenic to humans [49]. The two complexes more frequently involved in human infections are *F. solani* and *F. oxysporum*, with *F. solani* being the most virulent and common (40–60% of fusariosis) [50]. *Fusarium* spp. have a worldwide distribution, and they have an ability to adhere to different surfaces and form biofilm on water and plumbing systems [51]. The incidence of fusariosis has been increased due to the growing number of immunocompromised patients, so it is considered an emerging opportunistic fungal disease among this group of patients [52, 53].

6.2.3 Pathogenesis

The main route of transmission is the airway, followed by skin and the mucosal membranes. Skin involvement can be the primary site of infection or secondary to systemic fusariosis. Lesions are generally localized occurring after trauma or pre-existing onychomycosis. The invasive form of the disease occurs predominately among immunocompromised patients, especially in neutropenic and/or severe deficiency T-cell conditions. Patients with a hematological malignancy are more susceptible to the invasive form than SOTR [53, 54]. Among these patients, fusariosis is the second leading cause of fungal infection after aspergillosis [54].

6.2.4 Clinical Presentation (Fig. 24)

The most prevalent infections caused by *Fusarium* species occur on the eye (keratitis), nails (onychomycosis), and skin. In the disseminated forms also brain, lungs and bones are usually affected.

Fusarium spp. are considered as the main agent of onychomycosis (non-dermatophyte filamentous fungi) that presents as subungual distal onychomycosis

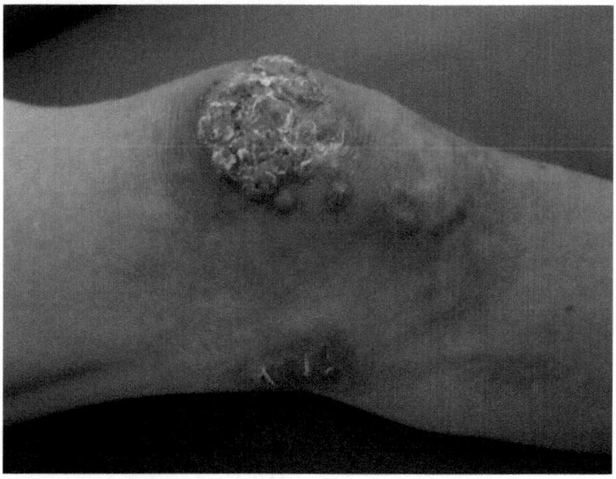

Fig. 24 Renal transplant recipient with a verrucous plaques and erythematous papules on the knee caused by *Fusarium* spp

or total dystrophic nail with paronychia and purulent discharge. Skin involvement is due primarily to the fungal dissemination in immunocompromised host, and the most typical lesions are disseminated painful papules and nodules with central necrosis.

6.2.5 Histopathology (Fig. 25)

The histopathological examination shows septate hyaline *hyphae* with typical branching at an acute or 90-degree angle that may invade blood vessels, forming clots, and tissue necrosis.

6.2.6 Diagnosis (Fig. 26)

Fusariosis is diagnosed based on mycology and histopathology exam by the isolation of fungi. The identification at the species level of *Fusarium* requires molecular methods.

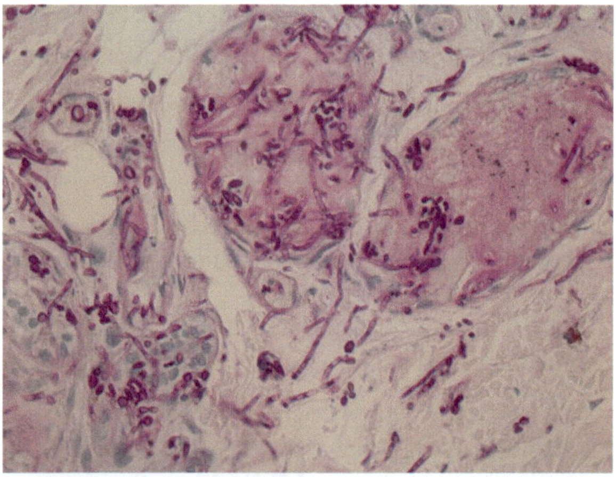

Fig. 25 Periodic acid–Schiff stain showed numerous hyaline hyphae inside the vascular lumen corresponding to cutaneous infection by *Fusarium* spp. (magnification 400×)

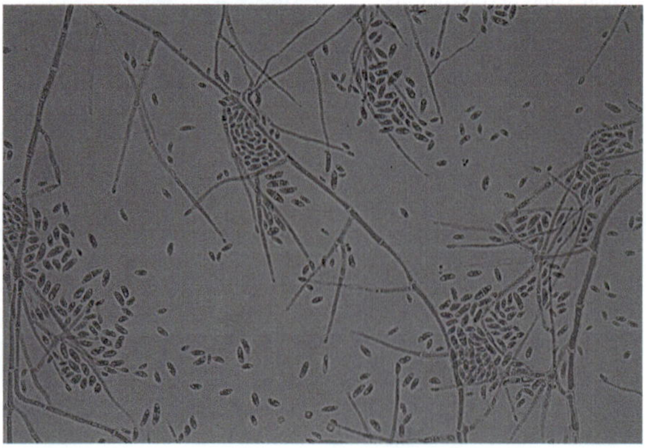

Fig. 26 Microscopic image of *Fusarium solani* complex with septated fusiform macroconidia and multiple cylindrical septated microconidia. (*Image courtesy of Patricio Christian Godoy Martinez, PhD, Universidad Austral de Chile*)

6.2.7 Treatment

Treatment is really a challenge since the fungus is resistant to most antifungal drugs demonstrated in vitro by a high MIC (minimal inhibitory concentration) to the most commonly used antifungals [55]. The drugs of choice are amphotericin B and voriconazole [56]. The treatment should be initiated as soon as fusariosis is suspected in order to prevent a disseminated form, with high mortality and severity rate.

6.3 *Cryptococcosis*

6.3.1 Introduction

Cryptococcosis is an opportunistic fungal infection that typically occurs only in severely immunocompromised patients, and it is specifically recognized as the second most common invasive fungal infection in renal transplant recipients in many countries [56, 57]. The incidence rates in SOTR varies between 0.3% and 5.5%, and overall mortality rates as high as 20–50% have been reported [39, 58, 59].

6.3.2 Epidemiology

The disease is caused by *Cryptococcus* spp., characterized as a species of encapsulated yeasts which is based on the capsule structure, and grouped into two species (*C. neoformans* and *C. gattii*). *C. neoformans* has a global occurrence and is known in every continent. *C. gattii* is reported as a globally occurring species with Australia being the more prevalent region.

6.3.3 Pathogenesis

Cryptococcal infection occurs primarily by inhalation of the infectious propagules (either poorly encapsulated yeast cells or basidiospores) from environmental reservoirs with deposition into pulmonary alveoli, which they encounter alveolar macrophages that play a central role in the immune response. Traumatic inoculation into tissues has been described, as well as via the gastrointestinal tract. Primary pulmonary infection is generally thought to be asymptomatic or minimally symptomatic despite high rates of serologic reactivity in children in certain urban settings. Clearance of the infection by the host may occur. When local immunity is suppressed, the yeast can grow and disseminate outside these pulmonary lymph node complexes similar to the pathophysiology that is observed in cases of reactivation tuberculosis or histoplasmosis [58, 59].

6.3.4 Clinical Presentation (Figs. 27, 28, 29, 30, and 31a, b)

C. neoformans and *C. gattii* have a major predilection for establishing clinical disease in the lungs and central nervous system (CNS). Other less frequent body sites of infection include skin, prostate, eyes, and bone/joints. However, it should be emphasized that this yeast can widely disseminate and infect most organs in severely immunosuppressed patients, and thus has the ability to appear at any human body site [39, 59, 60].

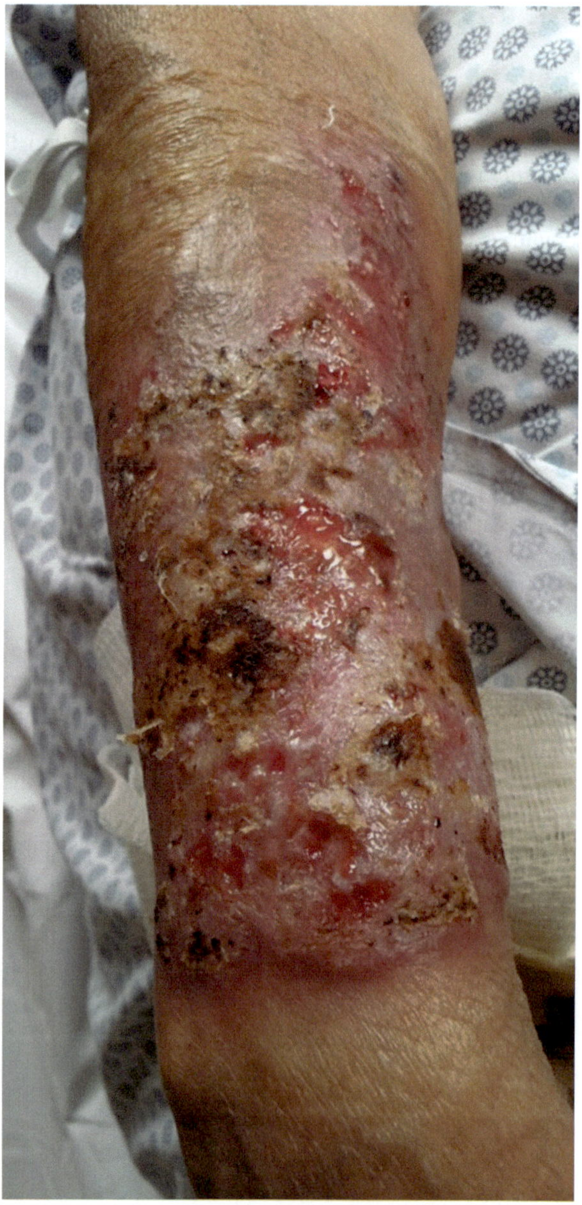

Fig. 27 Kidney-transplanted male that developed a large, ulcerated plaque on the right arm caused by *Cryptococcus neoformans*. Systemic spread compromising lung and meninges

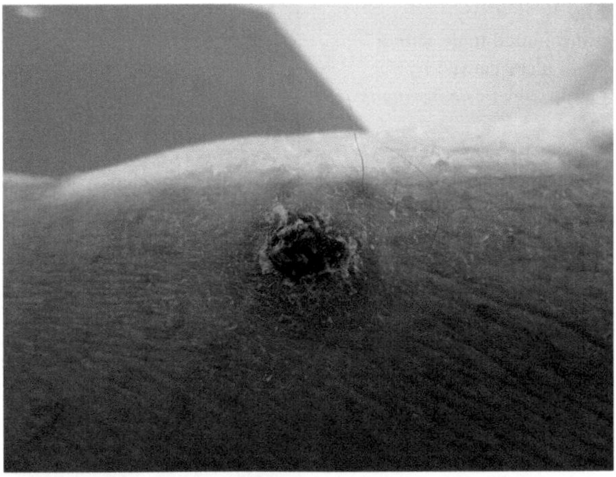

Fig. 28 Kidney-transplanted male that developed a verrucous plaque, with granulation tissue and elevation of the margins on his left arm caused by *Cryptococcus neoformans*. Systemic spread was detected only in lungs

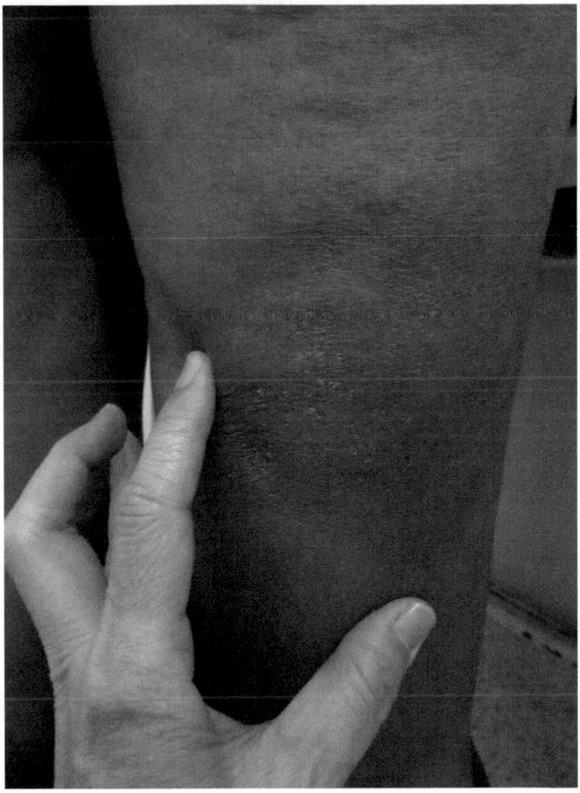

Fig. 29 Kidney-transplanted female that developed cellulitis on her left leg caused by *Cryptococcus neoformans*, with positive blood cultures for the same agent. Systemic spread was diagnosed with lung and central nervous system involvement

In transplant recipients, infection with cryptococcal species presents across a wide spectrum usually as meningoencephalitis and pneumonitis, with cutaneous infections appearing uncommonly. Cutaneous lesions have to be considered seriously because they may be the first clinical sign of cryptococcosis and may be an indicator of systemic dissemination. Cryptococcal skin involvement can occur in

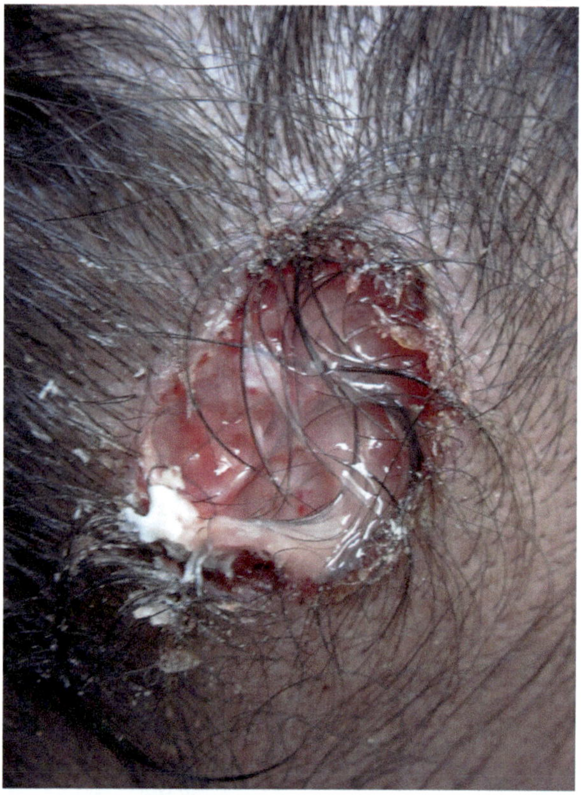

Fig. 30 Kidney-transplanted male with a scalp ulcer caused by *Cryptococcus neoformans*

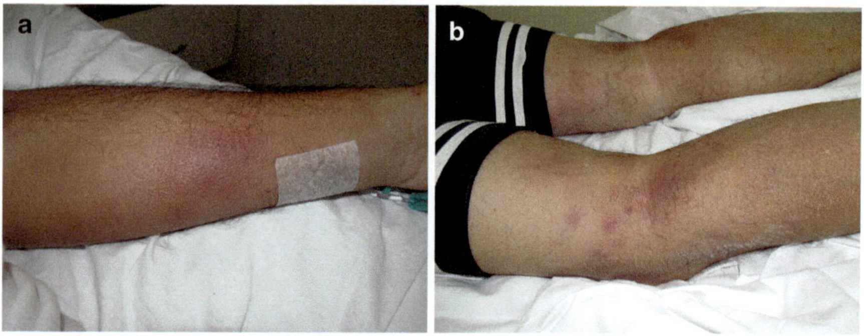

Fig. 31 Kidney-transplanted male that developed (**a**) erythematous plaque on the forearm (panniculitis) and (**b**) multiple plaques and erythematous nodules on the posterior region of the legs caused by *Cryptococcus neoformans*

disseminated disease and is known to be polymorphous in appearance. Classically, the hematogenous spread of *Cryptococcus* spp. is described as umbilicated papules similar to molluscum contagiosum. In SOTR, lesions can manifest as acneiform papules, pustular eruption, ulcers, subcutaneous nodules, cellulitis, and mimic other dermatological entities [61–63]. Involvement of bone or joint are described in some cases [64].

6.3.5 **Histopathology** (Fig. 32)

Cryptococcus spp. can be identified by histologic staining of tissues from the lung, skin, liver, bone marrow, brain, and other organs. The organism is observed as a yeast that reproduces by narrow-based budding, best identified by special stains that label the polysaccharide capsule including mucicarmine, periodic acid-Schiff, and Alcian blue stains. Fontana–Masson stain can identify melanin in the yeast cell wall [39, 58, 60].

6.3.6 **Diagnosis** (Fig. 33)

Cryptococcosis is defined as a patient who has: (a) isolation of *Cryptococcus neoformans* or *C. gattii* from positive culture obtained from any site; (b) direct detection of the fungus by means of India ink staining of body fluids; (c) cryptococcal antigen in cerebrospinal fluid or serum specimens with a compatible clinical and/or radiographic presentation; (d) biopsy specimens exhibiting encapsulated "yeast-like" forms consistent with *Cryptococcus* spp. Histopathologic methods and cryptococcal antigen testing cannot distinguish between *C. neoformans* and *C. gattii*. Patients with suspected or proven cryptococcosis should have a thorough evaluation for extrapulmonary disease, including lumbar puncture, blood, and other relevant tissue cultures. Cutaneous cryptococcus in immunocompromised patients is crucial to enable further investigations and effective management [39, 59, 60].

6.3.7 **Treatment**

There have been no randomized controlled trials of antifungal therapy for cryptococcosis in SOTR recipients. Current treatment recommendations are extrapolated from clinical trials among HIV patients and from data collected retrospectively in SOTR [65, 66].

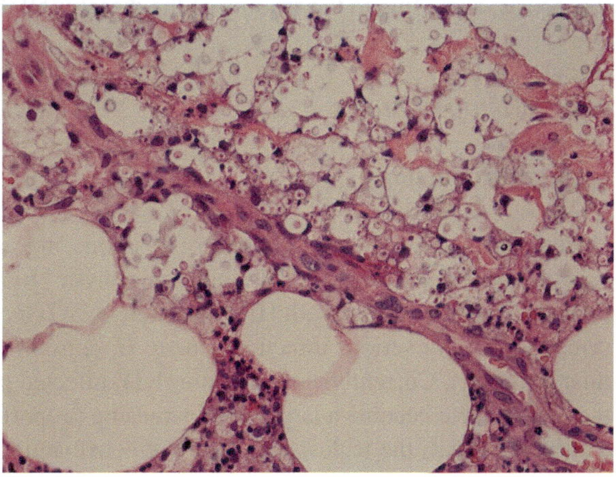

Fig. 32 Histological section of a skin fragment showing yeast-like structures with a thickened capsule, suggestive of *Cryptococcus* spp. (PAS stain, 400×)

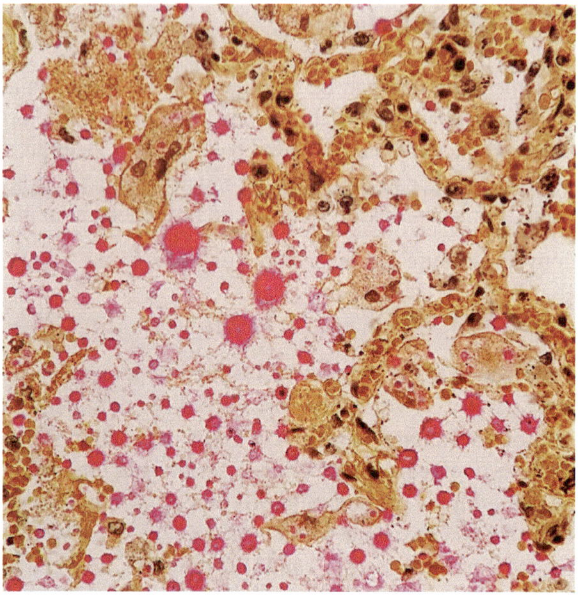

Fig. 33 Direct microscopic exam of *Cryptococcus* spp. with mucicarmine stain

The recommendation for the management of neurological disease, disseminated cryptococcosis, or severe pulmonary disease is induction therapy with liposomal amphotericin B (3–4 mg/kg/day) or amphotericin B lipid complex (5 mg/kg/day) plus flucytosine (100 mg/kg/day in four equally divided doses every 6 h based on creatinine clearance) for a minimum of 2 weeks followed by consolidation with fluconazole (400–800 mg/day) for 8 weeks and, finally maintenance therapy with fluconazole (200–400 mg/day) for 6–12 months. Fluconazole is preferred for consolidation and maintenance therapy for CNS disease for at least 1 year of treatment. Fluconazole is also the preferred therapy for asymptomatic or mild-to-moderate pulmonary disease. Newer triazoles should be reserved as alternative agents when fluconazole cannot be used or for patients with isolates that may be resistant to fluconazole. Reduction or withdrawn of immunosuppression should be performed at time of diagnosis of cryptococcosis, according to the severity of the disease [59, 65, 66].

6.4 Histoplasmosis

6.4.1 Introduction

Histoplasmosis is a potentially severe systemic mycosis caused by *Histoplasma capsulatum*, a dimorphic and soil saprophytic fungus. Immunocompromised patients, including those with HIV infection or SOTR, are more susceptible to disseminated and/or serious infections due to *H. capsulatum* because of impaired cellular immunity. Currently, however, non-HIV-infected patients, including transplant recipients, have become a larger and increasing proportion of these cases, in part as a consequence of the widespread use of effective antiretroviral therapy [67–69].

6.4.2 Epidemiology

In SOTR, T-cell immune dysfunction can also be significant although the incidence of clinical histoplasmosis is <0.5% in most studies. In endemic areas of US, histoplasmosis accounted for <5% of all invasive fungal infections in SOTR in two large centers, and its incidence is unknown in the majority of the organ transplant population in underdeveloped countries. In the European continent, the disease is considered an imported endemic mycosis. *H. capsulatum* var. *capsulatum* and *H. capsulatum* var. *duboisii* are the two subspecies that are pathogenic in humans. The geographical niche of the latter is confined to Africa and cutaneous and skeletal lesions distinctly dominate its clinical manifestation. *H. capsulatum* var. *capsulatum*, on the other hand, has a more global distribution, occurring mainly in specific endemic areas of North and South America, although it has been found on a large scale in countries like India, China, Pakistan, etc. [67–69].

6.4.3 Pathogenesis

The infection results from the inhalation of airborne conidia. After the small conidia are aerosolized into the lungs, they are phagocytized by alveolar macrophages and are transformed to the yeast phase. Inside the cells, it is disseminated widely through the lymphatics and the bloodstream. The majority of infections are asymptomatic although they can result in subclinical primary infections of the lungs or mild pneumonitis in immunocompetent hosts. However, in immunosuppressed hosts, cell-mediated immunity may not develop, the organism remains viable within macrophages, and disseminated infection ensues. Consequently, in immunosuppressed host, deep tissue disease may occur, involving the lung, with dissemination to liver, spleen, bone marrow, and CNS, either as a progression of the initial lymphohematogenous dissemination or as a reactivation of quiescent foci of past infections, or exceptionally, as a consequence of direct transmission from an infected graft [68–70].

6.4.4 Clinical Presentation (Figs. 34, 35a, b, and 36)

In a patient who is not markedly immunosuppressed, focal pneumonia can occur, presenting with fever, myalgias, dry cough, and dyspnea. More often, diffuse pneumonia with more severe dyspnea and hypoxemia is the presenting manifestation of pulmonary histoplasmosis in transplant recipients [71]. Disseminated histoplasmosis involves primarily the reticuloendothelial system: liver, spleen, bone marrow, and lymph nodes are commonly affected. Additionally, skin, gastrointestinal tract, adrenals, and CNS can be involved [71, 72].

Skin involvement is variable in SOTR. The highest surveillance study of histoplasmosis in SOTR showed cutaneous involvement in only 3% of cases [72, 73]. Faar et al. described in 1981, a review of 17 cases of histoplasmosis in SOTR,

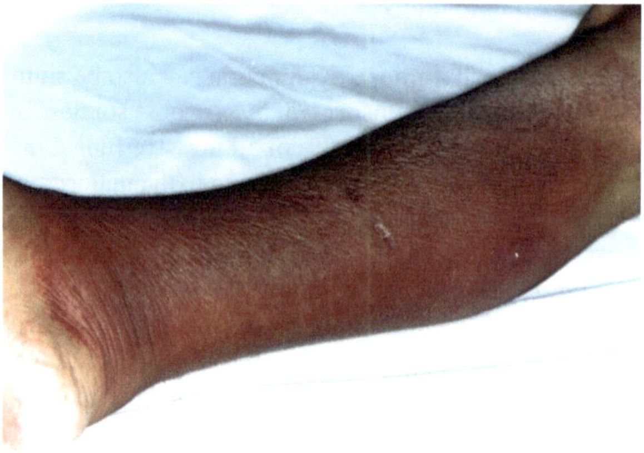

Fig. 34 Kidney-transplanted male that developed a cellulite on the right leg caused by *Histoplasma capsulatum*

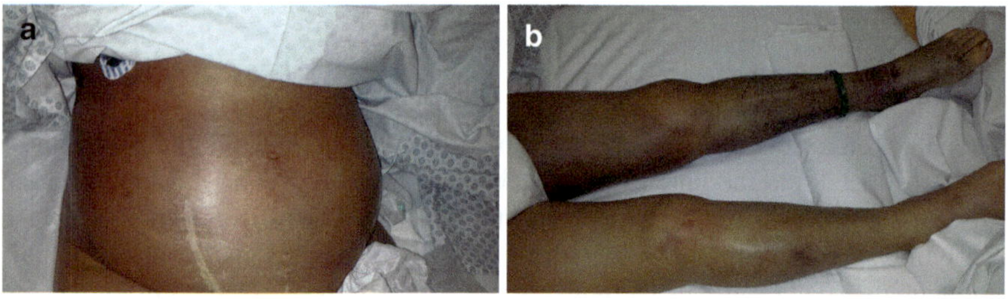

Fig. 35 Kidney-transplanted female that developed a cellulitis plaque (**a**) on the abdominal region and (**b**) on the left leg caused by *Histoplasma capsulatum*

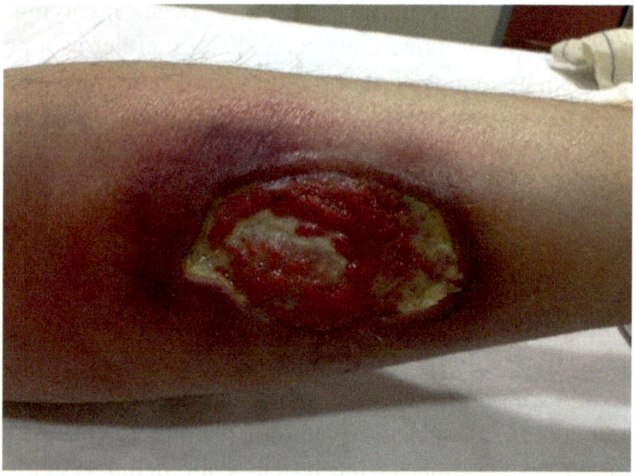

Fig. 36 Kidney-transplanted female that developed an ulcer with infiltrated borders on the right leg caused by *Histoplasma capsulatum*

showing 8 (47%) with cutaneous involvement [74]. In other recent review of cutaneous histoplasmosis in renal transplant recipients, the authors reported 22 cases of which 77% were associated with otherwise documented disseminated disease [75]. Multiple dermatological patterns are described in cutaneous histoplasmosis in

SOTR. Lesions can be solitary or multiple, showing aspects of cellulitis, subcutaneous, ulcers, plaques, nodules including panniculitis or even erythema nodosum. Unusual presentations such as necrotizing fasciitis and focal abscess have also been reported [75–79].

6.4.5 **Histopathology** (Fig. 37a, b)

Histopathologic examination shows a granulomatous response that is either necrotizing or non-necrotizing, with small narrow-ovoid yeast cells measuring 2–4 mm in greatest dimension in tissue and/or body fluid specimens morphologically consistent with *H. capsulatum*. Yeasts are localized within mononuclear phagocytic cells, such as macrophages and monocytes; however, in many preparations, extracellular yeast can also be observed. Special stains, such as the Grocott-Gomori methenamine–silver (GMS) and periodic acid–Schiff (PAS) stains are useful and provide contrast to yeast cells. The differential diagnosis for histoplasmosis includes other granulomatous disorders such as sarcoidosis, lymphoma, other fungal infections, and mycobacterial infections. Other fungi and microorganisms may be mistaken for *H. capsulatum*, especially *Candida glabrata*, *Blastomyces dermatitidis*, capsule-deficient strains of *C. neoformans* and *C. gattii*, *Talaromyces marneffei*, tiny shapes of *Paracoccidioides* spp. Some protozoa such as *Leishmania* spp., *Toxoplasma gondii*, and *Trypanosoma cruzi* are confounded with histoplasma yeast in the tissue [67, 70].

6.4.6 **Diagnosis** (Fig. 38)

The gold standard methods for the diagnosis of histoplasmosis include identification of yeast on histopathology or cytopathology of clinical specimens, and growth of mold in culture incubated at room temperature. Up to 4 weeks is required to

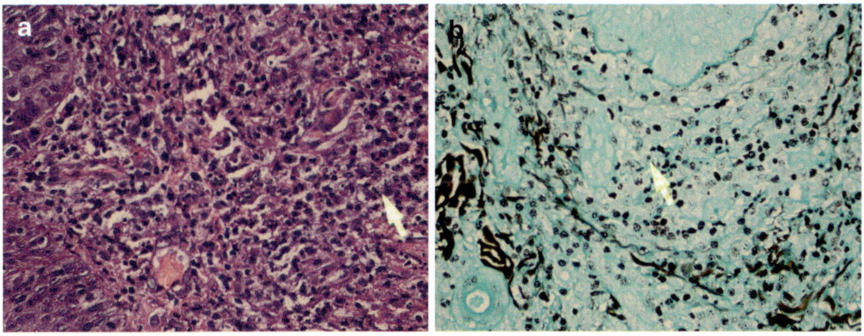

Fig. 37 Cutaneous infection by *Histoplasma capsulatum*. (**a**) Hematoxylin-eosin stain showed suppurative granulomatous inflammation and numerous budding yeast forms (400×). (**b**) Grocott methenamine stain revealed numerous yeasts stained in black

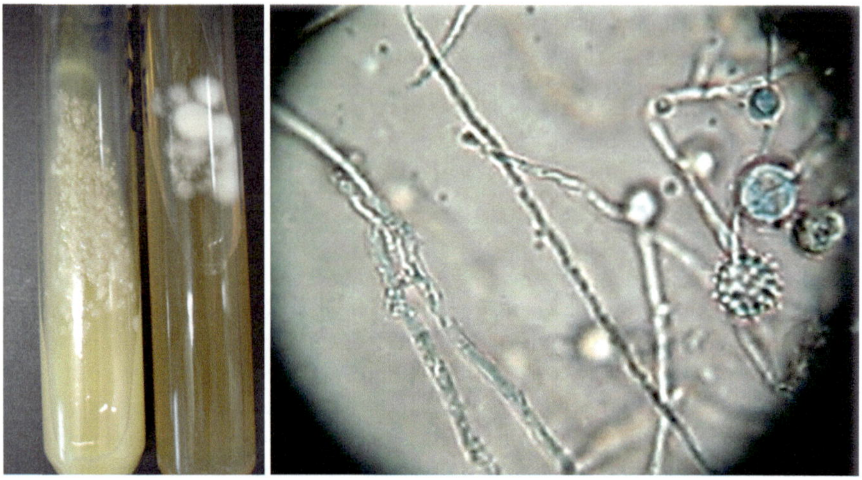

Fig. 38 Yeast (left tube) and mold form (right tube with white cottony mycelium) of *H. capsulatum*. Microscopic examination of mold growth reveals rounded tuberculate macroconidia originating from short, hyaline conidiophores. (*Image courtesy of Patricio Christian Godoy Martinez, PhD, Universidad Austral de Chile*)

isolate the organism in culture. The mold form of *H. capsulatum* usually grows as a white cottony mycelium. Microscopic examination of mold growth reveals characteristic large, rounded tuberculate macroconidia originating from short, hyaline conidiophores [67, 70, 71].

6.4.7 Treatment

There are no randomized controlled therapeutic trials in SOTR, and treatment recommendations are similar to those for HIV patients. In disseminated diseases, a lipid formulation of amphotericin B (liposomal amphotericin B at 3 mg/kg daily or amphotericin B lipid complex at 5 mg/kg daily) is first-line therapy for the first 2 weeks followed by oral itraconazole 400 mg daily for at least 1 year. In mild-to-moderate disease, oral itraconazole 400 mg daily is the preferred treatment [67–71].

6.5 Aspergillosis

6.5.1 Introduction

Aspergillus spp. is a ubiquitous environmental fungus that causes potentially lethal infections in immunocompromised hosts. Invasive aspergillosis is the second most frequent cause of invasive fungal infections after invasive candidiasis in

SOTR (first cause in lung transplantation). Annual incidence of invasive aspergillosis varies from 0.1% to 3.5% in SOTR. Risk factors for the development of aspergillosis within 3 months posttransplant included prolonged intensive care unit (ICU) stay, posttransplantation renal failure requiring hemodialysis, cytomegalovirus (CMV) disease, or one episode of bacterial infection. Older age, CMV disease, renal failure, chronic graft rejection, and immunosuppressive-related neoplasm were independent risk factors for aspergillosis after 3 months of transplantation [39, 80, 81].

6.5.2 Epidemiology

Aspergillus spp. are ubiquitous in the environment and found in the soil and in decaying vegetative material. Regional differences in precipitation, humidity, and temperature are thought to play a role in the environmental prevalence of *Aspergillus* spp., and a correlation with these factors and human infection has been suggested. *A. fumigatus complex* causes a majority of infections, followed by *A. flavus*, *A. niger*, and *A. terreus*. Additional cryptic species may be seen, particularly in highly immunocompromised patients [82–84].

6.5.3 Pathogenesis

Following inhalation or inoculation with *Aspergillus* conidia (spores), infection may develop locally or disseminate to contiguous or distant sites, particularly in those receiving immunosuppressive therapy or who are neutropenic following bone marrow transplantation or receipt of chemotherapy. In SOTR, lung transplant recipients are at the highest risk, with up to 10–15% of patients developing aspergillosis, particularly at the surgical anastomotic site. Small bowel, liver, heart, and kidney recipients also are prone to invasive aspergillosis and individual risk primarily is a result of the degree of immunosuppression, coinfection with CMV and metabolic disorders (renal disease, diabetes) [39, 80–84]. Cutaneous aspergillosis is a rare and uncommon disease. Primary cutaneous aspergillosis (PCA) is characterized when there is evidence of a cutaneous lesion infected with *Aspergillus* in the absence of infection elsewhere. This is in contrast to the most common form, the secondary cutaneous aspergillosis, which involves the hematogenous spread of *Aspergillus* infection from a distal site (lungs) to the skin. Particularly in SOT, primary disease as the potential to progress to systemic infection and is frequently lethal [82, 85].

Most cases have been reported in immunocompromised patients with hematologic or lymphoreticular malignancies or in organ transplant patients receiving long-term therapy with cytotoxic or chemotherapeutic agents, systemic glucocorticosteroids, broad-spectrum antibiotics, or a combination of these agents.

6.5.4 **Clinical Presentation** (Fig. 39a, b)

The category that manifests depends largely on the underlying host characteristics and the interaction between the fungus and the host. There are several dermatological patters of cutaneous aspergillosis, including ulcerative nodules, erythematous plaques, pustules, erythematous and violaceous nodules, hemorrhagic bullae, and ulcers [82, 85, 86].

6.5.5 **Histopathology** (Fig. 40)

Proved disease requires histopathologic, cytopathologic, or direct microscopic confirmation of tissue invasion. The finding of branching hyaline septate hyphae on microscopic examination is highly suggestive of invasive aspergillosis, but other hyaline molds also may exhibit these same findings, such as *Fusarium* spp., *Scedosporium* spp., and *Paecilomyces* spp. [82, 85, 86].

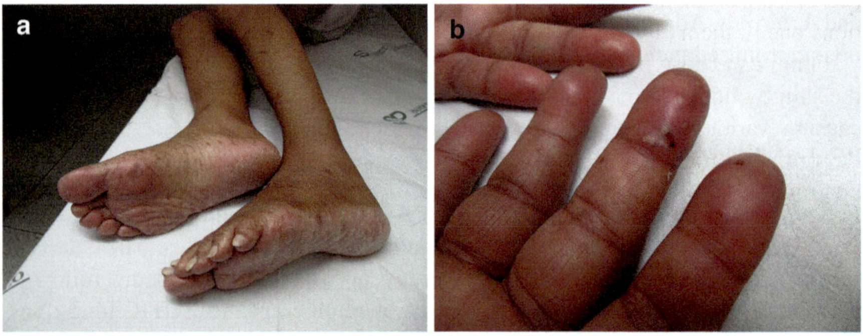

Fig. 39 Cutaneous spread of systemic infection by Aspergillosis in kidney transplant recipient. (**a**) Multiple purpuric lesions on the legs and plantar region. (**b**) Pustules and purpura on an erythematous base on the fingertips

Fig. 40 Periodic acid–Schiff (PAS) stain showed numerous hyaline hyphae with acute angulation corresponding to infection by *Aspergillus* spp. (100×)

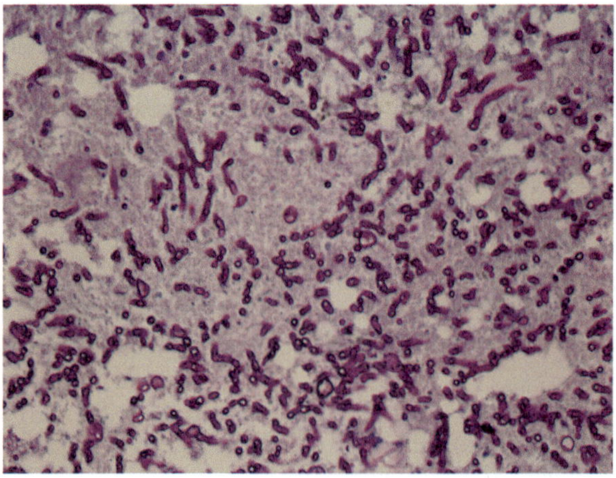

6.5.6 **Diagnosis** (Fig. 41a–d)

The diagnosis of cutaneous aspergillosis requires biopsy of the lesion with isolation of *Aspergillus* spp. in culture associated with the finding of hyaline hyphae in tissue. In the context of disseminated disease, detection of biomarkers such as serum galactomannan dosage may be useful [86].

6.5.7 Treatment

Treatment is a challenge and several antifungal treatment options now are available with activity against *Aspergillus* spp. The drug of choice is voriconazole or isavuconazole, orally or intravenously. Both are used for primary or secondary cutaneous forms, localized or disseminated diseases. Alternatively, lipid formulations of amphotericin B can be used. Surgical debridement is important when there is skin necrosis [87].

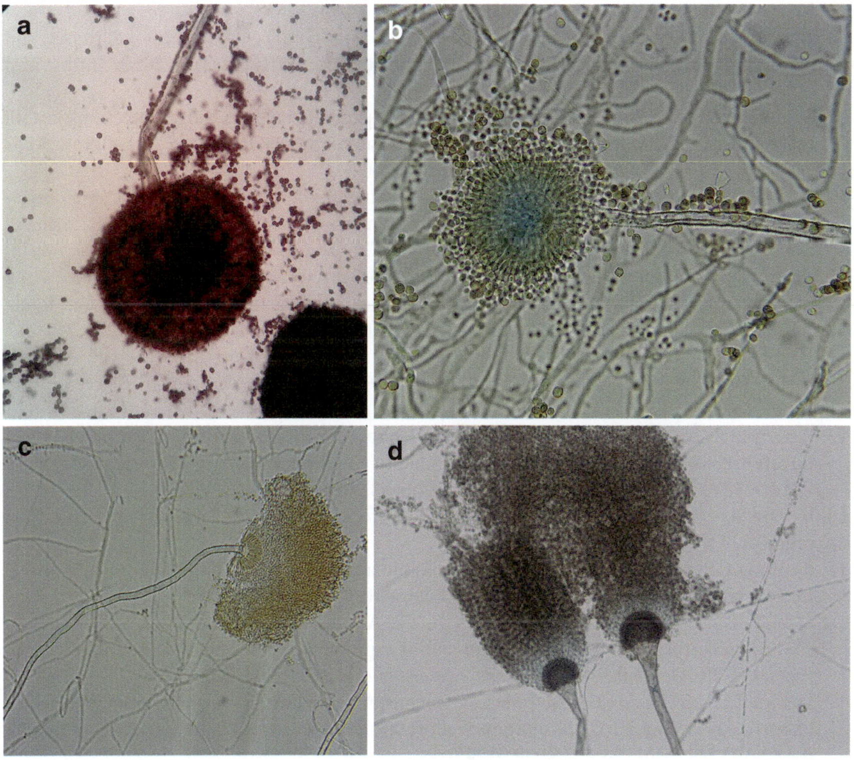

Fig. 41 (**a**) Microscopic images of *Aspergillus section nigri*. (**b**) Microscopic images of *Aspergillus section flavi*. (**c**) Microscopic images of *Aspergillus section terrei*. (**d**) Microscopic image of *Aspergillus section fumigatus*. (*Image courtesy of Patricio Christian Godoy Martinez, PhD, Universidad Austral de Chile*)

References

1. Skiada A, Petrikkos G. Cutaneous zygomycosis. Clin Microbiol Infect. 2009;15(Suppl 5):41–5. https://doi.org/10.1111/j.1469-0691.2009.02979.x.
2. Galezowski A, Delyon J, Le Cleach L, et al. Deep cutaneous fungal infections in solid-organ transplant recipients. J Am Acad Dermatol. 2020;83(2):455–62. https://doi.org/10.1016/j.jaad.2019.12.064.
3. Shoham S, Dominguez EA, AST Infectious Diseases Community of Practice. Emerging fungal infections in solid organ transplant recipients: Guidelines of the American Society of Transplantation Infectious Diseases Community of Practice. Clin Transplant. 2019;33(9):e13525. https://doi.org/10.1111/ctr.13525.
4. Virgili A, Zampino MR, Mantovani L. Fungal skin infections in organ transplant recipients. Am J Clin Dermatol. 2002;3(1):19–35. https://doi.org/10.2165/00128071-200203010-00003.
5. Tessari G, Cagalli A, Girolomoni G. Opportunistic deep cutaneous mycoses in solid organ transplant recipients. G Ital Dermatol Venereol. 2014;149(4):417–22.
6. Stelzmueller I, Lass-Floerl C, Geltner C, et al. Zygomycosis and other rare filamentous fungal infections in solid organ transplant recipients. Transpl Int. 2008;21(6):534–46. https://doi.org/10.1111/j.1432-2277.2008.00657.x.
7. Ferrándiz-Pulido C, Martin-Gomez MT, Repiso T, et al. Cutaneous infections by dematiaceous opportunistic fungi: diagnosis and management in 11 solid organ transplant recipients. Mycoses. 2019;62(2):121–7. https://doi.org/10.1111/myc.12853.
8. Boyce RD, Deziel PJ, Otley CC, et al. Phaeohyphomycosis due to Alternaria species in transplant recipients. Transpl Infect Dis. 2010;12(3):242–50. https://doi.org/10.1111/j.1399-3062.2009.00482.x.
9. Schieffelin JS, Garcia-Diaz JB, Loss GE, et al. Phaeohyphomycosis fungal infections in solid organ transplant recipients: clinical presentation, pathology, and treatment. Transpl Infect Dis. 2014;16(2):270–8. https://doi.org/10.1111/tid.12197.
10. Ogawa MM, Galante NZ, Godoy P, et al. Treatment of subcutaneous phaeohyphomycosis and prospective follow-up of 17 kidney transplant recipients. J Am Acad Dermatol. 2009;61(6):977–85. https://doi.org/10.1016/j.jaad.2009.03.037.
11. Santos DW, Camargo LF, Gonçalves SS, et al. Melanized fungal infections in kidney transplant recipients: contributions to optimize clinical management. Clin Microbiol Infect. 2017;23(5):333.e9–333.e14. https://doi.org/10.1016/j.cmi.2016.12.024.
12. Gilmour TK, Rytina E, O'Connell PB, Sterling JC. Cutaneous alternariosis in a cardiac transplant recipient. Australas J Dermatol. 2001;42(1):46–9. https://doi.org/10.1046/j.1440-0960.2001.00473.x.
13. Gonzalez Santiago TM, Pritt B, Gibson LE, Comfere NI. Diagnosis of deep cutaneous fungal infections: correlation between skin tissue culture and histopathology. J Am Acad Dermatol. 2014;71(2):293–301. https://doi.org/10.1016/j.jaad.2014.03.042.
14. Revankar SG. Dematiaceous fungi. Mycoses. 2007;50(2):91–101. https://doi.org/10.1111/j.1439-0507.2006.01331.x.
15. de Hoog GS. Evolution of black yeasts: possible adaptation to the human host. Antonie Van Leeuwenhoek. 1993;63(2):105–9. https://doi.org/10.1007/BF00872386.
16. Dang HX, Pryor B, Peever T, Lawrence CB. The Alternaria genomes database: a comprehensive resource for a fungal genus comprised of saprophytes, plant pathogens, and allergenic species. BMC Genomics. 2015;16:239. https://doi.org/10.1186/s12864-015-1430-7.
17. Duquia RP, de Almeida HL, Vettorato G, Rocha NM, de Castro LAS. Ecthyma-like phaeohyphomycosis caused by Cladosporium cladosporioides. Mycoses. 2010;53(6):541–3. https://doi.org/10.1111/j.1439-0507.2009.01745.x.
18. Gugnani HC, Sood N, Singh B, Makkar R. Case report. Subcutaneous phaeohyphomycosis due to Cladosporium cladosporioides. Mycoses. 2000;43(1–2):85–7. https://doi.org/10.1046/j.1439-0507.2000.00545.x.

19. Vieira MR, Milheiro A, Pacheco FA. Phaeohyphomycosis due to Cladosporium cladosporioides. Med Mycol. 2001;39(1):135–7. https://doi.org/10.1080/mmy.39.1.135.137.
20. Martínez-González MC, Verea MM, Velasco D, et al. Three cases of cutaneous phaeohyphomycosis by Exophiala jeanselmei. Eur J Dermatol. 2008;18(3):313–6. https://doi.org/10.1684/ejd.2008.0395.
21. Langfelder K, Streibel M, Jahn B, Haase G, Brakhage AA. Biosynthesis of fungal melanins and their importance for human pathogenic fungi. Fungal Genet Biol. 2003;38(2):143–58. https://doi.org/10.1016/s1087-1845(02)00526-1.
22. Nosanchuk JD, Casadevall A. The contribution of melanin to microbial pathogenesis. Cell Microbiol. 2003;5(4):203–23. https://doi.org/10.1046/j.1462-5814.2003.00268.x.
23. Gilaberte M, Bartralot R, Torres JM, et al. Cutaneous alternariosis in transplant recipients: clinicopathologic review of 9 cases. J Am Acad Dermatol. 2005;52(4):653–9. https://doi.org/10.1016/j.jaad.2004.10.875.
24. Almyroudis NG, Sutton DA, Linden P, Rinaldi MG, Fung J, Kusne S. Zygomycosis in solid organ transplant recipients in a tertiary transplant center and review of the literature. Am J Transplant. 2006;6(10):2365–74. https://doi.org/10.1111/j.1600-6143.2006.01496.x.
25. Schubach A, de Lima Barros MB, Wanke B. Epidemic sporotrichosis. Curr Opin Infect Dis. 2008;21(2):129–33. https://doi.org/10.1097/QCO.0b013e3282f44c52.
26. Queiroz-Telles F, Fahal AH, Falci DR, Caceres DH, Chiller T, Pasqualotto AC. Neglected endemic mycoses. Lancet Infect Dis. 2017;17(11):e367–77. https://doi.org/10.1016/S1473-3099(17)30306-7.
27. Chakrabarti A, Bonifaz A, Gutierrez-Galhardo MC, Mochizuki T, Li S. Global epidemiology of sporotrichosis. Med Mycol. 2015;53(1):3–14. https://doi.org/10.1093/mmy/myu062.
28. Rodrigues AM, de Hoog GS, de Camargo ZP. Sporothrix species causing outbreaks in animals and humans driven by animal-animal transmission. PLoS Pathog. 2016;12(7):e1005638. https://doi.org/10.1371/journal.ppat.1005638.
29. Fichman V, Marques de Macedo P, Francis Saraiva Freitas D, et al. Zoonotic sporotrichosis in renal transplant recipients from Rio de Janeiro, Brazil. Transpl Infect Dis. 2021;23(2):e13485. https://doi.org/10.1111/tid.13485.
30. Amirali MH, Liebenberg J, Pillay S, Nel J. Sporotrichosis in renal transplant patients: two case reports and a review of the literature. J Med Case Rep. 2020;14(1):79. https://doi.org/10.1186/s13256-020-02385-x.
31. Orofino-Costa R, de Macedo PM, Rodrigues AM, Bernardes-Engemann AR. Sporotrichosis: an update on epidemiology, etiopathogenesis, laboratory and clinical therapeutics. An Bras Dermatol. 2017;92(5):606–20. https://doi.org/10.1590/abd1806-4841.2017279.
32. Francesconi G, Valle AC, Passos S, Reis R, Galhardo MC. Terbinafine (250 mg/day): an effective and safe treatment of cutaneous sporotrichosis. J Eur Acad Dermatol Venereol. 2009;23(11):1273–6. https://doi.org/10.1111/j.1468-3083.2009.03306.x.
33. Borba-Santos LP, Rodrigues AM, Gagini TB, et al. Susceptibility of Sporothrix brasiliensis isolates to amphotericin B, azoles, and terbinafine. Med Mycol. 2015;53(2):178–88. https://doi.org/10.1093/mmy/myu056.
34. Mahajan VK. Sporotrichosis: an overview and therapeutic options. Dermatol Res Pract. 2014;2014:272376. https://doi.org/10.1155/2014/272376.
35. Gewehr P, Jung B, Aquino V, et al. Sporotrichosis in renal transplant patients. Can J Infect Dis Med Microbiol. 2013;24(2):e47–9. https://doi.org/10.1155/2013/603405.
36. Ottonelli Stopiglia CD, Magagnin CM, Castrillón MR, et al. Antifungal susceptibilities and identification of species of the Sporothrix schenckii complex isolated in Brazil. Med Mycol. 2014;52(1):56–64. https://doi.org/10.3109/13693786.2013.818726.
37. Vettorato R, Heidrich D, Fraga F, et al. Sporotrichosis by Sporothrix schenckii sensu stricto with itraconazole resistance and terbinafine sensitivity observed in vitro and in vivo: case report. Med Mycol Case Rep. 2018;19:18–20. https://doi.org/10.1016/j.mmcr.2017.10.001.

38. Waller SB, Dalla Lana DF, Quatrin PM, Ferreira MRA, Fuentefria AM, Mezzari A. Antifungal resistance on Sporothrix species: an overview. Braz J Microbiol. 2021;52(1):73–80. https://doi.org/10.1007/s42770-020-00307-z.
39. Husain S, Alexander BD, Munoz P, et al. Opportunistic mycelial fungal infections in organ transplant recipients: emerging importance of non-Aspergillus mycelial fungi. Clin Infect Dis. 2003;37(2):221–9. https://doi.org/10.1086/375822.
40. Teixeira MM, Theodoro RC, Nino-Vega G, Bagagli E, Felipe MSS. Paracoccidioides species complex: ecology, phylogeny, sexual reproduction, and virulence. PLoS Pathog. 2014;10(10):e1004397. https://doi.org/10.1371/journal.ppat.1004397.
41. Martinez R. Epidemiology of paracoccidioidomycosis. Rev Inst Med Trop Sao Paulo. 2015;57(Suppl 19):11–20. https://doi.org/10.1590/S0036-46652015000700004.
42. Martinez R. New trends in paracoccidioidomycosis epidemiology. J Fungi (Basel). 2017;3(1):E1. https://doi.org/10.3390/jof3010001.
43. Shikanai-Yasuda MA, Mendes RP, Colombo AL, et al. [Brazilian guidelines for the clinical management of paracoccidioidomycosis]. Epidemiol Serv Saude. 2018;27(spe):e0500001. https://doi.org/10.5123/S1679-49742018000500001.
44. de Oliveira Góes HF, Durães SMB, dos Santos Lima C, de Souza MB, Vilar EAG, Dalston MO. Paracoccidioidomycosis in a renal transplant recipient. Rev Inst Med Trop Sao Paulo. 2016;58:12. https://doi.org/10.1590/S1678-9946201658012.
45. Sinkos C, Grillo TG, Bonini ACM, et al. Mixed and disseminated paracoccidioidomycosis after liver transplantation: case report. Med Mycol Case Rep. 2021;32:25–9. https://doi.org/10.1016/j.mmcr.2021.02.004.
46. Peçanha-Pietrobom PM, Falqueto A, Rodrigues Gandarella AD, et al. Case report: paracoccidioidomycosis in solid organ transplantation: disseminated disease in a liver recipient and literature review. Am J Trop Med Hyg. 2019;101(5):1100–6. https://doi.org/10.4269/ajtmh.18-1008.
47. Abdala E, Miller R, Pasqualotto AC, Muñoz P, Colombo AL, Cuenca-Estrella M. Endemic fungal infection recommendations for solid-organ transplant recipients and donors. Transplantation. 2018;102(2S Suppl 2):S52–9. https://doi.org/10.1097/TP.0000000000002020.
48. Moreto TC, Marques MEA, de Oliveira MLSC, Moris DV, de Carvalho LR, Mendes RP. Accuracy of routine diagnostic tests used in paracoccidioidomycosis patients at a university hospital. Trans R Soc Trop Med Hyg. 2011;105(8):473–8. https://doi.org/10.1016/j.trstmh.2011.03.001.
49. Guarro J. Fusariosis, a complex infection caused by a high diversity of fungal species refractory to treatment. Eur J Clin Microbiol Infect Dis. 2013;32(12):1491–500. https://doi.org/10.1007/s10096-013-1924-7.
50. Nucci M, Anaissie E. Fusarium infections in immunocompromised patients. Clin Microbiol Rev. 2007;20(4):695–704. https://doi.org/10.1128/CMR.00014-07.
51. Costa-Orlandi CB, Sardi JCO, Pitangui NS, et al. Fungal biofilms and polymicrobial diseases. J Fungi (Basel). 2017;3(2):E22. https://doi.org/10.3390/jof3020022.
52. Douglas AP, Chen SC-A, Slavin MA. Emerging infections caused by non-Aspergillus filamentous fungi. Clin Microbiol Infect. 2016;22(8):670–80. https://doi.org/10.1016/j.cmi.2016.01.011.
53. Batista BG, de Chaves MA, Reginatto P, Saraiva OJ, Fuentefria AM. Human fusariosis: an emerging infection that is difficult to treat. Rev Soc Bras Med Trop. 2020;53:e20200013. https://doi.org/10.1590/0037-8682-0013-2020.
54. Mohanty NK, Sahu S. Fusarium solani infection in a kidney transplant recipient. Indian J Nephrol. 2014;24(5):312–4. https://doi.org/10.4103/0971-4065.133014.
55. Bansal Y, Singla N, Kaistha N, Sood S, Chander J. Molecular identification of Fusarium species complex isolated from clinical samples and its antifungal susceptibility patterns. Curr Med Mycol. 2019;5(4):43–9. https://doi.org/10.18502/cmm.5.4.2149.
56. Stanzani M, Vianelli N, Bandini G, et al. Successful treatment of disseminated Fusariosis after allogeneic hematopoietic stem cell transplantation with the combination of voricon-

azole and liposomal amphotericin B. J Infect. 2006;53(6):e243–6. https://doi.org/10.1016/j.jinf.2006.02.011.
57. Pappas PG, Alexander BD, Andes DR, et al. Invasive fungal infections among organ transplant recipients: results of the Transplant-Associated Infection Surveillance Network (TRANSNET). Clin Infect Dis. 2010;50(8):1101–11. https://doi.org/10.1086/651262.
58. Vilchez R, Shapiro R, McCurry K, et al. Longitudinal study of cryptococcosis in adult solid-organ transplant recipients. Transpl Int. 2003;16(5):336–40. https://doi.org/10.1007/s00147-002-0541-7.
59. Ponzio V, Camargo LF, Medina-Pestana J, Perfect JR, Colombo AL. Outcomes of cryptococcosis in renal transplant recipients in a less-resourced health care system. Transpl Infect Dis. 2018;20(4):e12910. https://doi.org/10.1111/tid.12910.
60. Maziarz EK, Perfect JR. Cryptococcosis. Infect Dis Clin N Am. 2016;30(1):179–206. https://doi.org/10.1016/j.idc.2015.10.006.
61. Nowak MA, Putynkowska A, Barańska-Rybak W, Czarnacka K, Dębska-Ślizień MA. Cutaneous cryptococcosis: an underlying immunosuppression? Clinical manifestations, pathogenesis, diagnostic examinations and treatment. Postepy Dermatol Alergol. 2020;37(2):154–8. https://doi.org/10.5114/ada.2020.94833.
62. Sun H-Y, Alexander BD, Lortholary O, et al. Cutaneous cryptococcosis in solid organ transplant recipients. Med Mycol. 2010;48(6):785–91. https://doi.org/10.3109/13693780903496617.
63. Anderson DJ, Schmidt C, Goodman J, Pomeroy C. Cryptococcal disease presenting as cellulitis. Clin Infect Dis. 1992;14(3):666–72. https://doi.org/10.1093/clinids/14.3.666.
64. Rerolle J-P, Szelag J-C, Diaconita M, Paraf F, Aldigier J-C, Le Meur Y. Intracranial granuloma and skull osteolysis: complication of a primary cutaneous cryptococcosis in a kidney transplant recipient. Am J Kidney Dis. 2005;46(6):e113–7. https://doi.org/10.1053/j.ajkd.2005.09.003.
65. Perfect JR, Dismukes WE, Dromer F, et al. Clinical practice guidelines for the management of cryptococcal disease: 2010 update by the infectious diseases society of America. Clin Infect Dis. 2010;50(3):291–322. https://doi.org/10.1086/649858.
66. Baddley JW, Forrest GN, AST Infectious Diseases Community of Practice. Cryptococcosis in solid organ transplantation—Guidelines from the American Society of Transplantation Infectious Diseases Community of Practice. Clin Transplant. 2019;33(9):e13543. https://doi.org/10.1111/ctr.13543.
67. Wheat LJ, Azar MM, Bahr NC, Spec A, Relich RF, Hage C. Histoplasmosis. Infect Dis Clin N Am. 2016;30(1):207–27. https://doi.org/10.1016/j.idc.2015.10.009.
68. Freifeld AG, Wheat LJ, Kaul DR. Histoplasmosis in solid organ transplant recipients: early diagnosis and treatment. Curr Opin Organ Transplant. 2009;14(6):601–5. https://doi.org/10.1097/MOT.0b013e3283329c9a.
69. Gajurel K, Dhakal R, Deresinski S. Histoplasmosis in transplant recipients. Clin Transplant. 2017;31:10. https://doi.org/10.1111/ctr.13087.
70. Azar MM, Loyd JL, Relich RF, Wheat LJ, Hage CA. Current concepts in the epidemiology, diagnosis, and management of histoplasmosis syndromes. Semin Respir Crit Care Med. 2020;41(1):13–30. https://doi.org/10.1055/s-0039-1698429.
71. Cuellar-Rodriguez J, Avery RK, Lard M, et al. Histoplasmosis in solid organ transplant recipients: 10 years of experience at a large transplant center in an endemic area. Clin Infect Dis. 2009;49(5):710–6. https://doi.org/10.1086/604712.
72. Kauffman CA, Freifeld AG, Andes DR, et al. Endemic fungal infections in solid organ and hematopoietic cell transplant recipients enrolled in the Transplant-Associated Infection Surveillance Network (TRANSNET). Transpl Infect Dis. 2014;16(2):213–24. https://doi.org/10.1111/tid.12186.
73. Assi M, Martin S, Wheat LJ, et al. Histoplasmosis after solid organ transplant. Clin Infect Dis. 2013;57(11):1542–9. https://doi.org/10.1093/cid/cit593.
74. Farr B, Beacham BE, Atuk NO. Cutaneous histoplasmosis after renal transplantation. South Med J. 1981;74(5):635–7. https://doi.org/10.1097/00007611-198105000-00036.

75. Sun NZ, Augustine JJ, Gerstenblith MR. Cutaneous histoplasmosis in renal transplant recipients. Clin Transplant. 2014;28(10):1069–74. https://doi.org/10.1111/ctr.12409.
76. Wagner JD, Prevel CD, Elluru R. Histoplasma capsulatum necrotizing myofascitis of the upper extremity. Ann Plast Surg. 1996;36(3):330–3. https://doi.org/10.1097/00000637-199603000-00019.
77. Kozusko SD, Riccio CA, Minor GM, Konofaos P. Cutaneous histoplasmosis in a renal transplant patient presenting with hand and forearm necrotizing myofasciitis. J Hand Surg Am. 2020;45(3):260.e1–5. https://doi.org/10.1016/j.jhsa.2019.04.003.
78. Dufresne SF, LeBlanc RE, Zhang SX, Marr KA, Neofytos D. Histoplasmosis and subcutaneous nodules in a kidney transplant recipient: erythema nodosum versus fungal panniculitis. Transpl Infect Dis. 2013;15(2):E58–63. https://doi.org/10.1111/tid.12052.
79. Rappo U, Beitler JR, Faulhaber JR, et al. Expanding the horizons of histoplasmosis: disseminated histoplasmosis in a renal transplant patient after a trip to Bangladesh. Transpl Infect Dis. 2010;12(2):155–60. https://doi.org/10.1111/j.1399-3062.2009.00466.x.
80. Farges C, Cointault O, Murris M, et al. Outcomes of solid organ transplant recipients with invasive aspergillosis and other mold infections. Transpl Infect Dis. 2020;22(1):e13200. https://doi.org/10.1111/tid.13200.
81. Gavalda J, Len O, San Juan R, et al. Risk factors for invasive aspergillosis in solid-organ transplant recipients: a case-control study. Clin Infect Dis. 2005;41(1):52–9. https://doi.org/10.1086/430602.
82. Cadena J, Thompson GR, Patterson TF. Aspergillosis: epidemiology, diagnosis, and treatment. Infect Dis Clin N Am. 2021;35(2):415–34. https://doi.org/10.1016/j.idc.2021.03.008.
83. Kanj A, Abdallah N, Soubani AO. The spectrum of pulmonary aspergillosis. Respir Med. 2018;141:121–31. https://doi.org/10.1016/j.rmed.2018.06.029.
84. Kousha M, Tadi R, Soubani AO. Pulmonary aspergillosis: a clinical review. Eur Respir Rev. 2011;20(121):156–74. https://doi.org/10.1183/09059180.00001011.
85. Walsh TJ. Primary cutaneous aspergillosis—an emerging infection among immunocompromised patients. Clin Infect Dis. 1998;27(3):453–7. https://doi.org/10.1086/514718.
86. Ozcan D, Güleç AT, Haberal M. Multiple subcutaneous nodules leading to the diagnosis of pulmonary aspergillosis in a renal transplant recipient. Clin Transplant. 2008;22(1):120–3. https://doi.org/10.1111/j.1399-0012.2007.00740.x.
87. Ullmann AJ, Aguado JM, Arikan-Akdagli S, et al. Diagnosis and management of Aspergillus diseases: executive summary of the 2017 ESCMID-ECMM-ERS guideline. Clin Microbiol Infect. 2018;24(Suppl 1):e1–e38. https://doi.org/10.1016/j.cmi.2018.01.002.

Parasitic Diseases

Marilia Marufuji Ogawa and Daniel Wagner de Castro Lima Santos

1 Introduction

Despite of the improvement of clinical management of solid organ transplant recipient (SOTR), infection is still the leading cause of morbidity and mortality among this group of patients. Even though viral, bacterial, and fungal infection are the main agents, the report of parasitic infections has been increased [1]. It might be explained by the increase of migration flow from poor rural areas to large cities and non-endemic countries as well as people traveling to endemic areas. SOTR may acquire the endemic parasitosis by three ways: transmission with the graft, de novo infection, and activation of dormant infection as a consequence of immunosuppression [2].

The aim of this chapter is to point out some of the parasitic infections with cutaneous manifestation that specialist in SOTR must be aware of: Chagas disease, leishmaniasis, and schistosomiasis. Chronic immunosuppression modifies the natural history of these diseases, especially the clinical features, that often are severe, and the management, that is frequently unfamiliar to clinicians. Moreover, a parasitic disease that is common and we should be aware of is scabies.

M. M. Ogawa
Department of Dermatology, Escola Paulista de Medicina, Universidade Federal de São Paulo, São Paulo, SP, Brazil

D. W. de Castro Lima Santos (✉)
Instituto D'or de Pesquisa e Ensino (IDOR), Rio de Janeiro, Brazil

Department of Infectious Diseases, Hospital Universitário Presidente Dutra da Universidade Federal do Maranhão (HUUFMA), São Luís, MA, Brazil

J. Tomimori et al. (eds.), *Atlas of Dermatologic Diseases in Solid Organ Transplant Recipients*, https://doi.org/10.1007/978-3-031-13335-0_9

2 Chagas Disease

2.1 Epidemiology

Chagas disease was discovered by a Brazilian physician called Carlos Chagas in 1909. It is caused by the parasite *Trypanosoma cruzi* that is transmitted to humans by an infected insect vector, triatomine bugs. People living in rural areas, especially those who live in poor housing conditions, are at greatest risk of getting infected since the triatomine bugs thrive in walls made of mud and thatched roof. It is an endemic disease in America (South America, Central America, and Mexico) and according to the World Health Organization, it is currently estimated at least 1 million people infected by *T. cruzi* in Brazil and 6–7 million people worldwide [3].

2.2 Pathogenesis

The life cycle of *T. cruzi* is the following: an infected triatomine insect vector (or "kissing bug") takes a blood meal and releases trypomastigotes in its feces near the site of the bite wound. Trypomastigotes enter the host through the wound or through intact mucosal membranes, such as the conjunctiva. Inside the host, the trypomastigotes invade cells near the site of inoculation, where they differentiate into intracellular amastigotes. The amastigotes multiply by binary fission and differentiate into trypomastigotes, and then are released into the circulation as bloodstream trypomastigotes. Trypomastigotes infect cells from a variety of tissues (predilection for the heart, gastrointestinal, and brain system) and transform into intracellular amastigotes in new infection sites. Clinical manifestations can result from this infective cycle. The bloodstream trypomastigotes do not replicate. The "kissing bug" becomes infected by feeding on human or animal blood that contains circulating parasites. The ingested trypomastigotes transform into epimastigotes in the vector's midgut. The parasites multiply and differentiate in the midgut and differentiate into infective metacyclic trypomastigotes in the hindgut [3].

The most common form of infection is through contact with feces of an infected insect. The infection can also occur though mother to child, contaminated blood products (transfusion), and organ transplanted from an infected donor. Transmission of parasite via contaminated food and drink is very rare, but it has been reported in the past 15 years in Brazil (Amazon region) due to the ingestion of contaminated açai palm products [3, 4].

In SOTR, Chagas disease may occur as a consequence of transmission of *T. cruzi* with the transplanted organ, through reactivation of dormant infection, and through de novo infection. In a review of 23 cases, 18.7% was due to transmission and 22.7% reactivation [5].

2.3 *Clinical Presentation* (*Fig. 1a, b*)

Chagas disease has an acute and a chronic phase. The acute phase occurs immediately after the bite of an infected triatomine bug and can last up to a few weeks or months. During this phase, the patient is asymptomatic or presents a mild symptom, as fever or an erythematous-violaceous nodule at the site of inoculation, known as chagoma. If the parasite entrance is the conjunctiva, the patient may present palpebral edema, conjunctivitis, and regional adenopathy (Romaña sign). In the acute phase, most of the patients resolve the infection and the parasitemia levels become negative. When this acute phase is not diagnosed, the infection can progress and the amastigotes can remain quiet inside the organs' cells. In the chronic phase, the majority of patients remain asymptomatic, however, 20–30% of infected people will develop severe problems over the course of their lives that may include: heart arrhythmia, dilated heart, dilated esophagus or colon [3].

In Chagas disease, reactivation means the passage from a chronic or latent state in which the patient is stable to an acute condition with increased levels of parasitemia and serological markers detected by parasitological and/or polymerase chain reaction

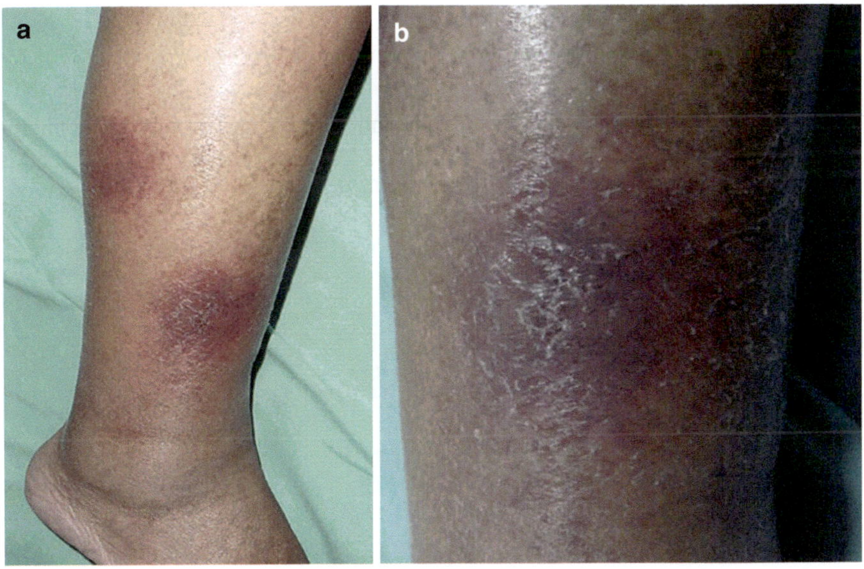

Fig. 1 (**a**) Chagas disease in a kidney transplant patient—presence of subcutaneous erythematous plaques on the leg. (**b**) Close-up view of the lesion. (Reproduced from Tomimori-Yamashita et al. 1997; Images collection, Department of Dermatology, EPM/Unifesp)

(PCR) techniques [6]. It occurs when the balance between infection and immunity breaks and the infection reappears and can be manifested in different clinical forms, such as fever, fatigue, anorexia, diarrhea, hepatosplenomegaly, cardiomyopathy, central nervous system, and cutaneous involvement [7–10]. The early diagnosis and prompt treatment are required to avoid the development of the disease to severe and even lethal forms [11, 12].

The cutaneous involvement of Chagas disease reactivation usually affects the hypodermis, so it manifests as subcutaneous nodules or panniculitis that may ulcerate, and it occurs specially during the first year posttransplantation because of intense immunosuppression [7, 8, 13–18].

Heart transplantation has become a usual indication for patients with end-stage chronic heart failure caused by Chagas cardiomyopathy in endemic countries. In this situation, Chagas disease should be routinely monitored because its reactivation may occur from 8% to 90% [19–21].

2.4 *Histopathology (Fig. 2a, b)*

Microscopic Chagas disease is characterized by diffuse lymphohistiocytic dermal infiltration with intracytoplasmic amastigotes of *T. cruzi* that can be confirmed by immunohistochemical analysis with anti-*T. cruzi* polyclonal antibody.

2.5 *Diagnosis*

The gold standard for the diagnosis of reactivation of Chagas disease is the microscopic identification of parasites from clinical specimens. Specific PCR in blood is also useful tool because of its high sensitivity [22].

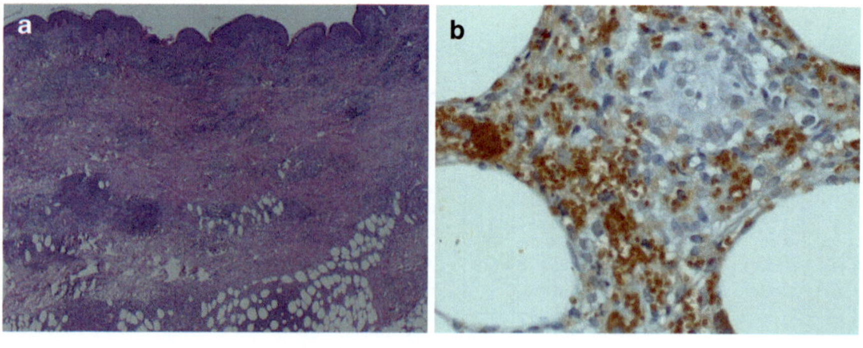

Fig. 2 (**a**) Skin biopsy of Chagas disease revealed diffuse dermal and hypodermal lymphohistiocytic infiltrate with compromise of lobular septa (Hematoxylin & eosin, 10×). (**b**) Ac polyclonal anti-*T. cruzi* revealed intracytoplasmic amastigotes. (Reproduced from Tomimori-Yamashita et al. 1997; Images collection, Department of Dermatology, EPM/Unifesp)

2.6 Treatment

Treatment of acute disease consists of either benznidazole (5 mg/kg daily) or nifurtimox (8–10 mg/kg daily), both drugs with significant toxicity, although the first is better tolerated. PCR should be performed weekly at least until two negative results are obtained. Follow-up should return to basal schedule of monitoring according to posttransplant time. Blood counts and hepatic enzymes should also be checked before treatment and 15–20 days after initiation because of bone marrow suppression and hepatotoxicity of the drug. Nifurtimox is preferred with resistant strains or benznidazole side effects, and it may cause peripheral polyneuritis and/or convulsions. Both treatments are suggested to be used for 30–60 days [5, 17]. Depending on the severity of Chagas disease reactivation, the treatment also requires lowering the doses, or switching to other immunosuppressant drugs especially if the patient is under mycophenolate mofetil because it showed a higher incidence of Chagas disease reactivation when compared to azathioprine [11].

2.7 Pre-transplant Screening for Chagas

According to Kocher et al. [11], the pre-transplant screening for Chagas disease in Europe should be done in patients originated from an endemic country (South and Central America, in the USA screening, Mexico is also included), those with a prolonged stay, over 6 months, in an endemic country, or extensive travel history to an endemic country. Without explicit travel history or migratory background from an endemic country, it is not standard to screen for Chagas disease, and specific procedures in a patient with a positive serology are yet to be defined. Considering the toxicity of trypanocidal drugs, a prophylactic treatment in all transplant recipients with positive serology does not seem to be justified, especially when taking into account the low number of disease reactivations and transmissions. No prospective data are available, but prophylactic treatment early after transplantation did not prevent reactivation in a small cohort [23].

The organ transplantation is possible even if the donor or recipient has a positive sorology for *T. cruzi* since a strategy of preventing reactivation and transmission has been established. On the other hand, the USA screening is against transplanting hearts from *T. cruzi*-infected donors, based on sparse data suggesting higher transmission risk and the known tropism of the parasite. Other organs (lung, pancreas, and intestines) can be considered with caution based on the anticipated degree of immunosuppression in the potential recipient and the urgency of the need for transplantation. All patients should provide appropriate informed consent concerning risks and benefits. The parameters that should be checked in a transplant recipient with a positive sorology for *T. cruzi* are: monthly specific *T. cruzi* PCR, even in the absence of symptoms; monthly blood smear for trypomastigote forms and clinical signs of Chagas disease reactivation. The USA screening recommends *T. cruzi*

PCR and microscopy of blood specimens weekly for the first 2 months, every 2 weeks during the third month, then monthly until at least 6 months posttransplantation [24].

3 Leishmaniasis

3.1 Epidemiology

Leishmaniasis is a protozoan disease transmitted through the bite of infected female sandflies of the genera Phlebotomus (Old World) and Lutzomyia (New World). Infection with *Leishmania* species may cause cutaneous, mucocutaneous, or visceral leishmaniasis (VL).

Visceral leishmaniasis (VL, kala-azar) occurs both in the "Old World" and in the "New World" and the causative agents are those in the *Leishmania donovani–L. infantum* complex. It is the most severe manifestation and it is estimated 50,000–90,000 new cases yearly [25]. Most cases occur in Brazil, East Africa, and in India. 60% of VL patients may present the post-kala-azar dermal (PKDL) manifestation and due to the presence of parasites in the skin, the patient may act as a human reservoir [26]. The PKDL is more common in India and less frequent in East Africa, rarely in Europe and America. The pathogenesis of PKDL is still unknown, several factors may be involved as genetic susceptibility, *Leishmania* species and the immune state of the host. The lesions appear from some months to 1–2 years after recovering from visceral leishmaniasis, demonstrating the failure of the cellular immunity in destroying the parasite at skin level [27].

Cutaneous leishmaniasis (CL) is the most common manifestation and more than 1 million new cases occur annually. It is endemic in more than 92 countries, in 2019 over 87% of new CL cases occurred in 10 countries: Afghanistan, Algeria, Brazil, Colombia, Iran (Islamic Republic of), Iraq, Libya, Pakistan, the Syrian Arab Republic, and Tunisia [25]. It is characterized by single or multiple skin ulcers and is associated with multiple species.

Mucocutaneous leishmaniasis (MCL) occurs in 1–10% in patients after a previous manifestation of leishmaniasis. It is often caused by *L. braziliensis* and *L. panamensis* and leads to metastasis of the disease to the mucosal tissues of the mouth and upper respiratory tract via lymphatic or hematogenous dissemination. Over 90% of mucocutaneous leishmaniasis cases occur in Bolivia, Brazil, Ethiopia, and Peru.

In immunocompromised patients, the VL is the most common manifestation associated with immunosuppression, followed by mucocutaneous presentation. Leishmaniasis is rare in SOTR but the publication of cases since 1990 has quadrupled [28] specially from the Mediterranean Basin, particularly in Spain, which is among the foremost in performing SOTR and is endemic for *L. infantum* transmission. However, in Brazil leishmaniasis among SOTR occurs 5.7 folds more frequent than in Spain since in Brazil the incidence of leishmaniasis is higher than in Spain [29]. So, the development of VL by SOTR is related to the degree of exposure to the infection [30]; moreover, the susceptibility of this group to develop the disease is 135 times higher than the immunocompetent patients living in the same endemic area [31]. It is relevant to know that over 1 billion people live in endemic areas of leishmaniasis, so they are at risk of infection [25]. Leishmaniasis may become symptomatic after natural infection through the bite of a sandfly, by reactivation of a dormant infection, or by introduction of the parasite through an organ graft, in the case of transplant patients.

3.2 Pathogenesis

Leishmania parasites are transmitted through the bites of infected female phlebotomine sandflies, which feed on blood to produce eggs. Approximately 30 species or subspecies of sandflies are proven vectors, however, more than 40 additional species are probably involved in transmission. The epidemiology of leishmaniasis depends on the characteristics of the parasite and sandfly species, the local ecological characteristics of the transmission sites, current and past exposure of the human population to the parasite, and human behavior. It is interesting to observe that the cutaneous leishmaniasis from the "Old World" (Africa, Asia, and Europe) occurs in open semi-arid or even desert conditions and the "New World" (Americas) is associated with forests [32], demonstrating the ability of sandfly to adapt in different setting of environments. Around 70 animal species have been found as natural reservoirs hosts of *Leishmania* parasite, however, with the ecological modifications made by men due to deforestation, agricultural practices, and urbanization caused the loss of this mammalian biodiversity forcing the sandfly to take blood from human beings. So, man is also becoming a natural reservoir of this parasite. The infected sandfly after biting their host regurgitate leishmania promastigotes into the skin which are phagocytosed mainly by macrophages where promastigotes transform in amastigotes. The amastigotes replicate and infect other macrophages. When the naïve sandflies feed on the blood of the infected host, the amastigotes transform back to promastigotes in the sandfly's gut and migrate to the proboscis, completing the leishmania life cycle. The development of the clinical manifestation of leishmaniasis will depend on the host, parasite, and the vector.

The pathogenesis of leishmaniasis is complex involves a set of interactions between host's innate and acquired immune responses and depending on these inflammatory responses will result in either asymptomatic or subclinical infection or chronic leishmaniasis. When the T-helper-1 cells predominate in response to leishmaniasis infection, it ensures clinical cure by activating macrophages and it also prevents recrudescence of latent chronic infection. Whereas the Th2 response deactivates macrophages and promotes intracellular infection.

In SOTR, the immunosuppressive drugs hamper the T cell activation and proliferation, consequently, facilitates the infection of intracellular microorganisms. There are two main possible pathogenic mechanisms for clinical manifestation of leishmaniasis in this group of patients, they can develop either from de novo acquisition of infection or reactivation of pre-existing latent leishmaniasis since the parasite can persist alive in the scar for years sustained by a persistent Th1 pattern of local immune response even after treatment [33, 34]. The reactivation can occur in the visceral form of the disease, and occasionally in the cutaneous form [28]. The mucosal reactivation is rare caused by a hyperimmune pattern of this form of the disease. The third possible pathogenic mechanism, the least common, is the iatrogenic transmission of leishmania by infected transplanted organ or following transfusion of infected blood products [28].

3.3 *Clinical Presentation (Figs. 3, 4, and 5)*

The clinical manifestation of tegumentary leishmaniasis is diverse and depends on the parasite and host immunity, although, most people who become infected with *Leishmania* spp. do not develop the disease [25]. The clinical presentation can be classified as the following:

(a) Localized Cutaneous Leishmaniasis: It is characterized by single or multiple ulcers located in one region of the body exposed to the bite of the phlebotomine sandfly. The ulcer presents well delimited and raised borders, with varied sizes and usually painless. Several species from New World and Old World are involved.
(b) Disseminated Leishmaniasis: This is a severe and emerging manifestation of *Leishmania (Viannia) braziliensis* characterized by multiple polymorphic lesions (>10) in different areas of the body, including nasal mucosal involvement in over 50% of cases [35].

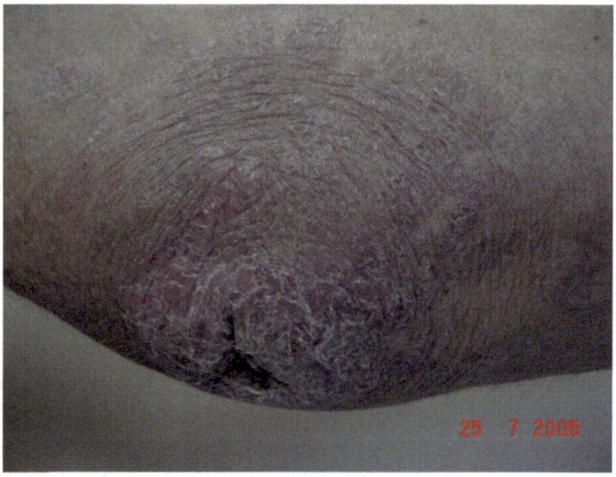

Fig. 3 Leishmaniasis in a kidney transplant receptor—erythematous scaling plaque on the elbow in a renal transplant receptor

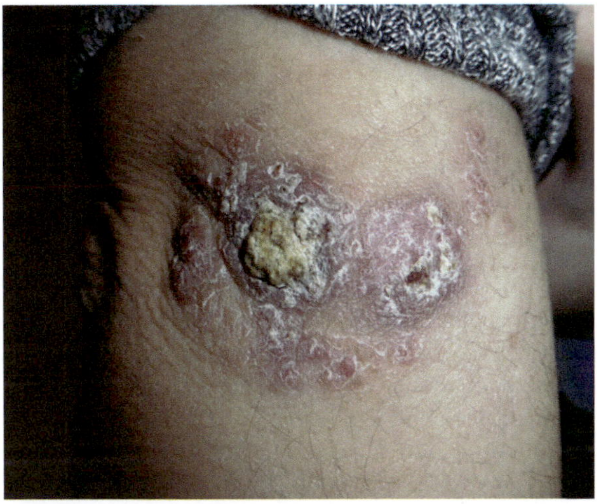

Fig. 4 Cutaneous leishmaniasis; verrucous plaque in a 24-year-old female patient iatrogenically immunosuppressed. (Courtesy of Dr. Maria Ubals, Vall d'Hebron University Hospital, Barcelona)

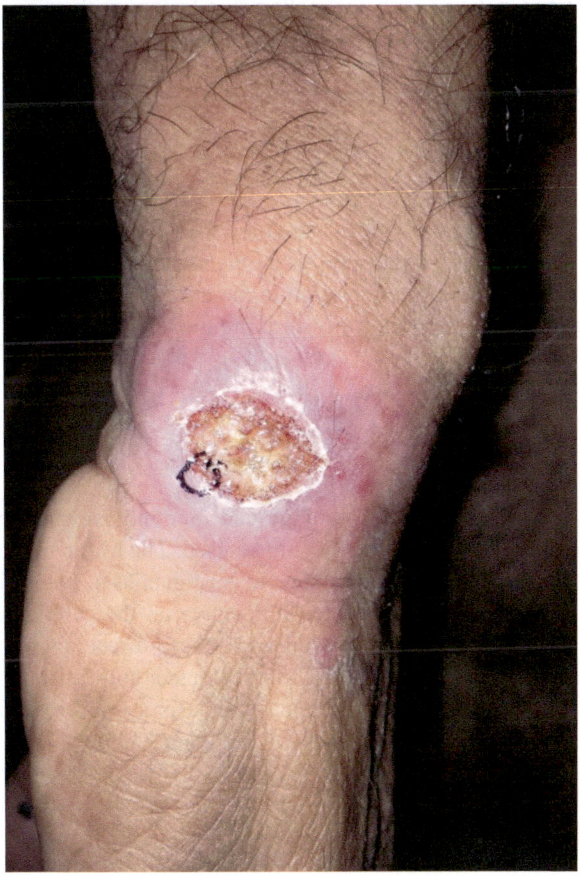

Fig. 5 Cutaneous leishmaniasis in a 72-year-old, immunosuppressed patient. (Courtesy of Dr. Maria Ubals, Vall d'Hebron University Hospital, Barcelona)

(c) Diffuse Cutaneous Leishmaniasis: This is a very rare form of leishmaniasis caused by *Leishmania (Leishmania) amazonensis* characterized by an inefficient parasite-specific cellular response and heavily parasitized macrophages. Clinical aspects are nodules, plaques, and vegetative/verrucous lesions disseminated on the body.
(d) Mucocutaneous Leishmaniasis: It is a very destructive form of leishmaniasis, especially of the nasal septum cartilage but can also affect the palate, lips, tongue, pharynx, and larynx. It usually manifests when localized cutaneous leishmaniasis was not treated or inadequately treated.

The cutaneous presentation among SOTR is uncommon and occurs as a late complication after transplantation. Clinical manifestation of cutaneous leishmaniasis is often similar to immunocompetent patients, but atypical forms have been reported, including erythematous papules and violaceous nodules or plaques [36, 37]; multiple, non-ulcerated, painful nodules [38]; progression of localized leishmaniasis to disseminated cutaneous leishmaniasis [39] or mucosal and cutaneous ulcer caused by visceral leishmaniasis [40]. Because of these different presentations, patients with nonhealing skin lesions with an epidemiology for leishmaniasis should be evaluated for leishmaniasis [41].

3.4 Histopathology *(Fig. 6a–c)*

The histopathology exam demonstrates chronic inflammation with tuberculoid granulomas, and the presence of leishmania amastigotes within macrophages. Plasmocytes are usually present in the inflammatory infiltration. Immunohistochemical exam is useful tool for confirming the diagnosis.

3.5 Diagnosis

It is based on histopathology and immunohistochemical exam, but if the microscopy is negative, a PCR could be used. The Montenegro skin test is a useful tool for detecting previous exposure to leishmaniasis, but in immunosuppressed patients does not have value since it depends on the cellular immunity. Serological tests, such as indirect immunofluorescence, direct agglutination, and enzyme-linked immunosorbent assay (ELISA) to detect anti-Leishmania antibodies are not commonly used in cutaneous leishmaniasis as well as in immunosuppressed patients because of reduced level of antibodies and variable specificity and sensitivity rates [42].

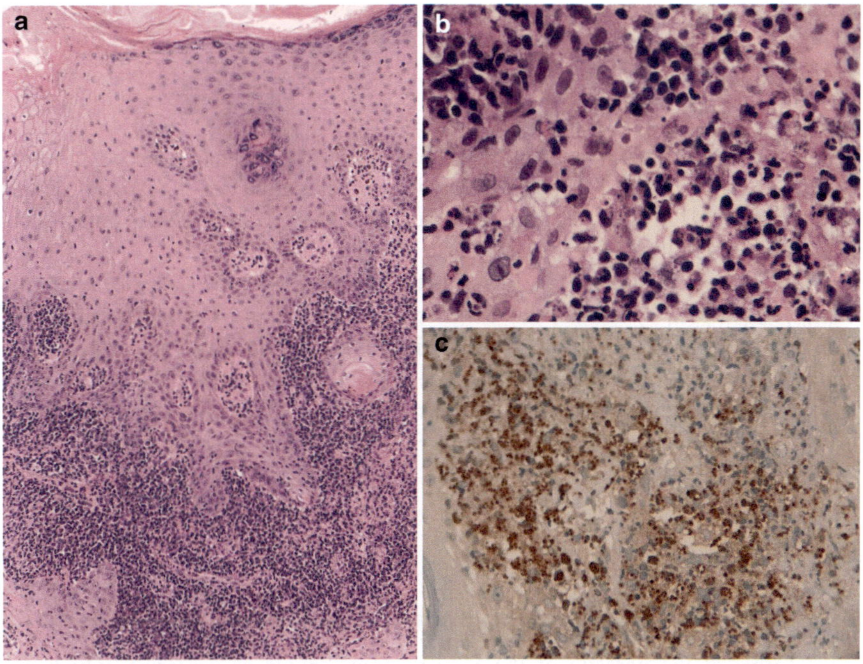

Fig. 6 Microscopic image of cutaneous Leishmaniasis. (**a**) Inflammatory granulomatous with dermal infiltrate and epidermal hyperplasia. (H&E). (**b**) Leishmania amastigotes in dermal infiltrate with histiocytes, plasma cells, and neutrophils (H&E). (**c**) Specific Immunohistochemistry for Leishmaniasis. (Courtesy of Dr. Maria Ubals, Vall d'Hebron University Hospital, Barcelona)

3.6 Treatment

The treatment of leishmaniasis in SOTR depends on patient's immune status, concomitant infections and liver, kidney, and cardiac functions; as well as on the type of Leishmania species and the severity of the clinical manifestation.

Liposomal amphotericin B is the first-line treatment for cutaneous and visceral leishmaniasis in SOTR since it shows high cure rates for cutaneous and mucocutaneous leishmaniasis. There are some side effects that should be considered, back pain during the infusion, electrolytes disturbances, infusion reactions, and nephrotoxicity.

Available data to determine the value of screening both donor and receptor of SOTR is still lacking. However, in case the SOTR at the time of transplantation is serologically positive for leishmaniasis, he should be closely monitored. Donor screening is not recommended due to the scarcity of data [41, 43].

4 Schistosomiasis

4.1 Epidemiology

Schistosomiasis is a parasitic chronic disease of poverty that causes severe morbidity, and it is one of the 17 neglected diseases classified by the World Health Organization [44]. It is caused by trematode flukes of the genus Schistosoma affecting around 300 million people each year.

Three main Schistosoma species affect human beings, *Schistosoma haematobium, Schistosoma mansoni*, and *Schistosoma japonicum. S. haematobium* and *S. mansoni* occur more frequently in Africa and Middle East. *S. mansoni* and *S. japonicum* in China and Philippines. The distribution of the parasite is defined by the host snails' habitat range. In Americas, Brazil has the largest endemic region, followed by other countries as Venezuela, Suriname, and Caribbean Islands [44].

4.2 Pathogenesis

Schistosomiasis is a parasitic disease acquired when people come into contact with larval forms of the parasite of the Schistosoma, known as cercariae, which are released by freshwater snails acting as intermediate hosts and penetrate the human's skin and develop into the mature worms. Usually, the first contact of the human with the parasite occurs by the age of 2 years reaching the highest prevalence in young adolescents, while wading, bathing, or washing in contaminated water. Humans are the definitive host of *Schistosoma* spp. and the mature worms live in humans from 3 to 10 years. The worms reach the liver where they mature and copulate. One female worm produces about 300 eggs daily. Half of these eggs are eliminated in the feces (*S. mansoni* and *S. japonicum*) or urine (*S. haematobium*) and part of them are retained in the tissue specially from liver and intestine provoking granuloma formation and leading to irreversible damage of the tissue. The infected person defecates near freshwater, the eggs are hatched and the larvae infects the intermediate snail host completing the life cycle of schistosomiasis [45].

There are few cases reported of transmission of schistosome through transplantation of an infected liver as well as posttranplant schistosomiasis that occurred with patients from endemic areas and in these cases the infection may be due to a reactivation of a prior infection in consequence of immunosuppression [46, 47]. There are also few reports of posttransplant schistosomiasis and these patients came from endemic area, and it might be due to a reactivation of a prior infection in consequence of immunosuppression [47]. If the live donor and recipient were correctly treated before transplantation, schistosomiasis infection is not considered a contraindication for transplantation [48, 49].

4.3 Clinical Presentation

The symptoms will depend on the body's reaction to the parasites' eggs. Most of the cases of schistosomiasis is asymptomatic at the initial stage. However, some patients may develop an itching dermatosis, cercarial dermatitis, characterized by small papules that lasts from 24 to 72 h at the site of the parasites' penetration. Some patients might develop within 1–2 months of infection skin rash with fever, chills, muscle ache, cough, diarrhea, abdominal pain, and hepatosplenomegaly (Katayama fever). Eosinophilia is frequent at this stage. If not treated, the schistosomiasis can persist for years. The symptoms and signs of chronic schistosomiasis include abdominal pain, blood in the stool or blood in the urine, and hepatomegaly. Complications of chronic schistosomiasis infection are liver fibrosis and bladder cancer.

Another manifestation that is not common is the cutaneous ectopic schistosomiasis that occurs when worms deposit their ova in a vein that irrigates the skin. It causes skin lesions characterized by grouped, erythematous, itchy, papular lesions, or nodules localized more often at the lower torso, periumbilical region, genital, and pelvic area. This clinical manifestation usually occurs 4 weeks to 2 years after infection [50, 51].

4.4 Histopathology (Fig. 7)

Microscopically, it is characteristic to observe in the dermis the schistosome egg surrounded by epithelioid granuloma.

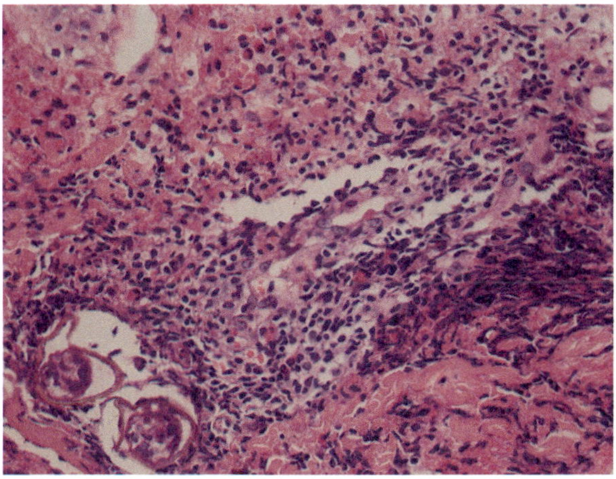

Fig. 7 The skin biopsy revealed the presence of a mixed inflammatory infiltrate with eosinophils. At inferior left corner, two eggs with lateral spike of *S. mansoni* are observed (Hematoxylin-eosin, 400×)

4.5 Diagnosis

Diagnosis is confirmed by microscopic exam of stool or urine for schistosome eggs (stool for *S. mansoni* or *S. japonicum* eggs and urine for *S. haematobium* eggs).

4.6 Treatment

Praziquantel is the drug of choice, 40 mg/kg per day orally for 1 day for *S. mansoni* and *S. haematobium* and 60 mg/kg per day orally for 1 day for *S. japonicum*.

5 Scabies

5.1 Epidemiology

Scabies is a highly contagious skin infestation caused by the mite, *Sarcoptes scabiei* var. *hominis*, an obligated human parasite. It has been considered as a mankind plague over 2500 years [52], and it is still a public health issue in all countries. Diagnosis of scabies is a challenge since pruritus is not an uncommon complain among SOTR since it can be related to drugs or to the transplant but physicians should consider scabies being one of the causes of pruritus in this population. Scabies affects annually 200–300 million people worldwide. In developing countries, the average incidence in children is around 5–10% and affects more children and elderly people [53, 54]. Transmission occurs after close skin-to-skin contact with infected person including sexual contact. Transmission through fomites may also occur. It is a worldwide disease, however, is more common in tropical countries. Outbreaks may occur in institutional settings, homeless people, immigrants, and after natural disasters [53].

5.2 Clinical Presentation (Figs. 8, 9, and 10)

Nocturnal pruritus is the hallmark of this disease with skin lesions characterized by multiple erythematous papules and burrows on finger webspace, wrist, axillae, waistline, areola (woman), and genital (man). Frequently, secondary lesions are seen such as excoriation, eczematous plaques, and impetigo. Scalp, palms, and soles are affected in infants, elderly, and immunocompromised patients.

In SOTR, as a consequence of the immunosuppressive regimen, are at high risk of getting the crusted scabies (also known as Norwegian scabies). This is a rare form

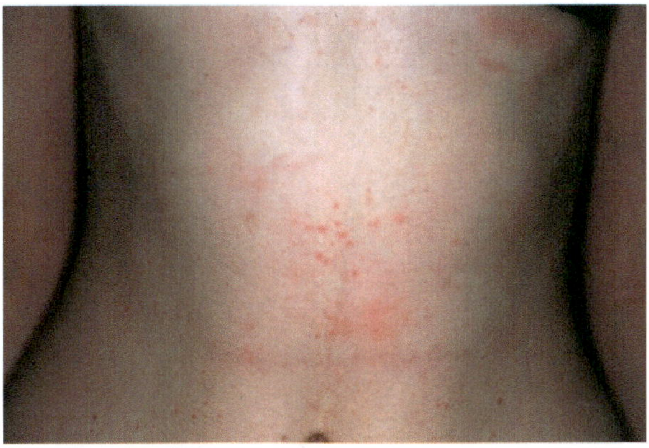

Fig. 8 Scabies in a renal transplant recipient—erythematous papules and excoriation on the abdomen

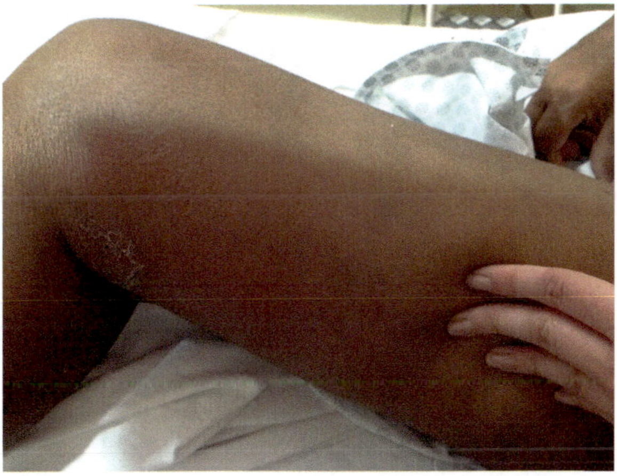

Fig. 9 Scabies in a renal transplant recipient—erythematous plaque with minimum scaling on lateral thigh

associated with T cell dysregulation characterized by high mite burden as high as 4700 mites/g of skin [55]. It presents clinically as thick crusted and hyperkeratotic plaques in an acral region as well as erythematous to gray scaly lesions on face, neck, scalp, and trunk. Concomitant bacterial or viral infection may occur, and it has been reported fatal cases due to the secondary infection [56, 57].

5.3 *Diagnosis (Figs. 11a, b, 12a, b, and 13a, b)*

The diagnosis of scabies is based on clinical findings. Scabies mites or eggs may be found by scraping the skin at the end of burrows and examined in a drop of 10% potassium hydroxide with the microscope (Müller Test). Dermoscopy is another method that helps localize the scabies mite allowing the skin scraping exam to be more accurate [58]. Biopsy may be performed and it reveals the presence of mite.

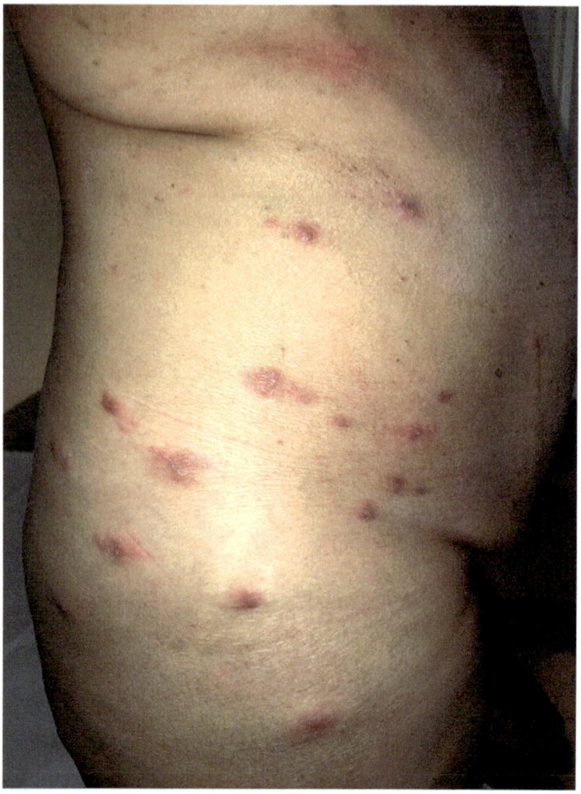

Fig. 10 Inflammatory scabies an inflammatory plaque was surrounding every burrow in a kidney transplant recipient. (Courtesy of Dr. Carla Ferrándiz-Pulido, Vall d'Hebron University Hospital, Barcelona)

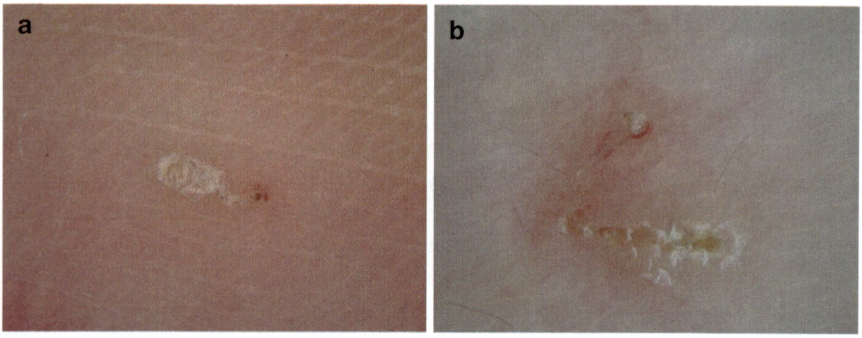

Fig. 11 (**a**) Dermatoscopic image of a track-like burrow with the typical delta wing sign (courtesy of Dr. Álvaro Gómez-Tomás, Vall d'Hebron University Hospital, Barcelona). (**b**) Dermatoscopic image of a track-like burrow with the typical delta wing sign. (Courtesy of Dr. Pablo Castro-Garcia, Vall d'Hebron University Hospital, Barcelona)

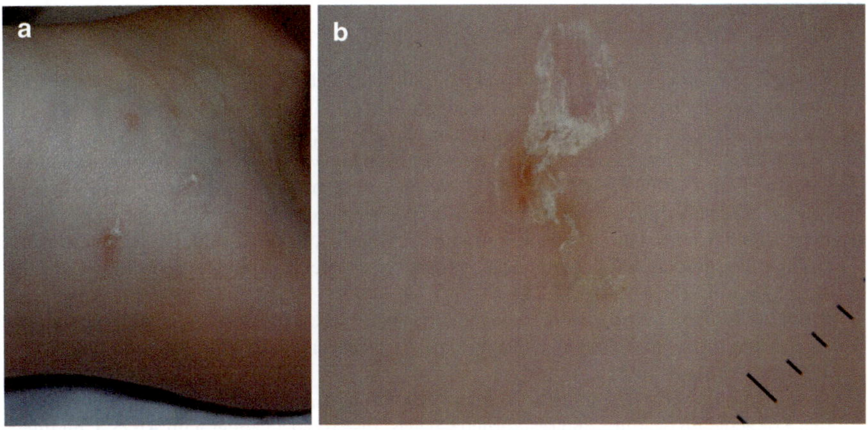

Fig. 12 (**a**) Clinical image of a track-like burrow on the wrist. (**b**) Corresponding dermatoscopic image Dr. Pablo Castro-Garcia, Vall d'Hebron University Hospital, Barcelona

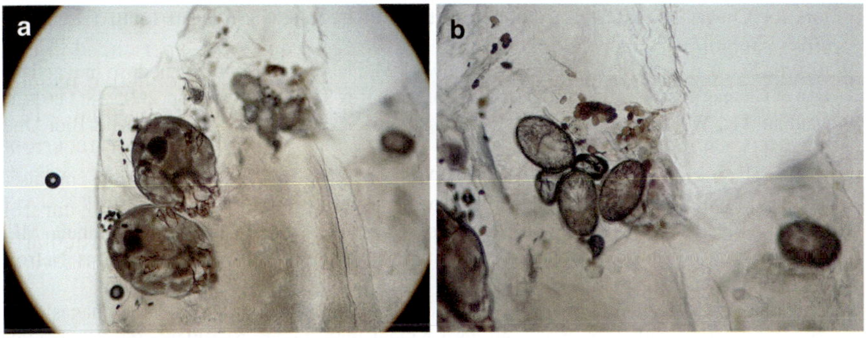

Fig. 13 (**a, b**) Mueller test. (Courtesy Dr. Pablo Castro-Garcia, Vall d'Hebron University Hospital, Barcelona)

5.4 Treatment

Ivermectin is a safe and effective drug for scabies treatment in SOTR. In crusted scabies, ivermectin has to be associated with topical treatment such as permethrin 5% and a keratolytic cream in order to reduce the crusting [59]. Ivermectin in this group of patients needs to be prolonged for more than 2 weeks [60], and in refractory cases 1-week course of daily ivermectin (0.2 mg/kg/dose) has been suggested. In this case, a close monitoring of liver function is required [61].

References

1. Silvia F, Simona F, Fabrizio B. Solid organ transplant and parasitic diseases: a review of the clinical cases in the last two decades. Pathogens. 2018;7(3):65–96.
2. Barsoum R. Parasitic infections in organ transplantations. Exp Clin Transplant. 2004;2:258–67.
3. World Health Organization. Chagas disease (also known as American trypanosomiasis). Geneva: WHO; 2020 [2020 Jun 15]. Available from: https://www.who.int/en/news-room/fact-sheets/detail/chagas-disease-(american-trypanosomiasis).
4. Ferreia RTB, Cabral ML, Martins RS, Araujo PF, Silva SA, Britto C, et al. Detection and genotyping of *Trypanosoma cruzi* from açai products commercialized in Rio de Janeiro and Pará, Brazil. Parasit Vectors. 2018;11:233–44.
5. Riarte A, Luna C, Sabatiello R, Sinagra A, Schiavelli R, De Rissio A, et al. Chagas' disease in patients with kidney transplants: 7 years of experience 1989-1996. Clin Infect Dis. 1999;29(3):561–7.
6. Sartori AM, Lopes MH, Caramelli B, Duarte MI, Pinto PL, Neto V, et al. Simultaneous occurrence of acute myocarditis and reactivated Chagas' disease in a patient with AIDS. Clin Infect Dis. 1995;21(5):1297–9.
7. Bocchi EA, Bellotti G, Uip D, Kalil J, de Lourdes HM, Stolfi N, et al. Long-term follow-up after heart transplantation in Chagas' disease. Transplant Proc. 1993;25(1 Pt 2):1329–30.
8. Campos SV, Strabelli TM, Amato Neto V, Silva CP, Bacal F, Bocchi EA, et al. Risk factors for Chagas' disease reactivation after heart transplantation. J Heart Lung Transplant. 2008;27(6):597–602.
9. d'Avila SC, d'Avila AM, Pagliari C, Goncalves VM, Duarte MI. Erythema nodoso in reactivation of Chagas' disease after cardiac transplantation. Rev Soc Bras Med Trop. 2005;38(1):61–3.
10. Vaidian AK, Weiss LM, Tanowitz HB. Chagas' disease and AIDS. Kinetoplastid Biol Dis. 2004;3(1):2–8.
11. Kocher C, Segerer S, Schleich A, Caduff R, Wyler LG, Muller V, et al. Skin lesions, malaise, and heart failure in a renal transplant recipient. Transpl Infect Dis. 2012;14(4):391–7.
12. Campos FP, Pansard HM, Arantes LC, Rodrigues AT, Daubermann MF, Azambuja MF, et al. A case of Chagas' disease panniculitis after kidney transplantation. J Bras Nefrol. 2016;38(1):127–31.
13. Gallerano V, Consigli J, Pereyra S, Zanni GS, Danielo C, Gallerano RH, et al. Chagas' disease reactivation with skin symptoms in a patient with kidney transplant. Int J Dermatol. 2007;46(6):607–10.
14. Navarro TC, Hidalgo PI, Enz P, Galimberti G, Galimberti RL. Chagas disease: cutaneous manifestation of a patient with liver transplantation. Reactivation. Med Cutan Iber Lat Am. 2007;35(1):25–8.
15. Riganti J, Maqueda MG, Piñero MC, Volonteri VI, Galimberti RL. Reactivation of Chagas' disease: cutaneous manifestations in two immunosuppressed patients. Int J Dermatol. 2012;51(7):829–34.
16. Fassi MV, Bosch MP, Garay IS, Kurpis M, Ruiz-Lascano A. Cellulite as unique expression of Chagas skin reactivation in a kidney transplant patient. Rev Argent Dermatol. 2014;95(2):21–4.
17. Ferraresso MG, Torre AC, Piva MMM, Barcan L. Chagas disease reactivation: cutaneous manifestations in a transplanted patient. An Bras Dermatol. 2018;93(6):890–2.
18. Oliveira WRP, Romero-Sandoval K, Magalhães TS, Giannotti MA, Tyring SK, da Costa PVA. Lobular panniculitis of the thigh as the only cutaneous manifestation of reactivation of Chagas disease in a renal transplant patient a case report. Rev Soc Bras Med Trop. 2021;54:e0269–2020.
19. Bacal F, Silva CP, Bocchi EA, Pires PV, Moreira LFP, Issa VS, et al. Mycophenolate mofetil increased Chagas disease reactivation in heart transplanted patients: comparison between two different protocols. Am J Transplant. 2005;5(8):2017–21.

20. Bestetti RB, Souza TR, Lima MF, Theodoropoulus TAD, Cordeirao JA, Burdmann EA. Effects of a mycophenolate mofetil-based immunosuppressive regimen in Chagas heart transplant recipients. Transplantation. 2007;84(3):441–2.
21. Bacal F, Silva CP, Pires PV, Mangini S, Fiorelli AI, Stolf NG, Bocchi EA. Transplantation for Chagas disease: an overview of immunosuppression and reactivation in the last two decades. Clin Transplant. 2010;24(2):E29–34.
22. Costa PA, Segatto M, Durso DF, Moreira WJC, Junqueira LL, Castilho FM, et al. Early polymerase chain reaction detection of Chagas disease reactivation in heart transplant patient. J Heart Lung Transplant. 2017;36(7):797–805.
23. Fiorelli AI, Santos RH, Oliveira JL Jr, Lourenço-Filho DD, Dias RR, Oliveira AS, et al. Heart transplantation in 107 cases of Chagas' disease. Transplant Proc. 2011;43(1):220–4.
24. Chin-Hong PV, Schwartz BS, Bern C, Montgomery SP, Kontak S, Kubak B, et al. Screening and treatment of Chagas' disease in organ transplant recipients in the United States: recommendation from the Chagas in transplant working group. Am J Transplant. 2011;11(4):672–80.
25. World Health Organization. Leishmaniasis Geneva: WHO; 2021 [2021 May 21]. Available from: https://www.who.int/news-room/fact-sheets/detail/leishmaniasis.
26. Zijlstra EE. PKDL and other dermal lesions in HIV co-infected patients with Leishmaniasis: review of clinical presentation in relation to immune responses. PLoS Negl Dis. 2014;8(11):e3258–70.
27. Roustan G, Jiménez JA, Gutiérrez-Solar B, Gallego JL, Alvar J, Patrón M. Post-kala-azar dermal leishmaniasis with mucosal involvement in a kidney transplant recipient: treatment with liposomal amphotericin B. Br J Dermatol. 1998;138(3):526–8.
28. Antinori S, Cascio A, Parravicini C, Bianchi R, Corbellino M. Leishmaniasis among organ transplant recipients. Lancet Infect Dis. 2008;8(3):191–9.
29. Clemente W, Vidal E, Girão E, Ramos AS, Govedic F, Merino E, et al. Risk factors, clinical features and outcomes of visceral leishmaniasis in solid-organ transplant recipients: a retrospective multicenter case-control study. J Clin Microbiol Infect. 2015;21(1):89–95.
30. Akuffo H, Costa C, van Griensven J, Burza S, Moreno J, Herrero M. New insights into leishmaniasis in the immunosuppressed. PLoS Negl Trop Dis. 2018;12(5):e0006375.
31. Carrasco-Anton N, Lopez-Medrano F, Fernandez-Ruiz M, Carrillo E, Moreno J, Garcia-Reyne A, et al. Environmental factors as key determinants for visceral leishmaniasis in solid organ transplant recipients, Madrid, Spain. Emerg Infect Dis. 2017;23(7):1155–9.
32. Reithinger R, Dujardin J-C, Louzir H, Pirmez C, Alexander B, Brooker S. Cutaneous leishmaniasis. Lancet Infect Dis. 2007;7(9):581–96.
33. Tuon FF, Amato VS, Floeter-Winter LM, de Andrade ZR, Amato Neto V, Siqueira França FO, et al. Cutaneous leishmaniasis reactivation 2 years after treatment caused by systemic corticosteroids—first report. Int J Dermatol. 2007;46(6):628–30.
34. Oliveira-Neto MP, Mattos M, Souza CS, Fernandes O, Pirmez C. Leishmaniasis recidiva cutis in New World cutaneous leishmaniasis. Int J Dermatol. 1998;37(11):846–9.
35. Machado GU, Prates FV, Machado PRL. Disseminated leishmaniasis: clinical, pathogenic, and therapeutic aspects. An Bras Dermatol. 2019;94:9–16.
36. Vinhal FA, Afonso-Cardoso SR, Silva AG, Pereira CG, Sousa W, Botelho SM, et al. Atypical presentation of cutaneous leishmaniasis after renal transplantation. Nephrol Dial Transpl. 2007;22(12):3674.
37. Yaich S, Charfeddine K, Masmoudi A, Masmoudi M, Zaghdhane S, Turki H, et al. Atypical presentation of cutaneous leishmaniasis in a renal transplant recipient successfully treated with allopurinol and fluconazole. Ann Saudi Med. 2013;33(2):187–91.
38. Mirzabeigi M, Farooq U, Baraniak S, Dowdy L, Ciancio G, Vincek V. Reactivation of dormant cutaneous Leishmania infection in a kidney transplant patient. J Cutan Pathol. 2006;33(10):701–4.
39. Zandieh A, Basira Zandieh B, Ladan D. Dissemination of localized cutaneous leishmaniasis in an organ transplant recipient: case report and literature review. Int J Dermatol. 2013;52(1):59–62.

40. Simon I, Wissing KM, Del Marmol V, Antinori S, Remmelink M, Nilufer BE. Recurrent leishmaniasis in kidney transplant recipients: report of 2 cases and systematic review of the literature. Transpl Infect Dis. 2011;13(4):397–406.
41. Clemente WT, Mourão PHO, Lolpez-Medarno F, Schwartz BS, García-Donoso C, Torre-Cisneros J. Visceral and cutaneous leishmaniasis recommendations for solid organ transplant recipients and donor. Transplantation. 2018;102(2S Suppl 2):S8–S15.
42. Anversa L, Tiburcio MGS, Richini-Pereira VB, Ramirez LE. Human leishmaniasis in Brazil: a general review. Rev Assoc Med Bras. 2018;64(3):281–9.
43. Schwartz BS, Mawhorter SD, AST Infectious Diseases Community of Practice. Parasitic infections in solid organ transplantation. Am J Transplant. 2013;13(Suppl 4):280–313.
44. World Health Organization. Schistosomiasis. Geneva: WHO; 2021 [2021 May 18]. Available from: https://www.who.int/news-room/fact-sheets/detail/schistosomiasis.
45. Colley DG, Bustinduy AL, Secor WE, King CH. Human schistosomiasis. Lancet. 2014;383(9936):2253–64.
46. Pannegeon V, Masini JP, Paye F, Chazouillères O, Girard PM. *Schistosoma mansoni* infection and liver graft. Transplantation. 2005;80(2):287.
47. Hoare M, Gelson WT, Davies SE, Curran M, Alexander GJ. Hepatic and intestinal schistosomiasis after orthotopic liver transplant. Liver Transpl. 2005;11(12):1603–7.
48. Mahmoud KM, Sobh MA, El-Agroudy AE, Mostafa FE, Baz ME, Shokeir AA. Impact of schistosomiasis on patient and graft outcome after renal transplantation: 10 years' follow-up. Nephrol Dial Transplant. 2001;16(11):2214–21.
49. Martín-Dávila P, Fortún J, López-Vélez R, Norman F, de Oca MM, Zamarrón P. Transmission of tropical and geographically restricted infections during solid-organ transplantation. Clin Microbiol Rev. 2008;21(1):60–6.
50. Vargas TJS, Lopes R, Palermo ML, Moraes FN, Azevedo KGP, Sousa MAJ. Ectopic cutaneous schistosomiasis. An Bras Dermatol. 2013;88(5):820–2.
51. van Dijk K, Starink MK, Bart A, Nijihuis EWP, van der Wal AC, van Thiel PPAM, et al. The potential of molecular diagnosis of cutaneous ectopic schistosomiasis. Am J Trop Med Hyg. 2010;83(4):958–9.
52. Hengge UR, Currie BJ, Jager G, et al. Scabies: a ubiquitous neglected skin disease. Lancet Infect Dis. 2006;6:769–79.
53. Thomas C, Coates SJ, Engelman D, Chosidow O, Chang AY. Part I—Ectoparasites: scabies. JAAD. 2020;82(3):533–48.
54. Leung AKC, Lam JM, Leong KF. Scabies: a neglected global disease. Curr Ped Rev. 2020;16(1):33–42.
55. Walton SF, McBroom J, Mathews JD, Kemp DJ, Currie BJ. Crusted scabies: a molecular analysis of Sarcoptes scabiei variety hominis populations from patients with repeated infestations. Clin Infect Dis. 1999;29(5):1226–30.
56. Mansy H, Somorin A, el-Sherif M, Eze C, al-Dusari S, Filobbos P. Norwegian scabies complicated by fatal brain abscess in a renal transplant patient. Nephron. 1996;72(2):323–4.
57. Abdo A, Kouri V, Burgos D, Urquiza A, Limonta D, Afonso C, et al. Norwegian scabies associated with herpes simplex infection in a renal transplant patient. Transplantation. 2009;87(6):943–4.
58. Fox G. Diagnosis of scabies by dermoscopy. BMJ Case Rep. 2009;2009:bcr06.2008.0279.
59. Centers for Disease Control and Prevention. CDC—scabies—resources for health professionals—medications. 2016. https://www.cdc.gov/parasites/scabies/healthprofessionals/meds.html.
60. Ortega-Loayza AG, McCall CO, Nunley JR. Crusted scabies and multiple dosages of ivermectin. J Drugs Dermatol. 2013;12(5):584–5.
61. Wang MK, Chin-Yee B, Lo CK, Lee S, El-Helow P, Alowami S, et al. Crusted scabies in a renal transplant recipient treated with daily ivermectin: a case report and literature review. Transpl Infect Dis. 2019;21(3):e13077–84.

Sexually Transmitted Infections

Isadora Zago Miotto and Walmar Roncalli Pereira de Oliveira

1 Human Papillomavirus

1.1 Epidemiology

Human papillomavirus (HPV) infection is one of the most common sexually transmitted diseases worldwide and can have an exuberant presentation in SOTRs. Risk factors for HPV infection include an increased number of lifetime sexual partners, long-term oral contraceptive use, history of chlamydia infection, and immunosuppression [1, 2].

An estimated 291 million women worldwide are carriers of HPV DNA, and high-risk genital HPVs have been reported in at least 10% of female liver transplant recipients [1]. There is also a high prevalence of HPV 16 in female renal transplant recipients. The prevalence of anal HPV infection ranges from 18% to 23% in SOTRs [3–5]. Anogenital invasive squamous cell carcinoma (SCC) related to HPV infection is 10 times more common in the immunosuppressed population, which is particularly associated with the high-risk HPVs 16 and 18 [6].

1.2 Pathogenesis

HPVs are small double-stranded DNA viruses with a tropism for the anogenital area that can induce a variety of mucocutaneous lesions and malignancies. HPVs are divided into two major groups: low-risk, non-oncogenic HPV types, associated with

I. Z. Miotto (✉) · W. R. P. de Oliveira
Department of Dermatology, Hospital of Clinics, University of São Paulo Medical School, São Paulo, SP, Brazil
e-mail: walmar.roncalli@hc.fm.usp.br

J. Tomimori et al. (eds.), *Atlas of Dermatologic Diseases in Solid Organ Transplant Recipients*, https://doi.org/10.1007/978-3-031-13335-0_10

anogenital warts and recurrent respiratory papillomatosis; and high-risk, oncogenic types, associated with vulvar, vaginal, cervical, anal, penile, and oropharyngeal malignancies [1, 7].

The vast majority of HPV infections are acquired via direct person-to-person contact. There are no reports of HPV transmission through organ transplantation; however, SOTRs are at a higher risk of infection compared to the general population [3].

The virus first infects the basal epithelial cells of keratinized skin, mucous membranes, and the transformation zone of the cervix [8]. T-cell immune response is crucial in preventing the development and progression of HPV infection. Immunocompromised individuals are unable to mount an adequate T-helper 1 (Th1) cell-mediated immune response against HPV infection. Therefore, they may develop multiple, extensive, and recalcitrant viral warts, which when associated with high-risk HPV subtypes facilitate malignant transformation [8, 9].

1.3 Clinical Presentation

Anogenital HPV infection may be subclinical or may present as genital warts, also known as condyloma acuminata, characterized by small hyperkeratotic skin colored papules that can emerge into plaques. SOTRs may present with larger, exuberant, and multifocal lesions [1, 3] (Fig. 1a–f).

Although anogenital warts are of low malignant potential, persistent infection can lead to malignant transformation into invasive SCC, particularly when associated with high-risk HPV types, such as HPVs 16, 18, 31, and 33, and immunosuppression [3, 9]. The incidence and persistence of HPV lesions in SOTRs are directly related to the immunosuppressant dose, regimen, and duration [6] (Fig. 2a–c).

Bowenoid papulosis is an uncommon sexually transmitted condition that tends to affect young sexually active people. It is clinically characterized by multiple well-demarcated red-brown to violaceous papules, usually less than 1 cm in size. The surface of the lesions can be flat, smooth, papillomatous, or verrucous. Some papules may coalesce into large plaques. Most lesions are associated with the oncogenic HPV 16 genotype but occasionally HPV 18, 31, 33, 34, 35, 39, 42, 48, 51, 52, 53, and 54 are detected. This condition is considered an intraepithelial neoplasia that may transform into invasive SCC, especially in SOTRs [10].

Verrucous carcinoma, also known as Buschke-Löwenstein tumor, is a highly differentiated verrucous carcinoma of the anogenital area associated with HPVs 6 and 11. It presents as a slow-growing, large, cauliflower-like tumor with locally destructive behavior [1] (Fig. 3).

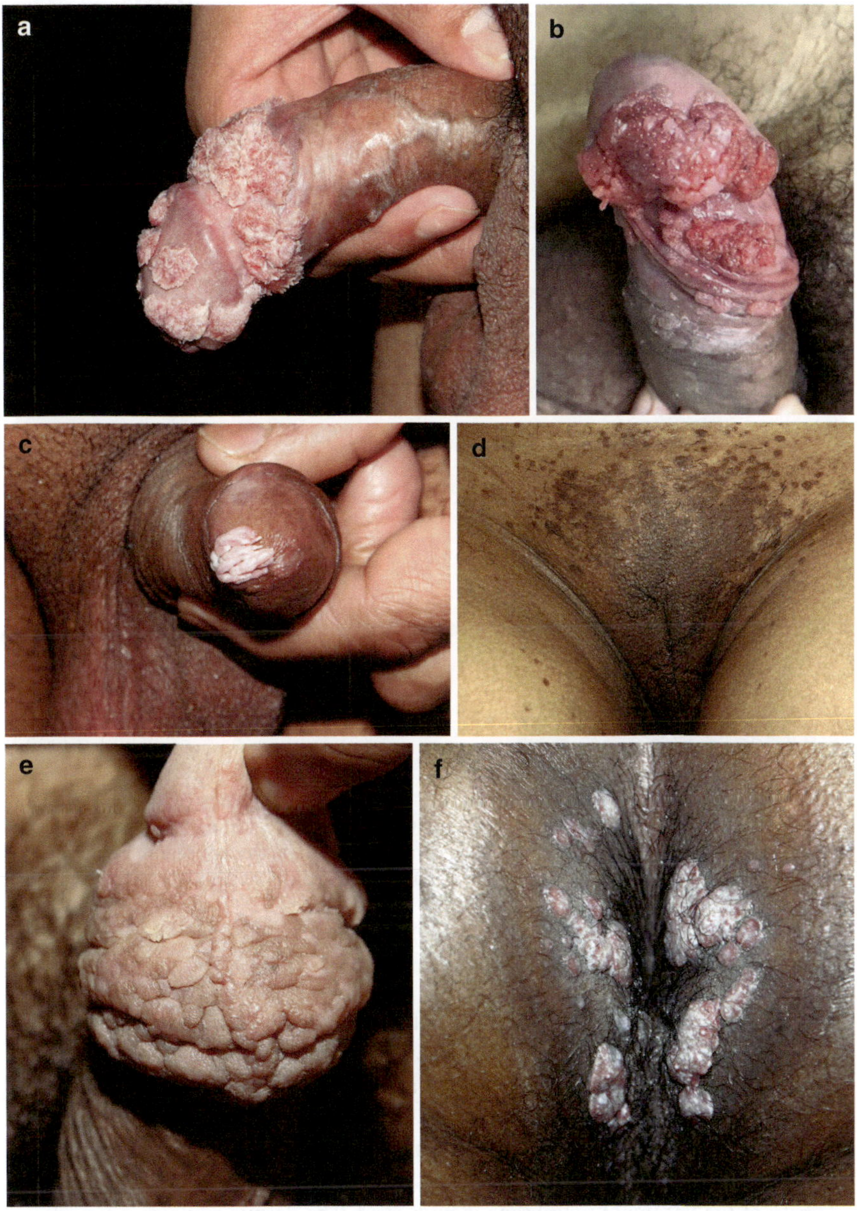

Fig. 1 Exuberant HPV genital infections on SOTRs. (**a**) Multiple erythematous keratotic papules on the glans and penis body. (**b**) Multiple confluent erythematous papules with a vegetating and friable surface on the glans and penis body. (**c**) Grouped filiform papules on the glans penis. (**d**) Confluent brownish papules on the pubic mound and vulva. (**e**) Multiple skin colored and confluent keratotic papules on the glans penis. (**f**) Multiple erythematous keratotic papules in the perianal region. (Images collection, Department of Dermatology, Hospital of Clinics, University of São Paulo Medical School (HC-FMUSP))

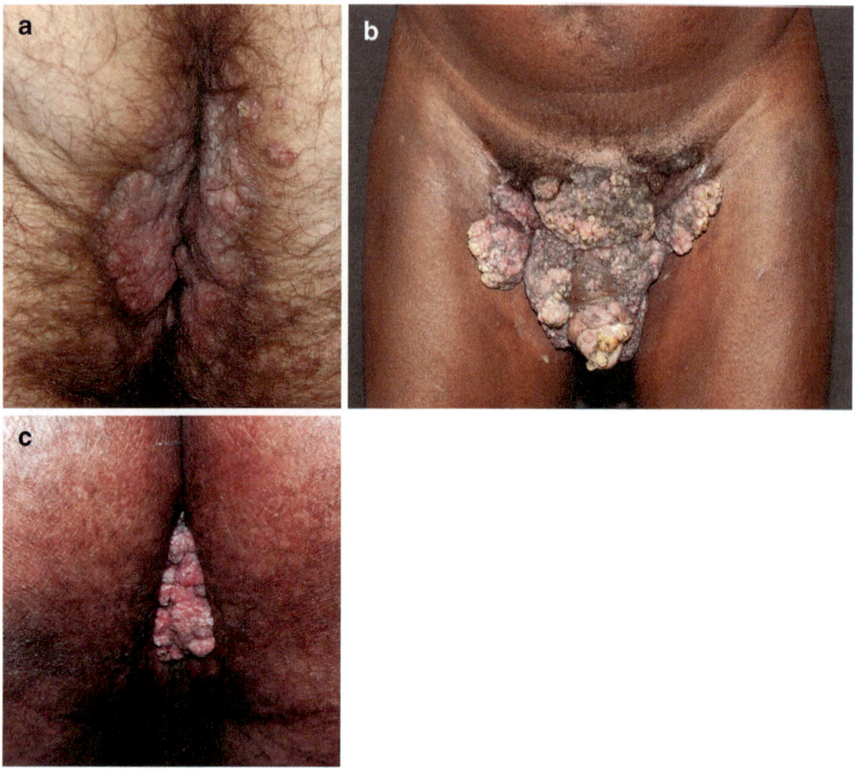

Fig. 2 Squamous cell carcinoma arising in a HPV positive area. (**a**) Extensive erythematous infiltrated plaque on the gluteal and perianal region. (**b**) Exuberant vegetating tumor on the genital area. (**c**) Vegetating erythematous tumor on the perianal region. (Images collection, Department of Dermatology, Hospital of Clinics, University of São Paulo Medical School (HC-FMUSP))

1.4 Histopathology

Classical histopathological features of condyloma acuminata include acanthosis, papillomatosis, hyperkeratosis, and parakeratosis. Superficial vacuolated keratinocytes, referred to as koilocytes, are a hallmark [11].

Bowenoid papulosis is characterized by acanthosis with full thickness epidermal atypia, known as bowenoid dysplasia. Multiple mitoses are usually visible above the basal layer as well as multinucleated keratinocytes with pleomorphism. The integrity of the basement membrane is preserved. The dermis contains a superficial lymphocytic infiltrate with perivascular accentuation. Immunohistochemistry for the p16 protein indicates strongly positive results for this disease [11].

Verrucous carcinoma has a tendency for endophytic growth without frank infiltration [11].

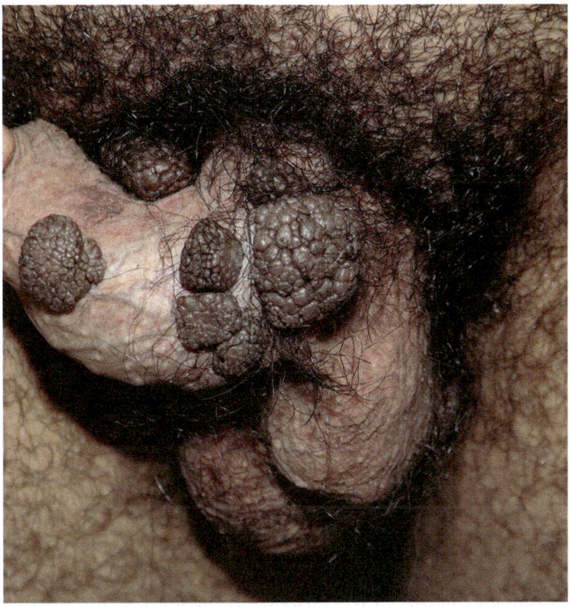

Fig. 3 Buschke-Löwenstein tumor: multiple brownish nodules with exophytic growth on the body of the penis. (Images collection, Department of Dermatology, Hospital of Clinics, University of São Paulo Medical School (HC-FMUSP))

1.5 Treatment

Treatment is mostly directed to destroy the lesions rather than the virus itself [1]. Cryotherapy, surgery, electrosurgery, salicylic acid, trichloroacetic acid, podophyllum, topical retinoids, 5-fluorouracil, intralesional bleomycin, imiquimod, and intralesional cidofovir are therapeutic options. These are viable options for reducing the size and number of genital warts, but recalcitrant lesions are very common in SOTRs. When possible, the immunosuppressive regimen may also be tapered down [3, 6, 12].

Imiquimod is a topical immune response modifier that exerts both antiviral and antitumor activities by activating a pro-inflammatory response mediated by IFN-α (interferon-α) release via Toll-like receptor 7 (TLR-7) [1]. The drug is a safe option for SOTRs in areas under 100 cm^2 [6]. It induces both innate and cell-mediated immune responses, with a dominant Th1 activity. Clearance rates after using imiquimod ranges from 40% to 70%, with a recurrence rate of 9–19% [8].

Cidofovir is a potent nucleoside analog that exerts its function by inactivating viral DNA polymerase and has been successfully used for the treatment of HPV infection. Topical or intralesional formulations are safe and effective, but systemic administration may induce nephrotoxicity and neutropenia and should be avoided on renal transplant recipients and patients with renal dysfunction [12].

Biopsy is recommended for exuberant and refractory lesions in order to exclude malignant transformation. Patients should also be referred to a gynecologist and proctologist since lesions can also occur in the vagina, cervix, and rectum [1].

Another important strategy focused on prevention is HPV vaccination. There are currently three vaccines subtypes available: bivalent (directed against HPVs 16 and 18), quadrivalent (directed against HPVs 6, 11, 16, and 18), and nine-valent HPV vaccine (directed against HPVs 6, 11, 16, 18, 31, 33, 45, 52, and 58). These vaccines elicit cell-mediated and/or humoral immune responses and are considered safe in SOTRs. They have been shown to prevent persistent HPV infection and to reduce the risk of malignant transformation [1].

2 Syphilis

2.1 Epidemiology

Syphilis is an endemic disease with a rising incidence in the past decades, largely due to the increased number of cases of human immunodeficiency virus (HIV) infection, drug abuse, and high-risk sexual behavior [11, 13]. More than 5 million cases are diagnosed every year worldwide. The prevalence is higher in low-income countries, while in developed countries the infection occurs disproportionately in minorities and in people with poor access to health care [13].

The disease can cause lifelong morbidity in those left untreated and in children born to infected mothers. Syphilis genital ulcers are densely infiltrated with lymphocytes (the primary target cells for HIV infection) and so provide a portal of entry for HIV acquisition [13].

Regarding SOTRs, potential donors are routinely tested for viral and bacterial infections, and because of this donor-derived infections contribute less than 1% overall incidence of post-transplant syphilis infection [14]. Evidence of donor active infection is not considered a contraindication for transplantation, as long as there is an appropriate antibiotic treatment of recipients in the early post-transplant phase [15, 16]. There are a few reports of organ transplantation from donors with serologic evidence of syphilis; in all cases, post-transplant treatment of the recipients with penicillin prevented progression of the infection [14].

2.2 Pathogenesis

Treponema pallidum is a slow growing spirochaeta capable of an undulating, corkscrew-like motion [15]. The microorganism can be visualized in material from a chancre with dark-field illumination, but cannot grow in conventional culture media [11].

With the exception of congenital syphilis, the disease is contagious mainly through direct sexual contact although some cases may spread via blood products (transfusions or needle sharing) and organ donation [11, 13, 17]. After inoculation, microorganisms disseminate through the lymphatic system and bloodstream to multiple organs, with central nervous system tropism. *T. pallidum* induces prominent humoral and cell-mediated immune responses, and there is an incubation period of about 3 weeks before the appearance of the primary lesion [13, 15].

2.3 Clinical Presentation

Syphilis can cause a series of highly variable clinical manifestations during the first 2–3 years of infection, followed by a prolonged latent stage that can evolve into a clinically apparent tertiary stage after several years or even decades. The disease presents a high potential of infection only during the early primary and secondary stages; however, congenital transmission can also occur at latency stage [13].

Primary syphilis or chancre is characterized by the presence of a painless, indurated, clean-based, and usually solitary ulcerative lesion that typically appears about 2–3 weeks after transmission. It can be accompanied by tender regional lymphadenopathy [11, 13]. Chancres can be located at nearly any place where the infection occurs; however, it is more frequent at the distal penis, vulva, vagina, cervix, and rectum (Fig. 4a, b). Without treatment, lesions spontaneously resolve in 3–6 weeks [13, 17, 18].

Secondary syphilis is the most commonly recognized clinical syndrome being a result of the hematogenous dissemination of *T. pallidum*. It usually appears 6–8 weeks after the development of the chancre and is highly contagious [11, 13]. Its classical manifestation is characterized by an erythematous or brownish macular rash that does not spare the palms of the hands or soles of the feet, and is extremely variable in appearance, justifying the term the great imitator. Mucous lesions may have an exuberant warty appearance and are referred to as condyloma lata [18]. Alopecia may be found, which is characterized by patchy and non-scarring diffuse hair loss of the scalp, often described as "moth-eaten" alopecia [19] (Fig. 5a–f).

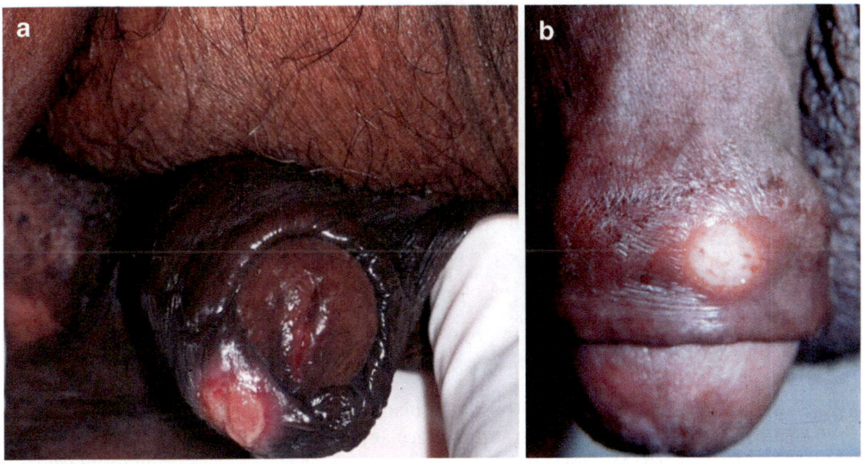

Fig. 4 Primary syphilis (chancre). (**a, b**) Indurated, clean-based, and solitary ulcerative lesion on the body of the penis. (Images collection, Department of Dermatology, Hospital of Clinics, University of São Paulo Medical School (HC-FMUSP))

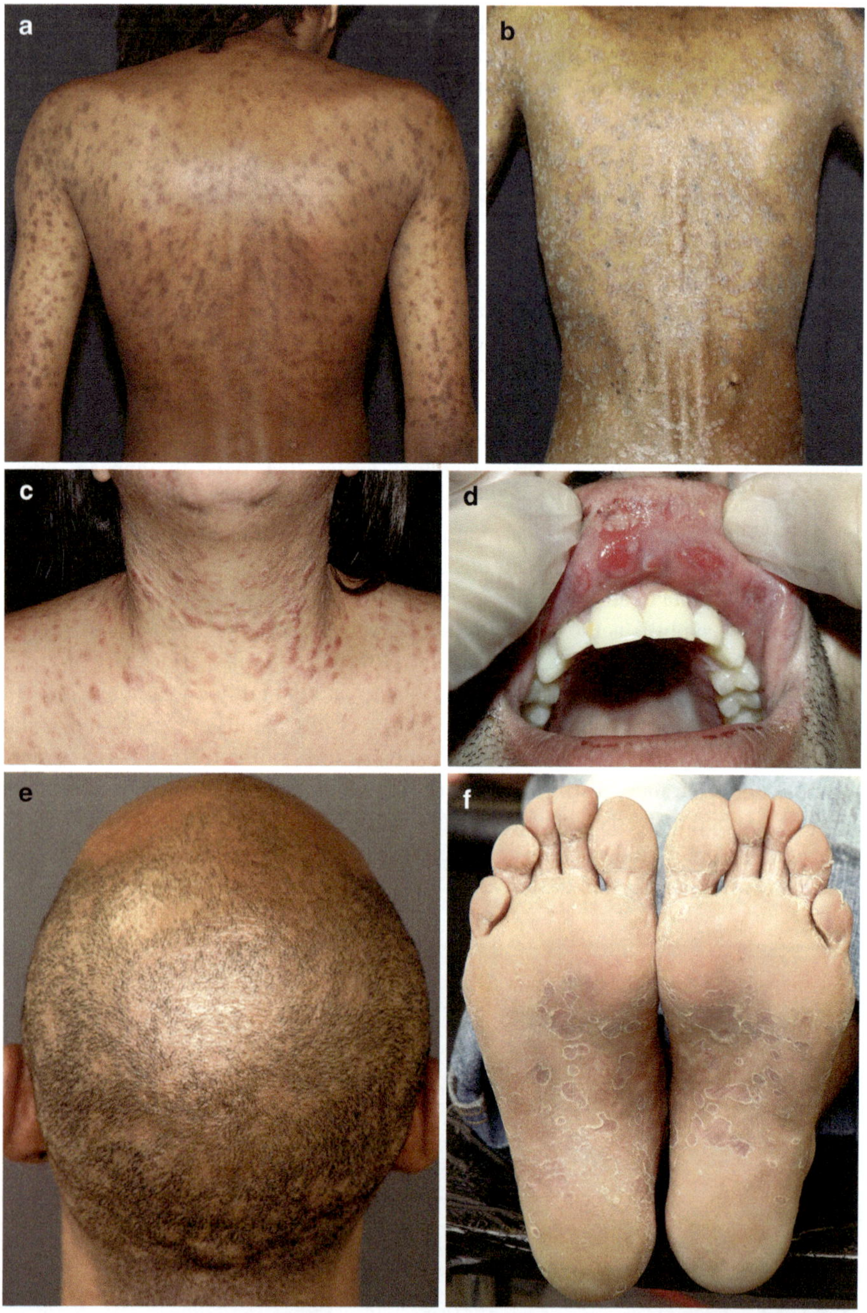

Fig. 5 Secondary syphilis. (**a**) Brownish macular rash on the upper trunk and arms. (**b**) Erythematous maculopapular rash with scaly surface. (**c**) Erythematous maculopapular rash on the upper trunk and neck. (**d**) Multiple erythematous plaques on the oral mucosa (condyloma lata). (**e**) Multiple non-scarring alopecia plaques with a "moth-eaten" pattern. (**f**) Multiple erythematous plaques with scaly collarette on the soles of the feet. (Images collection, Department of Dermatology, Hospital of Clinics, University of São Paulo Medical School (HC-FMUSP))

Myalgia, malaise, sore throat, low-grade fever, and diffuse lymphadenopathy are common in secondary syphilis. Hepatosplenomegaly, hepatitis, nephrotic syndrome, and ocular involvement such as uveitis and retinitis may occur [11]. Cutaneous lesions resolve spontaneously within a few weeks without treatment, but other manifestations may persist for several months [13].

With the resolution of the secondary lesions, untreated patients may enter into a latent stage characterized by the absence of signs and symptoms. In this latent stage, the infection can only be detected through serologic testing. After a variable length of time that can vary from years to decades, about one-third of untreated patients may develop tertiary syphilis [18]. Symptoms of this stage are mostly neurological (tabes dorsalis, cranial nerve palsies, general paresis, meningitis), cardiovascular (aneurysms, valvular insufficiency, coronary artery disease), and cutaneous (gummatous syphilis). Gumma can occur in any location and presents as noduloulcerative lesions with central necrosis and suppuration. When symptoms are present, they occur due to a mass effect or local inflammation [13] (Fig. 6).

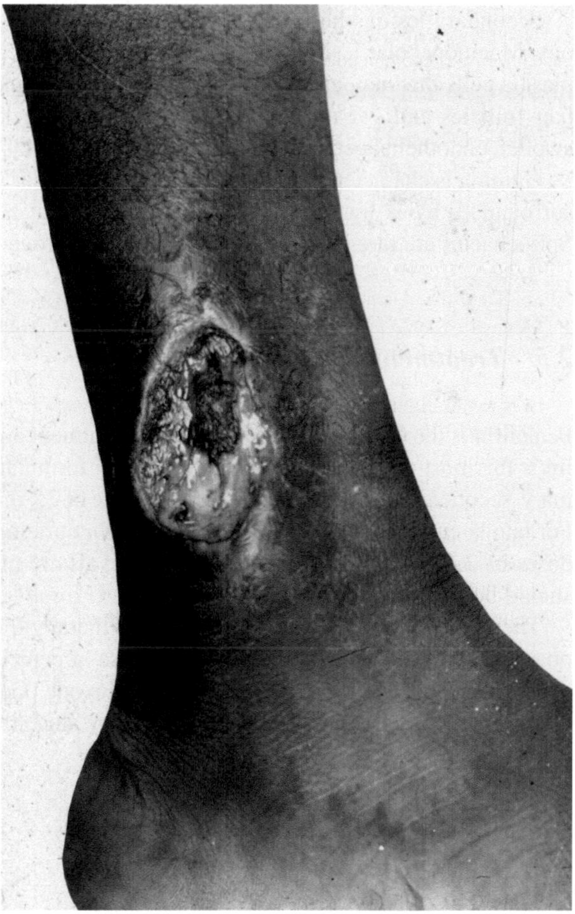

Fig. 6 Tertiary syphilis: noduloulcerative lesion with central necrosis and suppuration (gumma). (Images collection, Department of Dermatology, Hospital of Clinics, University of São Paulo Medical School (HC-FMUSP))

Diagnosis is often a challenge because of the high polymorphism of lesions and is mostly based on serological testing. There are two types of serological exams: non-treponemal tests, based on antigens synthesized from lecithin, cholesterol, and cardiolipin, which are employed mostly for triage and treatment follow-up, and treponemal tests, which are more specific and can detect different antibodies to treponemal antigens [13, 20].

2.4 Histopathology

Primary syphilis is histologically characterized by an ulceration of the epithelium, pseudoepitheliomatous hyperplasia of the adjacent epidermis and an intense lymphohistiocytic and neutrophil infiltrate in the dermis. Plasma cells are present but can be scarce. There is a large amount of mucoid substance responsible for the indurated aspect of the chancre. Microorganisms can be demonstrated by a silver stain, such as Warthin-Starry, or immunohistochemistry [11].

Secondary lesions have variable findings depending on their clinical morphology. Maculopapular lesions show a superficial and deep perivascular infiltrate with plasma cells that may adopt a band-like distribution and is often prominent around hair follicles and sweat glands. The presence of thick-walled blood vessels with swollen endothelial cells is a characteristic finding [11].

Gumma is characterized by central necrosis similar to caseation. The necrosis is surrounded by a lymphohistiocytic and plasma cell infiltrate with fibrosis. Spirochaetes are rare in this stage and not usually found with silver stains [11].

2.5 Treatment

Penicillin is the drug of choice for syphilis treatment and benzathine benzylpenicillin is the most commonly recommended drug formulation. For early syphilis (primary, secondary, and early latent), a single dose of 2.4 million units is recommended. For late latent syphilis, cases with an unknown duration and tertiary syphilis, three doses of 2.4 million units with weekly intervals are recommended. Neurosyphilis should be treated with intravenous penicillin G for at least 10 days [13, 21].

There are no recommendations to modify therapy for pregnant women or immunosuppressed patients such as SOTRs. In case of penicillin allergy, alternative therapy options include tetracyclines and ceftriaxone. Careful follow-up of patients receiving any alternative therapy is mandatory since there is a higher risk of drug resistance and treatment failure [11, 13, 21].

3 Molluscum Contagiosum

3.1 Epidemiology

Molluscum contagiosum virus (MCV) infection occurs worldwide and seems to be more prevalent in tropical areas. Skin lesions of molluscum contagiosum are called mollusca. It is a common condition, with a greater incidence in those aged between 1 and 4 years and in sexually active young adults [22]. It can affect up to 7% of SOTRs, in whom lesions larger than 1 cm can be found and are the so-called giant molluscum contagiosum. In SOTRs, lesions can also occur in atypical locations such as the palms of the hands and the soles of the feet [6, 20, 21].

3.2 Pathogenesis

MCV is a double-stranded DNA poxvirus transmitted through direct skin-to-skin (including sexual) or indirect (towels, underclothes, toys, razors, tattoo supplies) contact. MCV is a cytoplasmically replicating virus that produces proteins capable of inhibiting human antiviral immunity, thus preventing the development of innate immunity response and contributing to the persistence of skin lesions [6, 22].

The incubation period ranges from 2 weeks to 6 months. MCV has an affinity for follicular epithelium and only infects keratinocytes. Lesions are limited to the epidermis and the virus does not disseminate systemically [6, 22].

3.3 Clinical Presentation

Molluscum contagiosum lesions are firm, waxy, white or flesh-colored, and dome shaped with a central umbilication. Size can vary from 1 mm to 1 cm in diameter [6, 22].

The infection can occur in any part of the skin, but rarely affect the palms, soles, and mucous membranes, such as the lips, buccal mucosa, and conjunctiva. In children, lesions are usually located on the face, trunk, limbs, and axillary areas. In sexually transmitted cases, lesions are mainly observed on the anogenital area and inner thighs [6, 22–24]. Molluscum dermatitis is characterized by eczematous patches surrounding MCV lesions and occurs in up to 47% of infected patients [22] (Fig. 7a, b).

On immunocompromised individuals, such as SOTRs, MCV lesions may be atypical, larger, and/or mimic malignancies, such as basal cell carcinoma or keratoacanthoma, or other infectious diseases, such as cryptococcosis and histoplasmosis [6, 22–24].

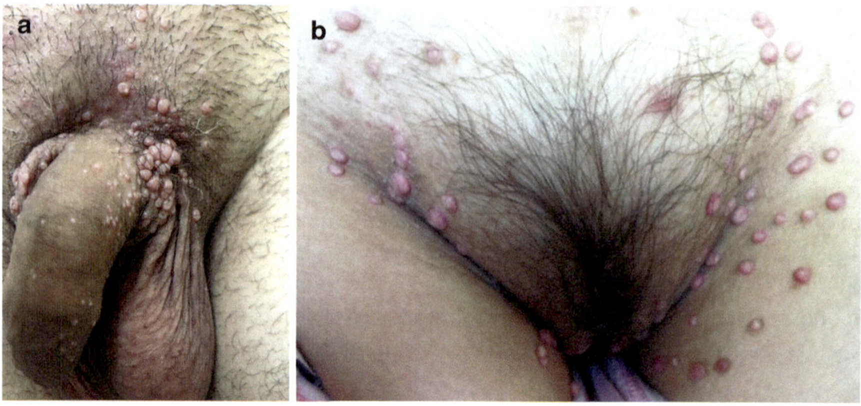

Fig. 7 Multiple exuberant molluscum contagiosum lesions on SOTRs. (**a**) Multiple umbilicated erythematous papules on the pubis and body of the penis. (**b**) Multiple umbilicated erythematous papules on the thighs and vulva. (Images collection, Department of Dermatology, Hospital of Clinics, University of São Paulo Medical School (HC-FMUSP))

Diagnosis is mostly based on clinical examination. Dermoscopy, reflectance confocal microscopy, and histopathology analysis may be useful as complementary tools [6].

3.4 *Histopathology*

MCV lesions have classic histopathologic features. A cup-shaped indentation of the epidermis into the dermis is usually observed. The proliferated rete ridges descend downwards and involve the dermis, while Henderson-Patterson bodies, which enclose virus particles, can be seen in the thickened epidermis [6, 22].

3.5 *Treatment*

Surgical removal, curettage, cryotherapy, and electrodessication are treatment options for MCV infection. However, destructive methods may not be suitable for immunocompromised patients, who are prone to secondary infections. Other therapeutic options include topical cidofovir, imiquimod, podophyllin, trichloroacetic acid, salicylic acid, tincture of iodine, topical retinoids, and intralesional interferon alpha [6, 25, 26].

The use of an immunomodulation regimen, such as imiquimod, has more feasibility and stronger evidence of treatment efficacy than traditional surgical methods in extensive disease. Local adverse effects are usually well tolerated and include erythema, itching, burning sensation, and pain [23].

4 Herpes Simplex

4.1 Epidemiology

Herpes simplex virus (HSV) has two subtypes: HSV-1 and HSV-2. HSV-1 usually causes herpes labialis (90%), whereas HSV-2 most often causes herpes genitalis (70–90% overall). Although HSV-2 remains the causal agent of most genital herpes infections, recent studies have shown an increasing proportion of cases related to HSV-1. It is estimated that approximately one-third of the world's population has experienced a symptomatic episode of HSV infection [11, 27].

Most of the symptomatic HSV disease in SOTRs results from the reactivation of a previously acquired virus. Compared to immunocompetent hosts, SOTRs shed viruses more frequently, even in the absence of lesions, and have more severe clinical manifestations [28].

Transplant recipients HSV IgG serostatus should be determined prior to transplant, and it is useful to determine the possibility of primary HSV acquisition, either from the allograft or from other sources after transplant [28]. In a large cohort of SOTRs, the incidence of symptomatic HSV infection during the first year after transplant was 3% in patients receiving antiviral prophylaxis, *versus* 9.8% without prophylaxis [29]. HSV viral shedding can be detected within 5–14 days after transplantation in 50–66% of seropositive renal allograft recipients although symptomatic lesions only develop in 15–45% of SOTRs [2].

4.2 Pathogenesis

The herpesvirus group consists of relatively large and enveloped DNA viruses that are categorized into three groups, α, β, and γ, according to genome similarities. HSV-1 and HSV-2 belong to the subfamily α-herpesviridae. The pathogenesis of herpesvirus infections follows the sequence of primary infection, latency, and reactivation. Latency enables the virus to exist in a relatively non-infectious state for a variable period of time [10].

Transmission of HSV can occur even during asymptomatic periods of viral shedding. The virus is spread primarily through direct contact with contaminated saliva or other infected secretions during sexual contact. The virus replicates at the mucocutaneous site of infection and then travels by retrograde axonal flow to the dorsal root ganglia, where it establishes latency until reactivation [6, 11].

Primary infection from the allograft in SOTRs is rare but can be severe due to the lack of immunologic memory. The association between HSV reactivation and specific immunosuppressive agents is hard to access due to the varied regimens and the use of multiple drugs simultaneously in the early post-transplant period, time when HSV reactivation is more common [28, 29].

4.3 Clinical Presentation

Most people with HSV infection have mild or subclinical disease. It can present with a diversity of mucocutaneous lesions, and when it occurs on the genital area, it is usually sexually transmitted. In primary infections, symptoms typically occur within 3–7 days after exposure and are preceded by a prodrome of tender lymphadenopathy, malaise, anorexia, and fever. Lesions appear as painful and grouped vesicles on the erythematous base, followed by progression to pustules, erosions, and/or ulceration and crusts (Fig. 8). Similar clinical manifestations can occur in recurrent lesions although fewer in number and with decreased severity and duration, when compared to a primary infection [11, 27, 29].

In female patients, genital lesions occur on the external genitalia and mucosae of the vulva, vagina, and cervix. Pain and dysuria can be present. In men, lesions typically occur on the glans or shaft of the penis. In male homosexuals, other common areas are the buttocks, perianal area, and rectum [28, 29].

HSV infections in SOTRs can be more persistent and may present as slow-healing mucocutaneous ulcerations on the oropharynx and genital area (Fig. 9a, b). Disseminated infection is uncommon but associated with a high mortality rate [30].

The infection may also have a chronic course in immunocompromised hosts. It can occur in SOTRs as well as in immunosuppressed patients due to other conditions such as HIV, chronic lymphocytic leukemia, hypogammaglobulinemia, chronic hepatitis C, and myeloproliferative disorders. The infection presents as atypical large ulcers, vegetative, and/or hyperkeratotic lesions that can affect large areas of the perianal and/or genital region, and usually persists for at least a

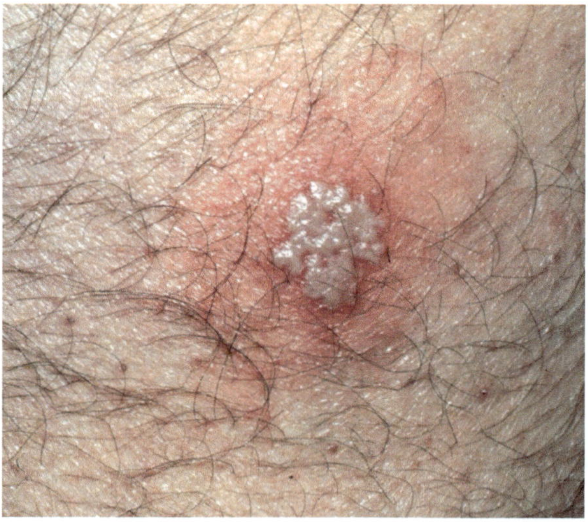

Fig. 8 Herpes simplex classic lesions: multiple grouped vesicles with an erythematous base. (Images collection, Department of Dermatology, Hospital of Clinics, University of São Paulo Medical School (HC-FMUSP))

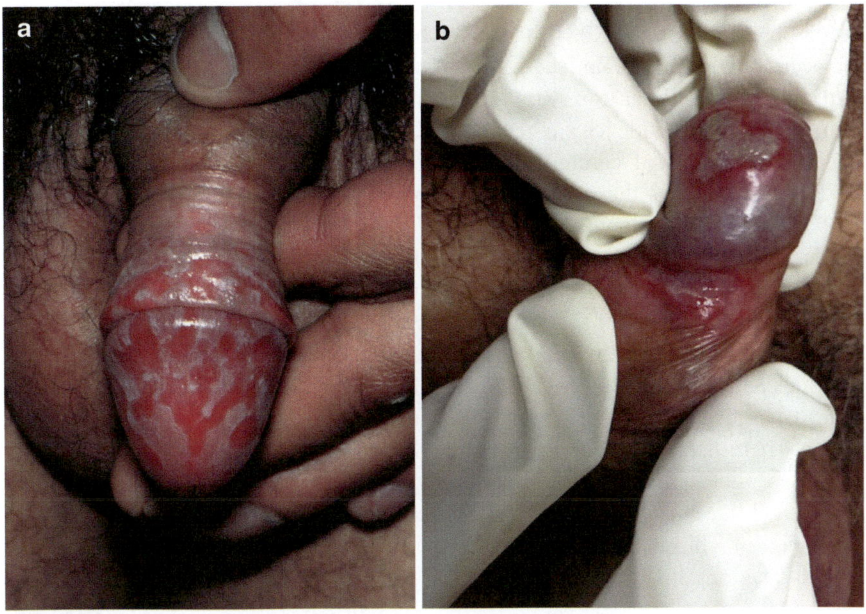

Fig. 9 Genital herpes lesions in SOTRs. (**a**, **b**) Multiple superficial erosions on the glans and body of the penis. (Images collection, Department of Dermatology, Hospital of Clinics, University of São Paulo Medical School (HC-FMUSP))

month. Lesions are highly polymorphic, can be single or multiple, and are extremely painful (Fig. 10a–d). The hyperkeratotic pattern may simulate SCC or other infections. Chronic herpes infections are apparently rare in immunocompetent patients [28–33].

Tzanck smear of a herpetic vesicle shows ballooned keratinocytes and giant cells (Fig. 11).

4.4 Histopathology

HSV infection is histologically characterized by edema, ballooning degeneration of keratinocytes, acantholysis, and the development of an irregular intraepidermal vesicle with large and multinucleated keratinocytes. The underlying dermis presents with an intense mixed inflammatory infiltrate [11].

Chronic herpes simplex lesions present with hyperplasia of the epidermis with multinucleated epithelial cells and dense mixed inflammatory infiltrate composed of lymphocytes, plasmocytes, and eosinophils [32, 33].

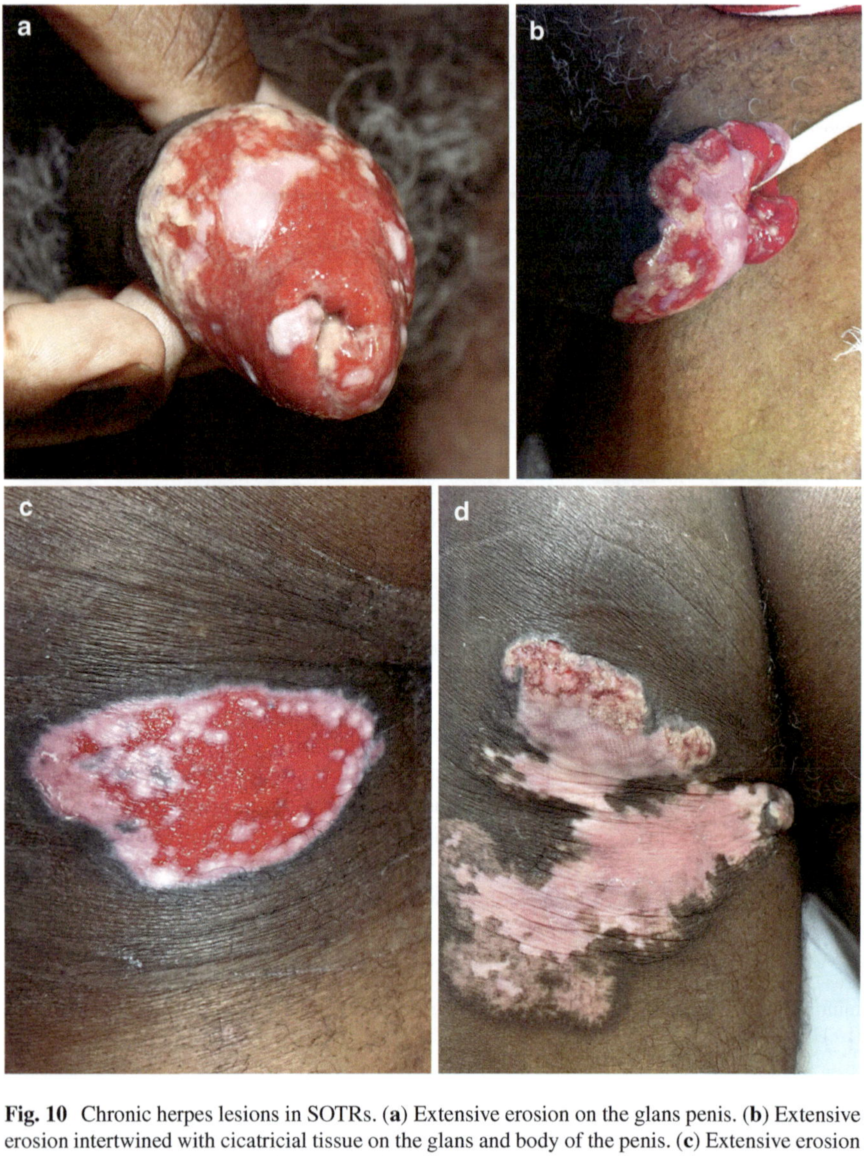

Fig. 10 Chronic herpes lesions in SOTRs. (**a**) Extensive erosion on the glans penis. (**b**) Extensive erosion intertwined with cicatricial tissue on the glans and body of the penis. (**c**) Extensive erosion on the buttocks. (**d**) Extensive hypochromic cicatricial lesion with a vegetant erythematous edge. (Images collection, Department of Dermatology, Hospital of Clinics, University of São Paulo Medical School (HC-FMUSP))

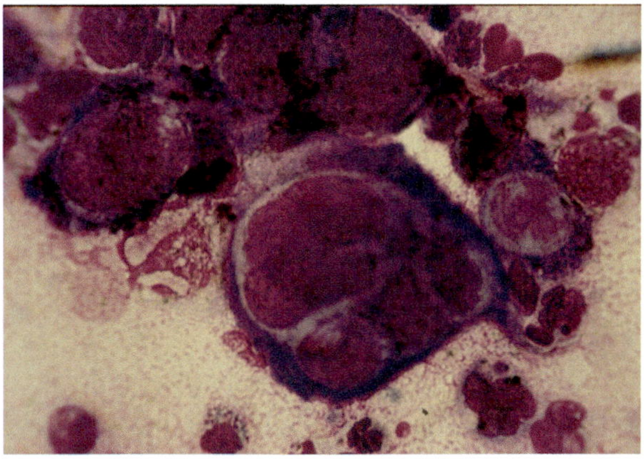

Fig. 11 Tzanck smear of a herpetic vesicle revealing ballooned keratinocytes and giant cells. (Images collection, Department of Dermatology, Hospital of Clinics, University of São Paulo Medical School (HC-FMUSP))

4.5 Treatment

Mucocutaneous herpes is a lifelong condition that can be treated with antiviral therapy, including acyclovir, famciclovir, penciclovir, and valacyclovir. However, response to treatment can be slower in immunocompromised individuals, and resistance to these agents varies between 4% and 7% [29, 32, 33]. In case of drug resistance, other therapeutic options include foscarnet, interferon-β, imiquimod, and cidofovir, with variable efficacy results [32, 33]. Susceptibility to antivirals is a dynamic process that varies with time, which allows the reintroduction of an antiviral drug associated with previous failure [32, 33].

Nucleoside analogs (acyclovir, famciclovir, penciclovir, and valacyclovir) are effective in reducing the duration and severity of a herpes simplex episode [27]. They can also be employed as prophylactic and suppressive regimens in patients with multiple recurrences per year, in order to prevent, delay, and shorten the duration of HSV outbreaks. In case of disseminated or severe infections, intravenous acyclovir should be used [6].

5 Chancroid

5.1 Epidemiology

Chancroid (soft chancre) is a very common sexually transmitted infection in some tropical areas of Southeast Asia, Africa, Central America, and the Pacific. Poor hygiene is a common feature of the endemic communities. The disease is associated with a higher risk of HIV acquisition [11, 34].

5.2 Pathogenesis

Chancroid is caused by *Haemophilus ducreyi*, a Gram-negative, facultative anaerobic coccobacillus. The disease is transmitted through minor abrasions during sexual contact and has an incubation period of 3 days to 2 weeks, with a median of 7 days [11, 27, 34].

5.3 Clinical Presentation

The initial lesion is seen as a soft painful papule surrounded by erythema that rapidly ulcerates with copious suppuration. The ulcer is sharply circumscribed, has an irregular ragged edge, and is typically not indurated (Fig. 12). It can be associated with unilateral tender inguinal lymphadenitis followed by suppuration (bubo formation) in nearly half of patients [11, 27, 34].

Multiple ulcers can be present, and there are many clinical variants of chancroid: giant, large serpiginous, transient, phagedenic, follicular, and papular [27]. Lesions are more commonly seen in men, and the prepuce, coronal sulcus, frenulum, and glans are the most affected sites [11].

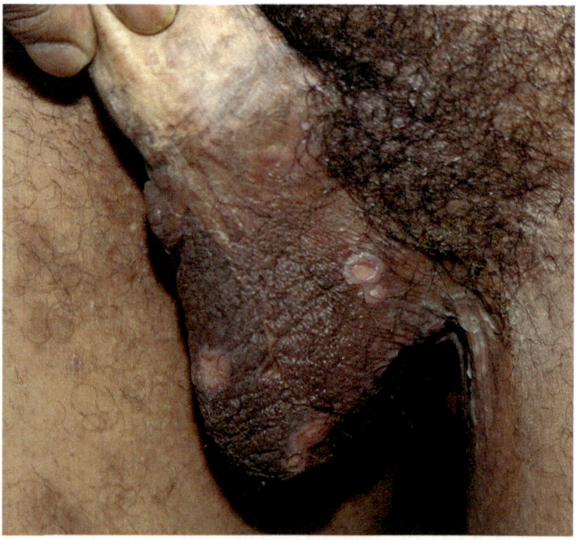

Fig. 12 Chancroid lesions—multiple circumscribed non-indurated ulcers on the scrotum. (Images collection, Department of Dermatology, Hospital of Clinics, University of São Paulo Medical School (HC-FMUSP))

5.4 Histopathology

Chancroid ulcers are histologically characterized by a superficial zone of neutrophils, bacteria and cell debris, a middle zone of granulation tissue, and an underlying infiltrate of histiocytes, lymphocytes, and plasma cells. The enlarged lymph nodes show central necrosis with a mixed inflammatory response of neutrophils and macrophages [10].

5.5 Treatment

Recommended treatment regimens for chancroid include ceftriaxone, azithromycin, ciprofloxacin, or erythromycin. Immunocompromised individuals have a higher rate of treatment failure [27].

References

1. Reusser N, Downing C, Guidry J, Tyring S. HPV carcinomas in immunocompromised patients. J Clin Med. 2015;4(2):260–81.
2. Tan H-H, Goh C-L. Viral infections affecting the skin in organ transplant recipients. Am J Clin Dermatol. 2006;7(1):13–29.
3. Chin-Hong PV, Reid GE. Human papillomavirus infection in solid organ transplant recipients: Guidelines from the American Society of Transplantation Infectious Diseases Community of Practice. Clin Transplant. 2019;33(9):1–15.
4. Rüdlinger R, Smith IW, Bunney MH, Hunter JAA. Human papillomavirus infections in a group of renal transplant recipients. Br J Dermatol. 1986;115(6):681–92.
5. Ogunbiyi OA, Scholefield JH, Raftery AT, Smith JHF, Duffy S, Sharp F, et al. Prevalence of anal human papillomavirus infection and intraepithelial neoplasia in renal allograft recipients. Br J Surg. 1994;81(3):365–7.
6. Ilyas M, Maganty N, Sharma A. Cutaneous infections from viral sources in solid organ transplant recipients. J Clin Virol. 2017;97:33–7.
7. Martelli-Marzagão F, Santos Junior GF, Ogawa MM, Enokihara MMSS, Porro AM, Tomimori J. Human papillomavirus detected in viral warts of renal transplant recipients. Transpl Infect Dis. 2016;18(1):37–43.
8. Harwood CA, Perrett CM, Brown VL, Leigh IM, Mcgregor JM, Proby CM. Imiquimod cream 5% for recalcitrant cutaneous warts in immunosuppressed individuals. Br J Dermatol. 2005;152(1):122–9.
9. Chin-Hong PV. Time to take on HPV in transplant clinic—warts and all. Am J Transplant. 2019;19(1):11–2.
10. Cardoso JC, Calonje E. Cutaneous manifestations of human papillomaviruses: a review. Acta Dermatovenerol Alp Pannonica Adriat. 2011;20(3):145–54.
11. Kee M. Pathology of the skin, vol. 51. London: Elsevier; 1999. p. 348–53.
12. Blouin MM, Cloutier R, Noël R. Intralesional cidofovir in the treatment of cutaneous warts in a renal transplant patient. J Cutan Med Surg. 2012;16(6):462–4.

13. Hook EW. Syphilis. Lancet. 2017;389(10078):1550–7.
14. Tariciotti L, Das I, Dori L, Perera MTPR, Bramhall SR. Asymptomatic transmission of Treponema pallidum (syphilis) through deceased donor liver transplantation. Transpl Infect Dis. 2012;14(3):321–5.
15. Cortez KJ, Greenwald MA. Current trends in donor testing to detect syphilis infection. Curr Infect Dis Rep. 2014;16(9):423.
16. Cortes NJ, Afzali B, MacLean D, Goldsmith DJA, O'Sullivan H, Bingham J, et al. Transmission of syphilis by solid organ transplantation. Am J Transplant. 2006;6(10):2497–9.
17. Ferrándiz-Pulido C, Ferrer B, Salcedo MT, Velasco M, Len O, Castells L. Secondary syphilis with liver involvement in a liver transplant recipient. Transpl Infect Dis. 2021;23(1):e13431.
18. Ghanem KG, Ram S, Rice PA. The modern epidemic of syphilis. N Engl J Med. 2020;382(9):845–54.
19. Çakmak SK, Tamer E, Karadağ AS, Waugh M. Syphilis: a great imitator. Clin Dermatol. 2019;37(3):182–91.
20. Arando Lasagabaster M, Otero Guerra L. Syphilis. Enferm Infecc Microbiol Clin. 2019;37(6):398–404.
21. Ghanem KG. Management of adult syphilis: key questions to inform the 2015 Centers for Disease Control and Prevention Sexually Transmitted Diseases Treatment Guidelines. Clin Infect Dis. 2015;61(Suppl 8):S818–36.
22. Chen X, Anstey AV, Bugert JJ. Molluscum contagiosum virus infection. Lancet Infect Dis. 2013;13(10):877–88.
23. Lin HY, Linn G, Bin LC, Chen CJ, Yu KJ. An immunocompromised woman with severe molluscum contagiosum that responded well to topical imiquimod: a case report and literature review. J Low Genit Tract Dis. 2010;14(2):134–5.
24. Allison TL. Immunosuppressive therapy in transplantation. Nurs Clin North Am. 2016;51(1):107–20.
25. Erickson C, Driscoll M, Gaspari A. Efficacy of intravenous cidofovir in the treatment of giant molluscum contagiosum in a patient with human immunodeficiency virus. Arch Dermatol. 2011;147(6):652–4.
26. Ha DL, Shin JO, Ryu HS, Lee HJ, Kim MB, Shin K. Molluscum contagiosum mimicking condyloma acuminata in a renal transplant patient: a unique presentation. Transpl Infect Dis. 2020;22(1):2–3.
27. Basta-Juzbašić A, Čeović R. Chancroid, lymphogranuloma venereum, granuloma inguinale, genital herpes simplex infection, and molluscum contagiosum. Clin Dermatol. 2014;32(2):290–8.
28. Wilck MB, Zuckerman RA. Herpes simplex virus in solid organ transplantation. Am J Transplant. 2013;13(Suppl 4):121–7.
29. Lee DH. Herpes simplex virus infections in solid organ transplantation: Guidelines from the American Society of Transplantation Infectious Diseases Community of Practice. Clin Transplant. 2019;33:e13526.
30. Carratalà J, Montejo M, Pérez-Romero P. Infections caused by herpes viruses other than cytomegalovirus in solid organ transplant recipients. Enferm Infecc Microbiol Clin. 2012;30(Suppl 2):63–9.
31. Weinrauch LA, D'Elia JA. Solid organ transplantation. JACC Heart Fail. 2018;6(4):348–9.
32. Wauters O, Lebas E, Nikkels AF. Chronic mucocutaneous herpes simplex virus and varicella zoster virus infections. J Am Acad Dermatol. 2012;66(6):e217–27.
33. Shim TN, Minhas S, Muneer A, Bunker CB. Atypical presentation of genital herpes simplex (HSV-2) in two patients with chronic lymphocytic leukemia. Acta Derm Venereol. 2014;94(2):246–7.
34. Lewis DA. Chancroid: clinical manifestations, diagnosis, and management. Sex Trans Infect. 2003;79:68–71.

Part III
Neoplasic Diseases

Precancerous Manifestations

Estella de Jong, Annemiek Leeman, and Jan Nico Bouwes Bavinck

1 Introduction

This chapter focuses on precancerous manifestations in solid organ transplant recipients (SOTRs). The terms precancerous, premalignant, and preneoplastic are often considered synonyms, yet there are different definitions stated in literature. In this chapter, the term precancerous manifestation is used for cutaneous lesions consisting of genetically and phenotypically altered cells that do not yet have the capacity to invade the surrounding tissues. They often precede skin malignancies such as cutaneous squamous cell carcinoma (cSCC).

Due to their impaired immune system and, therefore, the decreased ability to detect and destroy mutated cells, SOTRs are at increased risk of developing precancerous cutaneous growths. Moreover, many SOTRs develop lots of these lesions. As precancerous manifestations have an increased risk of evolution into invasive skin malignancies compared to the surrounding healthy skin, early detection, treatment, and management is especially important in this patient group. In this subchapter, common preneoplastic manifestations that present in SOTR will be discussed, including the pathophysiology, epidemiology, clinical presentation, histological characteristics, differential diagnosis, and treatment options.

E. de Jong (✉) · A. Leeman · J. N. Bouwes Bavinck
Department of Dermatology, Leiden University Medical Centre, Leiden, The Netherlands
e-mail: e.de_jong.huid@lumc.nl; a.leeman@lumc.nl; j.n.bouwes_bavinck@lumc.nl

J. Tomimori et al. (eds.), *Atlas of Dermatologic Diseases in Solid Organ Transplant Recipients*, https://doi.org/10.1007/978-3-031-13335-0_11

2 Actinic Keratosis

2.1 *Pathophysiology*

Actinic keratosis (AK) or solar keratosis is a cutaneous growth that results from the proliferation of atypical epidermal keratinocytes. The main cause for the development of AK is sun exposure. DNA mutations in the germinative basal layer of epidermal keratinocytes caused by ultraviolet radiation (mainly UVB and UVA to a lesser extent) lead to increased survival and proliferation of atypical cells. The role of mutations in the p53 tumor suppressor gene, a gene involved in cell cycle regulation, apoptosis, and DNA repair, has been studied extensively in the past. Besides p53, other tumor suppressor genes such as p16INK4a, p14ARF, and phosphatase and tensin homolog (PTEN) are often deregulated in AK [1].

2.2 *Epidemiology and Risk Factors*

AK is not rare. In fact, in the overall population in the United States it is one of the most common reasons to visit a dermatologist, with approximately 14% of all dermatology consultations. The overall prevalence of AK is estimated to vary between 6% and 26% dependent on different risk factors [2].

There are different genetic and environmental risk factors associated with AK development. Genetic risk factors for the development of AK in the immunocompetent population include increasing age, male gender, fair skin type (Fitzpatrick skin type I or II), and genetic disorders such as xeroderma pigmentosum. Environmental risk factors include high cumulative sun exposure and infection with the beta genus of the human papillomavirus (HPV). Research showed that the prevalence of AK increased with longer duration of immunosuppression, especially azathioprine.

AKs are dynamic lesions that have the ability to spontaneously go into regression. However, a small proportion (ca. 0.03–20%) of AK can develop into cSCC when left untreated [3, 4]. It is thought that approximately 70% of all cSCC are preceded by AK [5].

2.3 *The Role of HPV Infection*

Beta types of HPV have been closely linked with AK and cSCC development in immunocompetent patients [6–10] and in OTR [11]. Beta HPVs are found in the skin and hair follicles of more than 80% of healthy people. Colonization occurs from early childhood onwards. Increased viral load, number of infecting HPV genotypes and beta HPV-seropositivity have all been associated with AK and cSCC [6, 9, 10, 12]. The mechanisms involved in beta HPV-mediated skin carcinogenesis are fundamentally different from those occurring in the malignant transformation driven by the alpha HPV genotypes (HPV16, 18, etc.) [7]. Beta HPVs are thought to play a role at an early stage of carcinogenesis ("hit and run") at the time AK starts to develop. Beta HPVs exert pro-carcinogenic effects chiefly by enhancing accumulation of UVR-induced DNA damage in the skin [6, 8, 9, 13]. In normal cells, UVR up-regulates cellular defense processes, ultimately leading to p53 activation, cell cycle arrest, apoptosis, or DNA repair [14]. Expression of several genotypes beta HPV E6 and E7 (e.g., HPV5, 8, 38, and 49) deregulates many of these crucial pathways, mainly by directly targeting multiple transcription factors and/or transcriptional regulators, rendering infected cells highly susceptible to chromosomal instability and malignant transformation by UVR [6, 9, 10]. Other pro-carcinogenic properties include abrogation of NOTCH tumor suppression, repression of transforming growth factor (TGF) beta signaling, enhanced dermal invasion, and evasion of host immune surveillance [14].

After full establishment of the cSCC, the viral genome is often lost and the expression of the viral oncogenes is dispensable for the maintenance of the malignant phenotype. Hair follicles, followed by precursor lesions (AK, hyperkeratotic papilloma, and Bowen's disease) harbor the highest load of beta HPV DNA [15].

2.4 *Clinical Presentation*

AK present as non-indurated scaly, hyperkeratotic and/or erythematous papules, and plaques and are often present on sun-exposed areas such as the scalp, face, neck, upper chest, and distal arm (Figs. 1, 2, and 3). They are usually not painful.

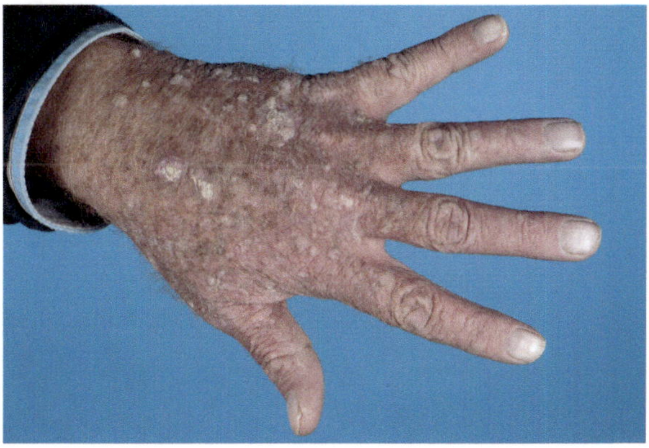

Fig. 1 Actinic keratosis on the dorsal side of the hand

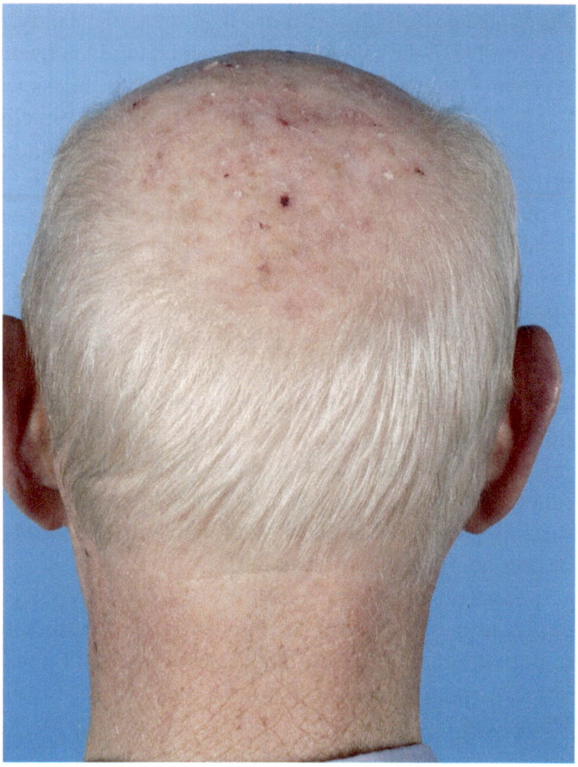

Fig. 2 Actinic keratosis on the sun-exposed area of the head

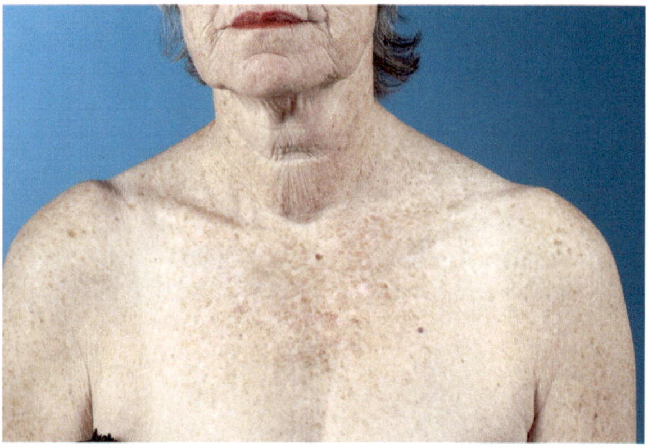

Fig. 3 Actinic keratosis on the sun-exposed area of the chest

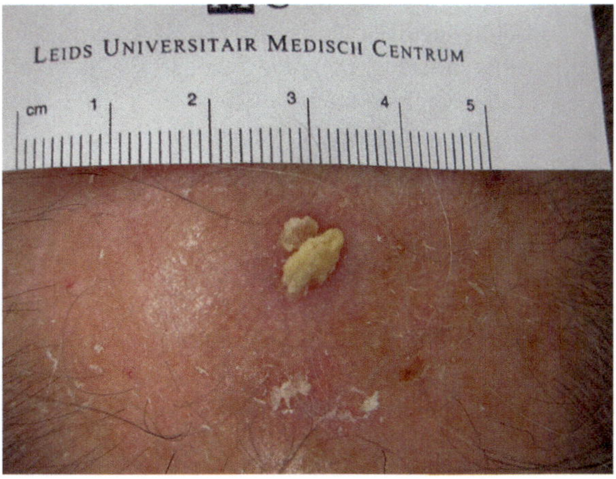

Fig. 4 Actinic keratosis of 1 cm with a cutaneous horn in the center

Dermoscopy shows erythematous to brown (pseudo)networks, dependent on the type of AK, and sometimes irregular hyperpigmented follicular openings or dotted vessels and rosettes.

There are different kinds of AK, including classic, hypertrophic, atrophic, pigmented AK, and AK with a cutaneous horn (Fig. 4). An important form of AK, which is located on the lips, is called actinic cheilitis (or solar cheilosis) and will be discussed separately.

2.5 *Histopathology*

Histological features of AK include intraepidermal atypia of basal keratinocytes which can extend to the mid or upper epidermal layers and along adnexal structures. Unlike Bowen's disease and cSCC, there is never full thickness atypia (Fig. 5a, b). The granular layer can be lost, attenuated, or mildly acanthotic. Depending on the type of AK, hyperkeratosis can be present (Fig. 6). Increased melanin in the basal keratinocytes and melanocytes may be present in pigmented AK. The term "Bowenoid AK" is given to lesions with focal near full thickness atypia. Dermal changes include solar elastosis and a mild (usually lymphocytic) inflammatory infiltrate.

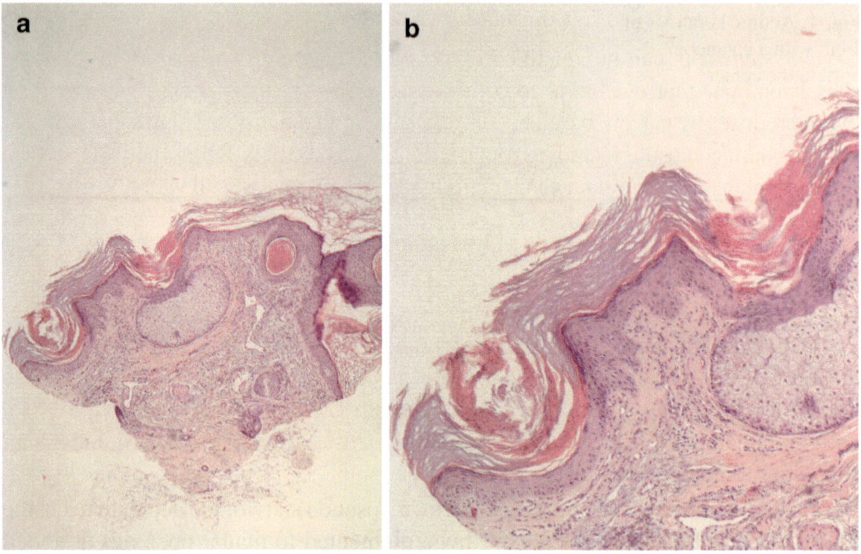

Fig. 5 (**a**, **b**) Histology of actinic keratosis. There is no full thickness atypia

Fig. 6 Histology of actinic keratosis with hyperkeratosis of the epidermis

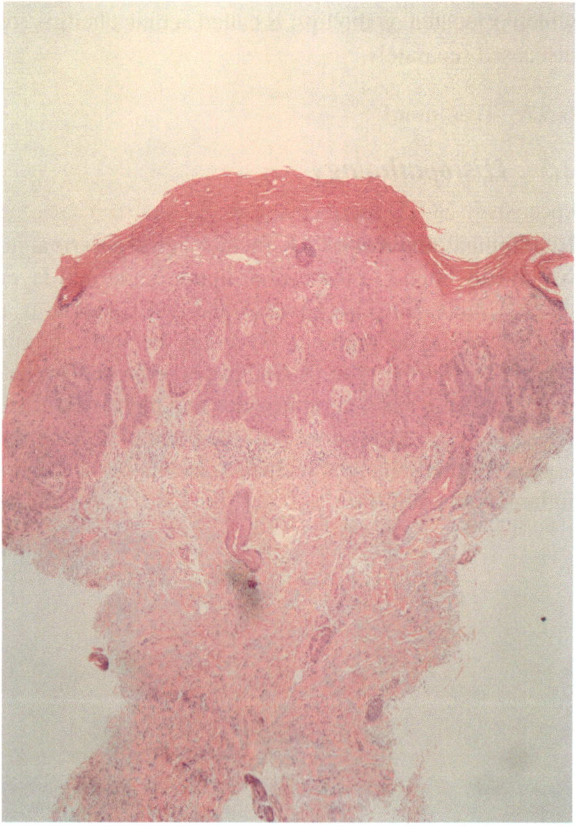

2.6 Detection of Actinic Keratosis in Solid Organ Transplant Recipients

AK is usually diagnosed clinically. However, in any doubt, for example in the presence of itch, pain, bleeding, ulceration, or uncertainty on induration, a biopsy should be taken to differentiate between AK and cSCC.

In sun-damaged skin, besides the clinical visible AK, there is the presence of subclinical atypia which cannot be seen with naked eye examination. The last years, more evidence and experience has been acquired on the role of reflectance confocal microscopy for subclinical lesions [16]. This method has revealed that cellular and nuclear atypia is found in AK in clinically unaffected appearing skin [17].

2.7 Classification Systems

A frequently used clinical classification system is developed by Olsen et al. and is based on the overall thickness of individual lesions [2]. In this scheme, grade I AK are slightly palpable, grade II lesions are moderately thick and grade III lesions are very thick and hyperkeratotic.

Roewert-Huber et al. introduced a histological classification system for grading AK and is based on the extent of atypical keratinocytes in the epidermis [18]. In grade I (mild), atypical keratinocytes are only present in the basal and suprabasal layers, limited to the lower third of the epidermis. In grade II (moderate), atypical keratinocytes extend to the lower two-thirds of the epidermis. In grade III (severe), full thickness atypia of the epidermis is found and is equivalent to lesions called in situ cSCC or Bowen's disease.

Schmitz et al. investigated the correlation between the clinical and histological classification system and found a match in only 53.8% [2]. Some Olsen grade I AK were already histologically grade III and, therefore, it has been suggested to treat all AK. Although 74% of AK regress within 12 months, this is important to realize when it comes to the treatment and management of multiple AK in SOTR [4]. One study explored risk factors for progression of AK in SOTR and found that cumulative sun exposure was associated with a lower rate of regression of AK in these patients. Other risk factors included increasing age, hair color, and recent treatment for AK.

2.8 Differential Diagnosis

The differential diagnosis of AK includes Bowen's disease, cSCC, verruca vulgaris, and benign lichenoid keratosis.

2.9 *Treatment and Management of Actinic Keratosis in SOTR*

Treatment options for AK are extensive and do not generally differ between immunocompetent and immunosuppressed patients [19, 20]. It is, however, important to realize that immunosuppressed patients including SOTR present with multiple lesions and field cancerization. Furthermore, they are less likely to undergo spontaneous or therapy-induced regression [21].

Cryotherapy is an easy and highly effective option for solitary lesions if performed correctly. Freeze time is an important determinant of treatment efficacy with complete cure rates of 83%, 69%, and 39% at 3 months with freeze times >20, 5–20, and <5 s, respectively [22]. However, longer freeze durations may also result in a higher chance of local reactions and scarring. SOTR often develop many AK and have heavily sun-damaged skin, which makes them a good candidate for field cancerization treatment. These field therapies are preferred because they address clinically visible as well as subclinical disease.

The most commonly used topical treatments include 5-Fluorouracil (5-FU) and imiquimod cream. 5-FU is a pyrimidine analog approved by the US Food and Drug Administration (FDA) for the treatment of AK and superficial basal cell carcinoma. 5-FU is proven to be superior to imiquimod in the treatment of AK [23]. There is evidence that the combination of 5-FU and calcipotriol significantly lowers the risk of cSCC compared to 5-FU alone in short treatment periods (a 4-day course) [24, 25]. Other field therapies for AK include chemowraps and photodynamic therapy (PDT).

A recent systematic review investigating local interventions for AK in SOTR stated that there is still limited evidence available for the best treatment and management of AK in SOTR [20]. Aminolevulinate PDT was the best studied intervention and showed the highest complete response rates. However, most studies had short follow-up periods. Furthermore, lesion-specific regimens may not be sufficient to achieve disease control. Field-directed regimens are preferable in this high-risk population.

3 Actinic Cheilitis

3.1 *Epidemiology*

An important form of AK is called actinic cheilitis (or solar cheilosis) and is present on the lip. Little is known about the exact incidence of actinic cheilitis in both immunocompetent and immunocompromised patients because premalignant lesions are often insufficiently documented. Small studies in immunocompetent patients show prevalence rates varying between 0.45% and 2.4% [26–28]. Risk factors for the development of actinic cheilitis are comparable with those in AK, with chronic sun exposure (e.g., fishermen and farmers) as the main risk factor. In these patient groups, the prevalence may be close to 40% [29]. There has been conflicting evidence as to whether alcohol and smoking independently increase the risk of actinic cheilitis [30].

When keeping in mind that SOTR have a 13–66-fold increased incidence of lip cancer compared with the general population, it is likely that their risk of premalignant lip lesions such as actinic cheilitis is highly increased as well [31]. Literature on the malignant transformation rate is scarce. In one study, a malignant transformation rate of actinic cheilitis to cSCC of 3.07% was mentioned [32].

3.2 Clinical Presentation

Actinic cheilitis is usually found on the lower lip and presents as a persistent scaly lesion. Patients often complain of a persistent dry lip. Atrophic changes (Fig. 7) as well as hyperkeratotic plaques or crusting may be present (Figs. 8, 9, and 10).

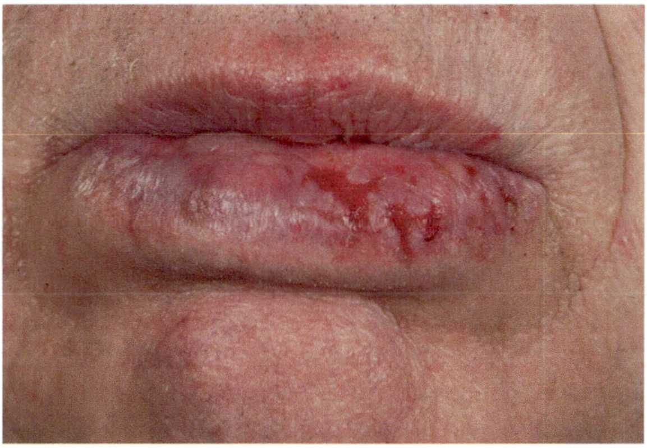

Fig. 7 Atrophic changes by actinic cheilitis

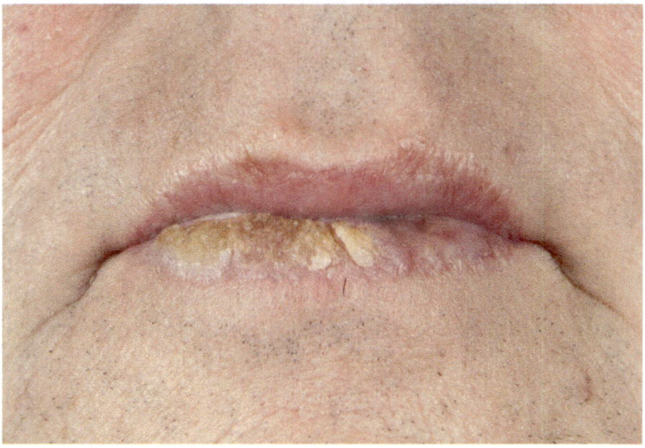

Fig. 8 Hyperkeratotic plaque by actinic cheilitis

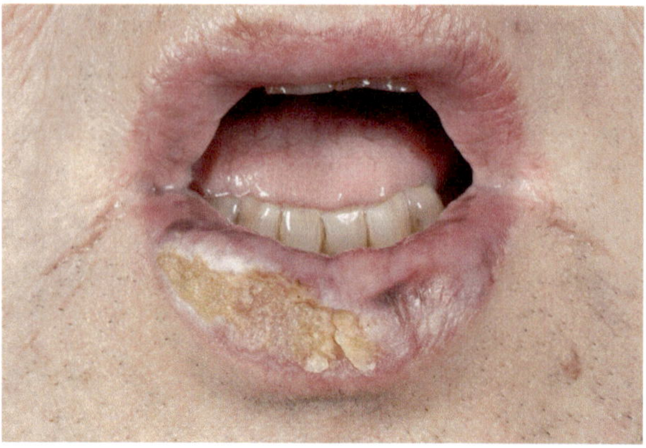

Fig. 9 Hyperkeratotic plaque by actinic cheilitis

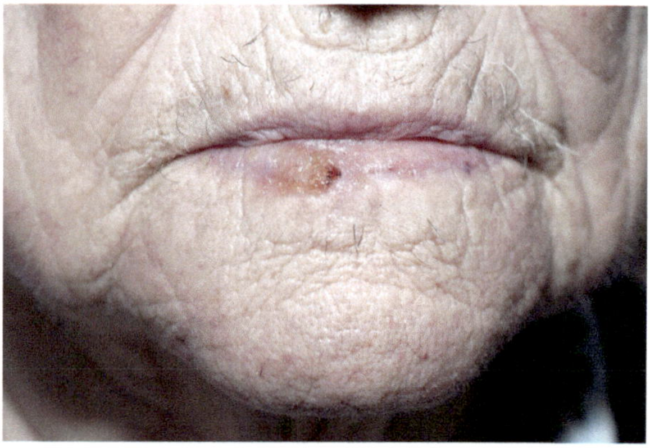

Fig. 10 Crusting by actinic cheilitis

Persistent fissures or ulceration on the lip may also indicate the presence of actinic cheilitis. In case of induration, pain, or persistent plaques that do not respond to treatment, a biopsy is needed to rule out cSCC.

Dermoscopic findings include ill-demarcated lesion borders, white-colored projections, "island"-like structures and radially arranged vascular telangiectasia surrounding ulcerated areas [33].

3.3 Histopathology

When in doubt of invasive growth, a punch biopsy can be performed. One must be aware that with punch biopsy, there is a chance of sample error [34]. When there is a high suspicion of cSCC, an elliptical incision biopsy in the thickest part of the lesion is preferred. Histopathological findings are comparable with those in AK

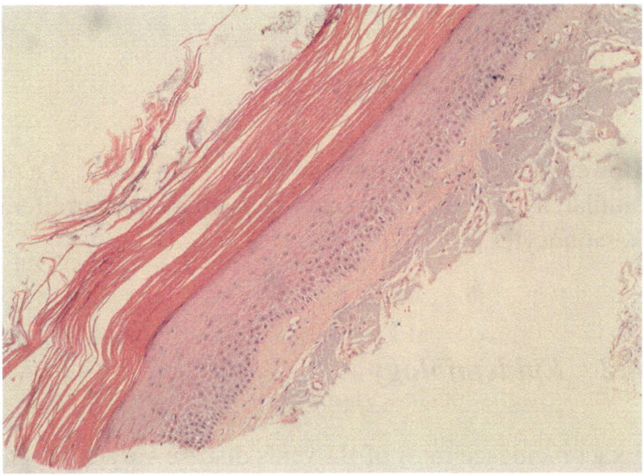

Fig. 11 Histology of actinic cheilitis

(Fig. 11). The most important histological finding is intraepidermal atypia of basal keratinocytes. Acanthosis, hyperkeratosis, and atrophy can be present. Within the dermis one might find an inflammatory infiltrate predominantly composed of lymphocytes as well as solar elastosis.

3.4 Differential Diagnosis

The differential diagnosis of actinic cheilitis includes cSCC of the lip, Bowen's disease, cheilosis, lichen planus, lupus erythematosus, cheilitis glandularis, and cheilitis granulomatosa.

3.5 Treatment and Management

The goal of therapy is to reduce the risk of malignant transformation from actinic cheilitis to cSCC while maintaining the functionality and appearance of the lips. A variety of therapies in the management of actinic cheilitis are available, including both surgical and non-surgical options. In 2019, a systematic review was published investigating the outcome of surgical and non-surgical treatment options and stated that the surgical treatment was more favorable than non-surgical treatment for actinic cheilitis [35]. An alternative with favorable outcomes is carbon dioxide laser ablation [36]. Chemical peel and PDT were associated with higher recurrence. Cryotherapy, 5-FU, and imiquimod are easy options and can be used for mild actinic cheilitis.

4 Bowen's Disease

4.1 *Pathophysiology*

Bowen's disease, also referred to as in situ cSCC, is a premalignant skin lesion that, similar as AK and cSCC, is caused by the proliferation of atypical epidermal keratinocytes.

4.2 *Epidemiology*

Exact incidence rates of Bowen's disease vary between demographic locations and are not investigated in large studies. Bowen's disease tends to be increasing. A Dutch study shows incidences of 8.1 per 100,000 individuals in 2003 to 68.9 per 100,000 in 2013 [37]. This increase was the highest in women. One study compared immunocompetent and immunocompromised patients with Bowen's disease and found that immunocompromised patients were significantly more likely to have multiple Bowen's disease (15% vs 33%, respectively) [38]. It is thought that approximately 3–5% of Bowen's disease will transform into cSCC; however, exact numbers are not available.

4.3 *Clinical Presentation*

Bowen's disease presents as an erythematous, well-demarcated, scaly patch, or plaque that is usually asymptomatic (unlike inflammatory diseases such as eczema and psoriasis which are often itching) (Figs. 12, 13, 14a, b, and 15). Bowen's disease can be pigmented and grows predominantly on sun-exposed areas. Nevertheless,

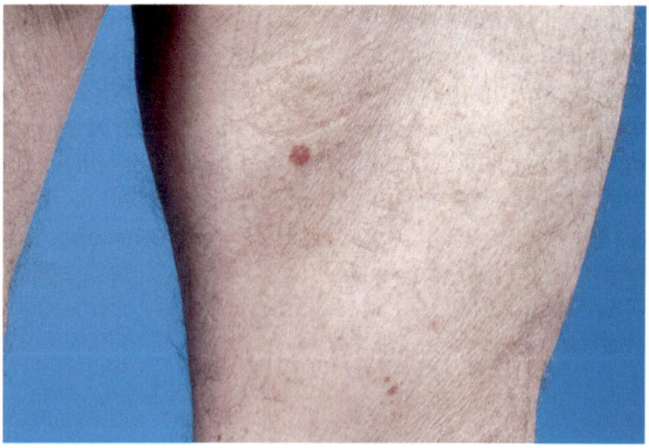

Fig. 12 Bowen's disease, shown as an erythematous, well-demarcated plaque

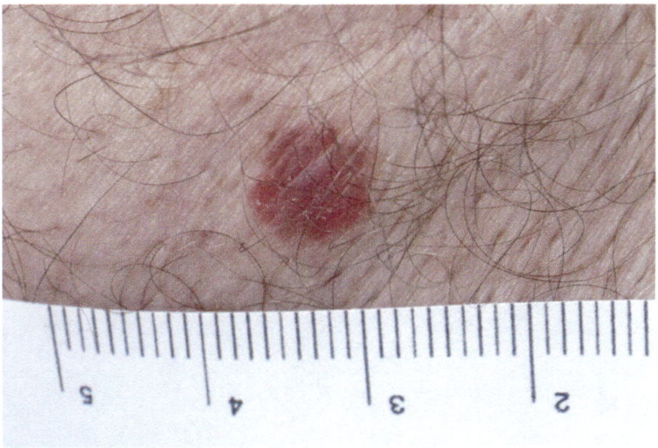

Fig. 13 Close-up of a Bowen's disease of 7 mm

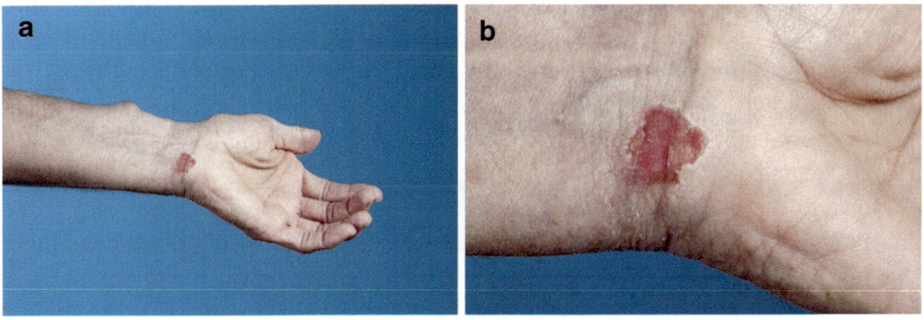

Fig. 14 (**a**) Bowen's disease on the wrist. (**b**) Close-up of Bowen's disease on the wrist

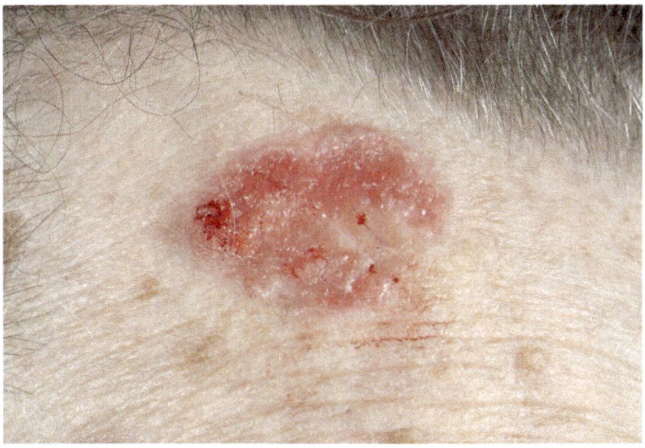

Fig. 15 Bowen's disease on the forehead

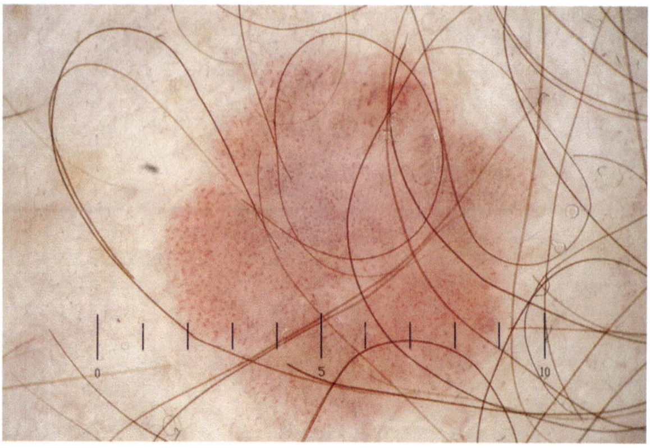

Fig. 16 Dermoscopy of Bowen's disease which displays dotted vessels

especially in SOTR, Bowen's disease can also be found on areas that are not sun-damaged, for example, the genital area, which will be discussed, separately. Dermoscopy of Bowen's disease displays dotted and/or glomerular vessels (Fig. 16), white to yellowish surface scales, and a red-yellowish background color. Pigmented lesions show a structureless, brown pattern with hypopigmented areas, often eccentrically located, and brown dots at the periphery [39].

Bowen's disease is a histological diagnosis and therefore a punch biopsy is the golden standard for differentiating between AK, Bowen's disease, cSCC, and other skin diseases.

4.4 Histopathology

Histological features of Bowen's disease are similar to AK with one important distinction: in contrast to AK, Bowen's disease requires full thickness keratinocyte atypia by definition (without infiltration of atypical cells into the dermis which makes it an invasive cSCC) (Fig. 17). Nuclear hyperchromasia, multinucleation, and numerous (atypical) mitotic figures are present. Bowen's disease may extend into eccrine sweat glands, which must not be confused with invasive disease.

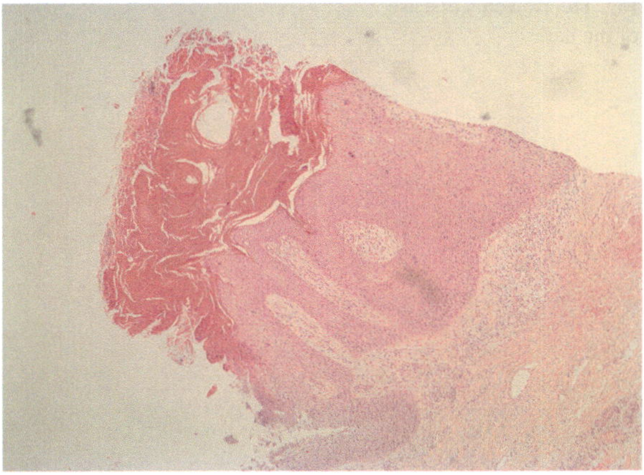

Fig. 17 Histology of Bowen's disease. There is no infiltration of atypical cells into the dermis present

4.5 *Differential Diagnosis*

The differential diagnosis of Bowen's disease includes AK, superficial invasive cSCC, nummular eczema, psoriasis, inflamed seborrheic keratosis, prurigo nodule, pyoderma gangrenosum, and necrobiosis lipoidica.

4.6 *Treatment and Management*

Treatment options for Bowen's disease include surgical excision, curettage and electrodessication, PDT, cryotherapy, topical 5-FU, and imiquimod. The decision on which treatment to use depends on multiple factors such as size and site of the lesion, comorbidity, and the patient's preference.

Surgical excision with a 5 mm margin has the most favorable outcome rate and complete excision rate is found in 94% for lesions excised with a 5 mm margin [40]. For difficult locations, curettage and electrodessication may be the treatment of choice. Recurrent rates largely depend on the experience of the clinician but are thought to be between 2% and 20%.

Another treatment of difficult locations such as nail Bowen's disease (Figs. 18 and 19) may be laser therapy. For now, there is little data regarding the use of lasers in treating Bowen's disease and the information that is available is limited to case reports and series. A clearance rate of 86% in one study has been found. PDT is especially suitable for larger lesions (>3 cm in diameter) [41].

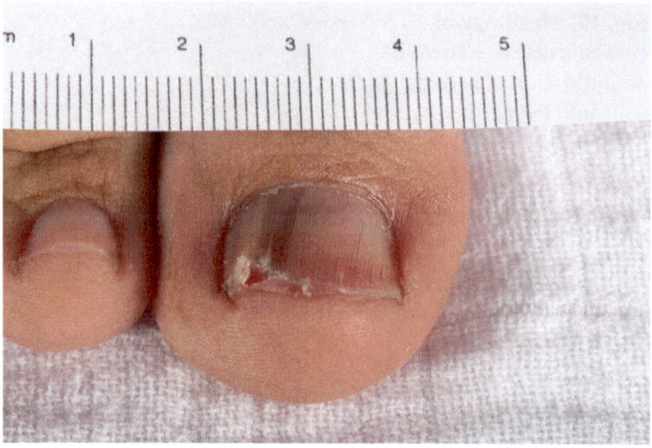

Fig. 18 Bowen's disease of the nail

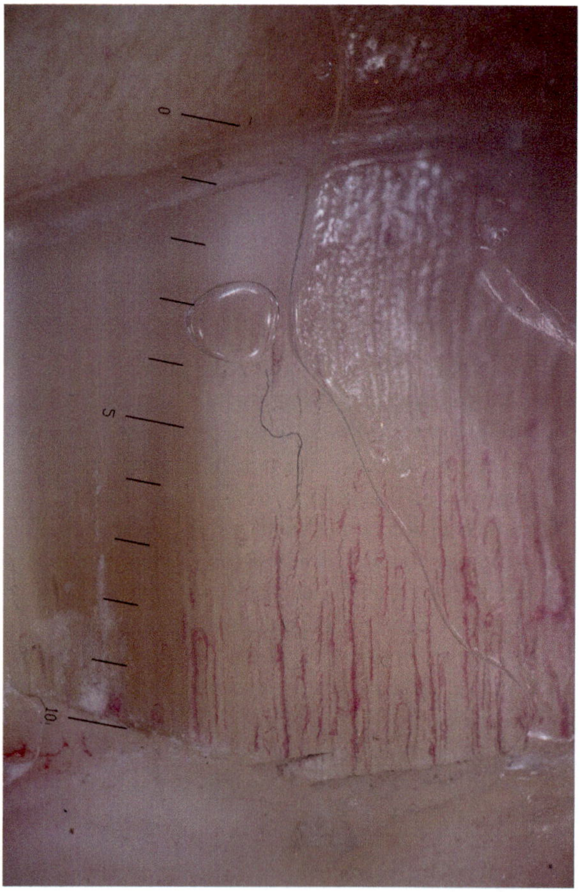

Fig. 19 Dermoscopy of Bowen's disease of the nail

Response rates of cryotherapy differ largely between clinicians. Cryotherapy may be a good option in SOTR with multiple small lesions that are not suitable for topical treatments such as 5-FU and imiquimod.

Local application of 5-FU implies daily use for a period of 3–4 weeks with a complete response in 48% to 83% of the cases, according to available evidence on immunocompetent patients [42]. Imiquimod, which is an antitumor and an antiviral agent, show complete response rates between 57% and 86% after 6 weeks of daily use.

5 Penile Intraepithelial Neoplasia

5.1 Terminology

Penile intraepithelial neoplasia (PeIN) is a precursor lesion with a progression rate to penile SCC of approximately 30%. Over the years, several terms have been used for precursor lesions of penile cancers, such as erythroplasia of Queyrat, penile Bowen's disease, bowenoid papulosis, and penile carcinoma in situ [43]. However, not all of these terms take into account the role of HPV in lesion origin, or lesion grade or severity. Therefore, it was suggested to use a model which uses a different classification for HPV-related (bowenoid, warty, basaloid, undifferentiated) PeIN and non-HPV-related (classic squamous, differentiated) PeIN.

5.2 Pathophysiology

Development of penile cancer through precursor lesions is thought to follow one out of two pathways which are similar to the pathways in vulvar carcinogenesis: the HPV-related pathway or the non-HPV-related pathway. Persistent infection with a high-risk human papillomavirus infection, mostly HPV16, can result in a warty, basaloid precursor lesion which can develop into undifferentiated SCC if not treated [44]. Clinical manifestations are Bowen's disease, erythroplasia of Queyrat, and bowenoid papulosis. The non-HPV-related precursor lesions are frequently associated with lichen sclerosus and can progress to a differentiated form of squamous cell carcinoma.

5.3 Epidemiology and Risk Factors

Penile cancer incidence rates are reported to be between 0.3 and 1.5 per 100,000 men in the western world and much higher in developing countries. High-risk HPV has been found to cause about 40% of penile cancer. The incidence rate of PeIN is not known.

Risk factors for developing HPV-related PeIN are persistent infection with a high-risk HPV type, mostly HPV16, number of sexual partners, history of genital warts (Figs. 20 and 21) or multizonal disease, and history of other sexually transmitted diseases. In the non-HPV-related pathway, the chronic inflammation found in lichen sclerosus (Fig. 22) seems to play a major role. Other consistently found risk factors for developing penile cancer are pore penile hygiene, smegma retention, phimosis, and unretractable foreskin otherwise, treatment with PUVA and smoking [45, 46]. SOTR and users of immunosuppressive drugs have a 7 and 5 times higher risk of penile cancer, respectively [47].

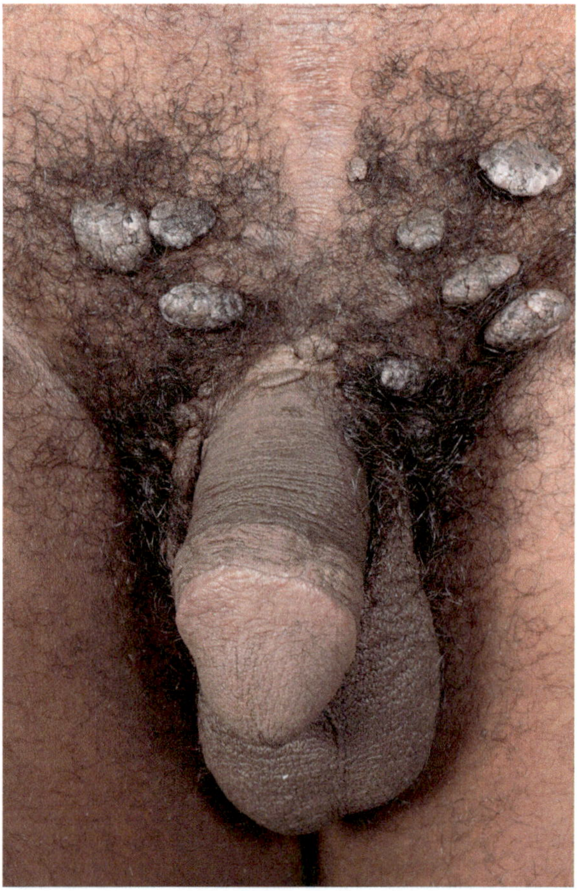

Fig. 20 Genital warts around the penis

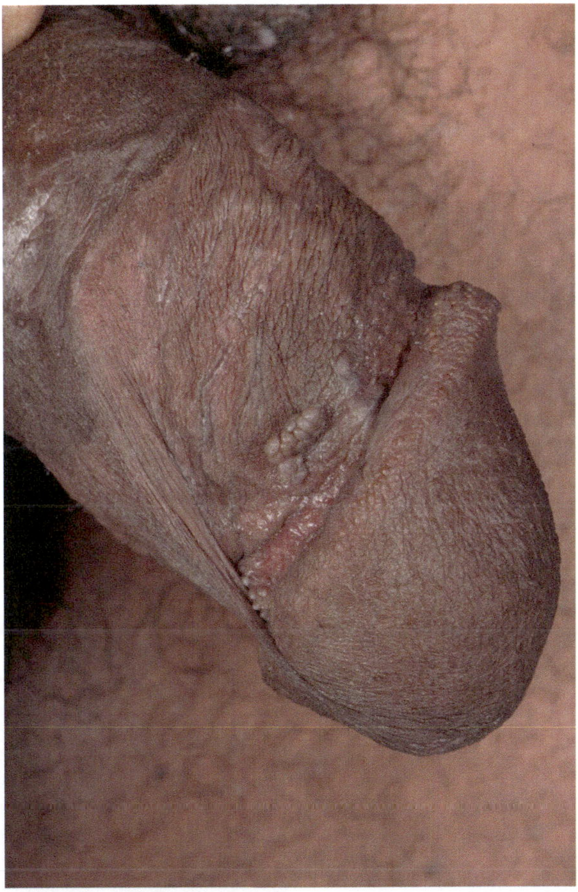

Fig. 21 Genital warts on the penis

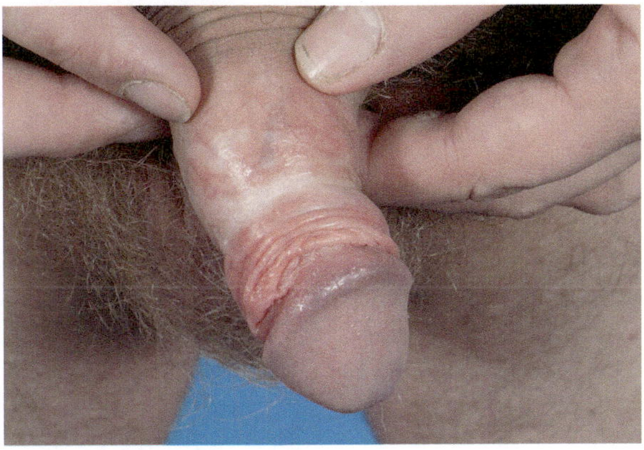

Fig. 22 Penile lichen sclerosus

5.4 Clinical Presentation

Although abandoned for the classification of PeIN, terms such Bowen's disease and bowenoid papulosis are still frequently used for clinical description. Erythroplasia of Queyrat (Fig. 23) presents as a well-defined, velvety, red plaque often on the glans and prepuce. Whitish areas in glans, coronal sulcus, or inner foreskin can be present as well as ulceration in some cases. Pain is uncommon. Bowenoid papulosis (Fig. 24) is characterized by multiple slightly elevated papules that are red to violet in color. Lesions are predominantly found on the penile shaft although the glans and prepuce may also be affected. HPV-related lesions can also present as warty papules.

As non-HPV-related differentiated PeIN is found in lichen sclerosus, white atrophic plaques may be seen on the glans and prepuce with sclerotic masses and adhesions in a later stage.

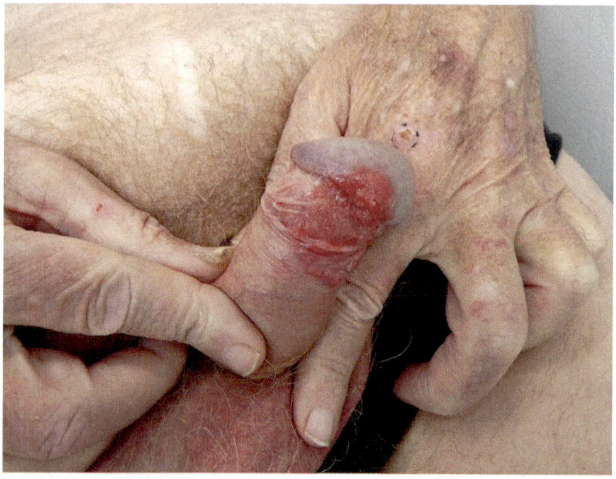

Fig. 23 Erythroplasia of Queyrat

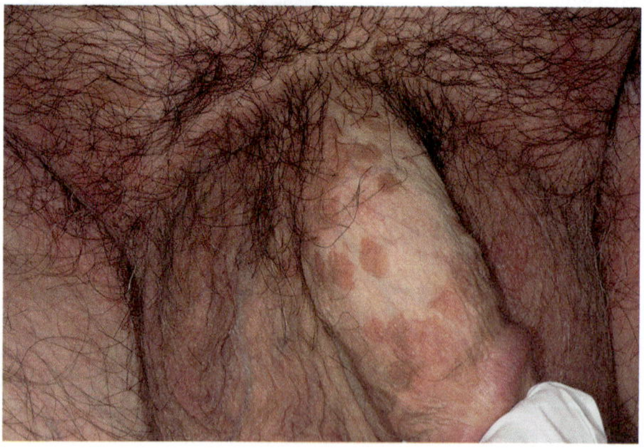

Fig. 24 Bowenoid papulosis of the penis

5.5 *Histopathology*

Precursor lesions of differentiated SCC, the classical type, is most often found as squamous hyperplasia. Microscopically, this squamous hyperplasia shows a flat, verrucous, pseudoepitheliomatous, or mixed patterns. The typical lesion is flat with acanthosis as the main feature, with hyperkeratosis of the orthokeratotic type. Normal squamous cell maturation with an orderly basal cell layer is seen [48].

HPV-related precursor lesions show low- or high-grade intraepithelial dysplasia with abnormal maturation, loss of polarity, nuclear atypia, and normal and abnormal mitoses. Low-grade lesions show dysplasia restricted to the lower one-third of the epithelium while high-grade lesions can show atypical cells in two-thirds or more of the squamous epithelium [48].

5.6 *Differential Diagnosis*

The differential diagnosis of PeIN includes penile SCC, balanitis (e.g., Zoon balanitis) (Fig. 25), lichen sclerosus, and lichen planus.

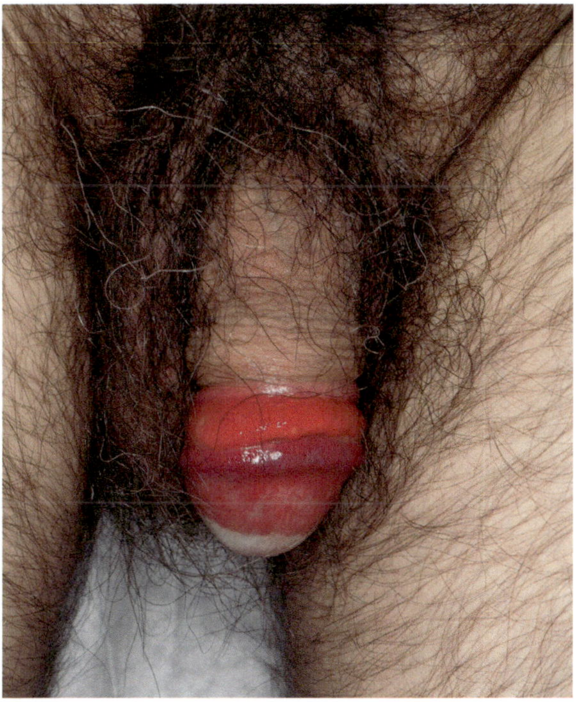

Fig. 25 Zoon balanitis

5.7 *Treatment and Management*

PeIN can be treated with local excision, laser therapy, radiotherapy, photodynamic therapy, and topical therapy with 5-FU or imiquimod cream according to severity. Penis-preserving strategies are recommended for the treatment of small lesions such as lesions historically called bowenoid papulosis, with a chance of spontaneous regression. Total glansectomy and prepuce has the lowest recurrence rate at 2% for the treatment of small lesions. Frequent follow-up is essential to enable early detection of recurrence and to assess proper treatment in an early stage.

6 Vulvar Intraepithelial Neoplasia

6.1 *Terminology*

Vulvar intraepithelial neoplasia (VIN) has many similarities with penile intraepithelial neoplasia in etiology and classification. In the currently used classification system, a distinction is made between HPV-related VIN which is also referred to as squamous intraepithelial lesion (SIL) and differentiated, non-HPV-related VIN (dVIN). The International Society for the Study of Vulvovaginal Disease (ISSVD) published this classification in 2015 [49]. HPV-related VIN or vulvar SIL can be classified as low-grade SIL (LSIL) and high-grade SIL (HSIL) [50]. Low-grade SIL is thought to represent productive HPV infections which are often self-limiting and caused by low-risk HPV genotypes (such as HPV6 and 11). High-grade SIL is caused by transforming infection with high-risk HPV (such as HPV16 and 18) and has a higher chance of progression to cancer. Differentiated VIN is frequently found adjacent to differentiated vulvar squamous cell carcinoma and is thought to develop in areas of chronic inflammation as found in lichen sclerosus [51].

6.2 *Pathophysiology*

The development of HSIL occurs through a persisting infection with a high-risk HPV genotype. About 15–25% of vulvar cancers are induced by high-risk HPV infection. In a recently published study, the 10-year risk of progression to vulvar squamous cell carcinoma was 9.7% [52].

The majority of vulvar cancer is HPV negative and is thought to be associated with lichen sclerosus (Fig. 26) [53, 54]. For differentiated VIN, progression risk is much higher, showing progression to cancer in 50% [52]. Differentiated VIN is thought to be highly proliferative and progresses over a shorter period of time.

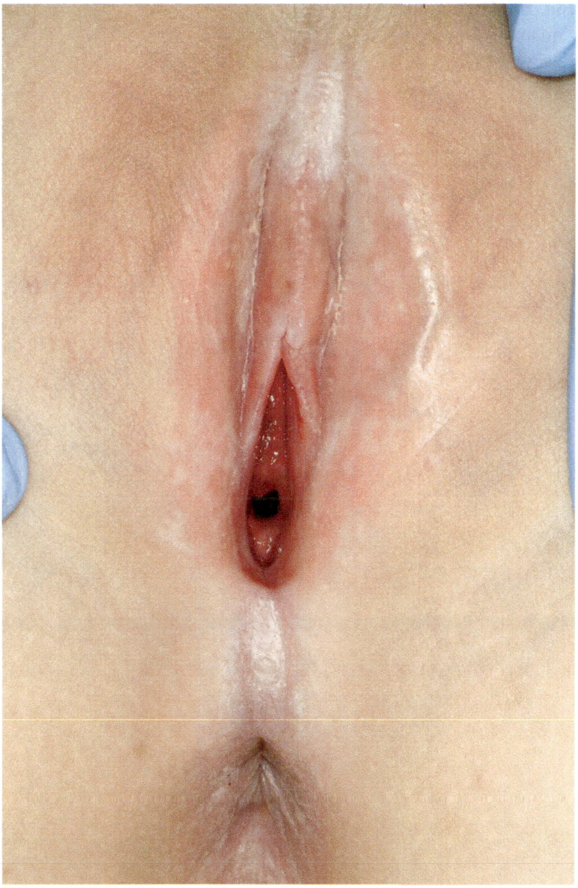

Fig. 26 Vulvar lichen sclerosus

6.3 Epidemiology and Risk Factors

HSIL (Fig. 27), which is caused by persisting infection with the sexually transmitted HPV infection, is more frequently found in younger women (30–50 years of age). Also, marital status, oral contraceptive use, smoking, and immunosuppression causes an increased risk of HSIL. The incidence between 1991–1995 and 2006–2011 has shown an increase from 2.39 to 3.26 [52].

dVIN is thought to develop in lichen sclerosus and is mostly found in women between 60 and 80 years of age. Mechanisms possibly involved in degeneracy include chronic inflammation, ischemic, and oxidative stress and mutations in p53 [55]. Over the past decades, the incidence has increased from 0.02 to 0.08 [52]. The risk of vulvar lichen planus (Fig. 28) in the development of vulvar SCC is unclear and differentiation between dVIN and erosive and hypertrophic lichen planus is difficult [56].

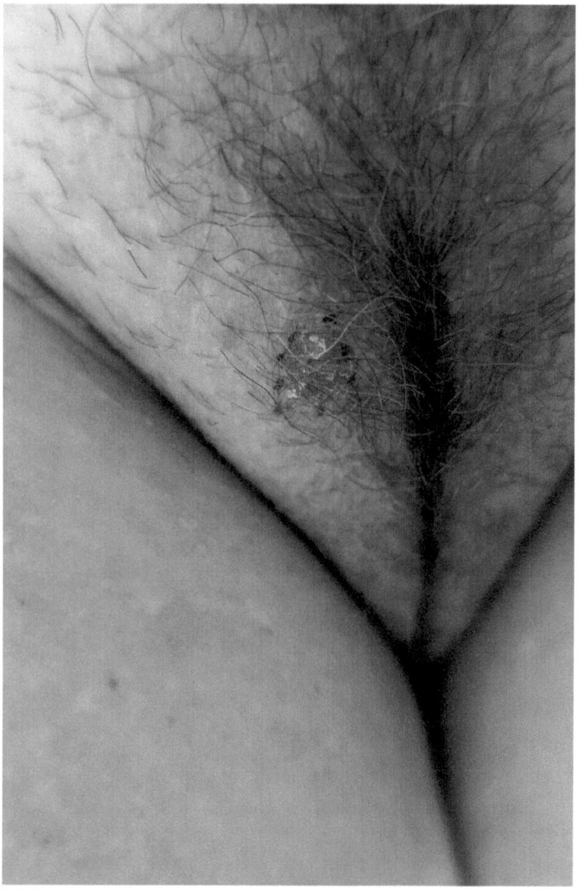

Fig. 27 High-grade Squamous Intraepithelial Lesion (HSIL)

6.4 Clinical Presentation

Most vulvar SCCs occur on the labia majora. The labia minora, clitoris, and perineum may also be primary sites.

VIN presents as an asymptomatic or pruritic lesion, which can sometimes cause pain, burning, or dysuria. Single lesions may be hard to identify as such. White, pink, brown, gray, or red macules or elevated plaques with a verrucous surface may be seen. dVIN is often found in women who are suffering from lichen sclerosus (Fig. 26) which can be identified by a combination of erythema, white skin changes (such as hyperkeratosis and sclerosis), fissures, or changes in anatomy such as flattened appearance of the labia minora and a buried clitoris.

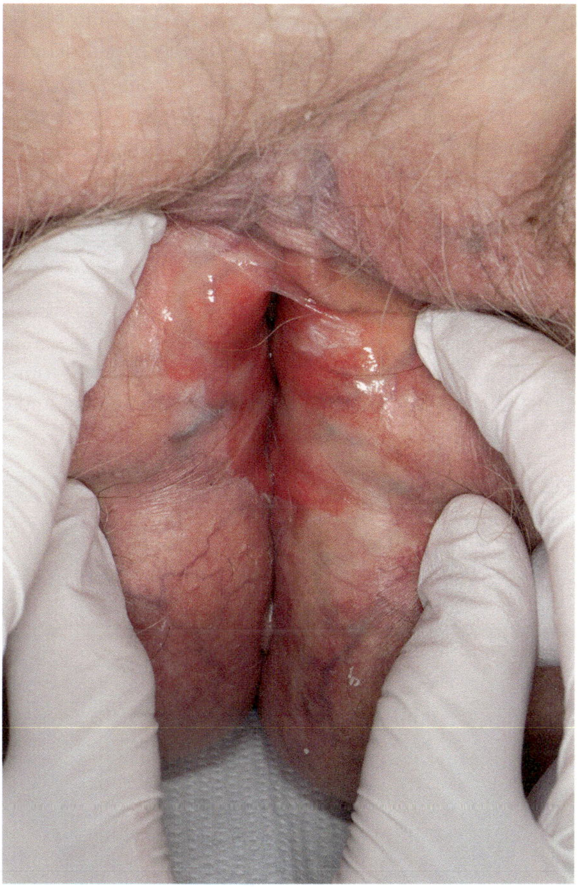

Fig. 28 Vulvar lichen planus

6.5 Histopathology

HSIL has well-defined histological characteristics which can be appreciated including hyperkeratosis and parakeratosis, acanthosis with club-shaped rete ridges, disorientation of the individual cells commencing above the basal cell layer and above at least the lower third of the epithelium and nuclear clumping with mitotic figures. High nuclear-to-cytoplasmic ratios, hyperchromasia, pleomorphism, increased number of mitoses above the parabasal cell layer and apoptotic bodies are common. The warty type of HSIL can display viral changes such as koilocytosis and multinucleated cells. The basaloid type is flat and has basaloid cells seen over the full thickness of the epithelium.

Differentiated VIN is a challenging histological diagnosis with morphologic similarities with dermatoses showing chronic inflammation. Acanthosis, parakeratosis, irregular elongation, and anastomoses of the rete ridges may be seen. A histological clue may be found in the hypereosinophilic appearance of a lesion, which is a result of accumulation of intracellular keratin and the juxtapositioning of the cells to the epidermal-dermal junction. Dyskeratosis, extracellular keratin, and abortive squamous pearls in the lower layers of the epidermis and prominent intercellular bridges in the absence of inflammation may be seen [51].

6.6 *Differential Diagnosis*

The differential diagnosis of VIN includes condylomata acuminate (genital warts) (Figs. 29 and 30), lichen sclerosus, lichen planus, and condylomata lata.

Fig. 29 Condylomata acuminate (genital warts)

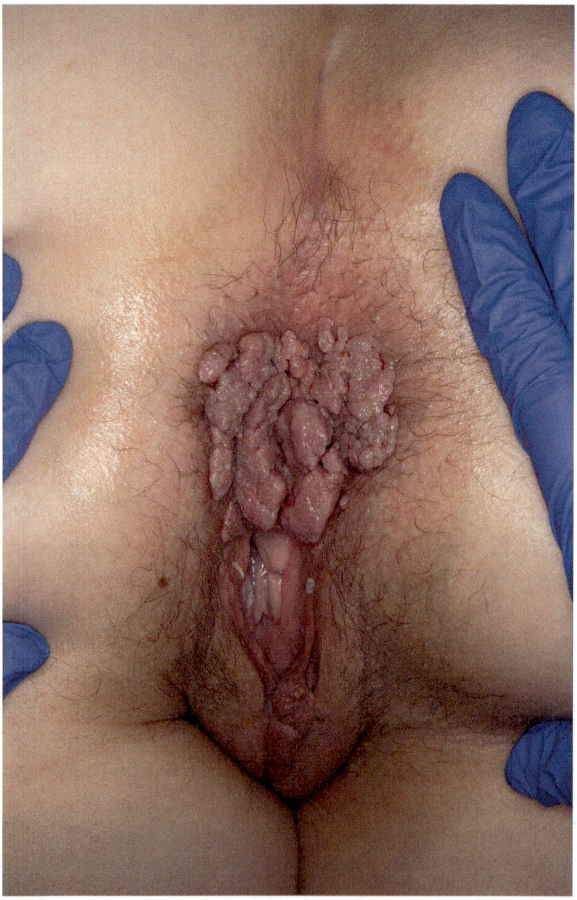

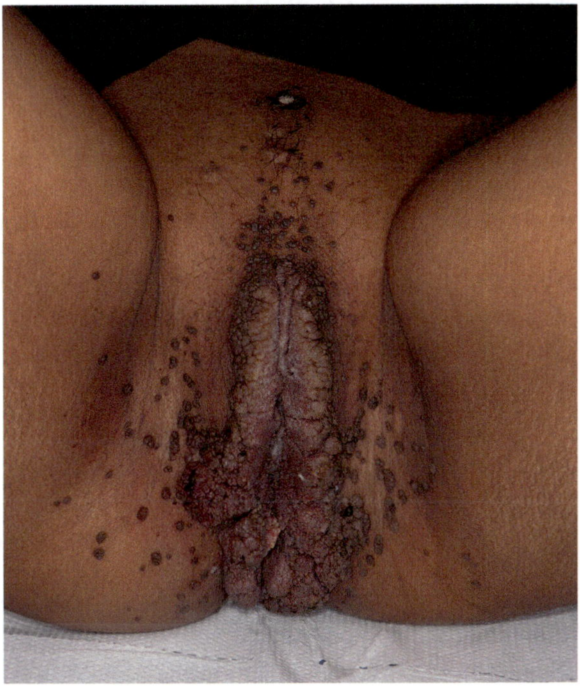

Fig. 30 Condylomata acuminate (genital warts)

6.7 Treatment and Management

The decision for the best treatment of VIN is dependent on different tumor characteristics, including the size, location, multifocality, multicentricity, possible signs of occult invasion, patient characteristics (age, general condition, comorbidities, reliability of follow-up), and availability of medical resources and expertise [55]. The goals of treatment are prevention of invasive vulvar cancer, prevention of recurrence, symptom relief, and preservation of vulvar anatomy and function and quality of life.

Treatment options for HSIL include surgery, ablative therapy with CO_2 laser, and topical treatment with imiquimod. Surgery is the preferred option in case of suspicion of invasion or for lesions resistant to less invasive treatment modalities such as ablative or topical treatment. In patients with dVIN, the recommended treatment modality is surgery.

In order to reduce the risk of VIN and prevent disease recurrence, patients should be encouraged to quit smoking. Factors that increase risk of recurrent disease are older age (>50 years) and multizonal HPV-related disease, persisting HPV infection and immunosuppression for HSIL, and underlying lichen sclerosus and immunosuppression for dVIN [57].

7 Anal Intraepithelial Neoplasia

7.1 Terminology

Anal intraepithelial neoplasia (AIN) is a precursor lesion in the intra-anal and perianal region. Unlike penile and vulvar intraepithelial neoplasia, AIN is virtually solely caused by HPV infection. It can be classified into anal low-grade squamous intraepithelial lesions (LSIL) and anal high-grade squamous intraepithelial lesions (HSIL). HSIL is considered to be premalignant with a higher risk of progression to anal cancer. LSIL consists of mostly productive HPV infections and has a higher chance of spontaneous regression.

7.2 Pathophysiology

AIN is a precursor of anal cancer and is caused by persistent infection with high-risk HPV. In over 90% of anal cancer, HPV16 is found [58]. However, anal HSIL can be caused by both low-risk HPV and high-risk HPV and vice versa as found in a study among HIV-positive men who have sex with men (MSM) [59]. Most knowledge about its pathophysiology comes from cervical cancer studies as both have great similarities. Micro-traumata to the mucosa can allow HPV virions to enter the basal layer of the epithelium. If not cleared by the immune system, cancer develops through a series of stages and a complex process of different events including chromosomal loss, somatic gene activation and suppression, somatic mutation, viral integration, and methylation [60]. However, it should not be assumed that the natural history of AIN is identical to that of cervical intraepithelial neoplasia.

In anal SIL, progression rates of HSIL to anal cancer have been reported up to at least 20% in HIV+ MSM [61]. A small proportion of anal LSIL will progress to HSIL [62].

7.3 Epidemiology

The exact incidence of AIN is unknown. It is most frequently found in high-risk populations such as MSM, immunocompromised patients and women with a history of cervical or vulvar cancer, among which incidences are rising. In the general population, the risk of anal cancer is estimated at 2 per 100,000 and tends to be rising [63]. The incidence of anal cancer ranges from 5 per 100,000 per year among HIV-negative MSM to 78 per 100,000 per year among HIV-positive MSM [64]. HIV infection is associated with an increased prevalence of HPV infection overall and an increased prevalence of the most frequent oncogenic HPV types, in both MSM and women.

Other risk factors that have been associated with the development of AIN in men include a history of genital warts, injection drug use, and current cigarette smoking. Additional risk factors in women include a history of cervical or vulvar cancer, high-grade cervical or vulvar intraepithelial neoplasia (multizonal disease) and immunosuppression [65].

7.4 Clinical Presentation

AIN (Fig. 31) can present in different forms. Bowenoid AIN resembles Bowenoid papulosis and is recognized as single or multiple, well-demarcated, brown or red, slightly elevated papules and plaques. Erythroplakic AIN presents as one or more erythematous, erosive, or scaly macules in the mucosal surface resembling

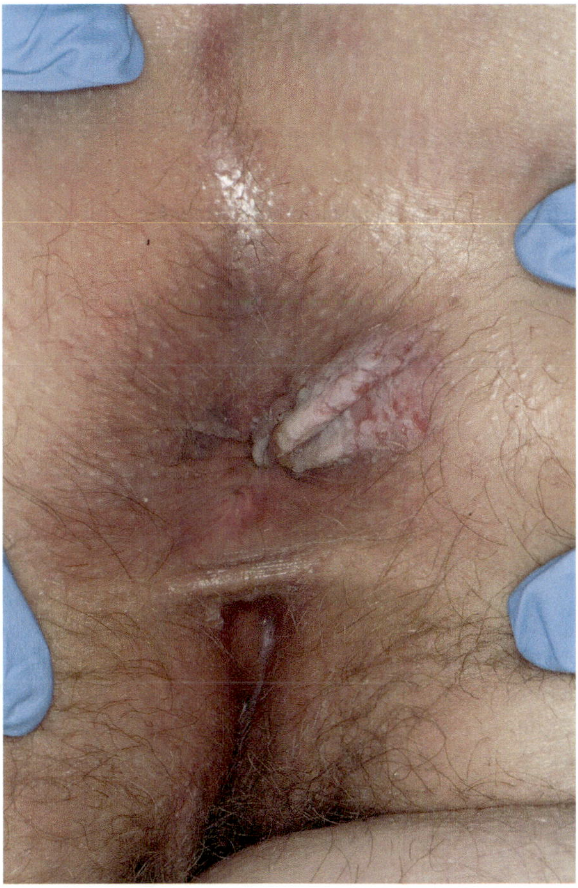

Fig. 31 Anal intraepithelial neoplasia

erythroplasia of Queyrat. Leukoplakic AIN can be recognized as white, flat, well-demarcated lesions with a punctuate vascular pattern and verrucous AIN are white or grey, exophytic lesions with irregular and hyperkeratinized or verrucous surface. AIN is usually asymptomatic.

7.5 *Histopathology*

Histological features of anal HSIL are identical to that of cervical HSIL and includes marked atypia and loss of maturation of at least one-third up to full thickness of the epithelium, increased number of mitoses and atypical mitoses. Diagnosis can be supported by use of p16 immunohistochemistry as a surrogate marker for hrHPV E7 transforming gene activity to confirm HSIL diagnosis in case of uncertainty or disagreement about LSIL vs. HSIL to show the presence of diffuse p16 positivity [50]. HPV E4 immunohistochemistry can be used as a marker of productive HPV infection [66].

7.6 *Differential Diagnosis*

The differential diagnosis of AIN includes condylomata acuminate (Fig. 32), lichen sclerosus (Fig. 33), lichen planus, psoriasis, atopic eczema, and seborrheic keratosis.

7.7 *Treatment and Management*

There are different treatment options for HSIL, including surgical excision, local ablation for small discrete lesions and topical treatment with imiquimod cream for more extensive lesions in the absence of invasive suspicion. For intra-anal HSIL, treatment with application of 80% trichloroacetic acid (TCA), infrared coagulation (IRC), radiofrequency ablation, or electrocautery/hyfrecation are mentioned in literature when the affected area represents less than 50% of the circumference of the anal transition zone (ATZ). For lesions that represent over 50% of the ATZ circumference, treatment may be IRC/hyfrecation or topical treatment with imiquimod to reduce the size. These approaches are not approved by the US Food and Drug Administration (FDA), as literature is scarce on this subject [67]. When there is suspicion of invasive squamous cell carcinoma, local excision is the treatment of choice. When this is not possible without mutilation of the anal sphincter, consider (chemo) radiotherapy can be considered.

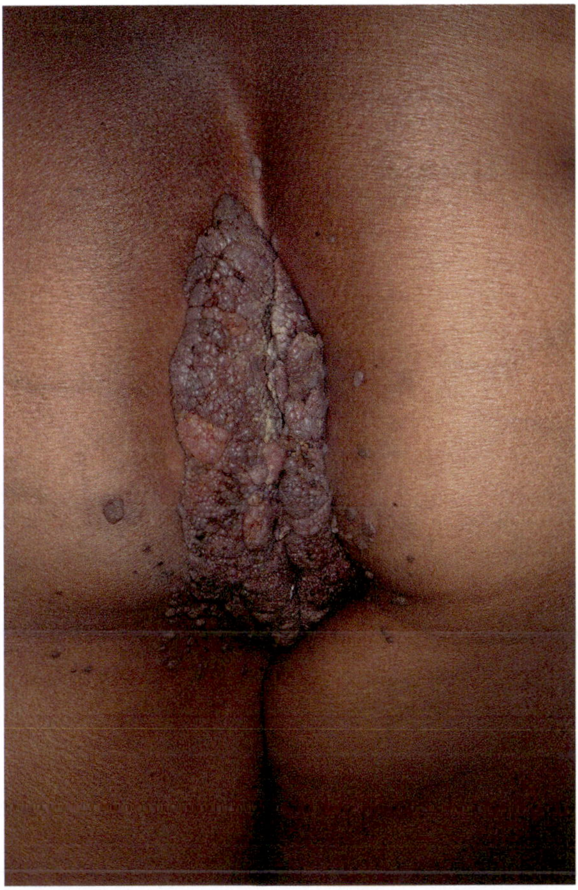

Fig. 32 Condylomata acuminate (genital warts)

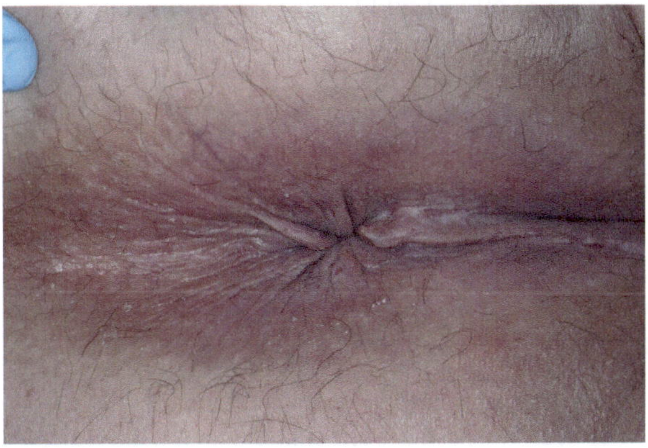

Fig. 33 Anal lichen sclerosus

8 Keratoacanthoma

8.1 Pathophysiology

Keratoacanthoma is a tumor that is believed to be derived from follicular infundibular keratinocytes [68]. They have a triphasic pattern of evolution: the proliferative (early) phase, the stabilized (well-developed) phase, and regressive (late) phase. Because of their strong clinical and histological resemblance with cSCC, there is little consensus on the exact classification of these tumors. Some dermatologists and pathologists see keratoacanthomas as a form of a very well-differentiated cSCC and not as a different entity. Therefore, the term "keratoacanthoma-like cSCC" can be found in literature and clinical practice. Others see keratoacanthoma as a benign tumor.

Literature states that changes in the expression of genes and proteins involved in epidermal cell proliferation, cell adhesion, and cell survival may play significant roles in keratoacanthoma [69]. Proposed contributors to lesion regression include the upregulation of factors that promote apoptosis, events related to normal cycling of the hair follicle, and activation of an immunologic response.

8.2 Epidemiology and Risk Factors

Keratoacanthoma is a common tumor with an incidence of approximately 1 per 1000 patients with fair skin type; however, exact incidences are hard to estimate due to their resemblance with cSCC. The vast majority of keratoacanthomas arises in people with Fitzpatrick skin type I or II. Keratoacanthoma can occur at any age, but it is usually found in middle-aged to elderly patients with a peak incidence between the ages of 50 and 69 [70]. It is more common in men than in women. Other risk factors for the development of keratoacanthoma include UV radiation, trauma, immunosuppression, and certain genetic diseases such as Muir Torre syndrome and xeroderma pigmentosum. The role of HPV in the development of keratoacanthoma is controversial.

8.3 Clinical Presentation

Keratoacanthoma presents as a fast growing (within a few weeks), dome-shaped nodule of 1 or 2 cm, and can predominantly be found on sun-exposed areas of the body such as the face, arms, and dorsal hands (Figs. 34, 35, 36, 37, and 38). It is characterized by exophytic growth and a central horn plug. Rare subtypes of keratoacanthoma include giant keratoacanthoma (>2 cm), subungual keratoacanthoma (which may present with pain, swelling, and inflammation), and mucosal

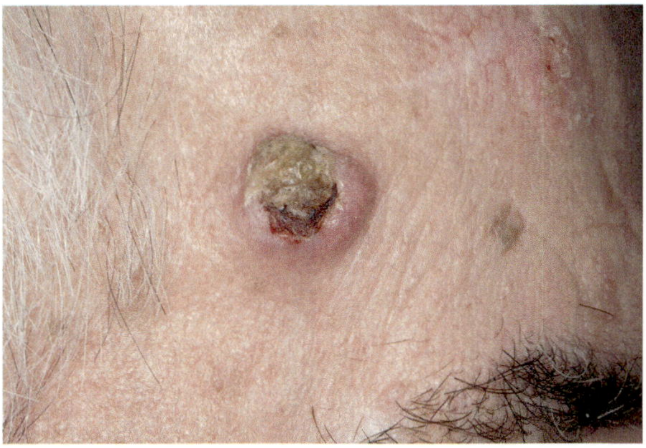

Fig. 34 Keratoacanthoma on the temporal side of the head

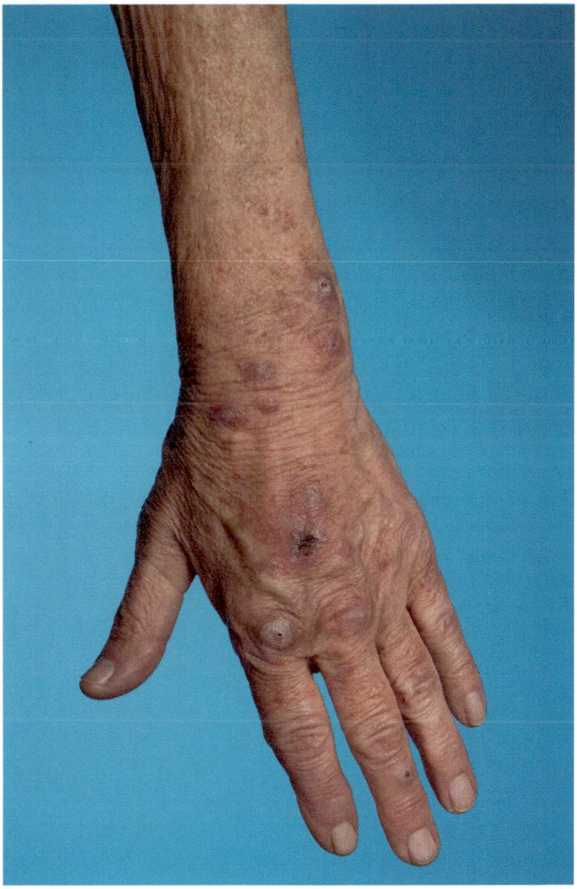

Fig. 35 Keratoacanthoma on the dorsal side of the hands

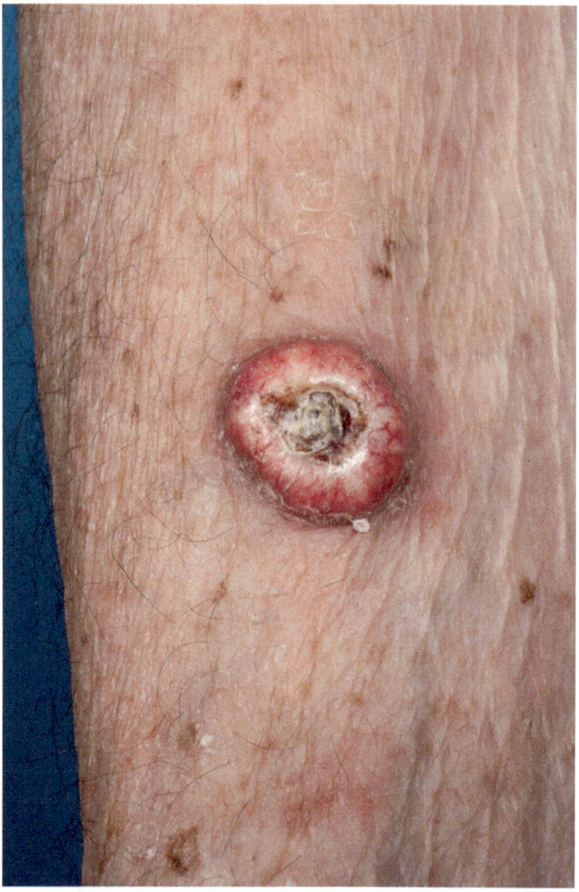

Fig. 36 Close-up of a keratoacanthoma on the anterior side of an arm

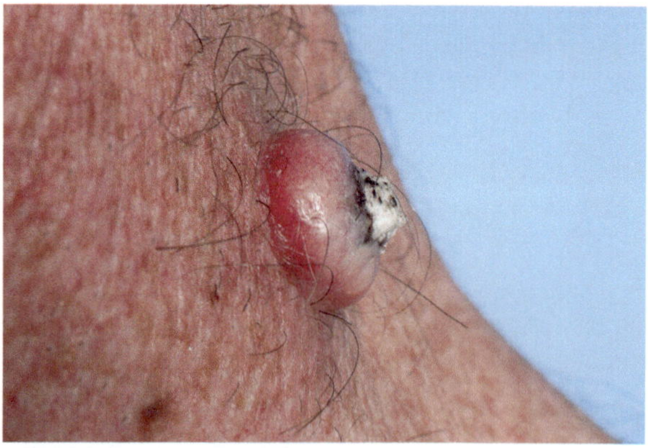

Fig. 37 Close-up of a dome-shaped keratoacanthoma, appreciate the central hornplug

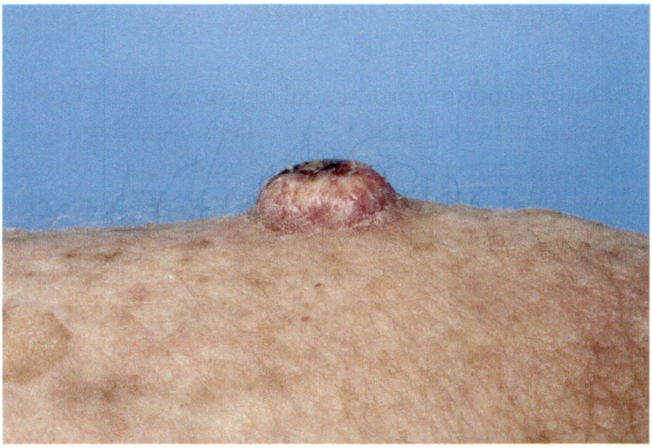

Fig. 38 Close-up of a dome-shaped keratoacanthoma

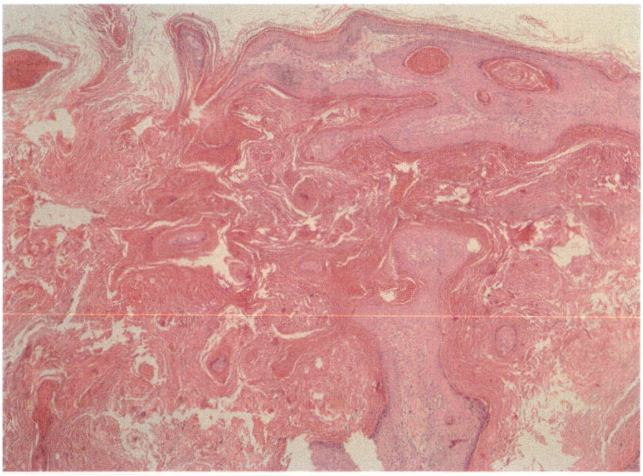

Fig. 39 Histology of keratoacanthoma with a keratin-filled crater and epithelial lipping

keratoacanthoma (oral mucosa, conjunctiva, genitalia, or nasal mucosa). Keratoacanthoma centrifugum marginatum is a rare form of keratoacanthoma which can be distinguished from giant keratoacanthoma by its horizontal growth pattern. Spontaneous regression is less common in these lesions.

8.4 Histopathology

The histology of keratoacanthoma resembles a well-differentiated cSCC. It is a large, well-differentiated symmetrical squamous tumor with abundant eosinophilic or glassy cytoplasm and enlarged hyperchromatic to vesicular appearing nuclei. It is furthermore characterized by a central keratin-filled crater, epithelial lipping, and a sharp demarcation from surrounding stroma (Fig. 39). An infiltrative growth pattern, mitotic activity, overt cytologic atypia, acantholysis, paradoxical maturation, and deep dermal or subcutaneous invasion supporting a diagnosis of cSCC.

8.5 Differential Diagnosis

The most important differential diagnosis is cSCC. Punch biopsies often do not differentiate between a cSCC and a keratoacanthoma, and therefore it is important to have good insight into the clinical presentation as well as histology from the whole lesion. Other differential diagnoses include basal cell carcinoma, Merkel cell carcinoma, Kaposi sarcoma, atypical fibrosarcoma or pleomorphic dermal sarcoma, giant molluscum contagiosum, prurigo nodule, deep fungal infection, and cutaneous metastases.

8.6 Treatment and Management

The preferred treatment for keratoacanthoma is complete surgical excision with a clinical margin of 3–5 mm. When there is no doubt about the clinical diagnosis and the lesion shows already signs of regression, it is accepted to perform curettage and electrodesiccation. This may solely be performed by clinicians experienced in this procedure. Alternative treatment options that have shown to be effective include cryotherapy, ablative laser treatment, radiotherapy, topical or intralesional 5-FU, isotretinoin, acitretin, and methotrexate (in patients with multiple or recurrent keratoacanthoma).

Until markers to differentiate keratoacanthoma from cSCC are identified, careful histopathologic evaluation, and close clinical follow-up are indicated, particularly with attention to the evolution of the lesion [71].

9 Porokeratosis

9.1 Pathophysiology

Porokeratosis is caused by a clonal proliferation of abnormal keratinocytes. It consists of a keratinization disorder, which may appear in several clinical forms and can undergo malignant transformation. However, the exact pathway that leads to this process remains unknown. A variety of factors have been proposed as potential contributors, including genetic susceptibility, ultraviolet radiation, and immunosuppression.

9.2 Epidemiology

Porokeratosis is poorly documented in literature. Dependent on the type of porokeratosis, it can occur at any age, but typically occurs in adults or older adults and is more common in men than it is in women.

Risk factors for the development of porokeratosis include genetic predisposition, ultraviolet radiation, and different therapies including the use of biologicals, phototherapy, and radiotherapy [72]. Immunosuppression is also associated with a higher chance of porokeratosis. Exact incidences vary widely in literature but may be as high as 11% in SOTR [73].

9.3 *Clinical Presentation and Risk Factors*

Porokeratosis is characterized by atrophic, sometimes annular macules or patches, with a well-defined ridge-like hyperkeratotic border which is called cornoid lamella (Figs. 40, 41, 42, and 43).

There are different clinical variants of porokeratosis. These include porokeratosis of Mibelli, disseminated superficial actinic porokeratosis (DSAP), disseminated superficial porokeratosis (DSP), linear porokeratosis, porokeratosis plantaris palmaris et disseminate (PPPD), punctuate palmoplantar porokeratosis, and porokeratosis ptychotropica. DSAP is the common form of porokeratosis and usually presents in elderly women with a history of sun exposure and presents at multiple lesions on sun-exposed areas of the body (mainly the dorsal sites of the underarms and lower legs). DSP resembles DSAP but can present on all locations. DSP often develops in childhood, most commonly between the ages of 5 and 10 years. Linear porokeratosis is a form of DSP which is more rare and has a higher chance of cSCC development [74]. Porokeratosis of Mibelli is also a frequent form of porokeratosis, which presents as solitary or multiple plaques or annular lesions from 1 to 2 mm and often begins in childhood. It affects males approximately twice as frequently as females. More rare forms of porokeratosis include PPPD and punctuate palmoplantar porokeratosis which start at hyperkeratotic papules on the hands and feet, and porokeratosis ptychotropica which presents in the buttock fold.

Fig. 40 One single lesion of porokeratosis. It shows a clear cornoid lamella

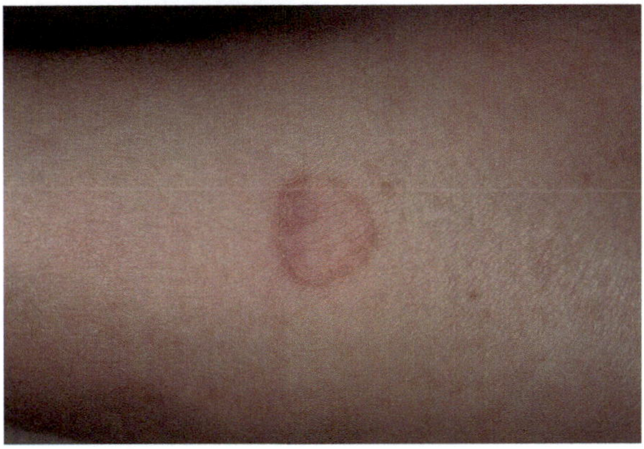

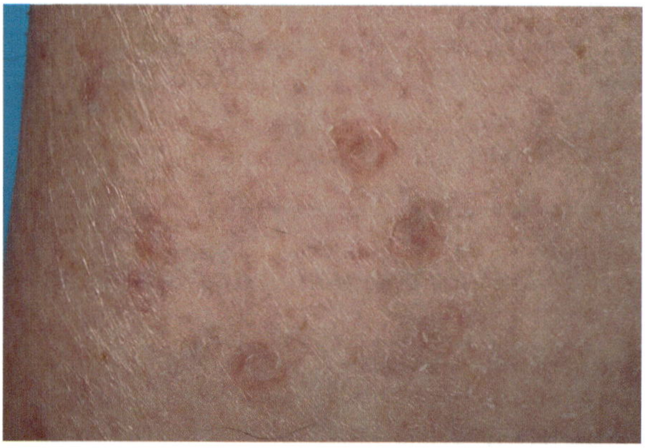

Fig. 41 Porokeratosis on the dorsal side of the leg, the cornoid lamella is evident

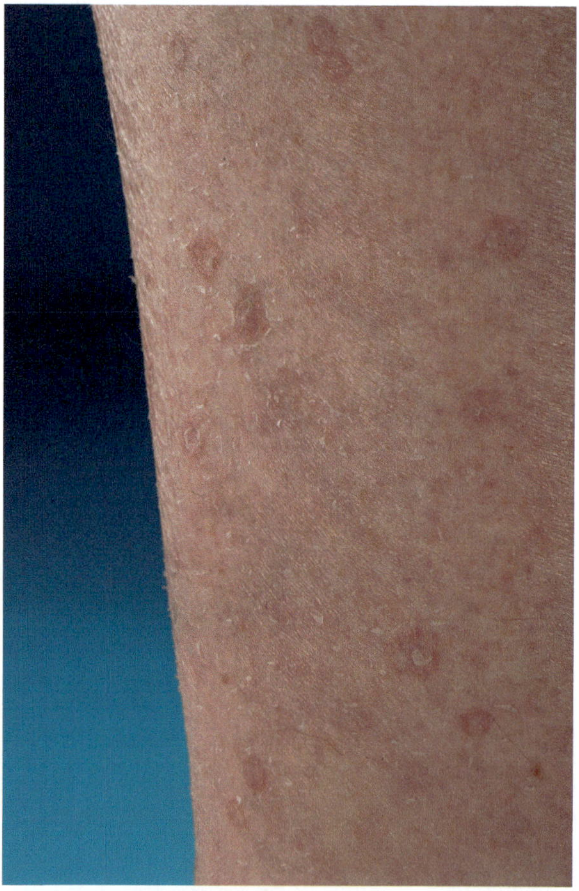

Fig. 42 Porokeratosis on the dorsal side of the leg

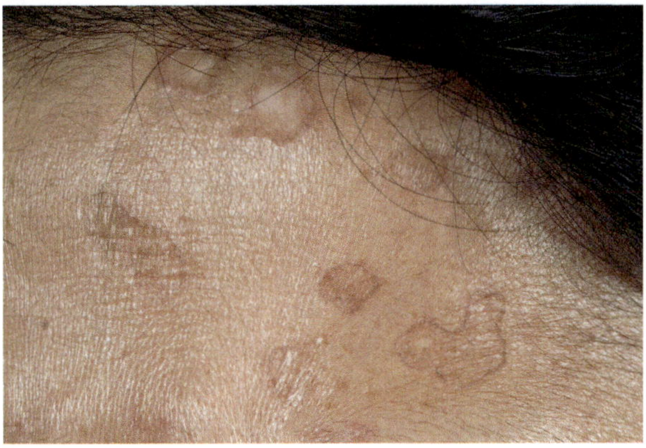

Fig. 43 Porokeratosis

9.4 *Histopathology*

Porokeratosis has a characteristic histology. It is advised to take a punch biopsy front the peripheral grooved ridge. Classic features for porokeratosis include a keratin-filled epidermal invagination with an angulated, parakeratotic tier which is called the cornoid lamella.

9.5 *Differential Diagnosis*

The differential diagnosis of DSAP and DSP includes AK, seborrheic keratosis, and inflammatory skin diseases such as (guttate) psoriasis, eczema, lupus erythematosus, pityriasis rosea, and lichen planus. Porokeratosis of Mibelli may clinically resemble AK, Bowen's disease, benign lichenoid keratosis, granuloma annulare, lichen simplex, and tinea corporis. The differential diagnosis of PPPD and punctuate palmoplantar porokeratosis includes palmoplantar keratodermas and arsenic keratoses and palmar pits in basal cell nevus syndrome.

9.6 *Treatment and Management*

There are different treatment options for porokeratosis; however, these are not based on guidelines. Options for the treatment of porokeratosis include topical treatments (5-FU, imiquimod, topical keratolytics, vitamin D analogs, emollients), cryotherapy, curettage and electrodesiccation, PDT, laser therapy, surgical excision, and oral retinoids. In some cases, radiotherapy may be considered. In 2017, a systematic review was published on the treatment of porokeratosis [75]. Available literature was, however, mostly based on case reports and randomized-controlled trials are needed to make an evidence-based decision on the best treatment options for the different kinds of porokeratosis. For now, the choice of treatment options should be based on different factors such as the size and number of lesions and patient preferences.

Patients should be followed annually to monitor for signs and symptoms of malignancy. Furthermore, patients with porokeratosis should be educated about sun protection and alarm symptoms because of the chance of malignant proliferation.

10 EV-Like Lesions

10.1 Pathophysiology and Epidemiology

Epidermodysplasia verruciformis (EV) is a rare autosomal recessive genodermatosis. It is associated with a high susceptibility to infection with particular genotypes of beta HPV (as has been discussed earlier in the section about AK) and has recently been classified in three subtypes [76]. Classic EV is associated with genetic mutations in the EVER (EVER1 and EVER2) genes. More recently, several other genes have been implicated in EV, including RHOH, MST-1, CORO1A, and ECM, which is now classified as non-classic EV. Since 2009, acquired forms of EV have been distinguished as an entity occurring in immunocompromised patients such as patients with HIV and SOTR [77]. Whereas classic and non-classic EV lesions present at young age, acquired EV by definition presents in adulthood or childhood in patients with a clear exogenous cause of immune impairment. Also, these patients lack a family history of EV. Besides genetic alterations, the pathogenesis is multifactorial, involving viral and environmental factors.

10.2 Clinical Presentation

EV is characterized by the development of red, skin colored, and hyperpigmented macules and papules usually on the trunk, neck, arms, and face during childhood, resembling flat warts of pityriasis versicolor-like lesions (Figs. 44, 45, and 46).

10.3 Histopathology

Mild to moderate acanthosis and hyperkeratosis are classic features in these lesions. An irregular granular layer with perinuclear halos (as signs of HPV infection), large cells with blueish cytoplasm and dysplastic changes may be present.

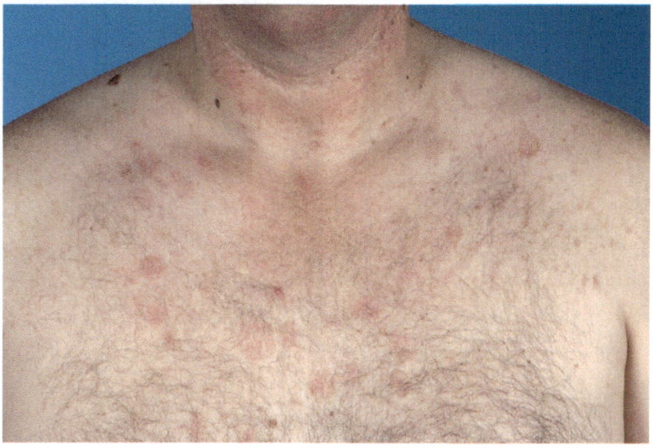

Fig. 44 Epidermodysplasia verruciformis on the chest

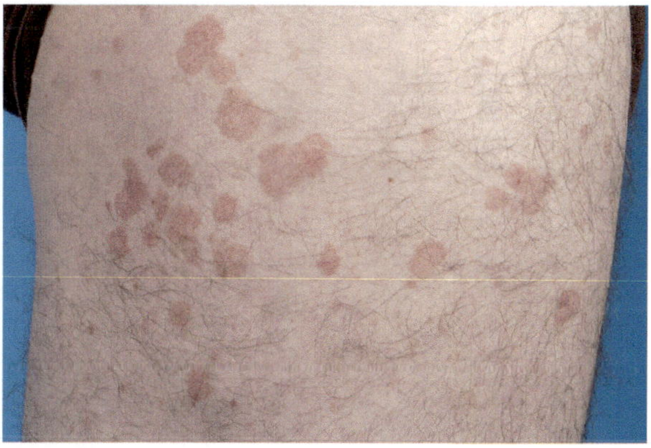

Fig. 45 Epidermodysplasia verruciformis on the leg

10.4 Treatment and Management

There is no curative therapy for EV, and therefore treatment options are symptomatic. There are different treatment options for EV-like lesions, including systemic retinoids, topical imiquimod, 5-FU, and PDT. However, the literature on these treatment options for EV is scarce and inconsistent.

It is recommended that patients with EV undergo lifelong annual or more frequent skin examinations, dependent on their history of skin malignancies. Education on the prevention and detection of skin cancer, especially cSCC, is especially important in EV patients. Treatment of cSCC with radiotherapy in patients with EV has been associated with aggressive tumor recurrence and should be avoided [78].

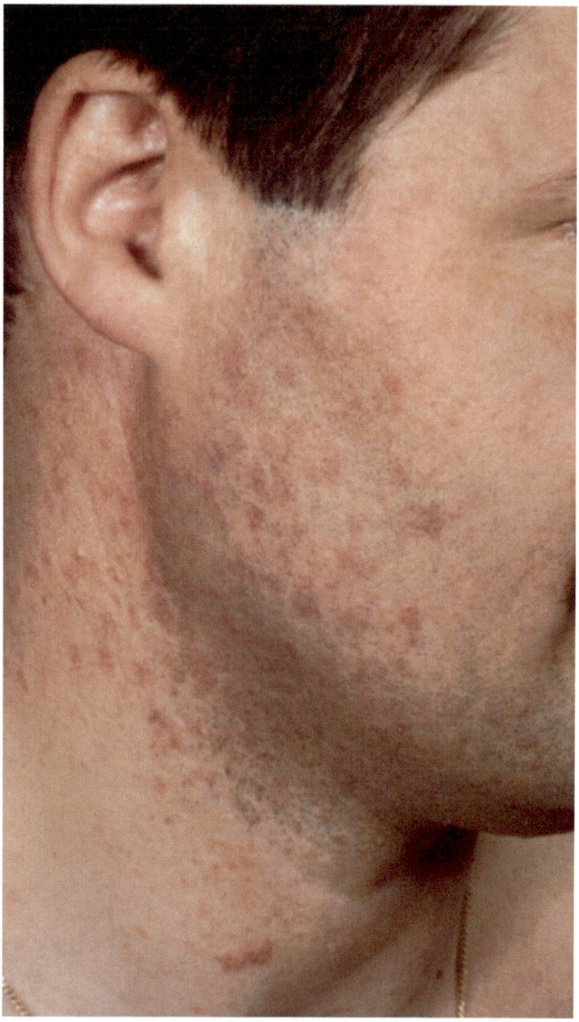

Fig. 46 Epidermodysplasia verruciformis in the face and neck region

11 Seborrheic Keratosis, Verruca Vulgaris, and Verruca Plana

11.1 Introduction and Pathophysiology

Besides all premalignant neoplasms as mentioned above, it is worth mentioning a few benign tumors that often present in SOTR and are often in the differential diagnosis of different premalignant neoplasms. The exact etiology of seborrheic keratosis (SK) is still unknown. Verruca vulgaris (VV) and verruca plana (VP) are associated with HPV infection.

11.2 Epidemiology

Seborrheic keratosis is the most common form of benign tumors in all patients, but especially in SOTR. A lot of patients develop multiple of these lesions and they tend to become more prevalent with aging (Fig. 47). Verruca vulgaris is more common in children; however, SOTR have a higher risk of these lesions (Figs. 48 and 49).

11.3 Clinical Presentation

Seborrheic keratosis presents as a sharply demarcated yellow, brown, or black verrucous papule and has a waxy appearance (Fig. 50). They usually appear on the head, neck, chest, or back, but not on the palms or soles. Classic dermoscopic features are milia-like cysts, comedo-like openings, a cerebriform of fingerprint pattern, and a jelly-like border (Fig. 51).

Fig. 47 Multiple seborrheic keratosis lesions on the temporal side of the head

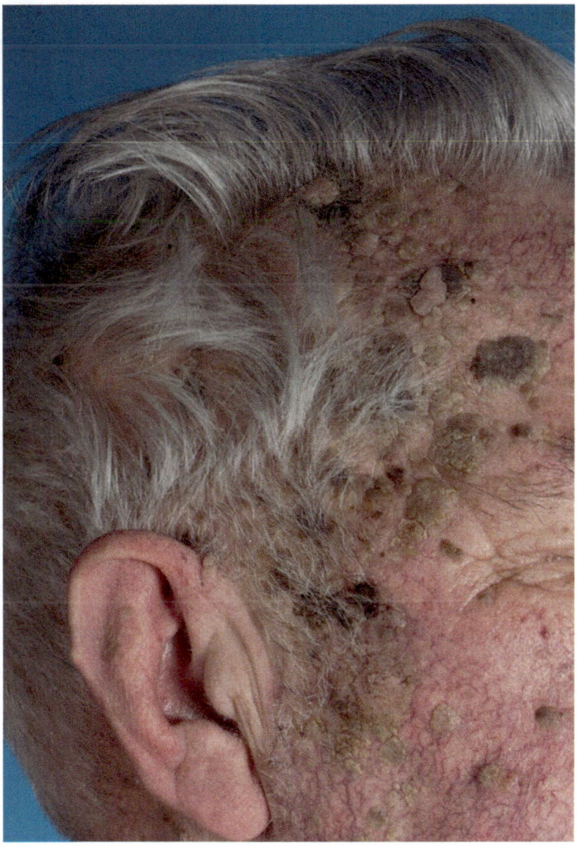

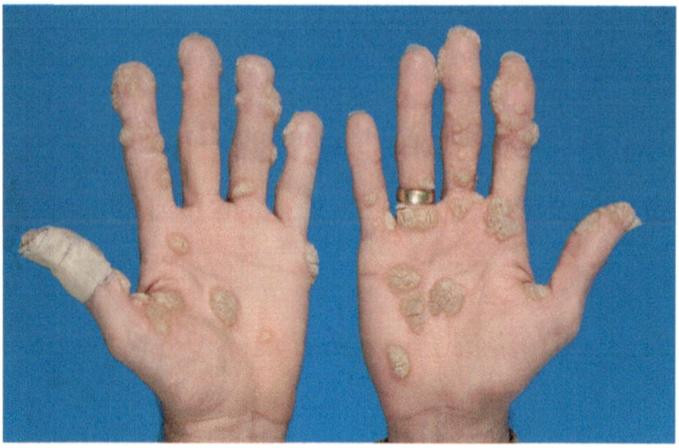

Fig. 48 Verruca vulgaris on the hands

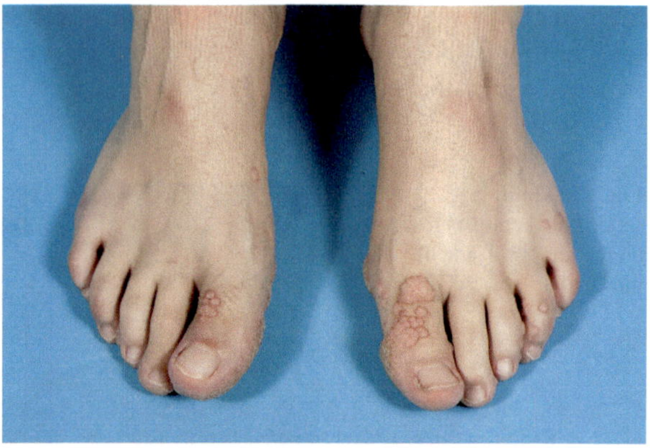

Fig. 49 Verruca vulgaris on the feet

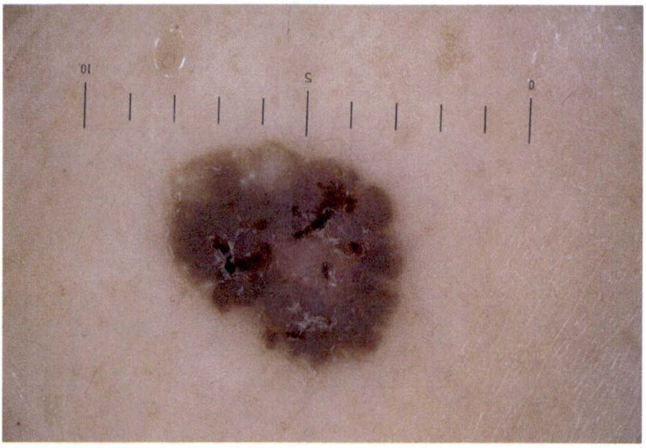

Fig. 50 Dermoscopy of a seborrheic keratosis. It shows a brown verrucous papule with a waxy appearance

Verruca vulgaris is usually present on the hands and foot soles (verruca plantaris) and appears as one or multiple skin-colored verrucous papules with a rougher surface. Verruca plana is a flat type of a verruca vulgaris and is usually found on the dorsal sides of the hands.

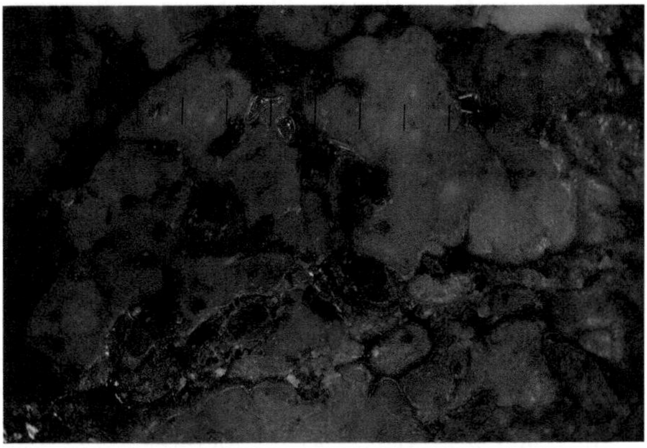

Fig. 51 Dermoscopy of a seborrheic keratosis. It shows milia-like cysts and comedo-like openings

11.4 Treatment and Management

Because these are benign lesions, no treatment is necessary. However, when these lesions give complaints such as irritation, itch or pain, different treatment options are available, including topical treatments (such as salicylic acid, imiquimod, 5-FU, and bleomycin or podophyllin), cryotherapy, and electrodessication.

Acknowledgments We would like to show our gratitude to Marjolein Lammerts, who contributed to the selection of the figures, and Koen Quint, who photographed the histology pictures.

References

1. Figueras Nart I, Cerio R, Dirschka T, Dréno B, Lear JT, Pellacani G, et al. Defining the actinic keratosis field: a literature review and discussion. J Eur Acad Dermatol Venereol (JEADV). 2018;32(4):544–63. https://doi.org/10.1111/jdv.14652.
2. Schmitz L, Kahl P, Majores M, Bierhoff E, Stockfleth E, Dirschka T. Actinic keratosis: correlation between clinical and histological classification systems. J Eur Acad Dermatol Venereol (JEADV). 2016;30(8):1303–7. https://doi.org/10.1111/jdv.13626.
3. Segura S, Gadea A, Nonell L, Andrades E, Sánchez S, Pujol R, et al. Identification of differentially expressed genes in actinic keratosis samples treated with ingenol mebutate gel. PLoS One. 2020;15(5):e0232146. https://doi.org/10.1371/journal.pone.0232146.
4. Jiyad Z, Marquart L, O'Rourke P, Green AC. Incidence and regression of actinic keratoses in organ transplant recipients. Acta Derm Venereol. 2018;98(1):77–81. https://doi.org/10.2340/00015555-2783.
5. Ackerman AB, Mones JM. Solar (actinic) keratosis is squamous cell carcinoma. Br J Dermatol. 2006;155(1):9–22. https://doi.org/10.1111/j.1365-2133.2005.07121.x.
6. Howley PM, Pfister HJ. Beta genus papillomaviruses and skin cancer. Virology. 2015;479-480:290–6. https://doi.org/10.1016/j.virol.2015.02.004.
7. Viarisio D, Gissmann L, Tommasino M. Human papillomaviruses and carcinogenesis: well-established and novel models. Curr Opin Virol. 2017;26:56–62. https://doi.org/10.1016/j.coviro.2017.07.014.

8. Tommasino M. The biology of beta human papillomaviruses. Virus Res. 2017;231:128–38. https://doi.org/10.1016/j.virusres.2016.11.013.
9. Quint KD, Genders RE, de Koning MN, Borgogna C, Gariglio M, Bouwes Bavinck JN, et al. Human Beta-papillomavirus infection and keratinocyte carcinomas. J Pathol. 2015;235(2):342–54. https://doi.org/10.1002/path.4425.
10. Tuttleton AS, Jennings L, Nindl I, Rosl F, Bouwes Bavinck JN, Seckin D, et al. Viral oncogenesis and its role in nonmelanoma skin cancer. Br J Dermatol. 2011;164(6):1201–13.
11. Bouwes Bavinck JN, Feltkamp MCW, Green AC, Fiocco M, Euvrard S, Harwood CA, et al. Human papillomavirus and posttransplantation cutaneous squamous cell carcinoma: a multicenter, prospective cohort study. Am J Transplant. 2018;18(5):1220–30. https://doi.org/10.1111/ajt.14537.
12. de Koning MNC, Struijk L, Bavinck JNB, Kleter B, Ter Schegget J, Quint WGV, et al. Betapapillomaviruses frequently persist in the skin of healthy individuals. J Gen Virol. 2007;88(Pt 5):1489–95. https://doi.org/10.1099/vir.0.82732-0.
13. Tommasino M. The human papillomavirus family and its role in carcinogenesis. Semin Cancer Biol. 2014;26:13–21. https://doi.org/10.1016/j.semcancer.2013.11.002.
14. South AP, Purdie KJ, Watt SA, Haldenby S, den Breems N, Dimon M, et al. NOTCH1 mutations occur early during cutaneous squamous cell carcinogenesis. J Invest Dermatol. 2014;134(10):2630–8. https://doi.org/10.1038/jid.2014.154.
15. Weissenborn SJ, Nindl I, Purdie K, Harwood C, Proby C, Breuer J, et al. Human papillomavirus-DNA loads in actinic keratoses exceed those in non-melanoma skin cancers. J Invest Dermatol. 2005;125(1):93–7. https://doi.org/10.1111/j.0022-202X.2005.23733.x.
16. Ulrich M, Krueger-Corcoran D, Roewert-Huber J, Sterry W, Stockfleth E, Astner S. Reflectance confocal microscopy for noninvasive monitoring of therapy and detection of subclinical actinic keratoses. Dermatology. 2010;220(1):15–24. https://doi.org/10.1159/000254893.
17. Nguyen KP, Peppelman M, Hoogedoorn L, Van Erp PE, Gerritsen MP. The current role of in vivo reflectance confocal microscopy within the continuum of actinic keratosis and squamous cell carcinoma: a systematic review. Eur J Dermatol. 2016;26(6):549–65. https://doi.org/10.1684/ejd.2016.2872.
18. Röwert-Huber J, Patel MJ, Forschner T, Ulrich C, Eberle J, Kerl H, et al. Actinic keratosis is an early in situ squamous cell carcinoma: a proposal for reclassification. Br J Dermatol. 2007;156(Suppl 3):8–12. https://doi.org/10.1111/j.1365-2133.2007.07860.x.
19. Cornejo CM, Jambusaria-Pahlajani A, Willenbrink TJ, Schmults CD, Arron ST, Ruiz ES. Field cancerization: treatment. J Am Acad Dermatol. 2020;83(3):719–30. https://doi.org/10.1016/j.jaad.2020.03.127.
20. Heppt MV, Steeb T, Niesert AC, Zacher M, Leiter U, Garbe C, et al. Local interventions for actinic keratosis in organ transplant recipients: a systematic review. Br J Dermatol. 2019;180(1):43–50. https://doi.org/10.1111/bjd.17148.
21. Werner RN, Nast A. 'Surprisingly little evidence' on how best to treat actinic keratosis in organ transplant recipients. Br J Dermatol. 2019;180(1):11–2. https://doi.org/10.1111/bjd.17326.
22. Thai KE, Fergin P, Freeman M, Vinciullo C, Francis D, Spelman L, et al. A prospective study of the use of cryosurgery for the treatment of actinic keratoses. Int J Dermatol. 2004;43(9):687–92. https://doi.org/10.1111/j.1365-4632.2004.02056.x.
23. Jansen MHE, Kessels J, Nelemans PJ, Kouloubis N, Arits A, van Pelt HPA, et al. Randomized trial of four treatment approaches for actinic keratosis. N Engl J Med. 2019;380(10):935–46. https://doi.org/10.1056/NEJMoa1811850.
24. Rosenberg AR, Tabacchi M, Ngo KH, Wallendorf M, Rosman IS, Cornelius LA, et al. Skin cancer precursor immunotherapy for squamous cell carcinoma prevention. JCI Insight. 2019;4(6) https://doi.org/10.1172/jci.insight.125476.
25. Cunningham TJ, Tabacchi M, Eliane JP, Tuchayi SM, Manivasagam S, Mirzaalian H, et al. Randomized trial of calcipotriol combined with 5-fluorouracil for skin cancer precursor immunotherapy. J Clin Invest. 2017;127(1):106–16. https://doi.org/10.1172/jci89820.

26. Savage NW, McKay C, Faulkner C. Actinic cheilitis in dental practice. Aust Dent J. 2010;55(Suppl 1):78–84. https://doi.org/10.1111/j.1834-7819.2010.01202.x.
27. de Souza Lucena EE, Costa DC, da Silveira EJ, Lima KC. Prevalence and factors associated to actinic cheilitis in beach workers. Oral Dis. 2012;18(6):575–9. https://doi.org/10.1111/j.1601-0825.2012.01910.x.
28. Ntomouchtsis A, Karakinaris G, Poulolpoulos A, Kechagias N, Kittikidou K, Tsompanidou C, et al. Benign lip lesions. A 10-year retrospective study. Oral Maxillofac Surg. 2010;14(2):115–8. https://doi.org/10.1007/s10006-009-0196-y.
29. Junqueira JL, Bönecker M, Furuse C, Morais Pde C, Flório FM, Cury PR, et al. Actinic cheilitis among agricultural workers in Campinas, Brazil. Community Dent Health. 2011;28(1):60–3.
30. Rodríguez-Blanco I, Flórez Á, Paredes-Suárez C, Rodríguez-Lojo R, González-Vilas D, Ramírez-Santos A, et al. Actinic cheilitis: analysis of clinical subtypes, risk factors and associated signs of actinic damage. Acta Derm Venereol. 2019;99(10):931–2. https://doi.org/10.2340/00015555-3237.
31. Laprise C, Cahoon EK, Lynch CF, Kahn AR, Copeland G, Gonsalves L, et al. Risk of lip cancer after solid organ transplantation in the United States. Am J Transplant. 2019;19(1):227–37. https://doi.org/10.1111/ajt.15052.
32. Dancyger A, Heard V, Huang B, Suley C, Tang D, Ariyawardana A. Malignant transformation of actinic cheilitis: a systematic review of observational studies. J Investig Clin Dent. 2018;9(4):e12343. https://doi.org/10.1111/jicd.12343.
33. Ito T, Natsuga K, Tanimura S, Aoyagi S, Shimizu H. Dermoscopic features of plasma cell cheilitis and actinic cheilitis. Acta Derm Venereol. 2014;94(5):593–4. https://doi.org/10.2340/00015555-1795.
34. Menta Simonsen Nico M, Rivitti EA, Lourenço SV. Actinic cheilitis: histologic study of the entire vermilion and comparison with previous biopsy. J Cutan Pathol. 2007;34(4):309–14. https://doi.org/10.1111/j.1600-0560.2006.00606.x.
35. Carvalho MV, de Moraes SLD, Lemos CAA, Santiago Júnior JF, Vasconcelos B, Pellizzer EP. Surgical versus non-surgical treatment of actinic cheilitis: a systematic review and meta-analysis. Oral Dis. 2019;25(4):972–81. https://doi.org/10.1111/odi.12916.
36. Trager MH, Farmer K, Ulrich C, Basset-Seguin N, Herms F, Geskin LJ, et al. Actinic cheilitis: a systematic review of treatment options. J Eur Acad Dermatol Venereol (JEADV). 2021;35(4):815–23. https://doi.org/10.1111/jdv.16995.
37. Jansen MHE, Özhan-Hasan H, Nelemans PJ, Winnepenninckx VJ, Mosterd K. Trends in the incidence of Bowen disease based on a single-center study in the Netherlands. Dermatol Surg. 2019;45(11):1353–8. https://doi.org/10.1097/dss.0000000000001980.
38. Drake AL, Walling HW. Variations in presentation of squamous cell carcinoma in situ (Bowen's disease) in immunocompromised patients. J Am Acad Dermatol. 2008;59(1):68–71. https://doi.org/10.1016/j.jaad.2008.03.028.
39. Wozniak-Rito AM, Rudnicka L. Bowen's disease in dermoscopy. Acta Dermatovenerol Croat. 2018;26(2):157–61.
40. Westers-Attema A, van den Heijkant F, Lohman BG, Nelemans PJ, Winnepenninckx V, Kelleners-Smeets NW, et al. Bowen's disease: a six-year retrospective study of treatment with emphasis on resection margins. Acta Derm Venereol. 2014;94(4):431–5. https://doi.org/10.2340/00015555-1771.
41. Morton CA, Whitehurst C, McColl JH, Moore JV, MacKie RM. Photodynamic therapy for large or multiple patches of Bowen disease and basal cell carcinoma. Arch Dermatol. 2001;137(3):319–24.
42. Neagu TP, Ţigliş M, Botezatu D, Enache V, Cobilinschi CO, Vâlcea-Precup MS, et al. Clinical, histological and therapeutic features of Bowen's disease. Romanian J Morphol Embryol. 2017;58(1):33–40.
43. Hoekstra RJ, Trip EJ, Ten Kate FJ, Horenblas S, Lock MT. Penile intraepithelial neoplasia: nomenclature, incidence and progression to malignancy in the Netherlands. Int J Urol. 2019;26(3):353–7. https://doi.org/10.1111/iju.13871.

44. Heideman DA, Waterboer T, Pawlita M, Delis-van Diemen P, Nindl I, Leijte JA, et al. Human papillomavirus-16 is the predominant type etiologically involved in penile squamous cell carcinoma. J Clin Oncol. 2007;25(29):4550–6. https://doi.org/10.1200/jco.2007.12.3182.
45. Bleeker MC, Heideman DA, Snijders PJ, Horenblas S, Dillner J, Meijer CJ. Penile cancer: epidemiology, pathogenesis and prevention. World J Urol. 2009;27(2):141–50. https://doi.org/10.1007/s00345-008-0302-z.
46. Daling JR, Madeleine MM, Johnson LG, Schwartz SM, Shera KA, Wurscher MA, et al. Penile cancer: importance of circumcision, human papillomavirus and smoking in in situ and invasive disease. Int J Cancer. 2005;116(4):606–16. https://doi.org/10.1002/ijc.21009.
47. Kristiansen S, Svensson Å, Drevin L, Forslund O, Torbrand C, Bjartling C. Risk factors for penile intraepithelial neoplasia: a population-based register study in Sweden, 2000-2012. Acta Derm Venereol. 2019;99(3):315–20. https://doi.org/10.2340/00015555-3083.
48. Cubilla AL, Velazquez EF, Young RH. Epithelial lesions associated with invasive penile squamous cell carcinoma: a pathologic study of 288 cases. Int J Surg Pathol. 2004;12(4):351–64. https://doi.org/10.1177/106689690401200408.
49. Bornstein J, Bogliatto F, Haefner HK, Stockdale CK, Preti M, Bohl TG, et al. The 2015 International Society for the Study of Vulvovaginal Disease (ISSVD) terminology of vulvar squamous intraepithelial lesions. Obstet Gynecol. 2016;127(2):264–8. https://doi.org/10.1097/aog.0000000000001285.
50. Darragh TM, Colgan TJ, Cox JT, Heller DS, Henry MR, Luff RD, et al. The lower anogenital squamous terminology standardization project for HPV-associated lesions: background and consensus recommendations from the College of American Pathologists and the American Society for Colposcopy and Cervical Pathology. Arch Pathol Lab Med. 2012;136(10):1266–97. https://doi.org/10.5858/arpa.LGT200570.
51. Hoang LN, Park KJ, Soslow RA, Murali R. Squamous precursor lesions of the vulva: current classification and diagnostic challenges. Pathology. 2016;48(4):291–302. https://doi.org/10.1016/j.pathol.2016.02.015.
52. Thuijs NB, van Beurden M, Bruggink AH, Steenbergen RDM, Berkhof J, Bleeker MCG. Vulvar intraepithelial neoplasia: incidence and long-term risk of vulvar squamous cell carcinoma. Int J Cancer. 2021;148(1):90–8. https://doi.org/10.1002/ijc.33198.
53. de Sanjosé S, Alemany L, Ordi J, Tous S, Alejo M, Bigby SM, et al. Worldwide human papillomavirus genotype attribution in over 2000 cases of intraepithelial and invasive lesions of the vulva. Eur J Cancer. 2013;49(16):3450–61. https://doi.org/10.1016/j.ejca.2013.06.033.
54. Hinten F, Molijn A, Eckhardt L, Massuger L, Quint W, Bult P, et al. Vulvar cancer: two pathways with different localization and prognosis. Gynecol Oncol. 2018;149(2):310–7. https://doi.org/10.1016/j.ygyno.2018.03.003.
55. Lebreton M, Carton I, Brousse S, Lavoué V, Body G, Levêque J, et al. Vulvar intraepithelial neoplasia: classification, epidemiology, diagnosis, and management. J Gynecol Obstet Hum Reprod. 2020;49(9):101801. https://doi.org/10.1016/j.jogoh.2020.101801.
56. Day T, Otton G, Jaaback K, Weigner J, Scurry J. Is vulvovaginal lichen planus associated with squamous cell carcinoma? J Low Genit Tract Dis. 2018;22(2):159–65. https://doi.org/10.1097/lgt.0000000000000384.
57. Satmary W, Holschneider CH, Brunette LL, Natarajan S. Vulvar intraepithelial neoplasia: risk factors for recurrence. Gynecol Oncol. 2018;148(1):126–31. https://doi.org/10.1016/j.ygyno.2017.10.029.
58. Hoots BE, Palefsky JM, Pimenta JM, Smith JS. Human papillomavirus type distribution in anal cancer and anal intraepithelial lesions. Int J Cancer. 2009;124(10):2375–83. https://doi.org/10.1002/ijc.24215.
59. Siegenbeek van Heukelom ML, Richel O, de Vries HJ, van de Sandt MM, Beck S, van den Munckhof HA, et al. Low- and high-risk human papillomavirus genotype infections in intra-anal warts in HIV-positive men who have sex with men. Br J Dermatol. 2016;175(4):735–43. https://doi.org/10.1111/bjd.14567.

60. Steenbergen RD, Snijders PJ, Heideman DA, Meijer CJ. Clinical implications of (epi)genetic changes in HPV-induced cervical precancerous lesions. Nat Rev Cancer. 2014;14(6):395–405. https://doi.org/10.1038/nrc3728.
61. Berry JM, Jay N, Cranston RD, Darragh TM, Holly EA, Welton ML, et al. Progression of anal high-grade squamous intraepithelial lesions to invasive anal cancer among HIV-infected men who have sex with men. Int J Cancer. 2014;134(5):1147–55. https://doi.org/10.1002/ijc.28431.
62. Jongen VW, Richel O, Marra E, Siegenbeek van Heukelom ML, van Eeden A, de Vries HJC, et al. Anal squamous intraepithelial lesions (SILs) in human immunodeficiency virus-positive men who have sex with men: incidence and risk factors of SIL and of progression and clearance of low-grade SILs. J Infect Dis. 2020;222(1):62–73. https://doi.org/10.1093/infdis/jiz614.
63. Deshmukh AA, Suk R, Shiels MS, Sonawane K, Nyitray AG, Liu Y, et al. Recent trends in squamous cell carcinoma of the anus incidence and mortality in the United States, 2001-2015. J Natl Cancer Inst. 2020;112(8):829–38. https://doi.org/10.1093/jnci/djz219.
64. Marra E, Siegenbeek van Heukelom ML, Leeman A, Waterboer T, Meijer C, Snijders PJF, et al. Virological and serological predictors of anal high-grade squamous intraepithelial lesions among human immunodeficiency virus-positive men who have sex with men. Clin Infect Dis. 2019;68(8):1377–87. https://doi.org/10.1093/cid/ciy719.
65. Tramujas da Costa e Silva I, de Lima Ferreira LC, Santos Gimenez F, Gonçalves Guimarães RA, Botinelly Fujimoto L, Barbosa Cabral CR, et al. High-resolution anoscopy in the diagnosis of anal cancer precursor lesions in renal graft recipients. Ann Surg Oncol. 2008;15(5):1470–5. https://doi.org/10.1245/s10434-007-9750-8.
66. Leeman A, Jenkins D, Marra E, van Zummeren M, Pirog EC, van de Sandt MM, et al. Grading immunohistochemical markers p16(INK4a) and HPV E4 identifies productive and transforming lesions caused by low- and high-risk HPV within high-grade anal squamous intraepithelial lesions. Br J Dermatol. 2020;182(4):1026–33. https://doi.org/10.1111/bjd.18342.
67. Richel O, de Vries HJ, van Noesel CJ, Dijkgraaf MG, Prins JM. Comparison of imiquimod, topical fluorouracil, and electrocautery for the treatment of anal intraepithelial neoplasia in HIV-positive men who have sex with men: an open-label, randomised controlled trial. Lancet Oncol. 2013;14(4):346–53. https://doi.org/10.1016/s1470-2045(13)70067-6.
68. Misago N, Takai T, Toda S, Narisawa Y. The changes in the expression levels of follicular markers in keratoacanthoma depend on the stage: keratoacanthoma is a follicular neoplasm exhibiting infundibular/isthmic differentiation without expression of CK15. J Cutan Pathol. 2014;41(5):437–46. https://doi.org/10.1111/cup.12317.
69. Ra SH, Su A, Li X, Zhou J, Cochran AJ, Kulkarni RP, et al. Keratoacanthoma and squamous cell carcinoma are distinct from a molecular perspective. Mod Pathol. 2015;28(6):799–806. https://doi.org/10.1038/modpathol.2015.5.
70. Schwartz RA. Keratoacanthoma: a clinico-pathologic enigma. Dermatol Surg. 2004;30(2 Pt 2):326–33; discussion 33. https://doi.org/10.1111/j.1524-4725.2004.30080.x.
71. Nagarajan P. Differentiating keratoacanthoma from squamous cell carcinoma-in quest of the holy grail. J Cutan Pathol. 2020;47(4):418–20. https://doi.org/10.1111/cup.13640.
72. Lu JD, Mufti A, Sachdeva M, Rahat S, Lansang RP, Yeung J. Drugs associated with development of porokeratosis: a systematic review. Dermatol Ther. 2021;34(1):e14560. https://doi.org/10.1111/dth.14560.
73. Herranz P, Pizarro A, De Lucas R, Robayna MG, Rubio FA, Sanz A, et al. High incidence of porokeratosis in renal transplant recipients. Br J Dermatol. 1997;136(2):176–9.
74. Sasson M, Krain AD. Porokeratosis and cutaneous malignancy. A review. Dermatol Surg. 1996;22(4):339–42. https://doi.org/10.1111/j.1524-4725.1996.tb00327.x.
75. Weidner T, Illing T, Miguel D, Elsner P. Treatment of porokeratosis: a systematic review. Am J Clin Dermatol. 2017;18(4):435–49. https://doi.org/10.1007/s40257-017-0271-3.
76. Huang S, Wu JH, Lewis DJ, Rady PL, Tyring SK. A novel approach to the classification of epidermodysplasia verruciformis. Int J Dermatol. 2018;57(11):1344–50. https://doi.org/10.1111/ijd.14196.

77. Gara S, Jones M, Litaiem N, Hedri H, Rammeh S, Zeglaoui F. Acquired epidermodysplasia verruciformis in renal-transplant recipients. Clin Case Rep. 2020;8(12):2678–81. https://doi.org/10.1002/ccr3.3251.
78. de Oliveira WR, da Cruz Silva LL, Neto CF, Tyring S. Deleterious effect of radiation therapy on epidermodysplasia verruciformis patients. J Cutan Med Surg. 2015;19(4):416–21. https://doi.org/10.1177/1203475415576859.

Squamous Cell Carcinoma

Roel Genders and Carla Ferrándiz-Pulido

1 Introduction

Cutaneous squamous cell carcinoma (cSCC) is a skin cancer originating from keratinocytes. It is the second most frequent form of keratinocyte carcinoma (KC) after basal cell carcinoma (BCC) and contributes to approximately 20% of all KC [1]. The incidence of cSCC varies globally, with a higher incidence in low skin phototype population living closer to the equator. Incidence trends of cSCC in low skin phototype populations shows geographic variation with the highest incidence rates in Spain (38.16 cases per 100,000 person-years) [2], the United Kingdom (31.7 per 100,000 person-years), and Switzerland (28.9 per 100,000 person-years) and the lowest in Croatia (8.9 per 100,000 person-years) [3]. In Australia, these numbers are reported to be 1035 for men and 472 for women per 100,000 person years, respectively [3]. With a lifetime incidence of cSCC between 7% and 14%, cSCC is considered a major health problem for the Caucasian population at high costs. The mortality from cSCC is likely to be underreported and may approach mortality rates in melanoma.

Improvements in surgical techniques and the increasingly better management of immunosuppressive therapy has led to very high long-term survival rates of solid organ transplant recipients (SOTR). However, this lifelong immunosuppression to

R. Genders
Department of Dermatology, Leiden University Medical Centre, Leiden, The Netherlands

Department of Dermatology, Roosevelt Clinic, Leiden, The Netherlands
e-mail: R.E.Genders@lumc.nl

C. Ferrándiz-Pulido (✉)
Department of Dermatology, Hospital Universitari Vall d'Hebron, Universitat Autònoma de Barcelona, Barcelona, Spain
e-mail: carla.ferrandiz@vallhebron.cat

J. Tomimori et al. (eds.), *Atlas of Dermatologic Diseases in Solid Organ Transplant Recipients*, https://doi.org/10.1007/978-3-031-13335-0_12

avoid graft rejection confers these patients a higher risk of developing different types of cancer, especially KC. The incidence of cSCC in SOTR is 60–250 times increased compared to the immunocompetent population [4]. In SOTR, cSCC occurs more frequently than BCC, with a decreased or even reversed ratio of cSCC to BCC compared to the general population (1:1–1:5 vs 4:1, respectively). Twenty to 75% of SOTR develop at least one cSCC within 20 years after transplantation. After a first invasive cSCC, within 3 years, multiple subsequent cSCCs will develop in 60–80% [5].

Because of this burden of numerous cSCC, the management of skin cancer in SOTR requires a dedicated transplant dermatology clinic with easy access to dermatologic care and more frequent surveillance for high-risk patients. Intervention with regular skin screening examinations may lessen morbidity associated with advanced skin cancer and improve overall quality of life posttransplantation [5, 6].

2 Pathogenesis and Risk Factors

The pathogenesis of cSCC is multifactorial and includes synergistic interplay between the carcinogenic effects of ultraviolet (UV) radiation, host genetic susceptibility factors and compromised immune surveillance. Other risk factors for cSCC are male sex, older age, smoking, human papillomavirus infection, exposure to ionizing radiation, and exposure to arsenic. There is also a higher risk for developing cSCC in scars, burn scars, and chronic ulcers or inflammation [7].

UV radiation, particularly among fair-skinned persons, is the primary risk factor for cSCC development. Cumulative or occupational sun exposure during lifetime is related to developing cSCC [7]. UV radiation appears to have dual effects in mutagenesis and immune suppression as well [8]. The molecular events taking place in cSCC carcinogenesis are most likely heterogenic, and current data argue for a multistep process frequently involving UV-induced p53 mutations [9]. UV radiation is a prevailing factor implicated in the etiology of actinic keratoses and cSCC as evidenced by the high frequency of UV-related mutations in both the p53 and p16 tumor suppressor genes.

Besides UV radiation, *immunosuppression* is an important risk factor for cSCC. Patients with hematologic malignancies, HIV (human immunodeficiency virus) infection or chronic diseases on immunosuppressive drugs are to a certain extent immunosuppressed and carry a higher risk for cSCC [10, 11].

There are *certain patient's characteristics* in SOTR that predispose them to an increased risk of developing cSCC. Some of them are inherent to the patient and cannot be modified including male sex, low Fitzpatrick skin phototype, a previous history of skin cancer, older age at transplantation, longer time since transplantation, or a high cumulative sun exposure before transplantation [12]. Considering this characteristics at the moment of transplantation will allow us to identify those patients at greater risk of developing posttransplant cSCC and prioritize their cutaneous screening after transplantation [13].

There are also other risk factors, which can be modified, such as the *type and dose of immunosuppressive therapy*. In SOTR, the long-term immunosuppressive therapy is an important risk factor for the development of cSCC. Available data suggest that cSCC burden is correlated to the level of immunosuppression and is the highest among heart and lung transplant recipients (TRs), intermediate in kidney TRs, and the lowest in liver TRs reflecting differences in level of immunosuppression required to prevent immunological graft-rejection [14]. The increased incidence of KC and inverted cSCC/BCC ratio in immunosuppressed compared with immunocompetent individuals suggests a central role of the immune system in the genesis of cSCC.

Immunosuppressive drugs (e.g., azathioprine, calcineurin inhibitors) are linked to aberrant production of cytokines that promote tumor growth, angiogenesis, and metastasis. Immunosuppressive drugs have a potential pro-oncogenic action in cells or by facilitating tumor cell escape from immunosurveillance [8, 9]. Azathioprine is an antimetabolite and purine analog, inhibiting purine and DNA synthesis. It is associated with an increased risk of cSCC in SOTR [15–17]. Mycophenolate mofetil (MMF) is an acid prolog and also anti-metabolite, inhibiting purine and DNA synthesis. It was introduced as an immunosuppressant after kidney transplantation in 1995 and has nowadays replaced azathioprine in many centers. Its use seems to be associated with a lower risk of cSCC in SOTR [18, 19]. Cyclosporin and tacrolimus are both calcineurin inhibitors, inhibiting phosphatase activity of calcineurin. First cyclosporine and from mid-1990s tacrolimus are used in SOTR. The research as to whether use of a calcineurin inhibitor would increase the risk of skin cancer in SOTR, and if tacrolimus would have a lower risk than cyclosporin is conflicting [16, 17, 20]. Traditionally, varying doses of azathioprine and cyclosporin, combined with corticosteroids were used. Nowadays, this has largely been replaced in more recent recipients by the modern MMF with tacrolimus [17]. *Mammalian Target of Rapamycin (mTOR) inhibitors (sirolimus and everolimus)* are another group of immunosuppressants that have been associated with a lower risk of cSCC development due to their antiproliferative and antiangiogenic properties. Several clinical trials have shown that conversion to an mTOR inhibitor at the expense of anticalcineurinic drugs after developing a cSCC, reduces the risk of developing successive cSCC, and delays the time until the development of a new cSCC, especially when the switch is performed after the development of the first cSCC [4]. A systematic review and meta-analysis of clinical trials evaluating the effect of sirolimus on malignancy rates in kidney TRs showed an impressive reduction in the risk of successive cSCC [17]. However, it also showed an increase in mortality rates in those exposed to sirolimus compared to controls, which was not due to a higher rejection rate, but to cardiovascular or infectious causes. This risk disappeared when high dose sirolimus group was excluded.

The prolonged immunosuppression leading to the development of numerous actinic keratoses and cSCC also makes a role for a viral pathogenesis very likely. *Cutaneous human papillomavirus (HPV)* of the beta genus (beta-HPV) has been most closely linked with cSCC [19]. Recent animal and human studies show that beta-HPV infection in combination with UV exposure significantly accelerates the development of cSCC [20]. It has been shown that beta-HPV infection facilitates the accumulation of UV-induced DNA mutations by different mechanisms, which in turn leads to cellular transformation and malignant transformation by UV radiation [19]. There is evidence suggesting that beta-HPV infection is involved in cSCC in the initial steps of carcinogenesis in both immunocompetent patients and in SOTR and increases the risk by a factor approximately of 1.5–3. However, beta-HPV is not transcriptionally active in cSCC, so the virus does not seem to play a role in maintaining the malignant phenotype of advanced cSCC [19, 21, 22].

Finally, *voriconazole* is a broad-spectrum antifungal drug from the triazole group, approved since 2002 for the prophylaxis and the treatment of fungal infections in lung TR. Among its adverse effects are changes in vision, elevated liver enzymes and photosensitivity that appears in up to 8–10% of patients [23]. In addition, it has been seen that it enhances damage to cellular DNA and prevents its repair. There are already several studies that have shown that this drug not only increases photosensitivity but is also an independent risk factor for developing cSCC, and that this risk is also greater the longer the exposure and the higher the dose (Fig. 1). Thus, it is recommended to suspend treatment with voriconazole if the patient develops cSCC [23].

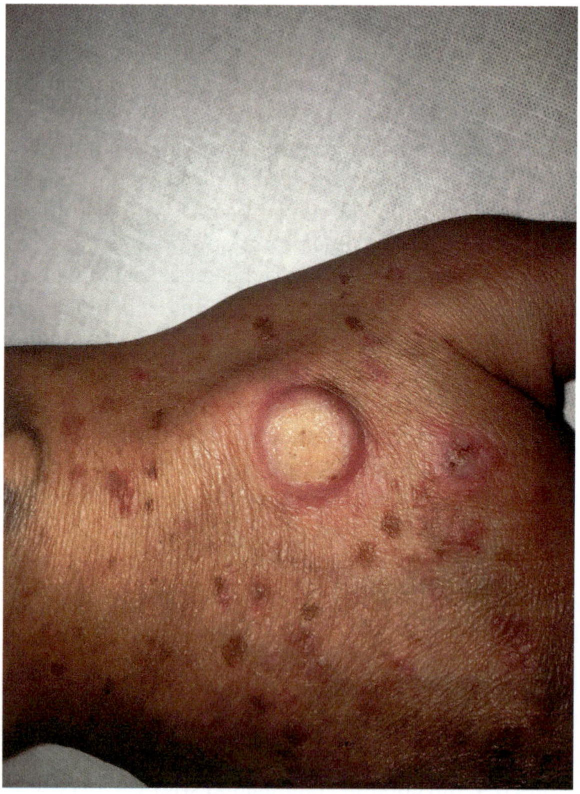

Fig. 1 35 years old, male, lung transplant recipient that developed a cutaneous squamous cell carcinoma on the dorsum of his hand. He had received treatment with voriconazole for 2 years

3 Clinical Presentation

cSCC can develop in the clinical spectrum of actinic keratosis and Bowen's disease, which are precursor lesions and has several clinical presentations (Fig. 2). The classical presentation of a cSCC is that of a skin-colored to erythematous tumor, nodule or elevated and infiltrated plaque with central erosion or hyperkeratosis with well-defined borders (Figs. 3, 4, and 5). However, sometimes a cSCC resembles an

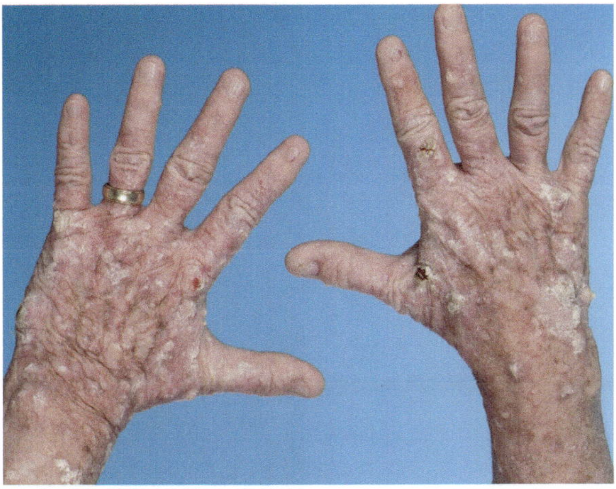

Fig. 2 Multiple verrucokeratotic lesions on the dorsum of the hands of a long-lasting kidney transplant recipient

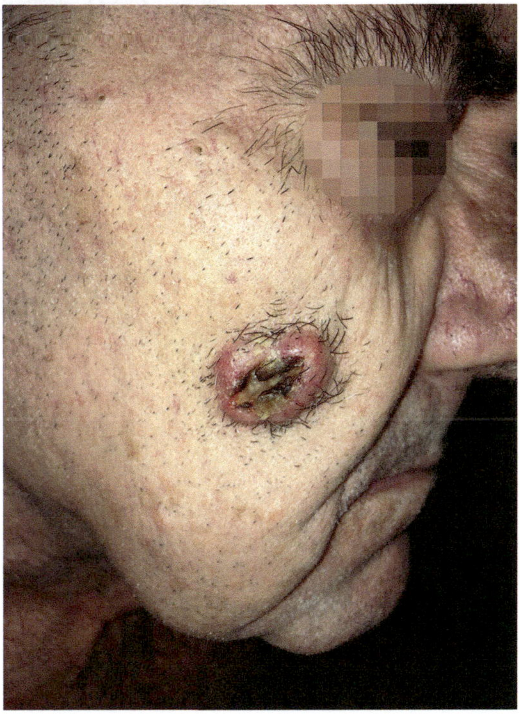

Fig. 3 A typical squamous cell carcinoma on the cheek of a 70-year-old lung transplanted patient; a 2 cm nodule with central ulceration and crusts, present since 2 months

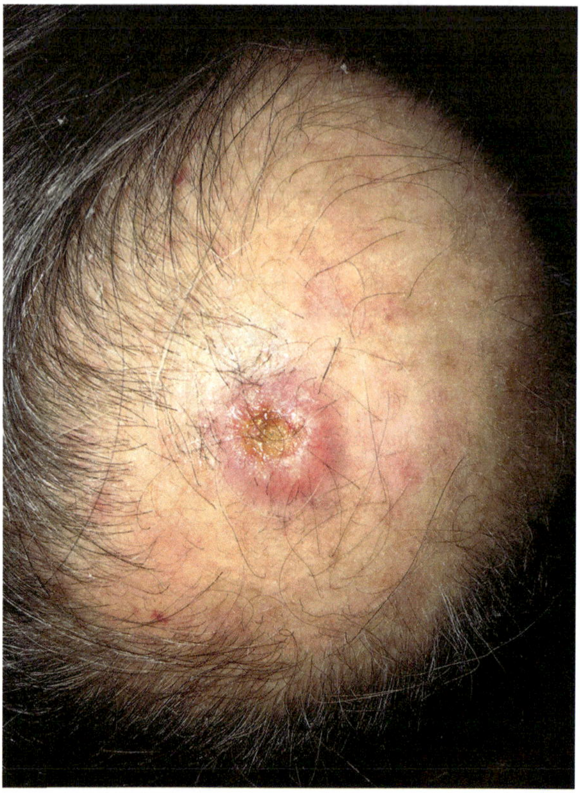

Fig. 4 A 63-year-old male that developed a moderately differentiated squamous cell carcinoma on his scalp 10 year after receiving a kidney transplantation. He was under treatment with tacrolimus and everolimus

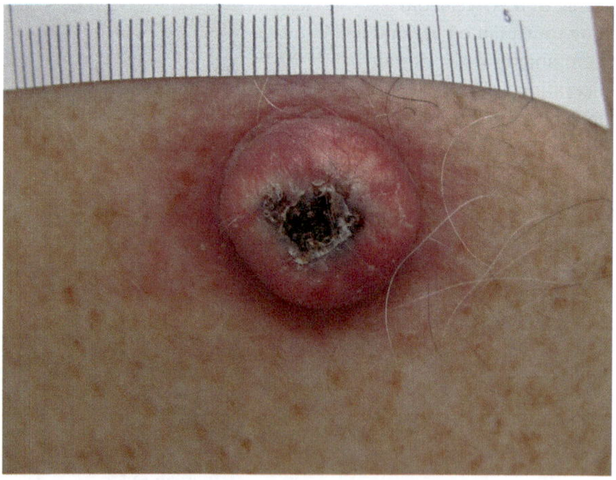

Fig. 5 An erythematous tumor with central hyperkeratosis and well-defined borders. Typical presentation of a cutaneous squamous cell carcinoma

actinic keratosis (precursor lesion) as a flat erythematous hyperkeratotic lesion with ill-defined borders (Fig. 6). It can also have other atypical presentations such as an ulceration with erythematous borders (Figs. 7, 8, and 9).

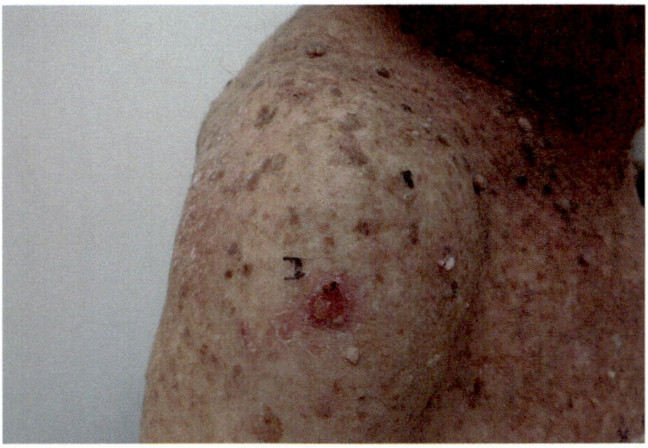

Fig. 6 A kidney transplant recipient with multiple keratotic lesions and a squamous cell carcinoma resembling a Bowen's disease

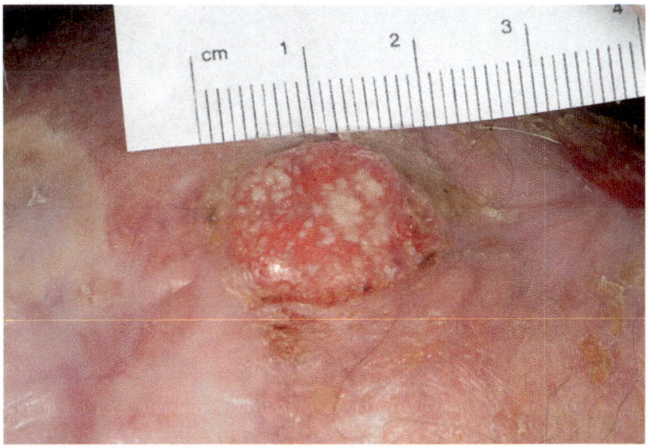

Fig. 7 A moderately differentiated and ulcerated squamous cell carcinoma with microscopically perineural invasion in a kidney transplant recipient

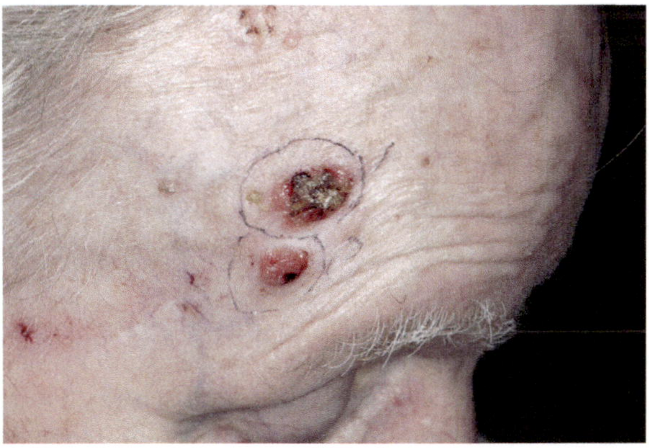

Fig. 8 Two simultaneous ulcerated squamous cell carcinomas on the forehead

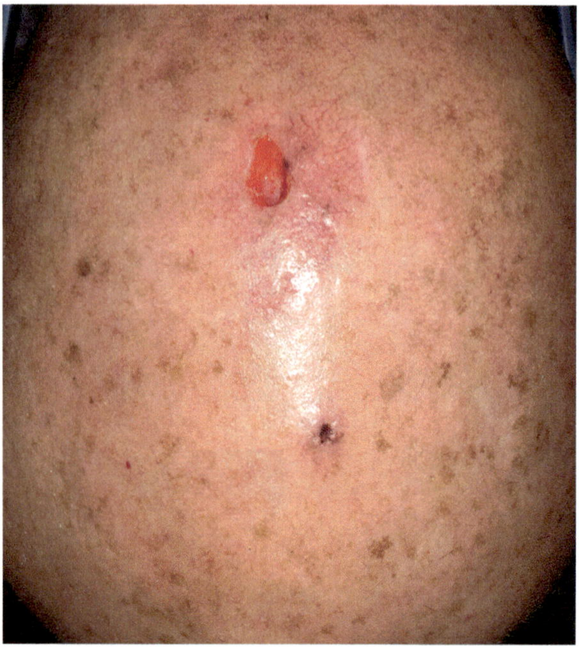

Fig. 9 Atypical presentation of a squamous cell carcinoma, with the appearance of a clean ulcer without infiltrated borders. The patient, a kidney transplant recipient, reported it as a trauma to his head

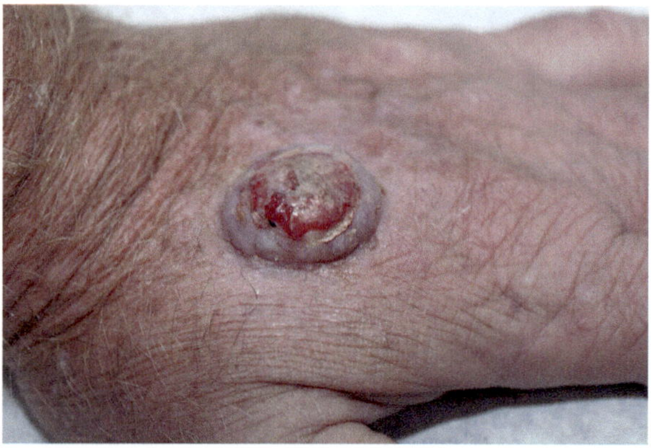

Fig. 10 Typical location for a squamous cell carcinoma on the dorsum of the hands from a kidney transplant recipient

Most cSCC are between 0.5 and 1.5 cm in diameter at time of presentation. The majority of cSCC arise in sun-exposed skin, like the scalp, ears, lips, back of the hands and lower legs (Figs. 10, 11, 12, and 13). The surrounding skin often shows evident sun damage (Fig. 14). However, this tumor can also be found in mucosal

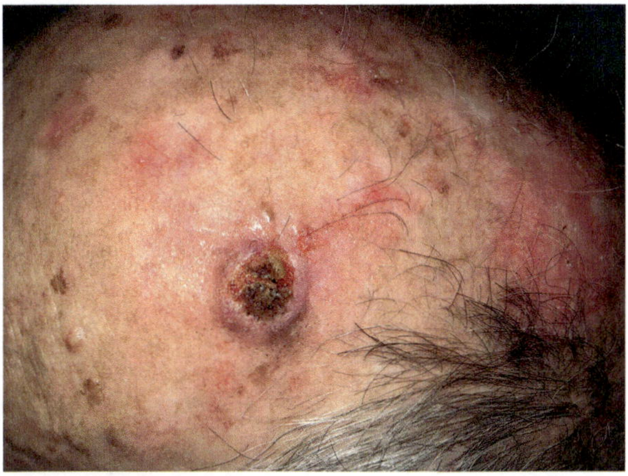

Fig. 11 A squamous cell carcinoma on the forehead of a liver transplant recipient with important sun-damage in the surrounding skin

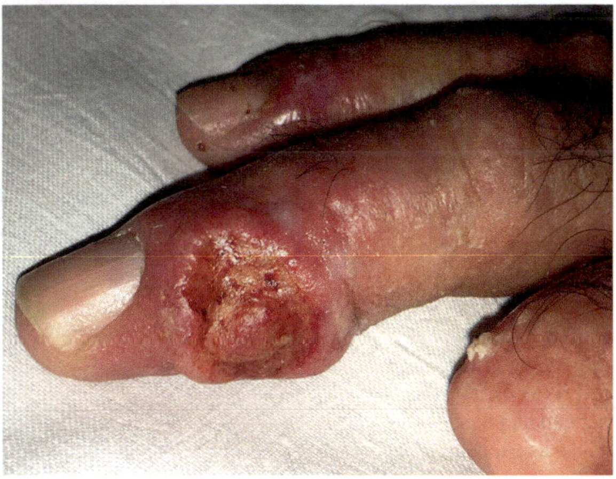

Fig. 12 An undifferentiated squamous cell carcinoma on the finger of a kidney transplant recipient treated with azathioprine for over 30 years

areas (oral or genital), in which case the alpha-human papillomavirus (α-HPV) may be more likely involved in its pathogenesis (Figs. 15 and 16). The clinical presentation often reflects the histopathological differentiation grade [24, 25].

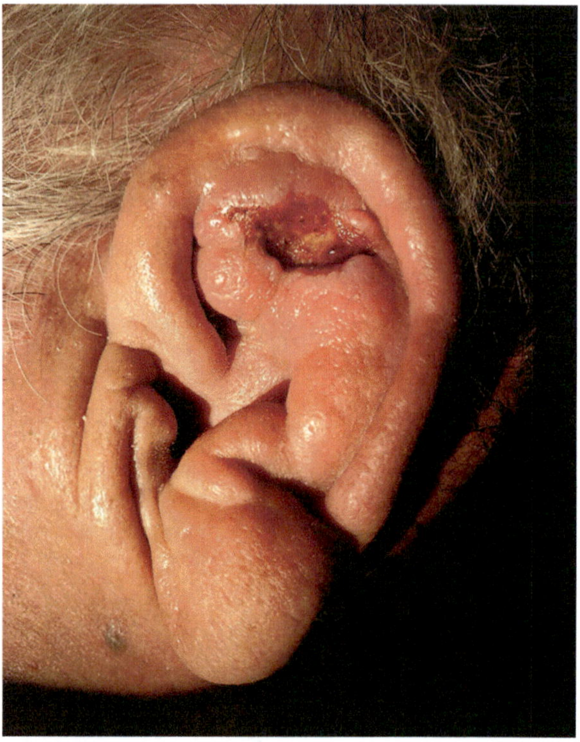

Fig. 13 An infiltrating squamous cell carcinoma on the ear of a kidney transplant recipient that required amputation of the pinna

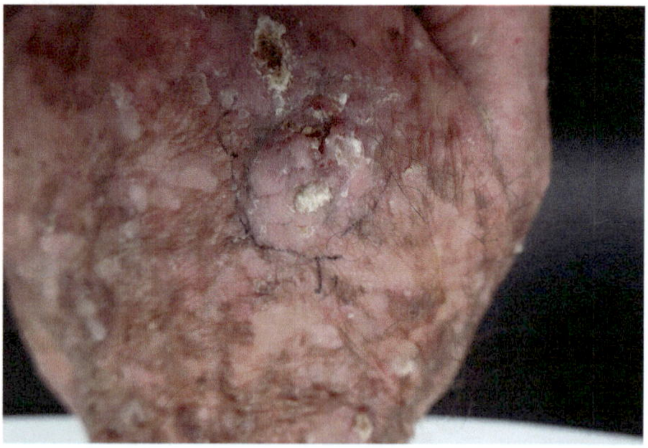

Fig. 14 A well-differentiated squamous cell carcinoma on the dorsum of a hand with evident surrounding sun-damaged skin

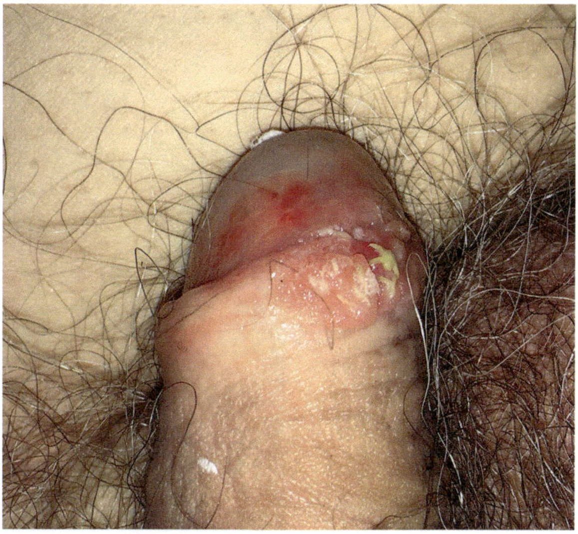

Fig. 15 A squamous cell carcinoma on the glans of a liver transplant recipient

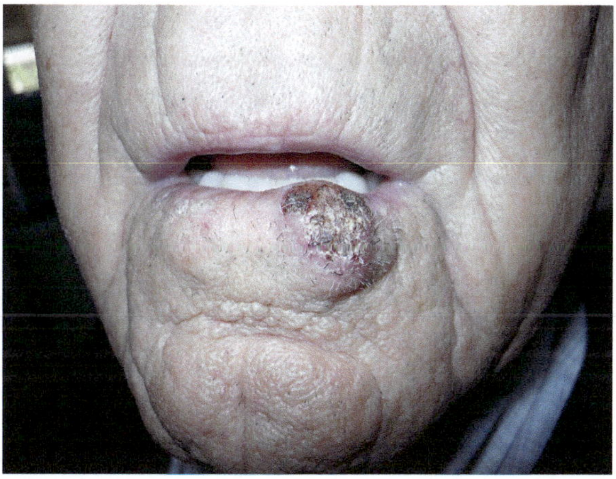

Fig. 16 A squamous cell carcinoma on the lip of a kidney transplant recipient

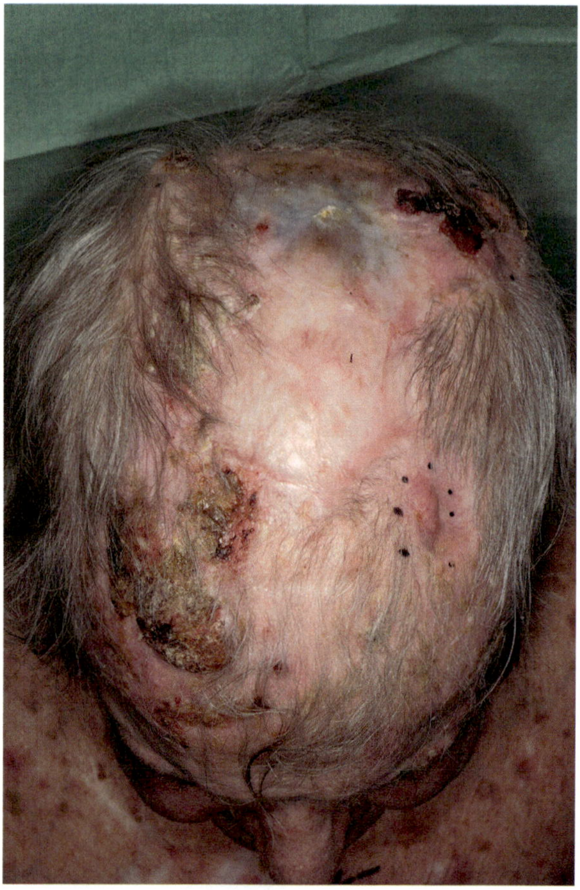

Fig. 17 Multiple simultaneous squamous cell carcinomas on the scalp of a long-lasting kidney transplant recipient

Besides being more frequent than in the general population, cSCC in SOTR has a series of peculiarities, such as its appearance at younger ages and the higher incidence of multiple cSCC (Figs. 17 and 18). This tumor arises 10–30 years earlier than in the general population, and it is not uncommon to find patients in their 40s or 50s who develop multiple cSCC. Moreover, SOTR with cSCC usually have numerous keratotic skin lesions, such as actinic keratoses, common warts, seborrheic warts, and hyperkeratotic papillomas, and they may mimic invasive cSCC hampering timely diagnosis making (Fig. 19) [26]. These lesions can be painful. Pain has been well studied in SOTRs, and this symptom has been found to be the most powerful patient-reported warning sign for identifying invasive cSCC, regardless of other variables such as perineural invasion or hyperkeratosis [27]. Especially

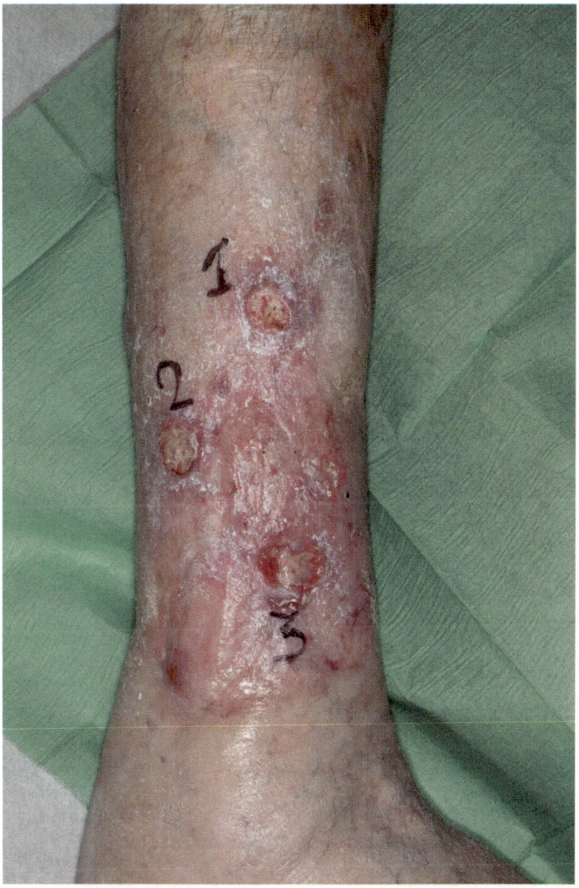

Fig. 18 Multiple simultaneous squamous cell carcinomas on the forearm of a kidney transplant recipient

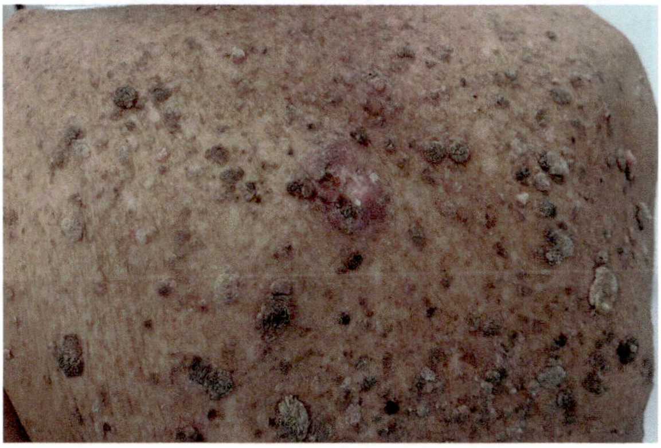

Fig. 19 Squamous cell carcinoma arising on the back of a kidney transplant recipient with severe cumulative sun-damage and multiples keratotic lesions

in patients with numerous skin lesions, pain can be helpful in differentiating cSCC from benign keratinocyte lesions. Finally, cSCC has a more aggressive course in SOTR that the general population. It may have a very rapid enlargement over 1–4 months and has also a higher risk of local recurrence, deeper infiltration depth, greater subclinical extension, and perineural or lymphovascular invasion and a higher risk of distant metastasis (Figs. 20, 21, and 22) [4].

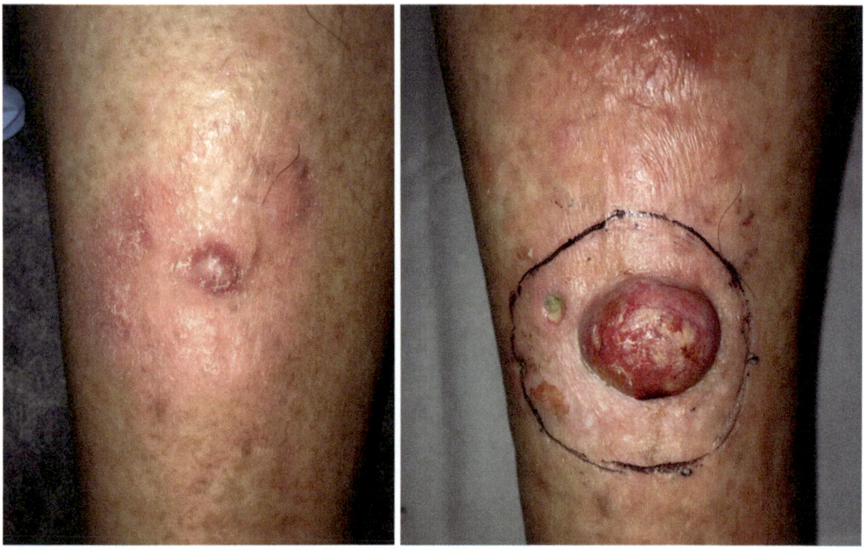

Fig. 20 A kidney transplant recipient with a squamous cell carcinoma on her leg, with rapid enlargement in 2 weeks (lesion at the moment of consultation, and 2 weeks after)

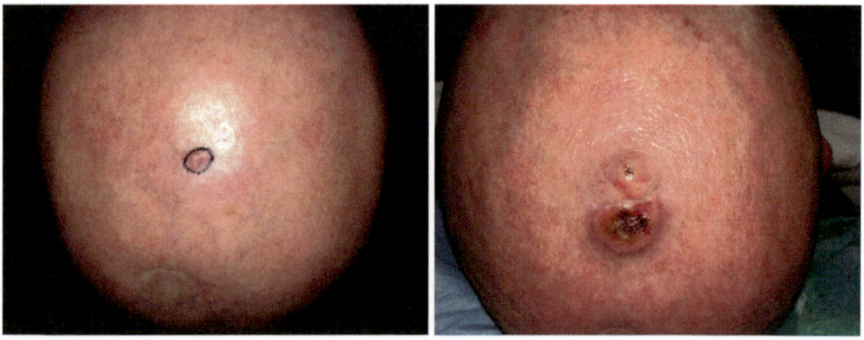

Fig. 21 A lung transplant recipient with a rapidly growing sarcomatous squamous cell carcinoma on his scalp (lesion at the moment of consultation, and 1 month after)

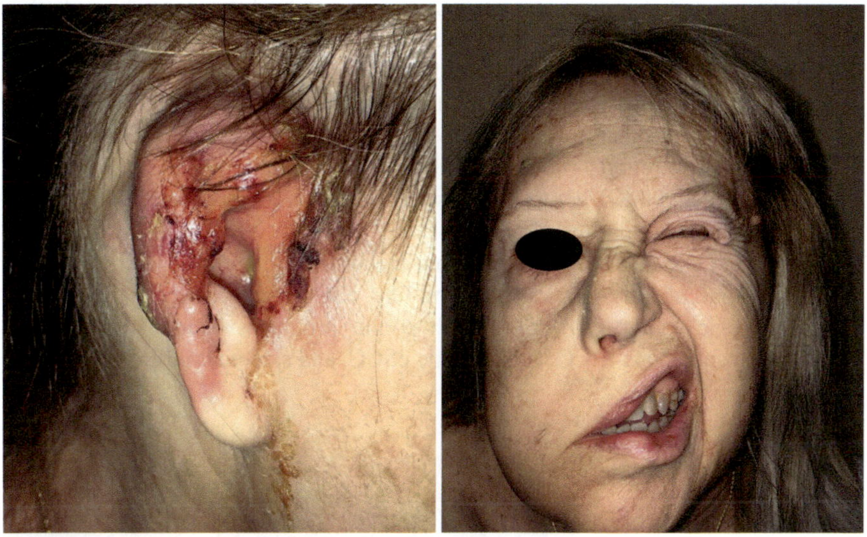

Fig. 22 A kidney transplant recipient with an undifferentiated squamous cell carcinoma on her right ear with associated facial paralysis

4 Diagnosis

4.1 Clinical Examination

Because of its importance as prognostic factors, the location and size (including induration) of the lesion should be noted. On palpation, attention is paid to the bottom layer to assess whether there may be growth in the deeper structures, such as muscle and bone. In an abnormality that is clinically suspicious for a cSCC, investigation of the regional lymph node stations is required. Inspection of the entire skin is warranted. Attention is also paid to other skin disorders appropriate to sunlight damage and skin type.

In case of clinical suspicion, histological examination is performed by means of a biopsy or excision of adequate depth (minimum subcutaneous). A shave biopsy does not assess the depth of invasive ingrowth, perineural or angio-invasive growth.

4.2 Histopathology

On histopathology, cSCC differentiation may vary from well to poorly differentiated. This is graded on a 4-tier system developed by Broders. In this classification, the grade reflects the ratio of differentiated cells to undifferentiated cells. Grade 1 is well differentiated (keratinized), grade 2 is moderately differentiated, grade 3 is poorly differentiated, and grade 4 is undifferentiated (unkeratinized) (Figs. 23 and 24). Well-differentiated tumors exhibit interconnecting follicular infundibular type squamous epithelium with keratinization. Mitosis may be rare or absent. Poor differentiation indicates that it is difficult to determine a keratinocyte lineage [7].

Histopathology reports should include the differentiation grade, the depth of invasion in mm and the structure of invasion, as well as the presence or not of perineural or lymphovascular invasion.

Histopathologic subtypes of cSCC that are well differentiated with low metastatic potential include keratoacanthoma-like cSCC and verrucous carcinoma. Histopathologic subtypes of cSCC with poorer prognosis include desmoplastic cSCC, adenosquamous cSCC, acantholytic cSCC, and sarcomatoid cSCC.

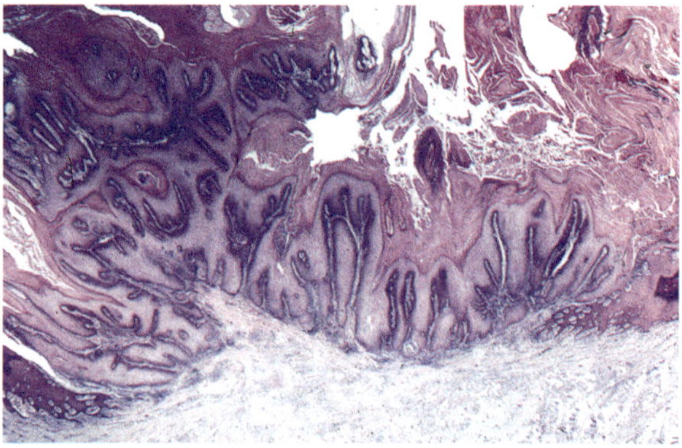

Fig. 23 A well-differentiated squamous cell carcinoma in a kidney transplant recipient (hematoxylin-eosin 10×)

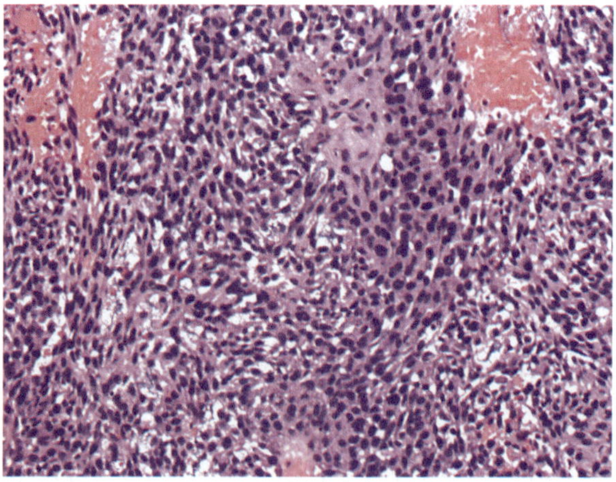

Fig. 24 Undifferentiated (sarcomatoid subtype) squamous cell carcinoma in a lung transplant recipient (hematoxylin-eosin 40×)

4.3 Imaging

In case of suspicion of lymph node involvement or diagnosis of high-risk cSCC (T2b BWH or T3 AJCC) or high-risk features not included in the staging systems such as lymphovascular invasion or high-risk locations (lip and ear), an imaging technique for initial staging is advised, including regional ultrasound or computed tomography (CT) with contrast. A magnetic resonance imaging (MRI) or CT scan may also be needed to evaluate the local invasion of deep structures before surgery when the clinical picture is suggestive of involvement of large-caliber nerves, muscle, or bone (Fig. 22) [28]. Sentinel lymph node biopsy can be used as an adjuvant method in detecting metastasis. However, it has to be established which patients benefit the most from this procedure, especially in high-risk populations like SOTR [29].

4.4 Staging

The challenge in daily practice is to identify high-risk cSCC and to detect a metastasis as early as possible [30]. A tumor staging system helps to accomplish this task. Three different systems are currently in use; the International Union Against Cancer (UICC), the American Joint Committee on Cancer (AJCC) classification and the Brigham and Women's Hospital (BWH) tumor staging system [31]. The AJCC staging system is the most commonly used. These staging systems are based upon defined series of major and minor criteria, which contain both clinical and histological features. High-risk features that are used for tumor staging are tumor size, depth of invasion, location on head and neck, differentiation grade, and perineural invasion.

Currently, the features that are correlated with worse prognosis are, namely larger tumors, poor differentiation grade, depth of invasion >6 mm or beyond subcutis, perineural invasion of nerves >0.1 μm, and lymphovascular invasion [24, 25]. Location on the central face, ear, and lip are high-risk locations, as well as rapid growth, recurrent tumor, prior radiation therapy, and immunocompromised status [32].

Not every high-risk factor is included in the current staging systems, like location lip and ear and poor differentiation, but are still considered as high-risk factors for cSCC to take into account as a prognostic factor for clinical practice. This also accounts for immunosuppression although immunosuppressed status is not included in the staging systems [33].

A recent systematic review and meta-analysis (17,248 patients with 23,421 cSCC) found immunosuppression to be a significant risk factor and tumor depth was associated with the highest risk of local recurrence and metastasis of cSCC [34]. Immunosuppressed patients have demonstrated in one report a higher risk of local recurrence and regional recurrence compared to immunocompetent patients (10.5%). Immunosuppressed patients with cSCC of the head and neck more frequently present with high-risk pathologic features and inferior outcomes [35]. Immunosuppression is also correlated with decreased disease-specific survival, either by metastasis or because of tumor growth by local infiltration [14].

4.5 *Metastasis Risk*

cSCC has the potential to metastasize, usually to the regional lymph nodes (Figs. 25, 26, 27, and 28). The overall incidence rate of cSCC metastasis is variable, ranging from 0.1% to 9.9%, with a tendency to a higher incidence in tertiary hospitals [36].

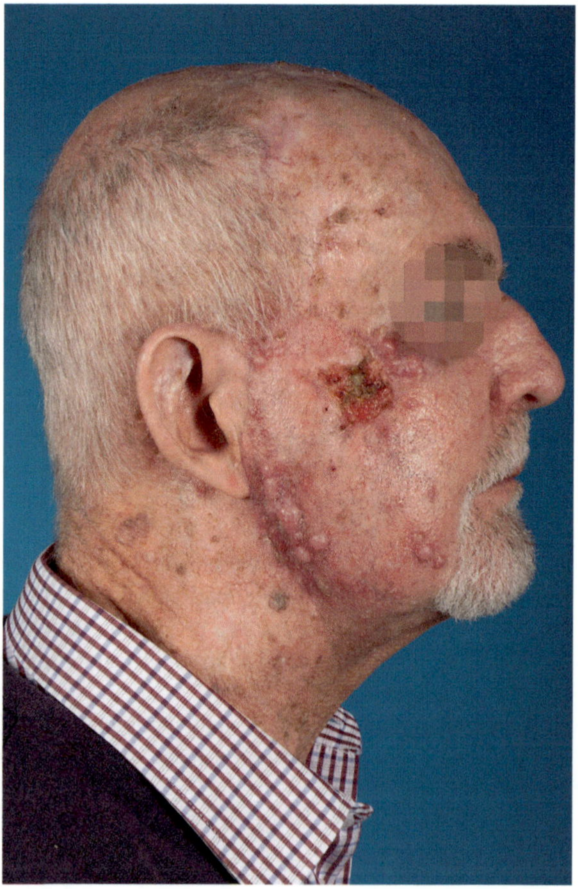

Fig. 25 Multiple in-transit metastasis from squamous cell carcinoma in a kidney transplant recipient

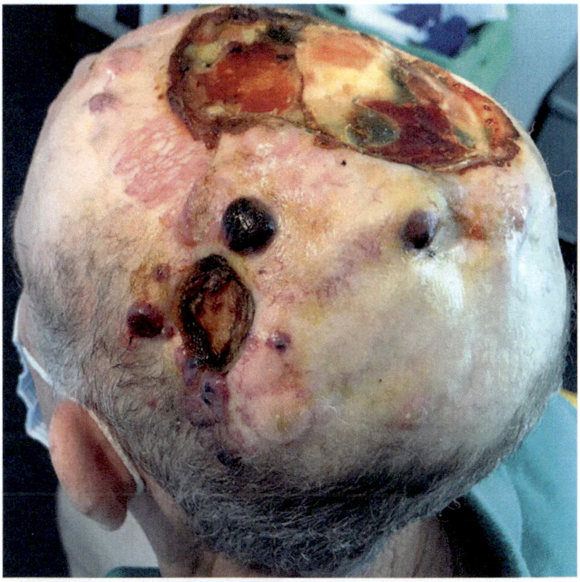

Fig. 26 Multiple in-transit metastasis after a local recurrence of a squamous cell carcinoma, sarcomatoid-type, in the scalp from a lung transplant recipient

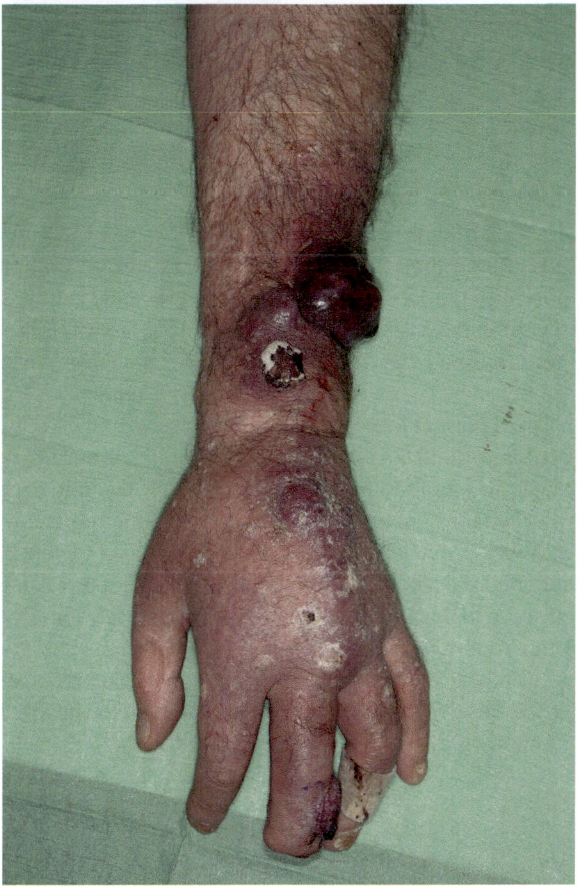

Fig. 27 Recurrent squamous cell carcinoma with multiple in-transit metastases

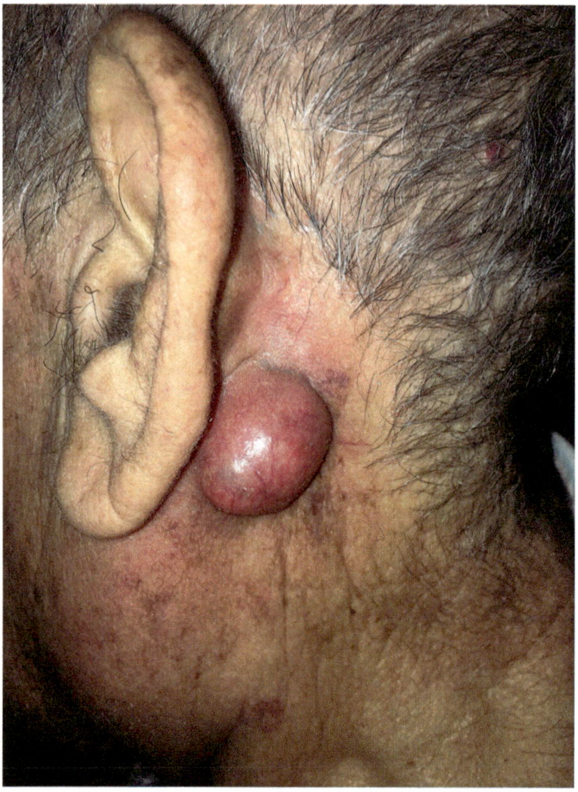

Fig. 28 Lymph-node metastasis from a squamous cell carcinoma primarily located on the scalp of a kidney transplant recipient

The risk of developing metastases of low-risk cSCC is 0–5% in the general population. Large tumors, recurrent tumors, deep infiltration, location on the lip or ear, poor differentiation grade and perineural and lymphovascular invasion increase the risk for metastasis up to 45% [37]. A 13% risk of metastatic disease in immunocompromised patients has been described, twice the risk in patients without immunosuppression [37]. Because of the large numbers of cSCC in individual patients, SOTRs present more often with aggressive cSCC (thicker tumors, poorly differentiated and infiltrative), with a higher predilection for metastasis [38]. Broadly, it is stated in literature that cSCC in SOTR frequently seems to exhibit a more aggressive behavior, irrespective of the size of the tumor, with more frequent metastases and worse outcome compared to immunocompetent patients [39, 40]. It has been reported that about 5–23% of all patients with metastatic cSCC are immunocompromised and in these studies investigating metastatic cSCC, immunosuppression is often reported as a risk factor [41].

A recent review showed pooled metastasis risk estimate for SOTR of 7.3% for cSCC on total body and 11.0% for cSCC of the head neck area, respectively. For the immunocompetent population showed a risk of 3.1% (95% CI 2.8–3.4) in total body cSCC and of 8.5% (95% CI 7.3–9.8) in cSCC of the head and neck area. Per single cSCC in SOTR were 1.3% (95% CI 1.0–1.7) in total body cSCC and 4.0% (95% CI 2.7–5.5) in cSCC of the head and neck area. In the immunocompetent population, these pooled risk estimates were 2.4% (95% CI 2.1–2.6) and 6.7% (95% CI 5.7–7.8), respectively [42]. Overall, immunosuppressed patients/SOTR carry a 1.6 to two-fold higher risk for metastasis [42].

5 Treatment

Treatment of choice in most countries is complete surgical excision [28]. The aim of surgical excision of cSCC should be complete histological clearance at peripheral and deep margins.

In SOTR with many cSCCs, curettage and electrodesiccation can be a safe therapy for appropriately selected low-risk cSCCs, on the trunk or extremities, with an acceptable overall rate of residual or recurrent cSCCs of 6%. However, most cSCC are surgically removed by conventional excision. Guidelines recommend excision margins of 4–6 mm for low-risk cSCC and from 6 to 10 mm or higher for high-risk cSCC [28, 43]. Wider excision should be performed when histologic margins appear more limited (debatable <1 or <2 mm) if high-risk features are present and if the benefits outweigh the risks. In case of incomplete excision, re-excision is recommended. Overall, the risk of incomplete excision can be minimized by determining adequate excision margins [7, 43, 44].

Excision with complete peripheral and deep-margin histologic margin control, like Mohs micrographic surgery (MMS), is more often recommended for high-risk cSCC, especially in anatomic sites where tissue conservation is desired [7, 43, 44]. Also techniques in paraffin block specimens, for example, Breuninger technique, can be used for 100% margin control. In cases deemed inoperable or when surgery is refused by the patient, primary radiation therapy (RT) can also provide high local cure rates with good cosmesis [45].

The benefit of adjuvant radiation therapy (ART) has not been directly studied in cSCC. In SOTR, ART is recommended when surgical margins are uncertain or cannot be re-excised or when there is a high risk of local recurrence (i.e., marked single-cell tumor spread at the periphery, lymphovascular invasion, in-transit metastasis, or the invasion of large-caliber nerves [>0.1 mm]).

After the development of the first cSCC, it is important to review the immunosuppressive regimen. Although, based on expert opinion panels, and with a limited high level of evidence data it is recommended to reduce the immunosuppression dose, according to the risk of each individual. Apart from reducing the dose, patients may also benefit from a switch of immunosuppressive drug, for instance, from calcineurin inhibitors to mTORi. Decisions need to be made in multidisciplinary committees including transplant physicians [45].

5.1 Systemic Treatments

Chemotherapy has been traditionally used to treat metastatic cSCC; however, data for systemic chemotherapy to treat cSCC is limited. Cisplatin alone or in combination with 5-FU has shown clinical efficacy [46]. However, since the irruption of immune-checkpoint inhibitors (ICPi) in the treatment of cSCC, the prognosis of these patients has radically changed. Cemiplimab, an anti-programmed cell death protein 1 (PD-1) was the first drug approved by the FDA (Food and Drug Administration) and EMA (European Medicines Agency) to treat locally advanced or metastatic cSCC, with overall response rates around 50% of cases [47]. Limited data are available on the efficacy and toxicity of ICPi in SOTR, as these patients were excluded from clinical trials testing these substances for safety and efficacy, despite the fact that they represent 30% of the patients who would require this treatment. The reason to exclude them came from the experience with other immunotherapies, where 40–50% of SOTR presented an acute graft rejection [48]. In fact, immunotherapy in transplant patients is a double-edged sword. On the one hand, they seem to be very effective because they unleash the immune response of T cells against the tumoral cells that are impaired because of the immunosuppressive medication; but at the same time, immunotherapy could also activate alloreactive T cells leading to acute rejection and graft loss [48]. Therefore, treatment with ICPi should be reserved only for non-life-threatening transplant patients, such as kidney transplant recipients. When using ICPi in SOTR, it is recommended to do immunosuppression minimization, especially calcineurin inhibitor withdrawal. The addition of sirolimus or everolimus may be helpful for mitigate rejections, along with low-dose prednisone [49].

Epidermal growth factor receptors, such as cetuximab, have been used off-label for cSCC [50]. The efficacy data come from observational studies. Generally used in elderly patients with little tolerance to chemotherapy, obtaining response rates of 30–40%, complete response less than 20% and a short response duration of 8 months on average. In general, targeted therapy in cSCC have relatively short progressive-free survival and overall survival [50]. Epidermal growth factor receptor inhibitors have shown to have satisfactory antitumor activity with acceptable side-effect profile. However, their place in the management of advanced cSCC alone or in combination with either radiation therapy and/or chemotherapy needs to be better characterized. The use of cetuximab for cSCC in SOTR is infrequent, and it is important to remark the risk of severe lung toxicity in lung transplanted organs, appearing 1 month after starting treatment. Therefore, lung transplantation is an absolute contraindication to the use of cetuximab [45, 51].

6 Prevention

Among the primary prevention measures, information and health education on photoprotection and self-examination measures are essential, and among secondary prevention measures, the detection, and early treatment of AKs and the field of cancerization to prevent their progression to invasive cSCC, as well as modification of the IS agents in those of greater risk should be considered [45].

In high-risk patients (i.e., patients who develop multiple cSCCs [more than five] every year or who have aggressive cSCCs or early onset of cSCCs) can be considered for oral chemoprophylaxis. Oral nicotinamide (500 mg/12 h) has been shown to be effective and safe in reducing the appearance of new KC in high-risk patients, and although the differences were not statistically significant in a trial with SOTR patients, we do know that it is a very well-tolerated and safe medication, so we should offer it to all our patients [52]. Oral retinoids (acitretin or etretinate) are also recommended in high-risk patients [45, 53]. There are few randomized clinical trials that support its efficacy in SOTR, and most of them include only a small number of patients and do not have a control arm. Despite the paucity of data, it is a widely used drug, and it can be said that the beneficial effects in the prevention of invasive AK and cSCC offered by oral retinoids occur only during treatment and that its mucocutaneous toxicity limits its long-term use. The starting dose should be low and progressively increased to the maximum dose tolerated by the patient. In addition, it is also necessary to consider that they have an immunostimulatory effect that could have consequences on the transplanted organ, in addition to having an effect on osteoporosis that must be added to the effect of corticosteroids and possible vitamin D deficiency [45, 53].

Finally, capecitabine is a chemotherapeutic drug that is converted to 5-fluoracil in the body. At low doses (1 g/m^2) on days 1 and 14 of 21-day cycles, a decrease in the incidence of cSCC and in the number of AK has been observed [54]. The adverse effects that included fatigue, nausea, hand-foot syndrome, and renal dysfunction of variable degree requires in some cases a dose readjustment. Although this treatment may be beneficial in some cases, there is a lack of randomized clinical trials to support its efficacy [54]. It is important to remember that before starting this treatment, a dihydropyrimidine DH deficiency must be ruled out and kidney function evaluated (it increases toxicity).

7 Future Perspectives

Because the incidence of KC is still rising, it is evident that prevention and early detection is of upmost importance in the management of these cancers. Also the challenge in daily practice is to identify cSCC, especially high-risk cSCC, and to detect a metastasis as early as possible. In clinical practice, pain is a helpful indicator in differentiating cSCC from benign lesions. Early detection and treatment of cSCC prevents it to grow deeper and therefore lowers the risk for metastasis. Early intervention for metastases can confer to a survival advantage and radiologic imaging in patients with high-risk cSCC may influence management.

Due to the ongoing insight in risk factors for cSCC, evidence-based guidelines for the care of cSCC will be periodically updated with the most recent published data. The improvements in staging systems leads to more precise risk stratification and identification of aggressive cSCC, allowing for an accurate framework for management based on these risk levels. Overall, due to higher risk of immunosuppression, it is most important to keep in mind that close and regular inspection of the skin with adequate and rapid diagnosis and treatment of cSCC is important to prevent metastasis in SOTR.

References

1. Madan V, Lear JT, Szeimies R-M. Non-melanoma skin cancer. Lancet (London, England). 2010;375(9715):673–85. https://doi.org/10.1016/S0140-6736(09)61196-X.
2. Tejera-Vaquerizo A, Descalzo-Gallego MA, Otero-Rivas MM, et al. Skin cancer incidence and mortality in Spain: a systematic review and meta-analysis. Actas Dermosifiliogr. 2016;107(4):318–28. https://doi.org/10.1016/j.ad.2015.12.008.
3. Xiang F, Lucas R, Hales S, Neale R. Incidence of nonmelanoma skin cancer in relation to ambient UV radiation in white populations, 1978-2012: empirical relationships. JAMA Dermatol. 2014;150(10):1063–71. https://doi.org/10.1001/jamadermatol.2014.762.
4. Euvrard S, Kanitakis J, Claudy A. Skin cancers after organ transplantation. N Engl J Med. 2003;348(17):1681–91. https://doi.org/10.1056/NEJMra022137.
5. O'Reilly Zwald F, Brown M. Skin cancer in solid organ transplant recipients: advances in therapy and management: part I. Epidemiology of skin cancer in solid organ transplant recipients. J Am Acad Dermatol. 2011;65(2):253–61. https://doi.org/10.1016/j.jaad.2010.11.062.
6. O'Reilly Zwald F, Brown M. Skin cancer in solid organ transplant recipients: advances in therapy and management: part II. Management of skin cancer in solid organ transplant recipients. J Am Acad Dermatol. 2011;65(2):263–79. https://doi.org/10.1016/j.jaad.2010.11.063.
7. Que SKT, Zwald FO, Schmults CD. Cutaneous squamous cell carcinoma: incidence, risk factors, diagnosis, and staging. J Am Acad Dermatol. 2018;78(2):237–47. https://doi.org/10.1016/j.jaad.2017.08.059.
8. Rangwala S, Tsai KY. Roles of the immune system in skin cancer. Br J Dermatol. 2011;165(5):953–65. https://doi.org/10.1111/j.1365-2133.2011.10507.x.
9. Boukamp P. Non-melanoma skin cancer: what drives tumor development and progression? Carcinogenesis. 2005;26(10):1657–67. https://doi.org/10.1093/carcin/bgi123.
10. Falchi L, Vitale C, Keating MJ, et al. Incidence and prognostic impact of other cancers in a population of long-term survivors of chronic lymphocytic leukemia. Ann Oncol. 2016;27(6):1100–6. https://doi.org/10.1093/annonc/mdw072.
11. Silverberg MJ, Leyden W, Warton EM, Quesenberry CP, Engels EA, Asgari MM. HIV infection status, immunodeficiency, and the incidence of non-melanoma skin cancer. J Natl Cancer Inst. 2013;105(5):350–60. https://doi.org/10.1093/jnci/djs529.
12. Madeleine MM, Patel NS, Plasmeijer EI, et al. Epidemiology of keratinocyte carcinomas after organ transplantation. Br J Dermatol. 2017;177(5):1208–16. https://doi.org/10.1111/bjd.15931.
13. Jambusaria-Pahlajani A, Crow LD, Lowenstein S, et al. Predicting skin cancer in organ transplant recipients: development of the SUNTRAC screening tool using data from a multicenter cohort study. Transpl Int. 2019;32(12):1259–67. https://doi.org/10.1111/tri.13493.
14. Garrett GL, Blanc PD, Boscardin J, et al. Incidence of and risk factors for skin cancer in organ transplant recipients in the United States. JAMA Dermatol. 2017;153(3):296–303. https://doi.org/10.1001/jamadermatol.2016.4920.
15. Wisgerhof HC, van der Boog PJM, de Fijter JW, et al. Increased risk of squamous-cell carcinoma in simultaneous pancreas kidney transplant recipients compared with kidney transplant recipients. J Invest Dermatol. 2009;129(12):2886–94. https://doi.org/10.1038/jid.2009.181.
16. Dantal J, Morelon E, Rostaing L, et al. Sirolimus for secondary prevention of skin cancer in kidney transplant recipients: 5-year results. J Clin Oncol. 2018;36(25):2612–20. https://doi.org/10.1200/JCO.2017.76.6691.

17. Knoll GA, Kokolo MB, Mallick R, et al. Effect of sirolimus on malignancy and survival after kidney transplantation: systematic review and meta-analysis of individual patient data. BMJ. 2014;349:g6679. https://doi.org/10.1136/bmj.g6679.
18. Howley PM, Pfister HJ. Beta genus papillomaviruses and skin cancer. Virology. 2015;479–480:290–6. https://doi.org/10.1016/j.virol.2015.02.004.
19. Quint KD, Genders RE, de Koning MNC, et al. Human Beta-papillomavirus infection and keratinocyte carcinomas. J Pathol. 2015;235(2):342–54. https://doi.org/10.1002/path.4425.
20. Hasche D, Stephan S, Braspenning-Wesch I, et al. The interplay of UV and cutaneous papillomavirus infection in skin cancer development. PLoS Pathog. 2017;13(11):e1006723. https://doi.org/10.1371/journal.ppat.1006723.
21. Genders RE, Mazlom H, Michel A, et al. The presence of betapapillomavirus antibodies around transplantation predicts the development of keratinocyte carcinoma in organ transplant recipients: a cohort study. J Invest Dermatol. 2015;135(5):1275–82. https://doi.org/10.1038/jid.2014.456.
22. Chahoud J, Semaan A, Chen Y, et al. Association between β-genus human papillomavirus and cutaneous squamous cell carcinoma in immunocompetent individuals-a meta-analysis. JAMA Dermatol. 2016;152(12):1354–64. https://doi.org/10.1001/jamadermatol.2015.4530.
23. Williams K, Mansh M, Chin-Hong P, Singer J, Arron ST. Voriconazole-associated cutaneous malignancy: a literature review on photocarcinogenesis in organ transplant recipients. Clin Infect Dis. 2014;58(7):997–1002. https://doi.org/10.1093/cid/cit940.
24. Cassarino DS, Derienzo DP, Barr RJ. Cutaneous squamous cell carcinoma: a comprehensive clinicopathologic classification—part one. J Cutan Pathol. 2006;33(3):191–206. https://doi.org/10.1111/j.0303-6987.2006.00516_1.x.
25. Cassarino DS, Derienzo DP, Barr RJ. Cutaneous squamous cell carcinoma: a comprehensive clinicopathologic classification—part two. J Cutan Pathol. 2006;33(4):261–79. https://doi.org/10.1111/j.0303-6987.2006.00516.x.
26. Bouwes Bavinck JN, Euvrard S, Naldi L, et al. Keratotic skin lesions and other risk factors are associated with skin cancer in organ-transplant recipients: a case-control study in The Netherlands, United Kingdom, Germany, France, and Italy. J Invest Dermatol. 2007;127(7):1647–56. https://doi.org/10.1038/sj.jid.5700776.
27. Bouwes Bavinck JN, Harwood CA, Genders RE, et al. Pain identifies squamous cell carcinoma in organ transplant recipients: the SCOPE-ITSCC PAIN study. Am J Transplant. 2014;14(3):668–76. https://doi.org/10.1111/ajt.12587.
28. Stratigos A, Garbe C, Lebbe C, et al. Diagnosis and treatment of invasive squamous cell carcinoma of the skin: European consensus-based interdisciplinary guideline. Eur J Cancer (Oxford, England: 1990). 2015;51(14):1989–2007. https://doi.org/10.1016/j.ejca.2015.06.110.
29. Genders RE, Bouwes Bavinck JN. Sentinel lymph node biopsy for cutaneous squamous cell carcinoma: valuable or not valuable? Br J Dermatol. 2015;172(4):854–5. https://doi.org/10.1111/bjd.13601.
30. Martorell-Calatayud A, Sanmartín Jimenez O, Cruz Mojarrieta J, Guillén BC. Cutaneous squamous cell carcinoma: defining the high-risk variant. Actas Dermosifiliogr. 2013;104(5):367–79. https://doi.org/10.1016/j.adengl.2011.12.012.
31. Karia PS, Jambusaria-Pahlajani A, Harrington DP, Murphy GF, Qureshi AA, Schmults CD. Evaluation of American Joint Committee on Cancer, International Union Against Cancer, and Brigham and Women's Hospital tumor staging for cutaneous squamous cell carcinoma. J Clin Oncol. 2014;32(4):327–34. https://doi.org/10.1200/JCO.2012.48.5326.
32. Nehal KS, Bichakjian CK. Update on keratinocyte carcinomas. N Engl J Med. 2018;379(4):363–74. https://doi.org/10.1056/NEJMra1708701.
33. Schmults CD, Karia PS, Carter JB, Han J, Qureshi AA. Factors predictive of recurrence and death from cutaneous squamous cell carcinoma: a 10-year, single-institution cohort study. JAMA Dermatol. 2013;149(5):541–7. https://doi.org/10.1001/jamadermatol.2013.2139.
34. Thompson AK, Kelley BF, Prokop LJ, Murad MH, Baum CL. Risk factors for cutaneous squamous cell carcinoma recurrence, metastasis, and disease-specific death: a systematic review and meta-analysis. JAMA Dermatol. 2016;152(4):419–28. https://doi.org/10.1001/jamadermatol.2015.4994.

35. Manyam BV, Garsa AA, Chin R-I, et al. A multi-institutional comparison of outcomes of immunosuppressed and immunocompetent patients treated with surgery and radiation therapy for cutaneous squamous cell carcinoma of the head and neck. Cancer. 2017;123(11):2054–60. https://doi.org/10.1002/cncr.30601.
36. Weinberg AS, Ogle CA, Shim EK. Metastatic cutaneous squamous cell carcinoma: an update. Dermatol Surg. 2007;33(8):885–99. https://doi.org/10.1111/j.1524-4725.2007.33190.x.
37. Rowe DE, Carroll RJ, Day CL. Prognostic factors for local recurrence, metastasis, and survival rates in squamous cell carcinoma of the skin, ear, and lip. Implications for treatment modality selection. J Am Acad Dermatol. 1992;26(6):976–90. https://doi.org/10.1016/0190-9622(92)70144-5.
38. Smith KJ, Hamza S, Skelton H. Histologic features in primary cutaneous squamous cell carcinomas in immunocompromised patients focusing on organ transplant patients. Dermatol Surg. 2004;30(4 Pt 2):634–41. https://doi.org/10.1111/j.1524-4725.2004.30149.x.
39. Carucci JA, Martinez JC, Zeitouni NC, et al. In-transit metastasis from primary cutaneous squamous cell carcinoma in organ transplant recipients and nonimmunosuppressed patients: clinical characteristics, management, and outcome in a series of 21 patients. Dermatol Surg. 2004;30(4 Pt 2):651–5. https://doi.org/10.1111/j.1524-4725.2004.30151.x.
40. Martinez J-C, Otley CC, Stasko T, et al. Defining the clinical course of metastatic skin cancer in organ transplant recipients: a multicenter collaborative study. Arch Dermatol. 2003;139(3):301–6. https://doi.org/10.1001/archderm.139.3.301.
41. Dinehart SM, Chu DZ, Maners AW, Pollack SV. Immunosuppression in patients with metastatic squamous cell carcinoma from the skin. J Dermatol Surg Oncol. 1990;16(3):271–4. https://doi.org/10.1111/j.1524-4725.1990.tb03963.x.
42. Genders RE, Osinga JAJ, Tromp EE, O'Rourke P, Bouwes Bavinck JN, Plasmeijer EI. Metastasis risk of cutaneous squamous cell carcinoma in organ transplant recipients and immunocompetent patients. Acta Derm Venereol. 2018;98(6):551–5. https://doi.org/10.2340/00015555-2901.
43. Stratigos AJ, Garbe C, Dessinioti C, et al. European interdisciplinary guideline on invasive squamous cell carcinoma of the skin: part 1. Epidemiology, diagnostics and prevention. Eur J Cancer (Oxford, England). 1990;2020(128):60–82. https://doi.org/10.1016/j.ejca.2020.01.007.
44. Work Group, Invited Reviewers, Kim JYS, et al. Guidelines of care for the management of cutaneous squamous cell carcinoma. J Am Acad Dermatol. 2018;78(3):560–78. https://doi.org/10.1016/j.jaad.2017.10.007.
45. Mittal A, Colegio OR. Skin cancers in organ transplant recipients. Am J Transplant. 2017;17(10):2509–30. https://doi.org/10.1111/ajt.14382.
46. Shao X-H, Xu Y-S, Zhang X-Q, Li W-F. Evidence based analysis of cisplatin for treating patients with cutaneous squamous cell carcinoma. Asian Pac J Cancer Prev (APJCP). 2014;15(22):9813–5. https://doi.org/10.7314/apjcp.2014.15.22.9813.
47. Migden MR, Rischin D, Schmults CD, et al. PD-1 blockade with cemiplimab in advanced cutaneous squamous-cell carcinoma. N Engl J Med. 2018;379(4):341–51. https://doi.org/10.1056/NEJMoa1805131.
48. Abdel-Wahab N, Safa H, Abudayyeh A, et al. Checkpoint inhibitor therapy for cancer in solid organ transplantation recipients: an institutional experience and a systematic review of the literature. J Immunother Cancer. 2019;7(1):106. https://doi.org/10.1186/s40425-019-0585-1.
49. Barnett R, Barta VS, Jhaveri KD. Preserved renal-allograft function and the PD-1 pathway inhibitor nivolumab. N Engl J Med. 2017;376(2):191–2. https://doi.org/10.1056/NEJMc1614298.
50. Reigneau M, Robert C, Routier E, et al. Efficacy of neoadjuvant cetuximab alone or with platinum salt for the treatment of unresectable advanced nonmetastatic cutaneous squamous cell carcinomas. Br J Dermatol. 2015;173(2):527–34. https://doi.org/10.1111/bjd.13741.
51. Leard LE, Cho BK, Jones KD, et al. Fatal diffuse alveolar damage in two lung transplant patients treated with cetuximab. J Heart Lung Transplant. 2007;26(12):1340–4. https://doi.org/10.1016/j.healun.2007.09.019.

52. Drago F, Ciccarese G, Cogorno L, Calvi C, Marsano LA, Parodi A. Prevention of non-melanoma skin cancers with nicotinamide in transplant recipients: a case-control study. Eur J Dermatol (EJD). 2017;27(4):382–5. https://doi.org/10.1684/ejd.2017.3025.
53. Hardin J, Mydlarski PR. Systemic retinoids: chemoprevention of skin cancer in transplant recipients. Skin Ther Lett. 2010;15(7):1–4.
54. Endrizzi B, Ahmed RL, Ray T, Dudek A, Lee P. Capecitabine to reduce nonmelanoma skin carcinoma burden in solid organ transplant recipients. Dermatol Surg. 2013;39(4):634–45. https://doi.org/10.1111/dsu.12049.

Basal Cell Carcinoma

Edit B. Olasz Harken and Justin Fazio

1 Introduction

Basal cell carcinoma (BCC) is the most common malignancy worldwide [1]. The risk of developing BCC is related to multiple factors, including: excessive-UV radiation, sex, age, geographic location, UV susceptibility, immunosuppression, and genetic variations [2]. In solid organ transplant recipients (SOTRs), there is a significantly increased incidence of BCC compared to the general population. BCCs present at sites of sun damaged skin and require further classification based on their histologic characteristics for appropriate management. The treatment of choice for low-risk BCC is a wide local excision with postoperative margin evaluation. Mohs micrographic surgery (MMS) is generally reserved for high-risk BCC or low-risk BCC on the head and neck. Overall, BCC has an excellent outcome if treated appropriately [3–5].

2 Epidemiology

Basal cell carcinoma (BCC) is the most common malignancy worldwide [1]. Most cancer registries do not collect data on BCC due to the overall benign nature, making the exact incidence and prevalence challenging to estimate. The American Cancer Society (ACS) estimates that 5.4 million BCCs and squamous cell carcinomas (SCCs) are diagnosed each year in approximately 3.3 million

E. B. Olasz Harken (✉) · J. Fazio
Medical College of Wisconsin, Milwaukee, WI, USA
e-mail: ebolasz@mcw.edu; jfazio@mcw.edu

J. Tomimori et al. (eds.), *Atlas of Dermatologic Diseases in Solid Organ Transplant Recipients*, https://doi.org/10.1007/978-3-031-13335-0_13

people in the United States [2]. In this group, approximately 80% of lesions are diagnosed as BCC [2]. The risk of developing BCC is related to multiple factors, including: excessive-UV radiation, sex, age, geographic location, UV susceptibility, immunosuppression, and genetic variations [3]. For white patients, the lifetime risk for developing a BCC is approximately 33–39% for men and 23–28% for women [2]. Additional studies have estimated that the lifetime risk for the development of any skin cancer is 1 in 5 with more than 97% being keratinocyte carcinoma [4].

In solid organ transplant recipients (SOTRs), there is a significantly increased incidence of both BCC and SCC, proportional to the duration and type of immunosuppressive therapy [5]. SCC is reported to occur 65–250 times more frequently compared to the general population. Similarly, BCC is reported to occur 10–20 times the rate seen in the general population [5]. Thus, the ratio of SCC to BCC is approximately 2.5–1, which is reversed compared to the general population [3].

The risk of development of keratinocyte carcinoma following solid organ transplant is largely impacted by the type of organ transplanted, the type/intensity and duration of immunosuppression, white race, pretransplant invasive skin cancer, and the age of the patient at the time of transplantation [6]. A recent study evaluating 10,198 transplant recipients noted posttransplant keratinocyte carcinoma in 16.6% of the patients after a median of 3.96 years [6]. The highest 10-year cumulative incidence was in the subset of patients with a history of pretransplant skin cancer (66.5%), older than 50 years at the time of transplant (27.5% for 51–65 years; 40.5% for >65 years), and of the white race (24.1%) [6].

Although SOTRs are at significantly increased risk for the development of keratinocyte carcinoma, the incidence in this population seems to be declining. A study of 3580 SOTRs transplanted between 1994 and 2012 noted the overall standardized incidence ratios (SIRs) for SCC and BCC were 19.7 and 7.0, respectively [7]. There was a progressive fall in the SIRs for SCC and BCC from peak SIRs (95% confidence intervals) in 1994–1996 of 26.4 (21.5–32.4) and 9.1 (7.4–11.3) to 6.3 (2.3–16.7) and 3.2 (1.4–7.1) in 2012–2014, respectively [7]. Importantly, the SCC to BCC ratio was maintained, demonstrating that both are declining equally [7]. The declining incidence is likely related to improved immunosuppressive protocols and underscores the important role immunosuppressive treatments play in the pathogenesis of keratinocyte carcinoma.

Immunosuppression following solid organ transplant increases patient susceptibility to UV-induced DNA damage and promotes mutagenic changes [8]. Patients with heart and lung transplants require the most immunosuppression, followed by kidney, and liver transplants requiring the least amount of immunosuppression [3]. Compared with kidney transplant recipients, lung transplant recipients have an increased rate of keratinocyte carcinoma, whereas liver transplant are associated with a reduced rate [6]. Additionally, BCCs are noted to occur earlier and more frequently in heart and lung transplant recipients compared to other SOTRs. A study of 176 cases of BCC following solid organ transplant noted the average time to diagnosis was 6.9 years, with earlier diagnosis noted in heart transplant patients compared to kidney transplant [9]. Lastly, a retrospective cohort study evaluated the risk of skin cancer associated with different immunosuppressive treatment regimens [10]. One hundred and eighty-two SOTRs were followed for 1000 person-years and the results showed skin cancer developed in patients exposed to higher cumulative doses of cyclosporine, azathioprine, prednisone, and mycophenolate mofetil.

3 Pathogenesis

BCC development is due to mutations in several key tumor suppressors and proto-oncogenes [11]. Intermittent and intense UV exposure is associated with overactivation of the Hedgehog signaling pathway and mutagenesis of protein patched homolog 1 (PTCH1) and tumor protein 53 (TP53) genes [11]. The Hedgehog signaling pathway normally functions in tissue development by activating genes through the signaling pathway, utilizing the Patched cell surface receptor, Smoothened cell surface protein, and glioma-associated oncogene (GLI) intracellular signaling protein [11]. When Patched is not bound to hedgehog ligand, smoothened is inactive and no cell signaling occurs. Inactivating mutations in PTCH1 leads to a dysfunctional Patched receptor and constitutively active smoothened at the cell surface. This leads to further downstream activation of GLI and turning on multiple targeted genes in the nucleus [11]. Additionally, TP53, a gene coding the p53 protein of the cell cycle, is the second most common mutations seen in BCC [11].

4 Clinical Presentation

BCCs present at sites of sun damaged skin and are classically described as an enlarging, pink, shiny, ulcerated, non-healing, papules that bleeds intermittently [12]. The histologic patterns of BCC include nodular BCC (nBCC), superficial BCC (sBCC), morpheaform BCC, fibroepithelial BCC, infiltrative BCC, infundibulocystic BCC, and basosquamous BCC [12]. Majority of BCCs will have a single histologic pattern; however, studies have shown that up to 40% of lesions will display greater than one histologic pattern [13].

nBCC is the most common subtype, making up ~80% of lesions biopsied [14]. The prototypical nBCC is located on the head and neck and described as a shiny, pearly, papule or nodule, with a smooth surface, rolled borders, and arborizing vessels (Figs. 1, 2, 3, and 4) [15–17]. Typically, nBCCs are indolent and grow slowly

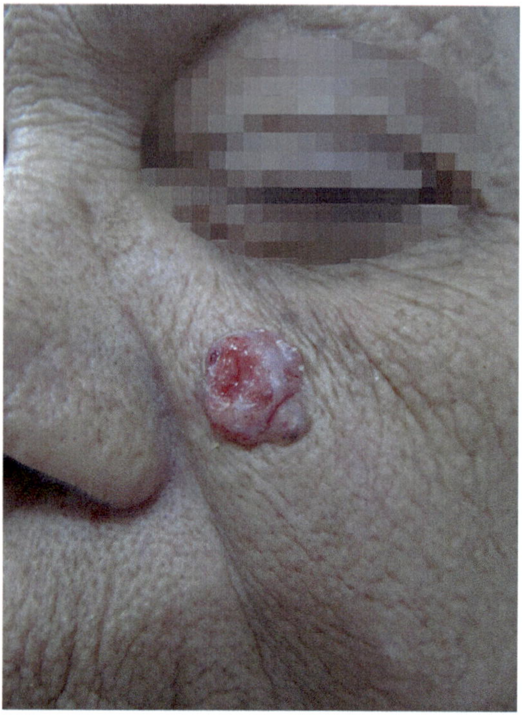

Fig. 1 Left malar cheek nodular BCC
Female, 61-year-old, kidney transplant (7 years), deceased donor, hypertension

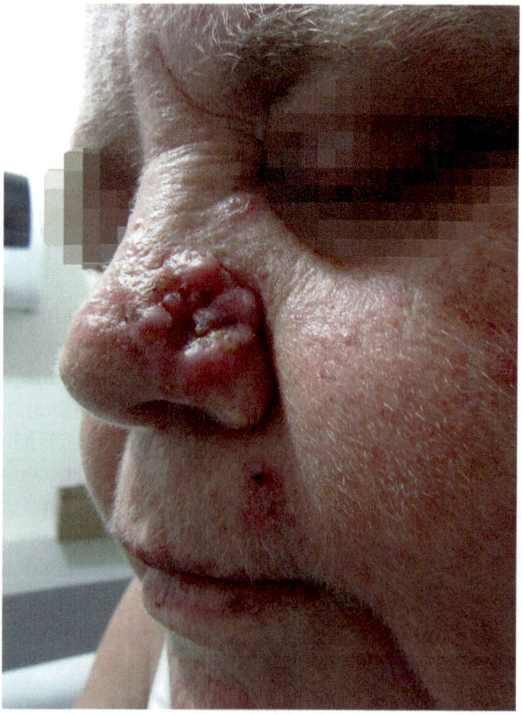

Fig. 2 Multiple nodular and superficial BCCs
Female, 60-year-old, kidney transplant (12 years), living donor (brother), hypertension

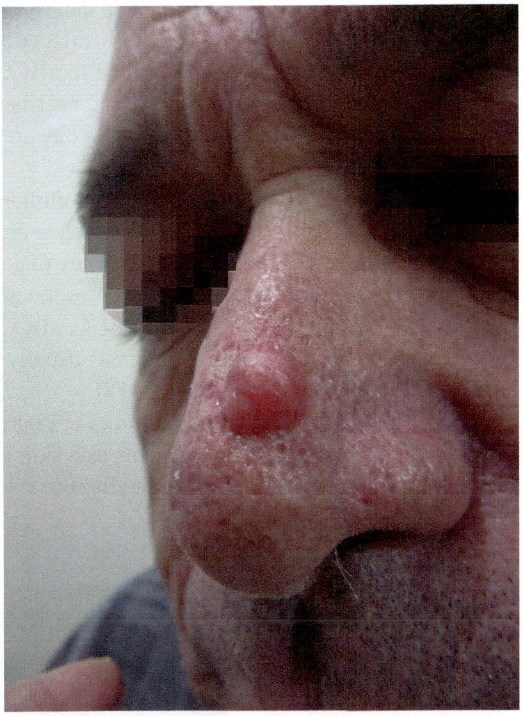

Fig. 3 Nodular BCC
Male, 56-year-old, kidney transplant (1 year), deceased donor, hypertension

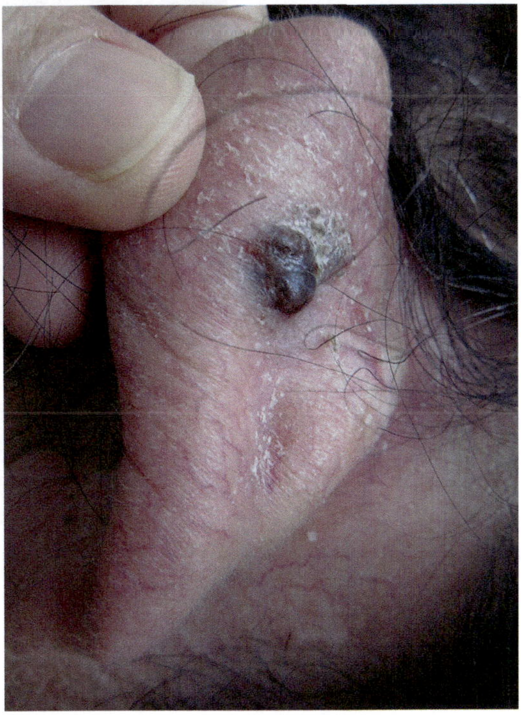

Fig. 4 Left ear pigmented nodular BCC
Male, 70-year-old, kidney transplant (15 years), deceased donor, hypertension

over multiple years, with rare cases of metastasis [12]. The morbidity associated with neglected nBCC is destruction of local anatomic structures. Another variant of BCC that can appear clinically identical to nBCC is the infundibulocystic subtype (Fig. 5) [12]. These tumors are well-circumscribed, pink, pearly papules or nodules on the head and neck of elderly patients. They are differentiated from nBCCs based on their distinct histologic characteristics.

Superficial BCCs are the second most common subtype of BCC and present as a well-circumscribed, erythematous, thin plaque or patch with scale, central clearing, and rolled borders (Figs. 6 and 7) [17]. They make up approximately 10–30% of all BCCs diagnosed, with an earlier age of onset, and occurring more often in females than males [12, 14, 18, 19]. Unlike nBCC, sBCCs are most seen on the trunk and extremities and the differential diagnosis usually includes inflammatory lesions or squamous cell carcinoma in situ [12, 14].

Fibroepithelial BCC (fibroepithelioma of Pinkus) is another less common variant of BCC that characteristically presents as a skin colored to pink pedunculated papule on the central lower back. Clinically, these lesions can resemble an acrochordon [20].

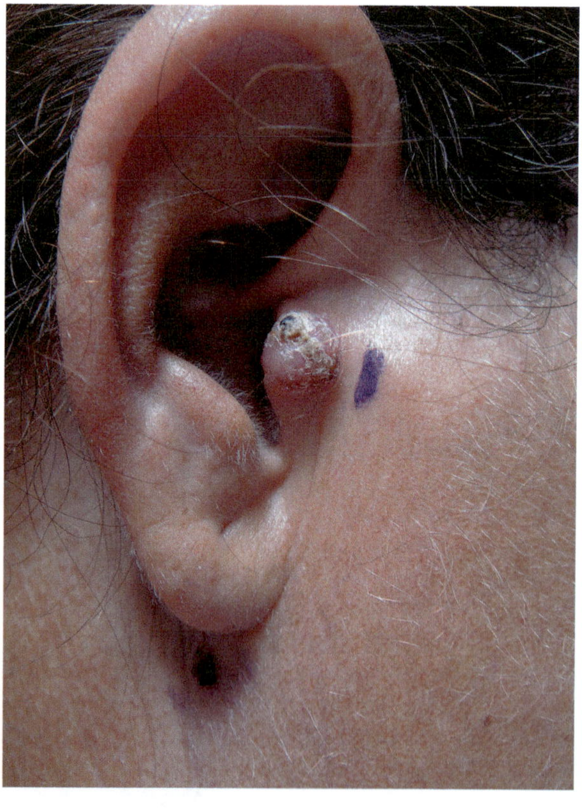

Fig. 5 Right ear infundibulocystic BCC Female, 50-year-old, kidney transplant

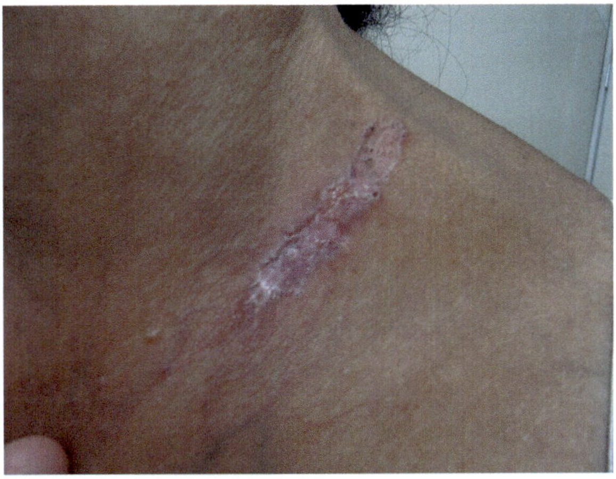

Fig. 6 Left neck superficial BCC Female, 54-year-old, kidney transplant (12 years), deceased donor, hypertension

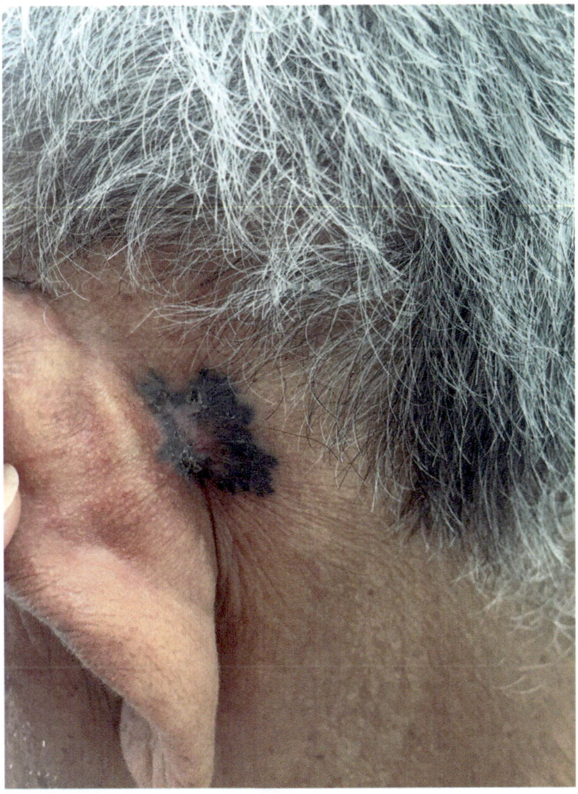

Fig. 7 BCC superficial and pigmented left ear Male, 74-year-old, kidney transplant (2 years), deceased donor, hypertension

Morpheaform BCC are different from the other subtypes in that they have infiltrative growth patterns, subclinical extension, and higher rates of local recurrence [17, 20]. They present as a firm, shiny, scar like, white to pink plaque with poorly defined borders on sun exposed sites [17]. Although considered biologically aggressive based on the infiltrative features seen in histology, they have excellent outcomes with appropriate treatment.

Micronodular BCC is an infiltrative histologic subtype of BCC that clinically appears identical to nBCC [12]. They often occur in combination with other histologic variants of BCC and comprise approximately 13% of all BCC diagnosed [13].

Basosquamous carcinoma, also called metatypical carcinoma, makes up less than 2% of all BCCs diagnosed. These tumors are clinically identical to nBCC but are biologically aggressive. Perineural invasion, higher rates of recurrence, and cases of metastasis are all noted in basosquamous carcinoma [21].

5 Histology

BCCs appear clinically similar and require further classification based on their histologic characteristics for appropriate management. The histologic patterns of BCC include nodular BCC, superficial BCC, micronodular BCC, morpheaform BCC, fibroepithelial BCC, infiltrative BCC, infundibulocystic BCC, and basosquamous [12].

nBCC is characterized by a basophilic rounded nests in the dermis with prominent peripheral palisading, mucinous retraction, and myxoid stroma around the neoplasm (Figs. 8 and 9) [13]. In cases of superficial BCC, there are one or more tumor foci that extend from the epidermis or adnexae and impinge on or enter the papillary dermis [13]. A band-like lichenoid infiltrate can be seen in addition to peripheral palisading and mucinous retraction [12]. Micronodular BCC is an infiltrative pattern that is characterized by small rounded basaloid nodules in the dermis with less

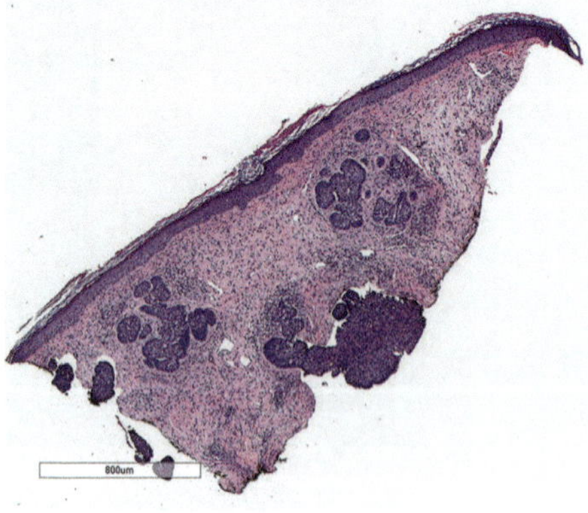

Fig. 8 Nodular BCC Characterized by basophilic rounded nests in the dermis with prominent peripheral palisading, mucinous retraction, and myxoid stroma around the neoplasm

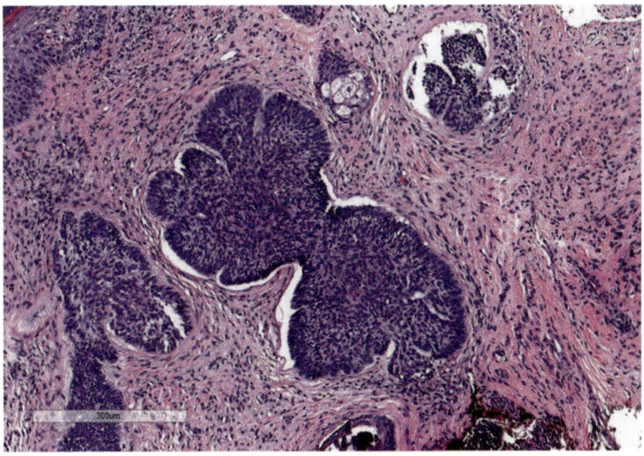

Fig. 9 Nodular BCC Characterized by prominent peripheral palisading, mucinous retraction, and myxoid stroma around the neoplasm

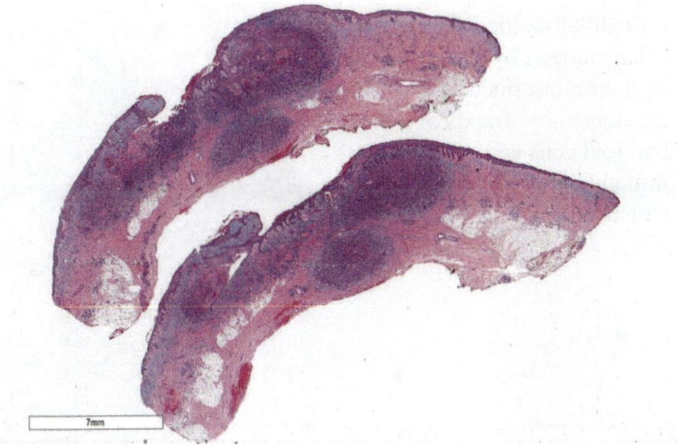

Fig. 10 Micronodular BCC Characterized by infiltrative pattern that is characterized by small rounded basaloid nodules in the dermis with less apparent peripheral palisading and retraction artifact compared to nodular BCC

apparent peripheral palisading and retraction artifact compared to nodular BCC (Fig. 10) [13]. The surrounding stroma is more collagenous compared to the characteristic myxoid stroma of nodular BCC [13]. Fibroepithelial BCCs are characterized by multiple trabecular, elongated, and branched thin strands of basaloid cells extending from the epidermis into the dermis (Fig. 11) [22]. The surrounding stroma is usually a dense spindle cell [12].

Infundibulocystic BCCs are characterized by well-circumscribed, anastomosing strands of basaloid cells and scattered infundibulum-like cystic structures (Fig. 12) [12].

Morpheaform BCCs consist of multiple small basaloid tumor islands in the dermis with sharp and angulated ends (Fig. 13) [13]. The tumor islands infiltrate into the dermis as narrow stands or cords of cells [13]. Peripheral palisading and retraction are not seen as readily compared to nodular BCCs [13]. The accompanying sclerotic stroma is a helpful identifying histologic characteristic but is not necessary for the diagnosis [13].

Infiltrative BCCs are characterized by basaloid tumor islands of varying sizes that closely resemble the morpheaform classification; however, infiltrative BCCs

Fig. 11
Fibroepithelial BCC
Characterized by multiple trabecular, elongated, and branched thin strands of basaloid cells extending from the epidermis into the dermis

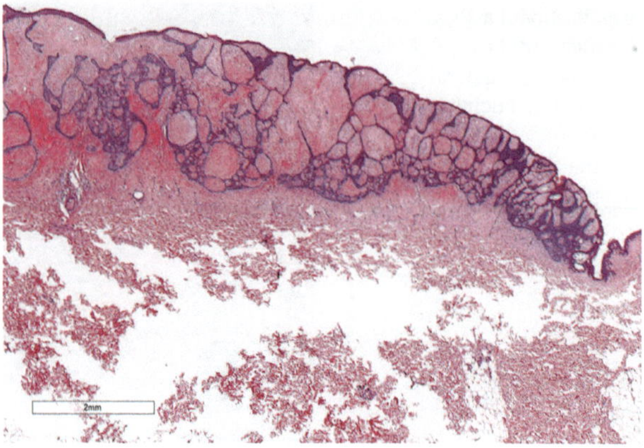

Fig. 12
Infundibulocystic BCC
Characterized by well-circumscribed, anastomosing strands of basaloid cells and scattered infundibulum-like cystic structures

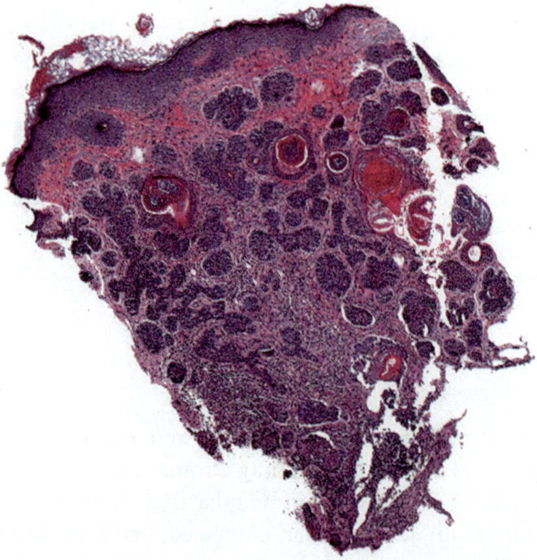

Fig. 13
Morpheaform BCC
Characterized by multiple small basaloid tumor islands in the dermis with sharp and angulated ends

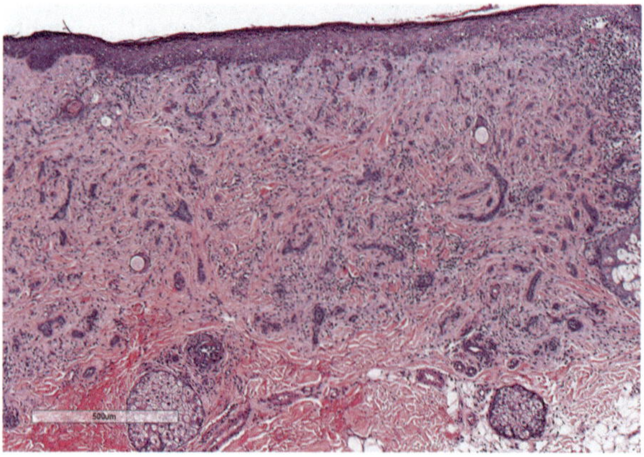

are defined by their irregular, jagged, and spiked configuration of their peripheral border, with limited retraction, and palisading. The tumor stroma is more collagenous compared to the classic myxoid stroma seen in nodular BCC [13].

Basosquamous or metatypical BCC are rare tumors with both basaloid and squamoid cells. Typically, there are areas of basaloid cells that are larger, paler, and rounder than nodular BCC combined with areas of eosinophilic squamoid cells with a transition zone [23]. Peripheral palisading and stromal retraction are both uncommon [23].

Histologically, there are areas of BCC with typical basaloid cells that are larger, paler, and rounder than solid BCC, and areas of SCC with squamoid cells that have abundant eosinophilic cytoplasm. A transition zone with intermediate cells is evident between the area of BCC and SCC tumor cells. Peripheral palisading is rare and there is minimal stromal retraction.

6 Treatment

A punch or shave skin biopsy is the standard of care for diagnosing BCC [12]. Both approaches have been evaluated and have similar diagnostic accuracy, approximately 80%; however, some studies have reported an overall concordance between the BCC subtype identified in the biopsy specimen and the subsequent excision as low as 54% [24]. Dermoscopy improves diagnostic accuracy and may aid the clinician in determining BCC subtype prior to the skin biopsy [7].

BCC has an excellent outcome if treated appropriately. The morbidity associated with poorly treated or neglected BCCs is destruction of local anatomic structures and metastasis on rare occasions. BCC is classified as low or high risk based on patient and tumor factors per the National Comprehensive Cancer Network (NCCN) guidelines [25]. Factors for the clinician to consider when choosing treatment options include immunosuppression status, primary or recurrent tumor, previous radiation at the site of the tumor, size of the tumor, anatomic location, tumor borders, histological subtype, and perineural involvement [25]. For low-risk BCC, the treatment of choice is a wide local excision with postoperative margin evaluation [12]. The NCCN recommends a 4-mm clinical margin when performing a wide local excision [25]. The margin recommendations given by the NCCN are based on data from a 2010 meta-analysis, which evaluated 16,066 low-risk nodular BCCs treated with surgical excision and found the recurrence rates for BCCs excised with 5, 4, 3, and 2 mm surgical margins were 0.4%, 1.6%, 2.6%, and 4%, respectively [26].

Mohs micrographic surgery (MMS) is generally reserved for high-risk BCC or low-risk BCC on the head and neck. This surgical technique provides complete margin evaluation, with the lowest rates of recurrence for BCC, and optimum cosmetic outcomes [12]. A randomized control trial compared wide local excision (WLE) to MMS for the treatment of 408 primary facial BCCs and 204 recurrent facial BCCs. MMS had lower rates of recurrence for both the primary and recurrent tumor groups [27]. Importantly, an extended 10-year follow-up showed that recurrent tumors had a 11.5% recurrence rate compared to 3.9% recurrence rate for WLE and MMS, respectively [28].

For nonsurgical candidates other treatment options include: electrodessication and curettage (ED&C), topical chemotherapy, intralesional chemotherapy, photodynamic therapy (PDT), radiation therapy, and systemic targeted therapy [12].

Electrodessication and curettage (ED&C) is an appropriate treatment option of low-risk BCC. Many clinicians prefer ED&C treatment because it is convenient for patients, but the recurrence rates are approximately 5–9% and have been reported as high as 25% in high-risk BCC [25]. ED&C is limited by the experience of the clinician performing the procedure and potential for mixed histology not observed in the sample biopsy. If the clinician enters the subcutaneous fat during the curettage, the procedure should be converted to a WLE to ensure complete tumor extirpation [12].

Topical 5-fluorouracil 5% (5-FU) and imiquimod 5% cream are FDA approved as appropriate treatment options for low-risk sBCCs. Imiquimod 5% cream activates the adaptive and innate immune system, causing tumor infiltration by inflammatory cells and apoptosis [12]. There is a theoretical risk that imiquimod can induce a systemic immunostimulation, thereby jeopardizing the viability of a transplanted organ. Overall, studies using imiquimod up to 100 cm^2 of area are rather reassuring since to date neither clinically relevant systemic alterations of immune function nor adverse effects on transplanted organs have been reported [29]. For BCC, it is applied once daily five or seven times per week for 6 weeks and is reported to have 5-year clearance rates of 77.9% and 80.4% [12, 30, 31]. 5-FU inhibits DNA synthesis and cell proliferation causing tumor necrosis [12]. It is applied twice daily for 6 weeks and has similar efficacy to imiquimod 5% cream for treating sBCCs [32]. Data from extended follow-up may point towards imiquimod 5% cream being a superior treatment [33]. A study with 3-year follow-up showed a clearance rate of 79.7% and 68.2% for imiquimod 5% cream and 5-FU, respectively [33]. The challenges with topical treatment are failure of treatment completion due to associated irritation and discomfort or perceived resolution of the skin cancer with subclinical spread. Tumors that recur after topical treatment are often more aggressive and challenging to treat given their discontinuous nature [34].

PDT is a commonly used treatment for actinic keratoses but is not FDA approved for the treatment of sBCC. The procedure involves applying a topical photosensitizer (methyl aminolevulinate or 5-aminolevulinic acid), allowing for a 1–3 h incubation period, completed with irradiation with a red or blue light [35]. A meta-analysis looking at 1383 BCCs noted complete clearance of 86.4% and 98.2% of tumors treated with PDT and WLE, respectively [36]. PDT is a reasonable treatment option for low-risk BCC and is commonly used for field treatment in SOTRs with heavy tumor burden.

Primary radiotherapy (RT) is considered in patients wanting to avoid surgery or non-surgical candidates. Recurrence rates of BCC are higher following treatment with RT compared to WLE. A randomized controlled trial compared BCCs treated with WLE vs RT with noted recurrence rates of 0.7% and 7.5% at 4 years after treatment for WLE and RT, respectively [37].

Systemic treatment is considered in patients with BCC that metastasized beyond the regional lymph node basin or are not candidates for surgery or RT [12]. Vismodegib and sonidegib are oral medications that target the hedgehog pathway and are approved by the FDA for the treatment of metastatic or locally advanced BCC [38]. These medications have response rates that are less than 50%, with a duration of 7–9 months, and poor side effect profile [12].

In 2021, the Food and Drug Administration granted regular approval to cemiplimab-rwlc for patients with locally advanced basal cell carcinoma (laBCC) previously treated with a hedgehog pathway inhibitor (HHI) or for whom a HHI is not appropriate and granted accelerated approval to cemiplimab-rwlc for patients with metastatic BCC (mBCC) previously treated with a HHI or for whom a HHI is not appropriate. Immune checkpoint inhibitors need to be used with extreme caution in SOTR due to the high allograft rejection rate. A systematic review of the safety of immune checkpoint inhibitors in SOTR showed that allograft rejection occurred in 41% of patients (11/23 renal, 4/11 hepatic, and 1/5 cardiac transplantations), at similar rates for anti-CTLA-4 and anti-PD-1 therapy. The median time to rejection was 21 days (95% confidence interval 19.3–22.8 days). Overall, 31% of patients permanently discontinued CPIs because of allograft rejection. Graft loss occurred in 81%, and death was reported in 46% [39].

6.1 Chemoprevention in SOTR

The chemotherapeutic drug capecitabine has been used off label as a chemopreventive modality to suppress the development of precancerous skin lesions and squamous cell carcinomas (SCCs) [40]. In the authors unpublished study of ten renal and kidney transplant patients, using low-dose capecitabine reduced the number of new SCCs while it had no effect on the number of new BCCs. The authors hypothesize that the lack of response may be due to decreased expression of thymidine phosphorylase in BCC compared to SCC. However, a 15-patient case series documented a significant reduction in BCC incidence rates when using capecitabine chemoprevention, from a mean (SD) of 0.06 (0.09) BCCs per month before capecitabine to 0.02 (0.05) during treatment [41].

6.2 Reduction of Immunosuppression

Although evidence supports the efficacy of reducing immunosuppression for transplant-associated skin cancer [42], to the authors' knowledge the effect of reduction of immunosuppression has not been specifically studied for BCCs in SOTR.

References

1. Miller SJ. Etiology and pathogenesis of basal cell carcinoma. Clin Dermatol. 1995;13(6):527–36.
2. Basal and Squamous Cell Skin Cancer Statistics. cancer.org. 2021. Available from https://www.cancer.org/cancer/basal-and-squamous-cell-skin-cancer/about/key-statistics.html.
3. Madeleine MM, Patel NS, Plasmeijer EI, Engels EA, Bouwes Bavinck JN, Toland AE, et al. Epidemiology of keratinocyte carcinomas after organ transplantation. Br J Dermatol. 2017;177(5):1208–16.
4. Rigel DS, Friedman RJ, Kopf AW. Lifetime risk for development of skin cancer in the U.S. population: current estimate is now 1 in 5. J Am Acad Dermatol. 1996;35(6):1012–3.
5. Euvrard S, Kanitakis J, Claudy A. Skin cancers after organ transplantation. N Engl J Med. 2003;348(17):1681–91.
6. Park CK, Fung K, Austin PC, Kim SJ, Singer LG, Baxter NN, et al. Incidence and risk factors of keratinocyte carcinoma after first solid organ transplant in Ontario, Canada. JAMA Dermatol. 2019;155(9):1041–8.
7. Menzies S, O'Leary E, Callaghan G, Galligan M, Deady S, Gadallah B, et al. Declining incidence of keratinocyte carcinoma in organ transplant recipients. Br J Dermatol. 2019;181(5):983–91.
8. Krynitz B, Edgren G, Lindelof B, Baecklund E, Brattstrom C, Wilczek H, et al. Risk of skin cancer and other malignancies in kidney, liver, heart and lung transplant recipients 1970 to 2008—a Swedish population-based study. Int J Cancer. 2013;132(6):1429–38.
9. Kanitakis J, Alhaj-Ibrahim L, Euvrard S, Claudy A. Basal cell carcinomas developing in solid organ transplant recipients: clinicopathologic study of 176 cases. Arch Dermatol. 2003;139(9):1133–7.
10. Colegio OR, Billingsley EM. Skin cancer in transplant recipients, out of the woods. Scientific retreat of the ITSCC and SCOPE. Am J Transplant. 2011;11(8):1584–91.
11. Bustami RT, Ojo AO, Wolfe RA, Merion RM, Bennett WM, McDiarmid SV, et al. Immunosuppression and the risk of post-transplant malignancy among cadaveric first kidney transplant recipients. Am J Transplant. 2004;4(1):87–93.
12. Cameron MC, Lee E, Hibler BP, Giordano CN, Barker CA, Mori S, et al. Basal cell carcinoma: contemporary approaches to diagnosis, treatment, and prevention. J Am Acad Dermatol. 2019;80(2):321–39.
13. Sexton M, Jones DB, Maloney ME. Histologic pattern analysis of basal cell carcinoma. Study of a series of 1039 consecutive neoplasms. J Am Acad Dermatol. 1990;23(6 Pt 1):1118–26.
14. Scrivener Y, Grosshans E, Cribier B. Variations of basal cell carcinomas according to gender, age, location and histopathological subtype. Br J Dermatol. 2002;147(1):41–7.
15. Pinkus H. Premalignant fibroepithelial tumors of skin. AMA Arch Derm Syphilol. 1953;67(6):598–615.
16. de Eusebio E, Sanchez Yus E, Lopez Bran E, Rojo S, Rueda M, del Cerro M. Infundibulocystic basaloid neoplasm. J Cutan Pathol. 1996;23(2):147–50.
17. Sloane JP. The value of typing basal cell carcinomas in predicting recurrence after surgical excision. Br J Dermatol. 1977;96(2):127–32.
18. Betti R, Inselvini E, Carducci M, Crosti C. Age and site prevalence of histologic subtypes of basal cell carcinomas. Int J Dermatol. 1995;34(3):174–6.
19. Bastiaens MT, Hoefnagel JJ, Bruijn JA, Westendorp RG, Vermeer BJ, Bouwes Bavinck JN. Differences in age, site distribution, and sex between nodular and superficial basal cell carcinoma indicate different types of tumors. J Invest Dermatol. 1998;110(6):880–4.
20. Litzow TJ, Perry HO, Soderstrom CW. Morpheaform basal cell carcinoma. Am J Surg. 1968;116(4):499–505.
21. Costantino D, Lowe L, Brown DL. Basosquamous carcinoma-an under-recognized, high-risk cutaneous neoplasm: case study and review of the literature. J Plast Reconstr Aesthet Surg. 2006;59(4):424–8.

22. Dourmishev LA, Rusinova D, Botev I. Clinical variants, stages, and management of basal cell carcinoma. Indian Dermatol Online J. 2013;4(1):12–7.
23. Leibovitch I, Huilgol SC, Selva D, Richards S, Paver R. Basosquamous carcinoma: treatment with Mohs micrographic surgery. Cancer. 2005;104(1):170–5.
24. Sun MT, Wu A, Huilgol SC, Selva D. Accuracy of biopsy in subtyping periocular basal cell carcinoma. Ophthalmic Plast Reconstr Surg. 2015;31(6):449–51.
25. NCCN Clinical Practice Guidelines in Oncology, Basal Cell Skin Cancer. 2021.
26. Gulleth Y, Goldberg N, Silverman RP, Gastman BR. What is the best surgical margin for a Basal cell carcinoma: a meta-analysis of the literature. Plast Reconstr Surg. 2010;126(4):1222–31.
27. Smeets NW, Krekels GA, Ostertag JU, Essers BA, Dirksen CD, Nieman FH, et al. Surgical excision vs Mohs' micrographic surgery for basal-cell carcinoma of the face: randomised controlled trial. Lancet. 2004;364(9447):1766–72.
28. van Loo E, Mosterd K, Krekels GA, Roozeboom MH, Ostertag JU, Dirksen CD, et al. Surgical excision versus Mohs' micrographic surgery for basal cell carcinoma of the face: a randomised clinical trial with 10 year follow-up. Eur J Cancer. 2014;50(17):3011–20.
29. Trakatelli M, Katsanos G, Ulrich C, Kalabalikis D, Sotiriadis D, Stockfleth E. Efforts to counteract locally the effects of systemic immunosuppression: a review on the use of imiquimod, a topical immunostimulator in organ transplant recipients. Int J Immunopathol Pharmacol. 2010;23(2):387–96.
30. Gollnick H, Barona CG, Frank RG, Ruzicka T, Megahed M, Maus J, et al. Recurrence rate of superficial basal cell carcinoma following treatment with imiquimod 5% cream: conclusion of a 5-year long-term follow-up study in Europe. Eur J Dermatol. 2008;18(6):677–82.
31. Quirk C, Gebauer K, De'Ambrosis B, Slade HB, Meng TC. Sustained clearance of superficial basal cell carcinomas treated with imiquimod cream 5%: results of a prospective 5-year study. Cutis. 2010;85(6):318–24.
32. Arits AH, Mosterd K, Essers BA, Spoorenberg E, Sommer A, De Rooij MJ, et al. Photodynamic therapy versus topical imiquimod versus topical fluorouracil for treatment of superficial basal-cell carcinoma: a single blind, non-inferiority, randomised controlled trial. Lancet Oncol. 2013;14(7):647–54.
33. Roozeboom MH, Arits A, Mosterd K, Sommer A, Essers BAB, de Rooij MJM, et al. Three-year follow-up results of photodynamic therapy vs. imiquimod vs. fluorouracil for treatment of superficial basal cell carcinoma: a single-blind, noninferiority, randomized controlled trial. J Invest Dermatol. 2016;136(8):1568–74.
34. van Delft LCJ, Nelemans PJ, Jansen MHE, Arits A, Roozeboom MH, Hamid MA, et al. Histologic subtype of treatment failures after noninvasive therapy for superficial basal cell carcinoma: an observational study. J Am Acad Dermatol. 2019;80(4):1022–8.
35. Hasan T, Ortel B, Solban N, Pogue B. Photodynamic therapy of cancer. Cancer Med. 2003;7:537–48.
36. Wang H, Xu Y, Shi J, Gao X, Geng L. Photodynamic therapy in the treatment of basal cell carcinoma: a systematic review and meta-analysis. Photodermatol Photoimmunol Photomed. 2015;31(1):44–53.
37. Avril MF, Auperin A, Margulis A, Gerbaulet A, Duvillard P, Benhamou E, et al. Basal cell carcinoma of the face: surgery or radiotherapy? Results of a randomized study. Br J Cancer. 1997;76(1):100–6.
38. Wahid M, Jawed A, Mandal RK, Dar SA, Khan S, Akhter N, et al. Vismodegib, itraconazole and sonidegib as hedgehog pathway inhibitors and their relative competencies in the treatment of basal cell carcinomas. Crit Rev Oncol Hematol. 2016;98:235–41.
39. Abdel-Wahab N, Safa H, Abudayyeh A, Johnson DH, Trinh VA, Zobniw CM, et al. Checkpoint inhibitor therapy for cancer in solid organ transplantation recipients: an institutional experience and a systematic review of the literature. J Immunother Cancer. 2019;7(1):106.

40. Schauder DM, Kim J, Nijhawan RI. Evaluation of the use of capecitabine for the treatment and prevention of actinic keratoses, squamous cell carcinoma, and basal cell carcinoma: a systematic review. JAMA Dermatol. 2020;156(10):1117–24.
41. Jirakulaporn T, Endrizzi B, Lindgren B, Mathew J, Lee PK, Dudek AZ. Capecitabine for skin cancer prevention in solid organ transplant recipients. Clin Transpl. 2011;25(4):541–8.
42. Otley CC, Griffin MD, Charlton MR, Edwards BS, Neuburg M, Stasko T, et al. Reduction of immunosuppression for transplant-associated skin cancer: thresholds and risks. Br J Dermatol. 2007;157(6):1183–8.

Melanoma

Alexandra Geusau and Julia Maria Ressler

1 Introduction

Long-term immunosuppression (IS) in solid organ transplant recipients (SOTR) increases the risk not only of keratinocyte carcinomas (KC) but also of developing melanoma [1]. The risk of developing a melanoma in SOTR is 2–8 times higher than in the general population [2, 3]. There are three clinical scenarios of concern for transplant patients. The first—theoretical issue—is the development of melanoma as a result of transmission from the organ donor, as a potential donor with the history of melanoma is out of question; generally, current or recent malignancy is a contraindication to organ donation because of the risk of transmission. The second scenario is a melanoma in the patient's medical history—it may be grounds for exclusion from a transplant listing. And the third clinical scenario is a de novo development of melanoma after transplantation [4]. In making clinical decisions for patients with each scenario, a basic understanding of the pathogenesis of melanoma, with its prognostic variables, treatment outcomes, and survival in the general population as well as the transplant population is required.

The incidence of the melanoma in the general population is increasing and varies by geographic location, with an incidence of 22.7/100,000 in the USA [5]. Melanoma is a very aggressive type of cancer and responsible for almost 90% of the morbidity of all skin cancers and can vary by its clinical presentation. The cutaneous melanoma makes up to 90% of all melanomas, the most relevant subtypes are the lentigo maligna melanoma, the superficial spreading melanoma, the nodular melanoma, and the acral lentiginous melanoma. A collection of clinical and dermoscopy images of different melanoma subtypes is presented in Figs. 1, 2, 3, 4, 5, 6, 7, and 8a, b. The

A. Geusau (✉) · J. M. Ressler
Department of Dermatology, Medical University of Vienna, Vienna, Austria
e-mail: Alexandra.geusau@meduniwien.ac.at; julia.ressler@meduniwien.ac.at

J. Tomimori et al. (eds.), *Atlas of Dermatologic Diseases in Solid Organ Transplant Recipients*, https://doi.org/10.1007/978-3-031-13335-0_14

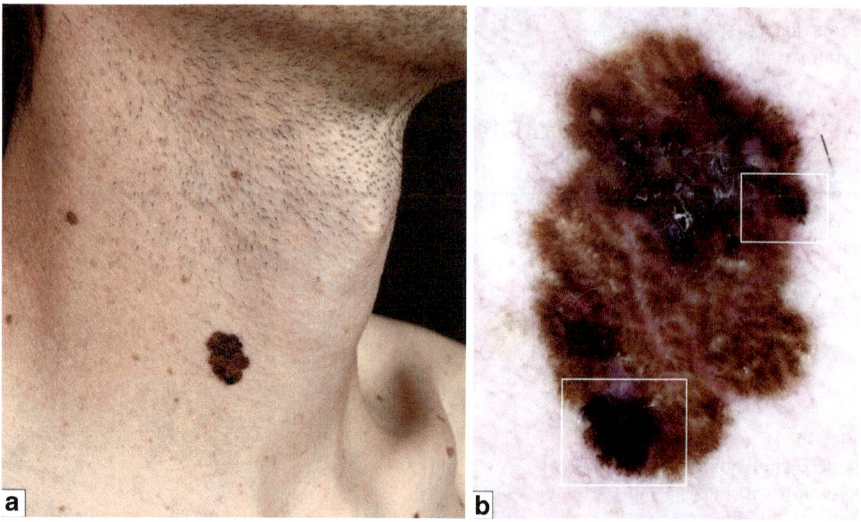

Fig. 1 (**a**) Primary superficial spreading melanoma (SSM) on the neck; (**b**) dermoscopy, pseudopods are located on the periphery. (*Image courtesy of the Department of Dermatology, Medical University of Vienna*)

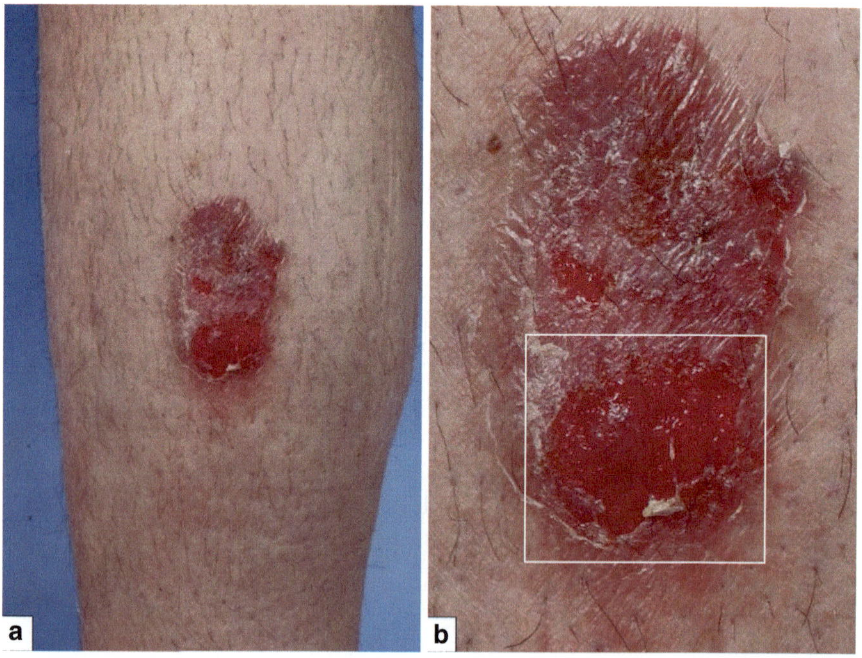

Fig. 2 (**a**) Amelanotic malignant melanoma (AMM) on the right leg; (**b**) close up, AMM with a nodular and a flat portion with an ulceration on the caudal part. (*Image courtesy of the Department of Dermatology, Medical University of Vienna*)

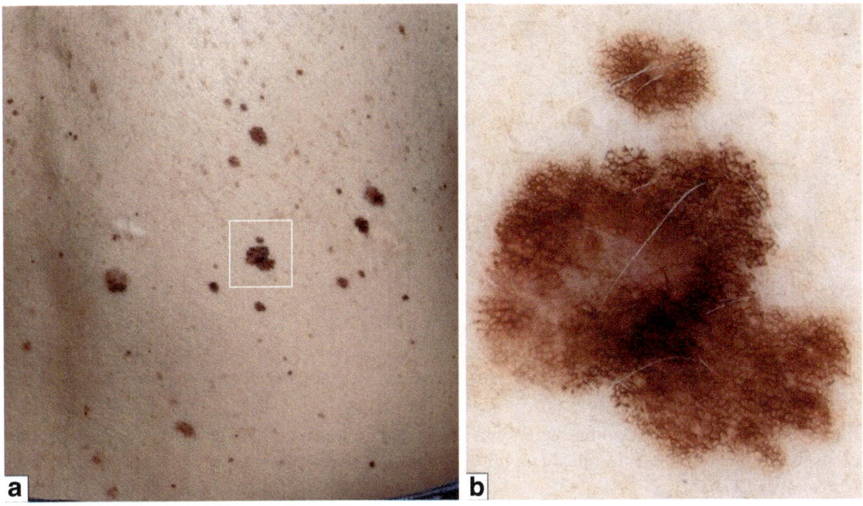

Fig. 3 (**a**) Patient with multiple nevi and one SSM in the right infrascapular region; (**b**) dermoscopy, pseudopods are located on the periphery. (*Image courtesy of the Department of Dermatology, Medical University of Vienna*)

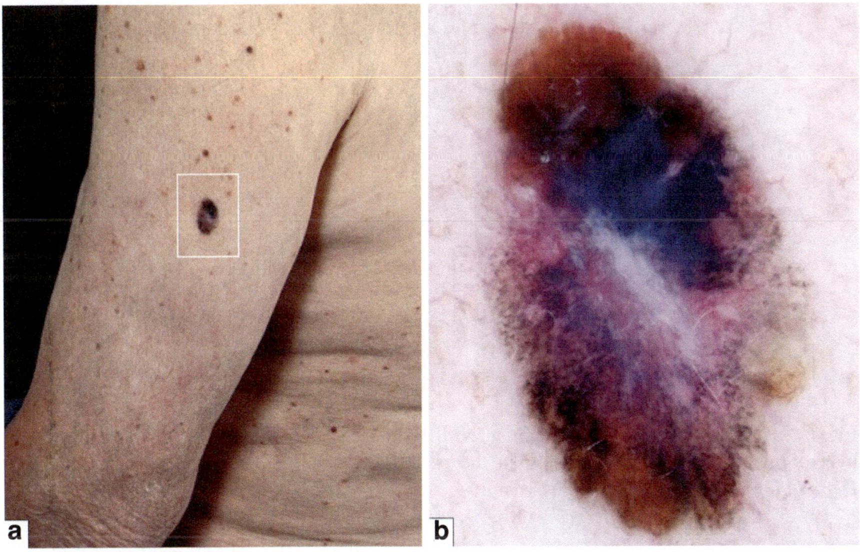

Fig. 4 (**a**) Nodular malignant melanoma (NMM) on the left upper arm; (**b**) dermoscopy, more than one colour, white lines, structureless eccentric area. (*Image courtesy of the Department of Dermatology, Medical University of Vienna*)

rest are the uveal, the mucosal melanoma and the rarely occurring melanoma of inner organs and central nervous system. Diagnosis is based on histopathologic criteria: the Breslow Index (BI) (mm), Clark Level (I–V), ulceration, and mitotic rate

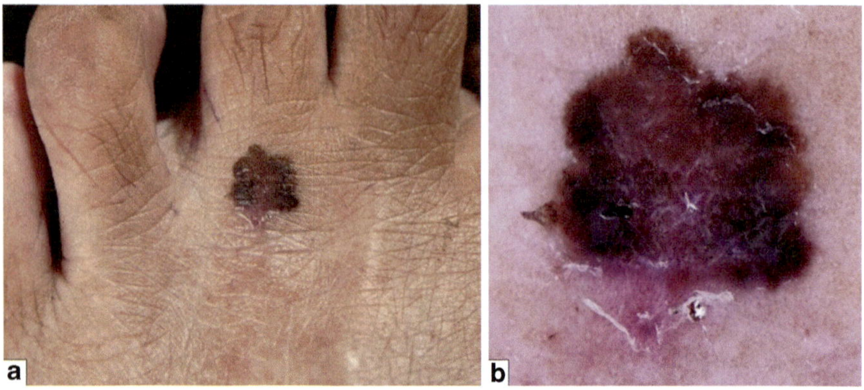

Fig. 5 (**a**) Superficial spreading melanoma (SSM) on the right arch of the foot; (**b**) dermoscopy, more than one colour, white lines. (*Image courtesy of the Department of Dermatology, Medical University of Vienna*)

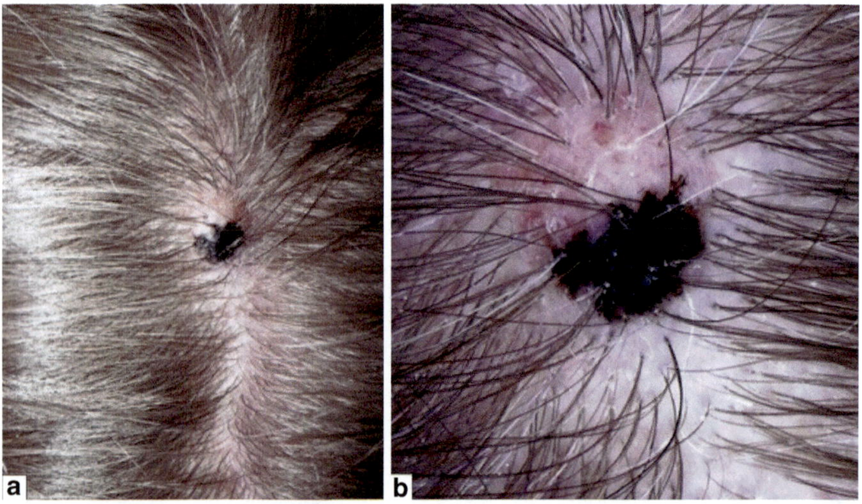

Fig. 6 (**a**) Nodular malignant melanoma (NMM) on the scalp; (**b**) dermoscopy, eccentric black hyperpigmentation with pseudopods on the periphery. (*Image courtesy of the Department of Dermatology, Medical University of Vienna*)

[6]. Melanoma is considered a highly immunogenic tumour, characterized by the development of early metastasis with lymphatic and/or haematogenous spread. According to the American Joint Committee of Cancer (AJCC) Version 8.0, melanoma is classified in four tumour stages. The prognosis depends on the tumour stage [7]. Long-term IS in case of SOTR—necessary for the maintenance of the transplanted organ—affects the prognosis and course of a melanoma.

Nowadays, SOTRs live longer, thanks to advances in surgical techniques and in the management of post-surgery complications; in addition, more patients are

4 De Novo Melanoma in an Organ Transplant Recipient

KC account for 40% of all de novo cancers, and for 90% of all skin tumours in SOTR [29]. The scientific literature presents varying data on the melanoma incidence and the potentially increased risk of a post-transplant melanoma in the context of organ transplantation. Lindelöf studied what was until recently the largest collective group of 5356 SOTR; patients were observed for a median period of 5.6 years after transplantation. The study, published in 2000, found no increased risk of melanoma in comparison to the general population [30]. Subsequent publications, all based on information from large databases, state a 2.2 to 8-fold increased melanoma risk for SOTR [31]. Therefore, pigmented skin lesions should be in the focus of skin examination after transplantation. As with immunocompetent patients, melanomas may occur at any site (Figs. 9, 10, 11, and 12a, b) and may be, as in the case of an amelanotic melanoma (Fig. 13), easily overlooked. In the worst scenario, the patients present with already advanced or metastatic disease (Figs. 14a, b and 15).

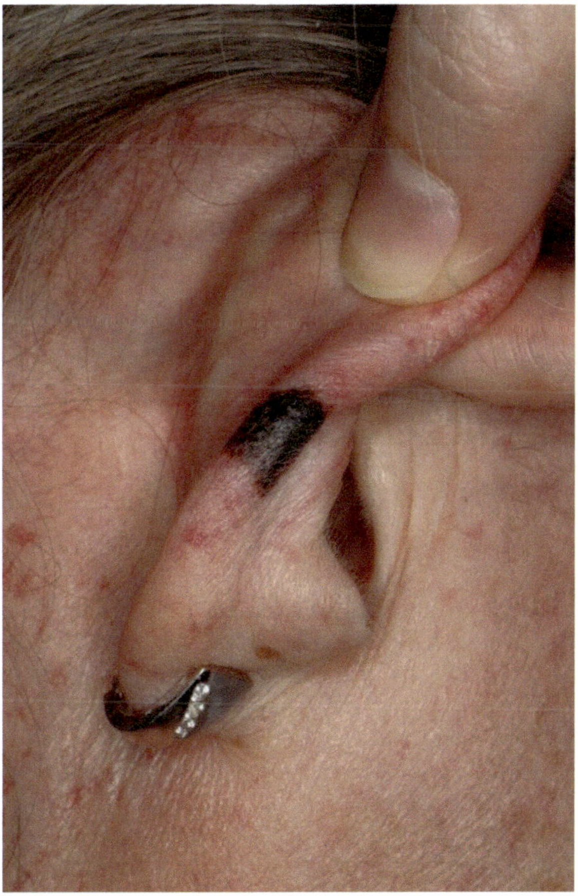

Fig. 9 Stage 1A superficial spreading melanoma on the ear of a 56-year-old lung-transplanted female diagnosed 6 months after transplantation . (*Image courtesy of Dra. Carla Ferrándiz-Pulido, MD, PhD, Vall d'Hebron Hospital, Barcelona*)

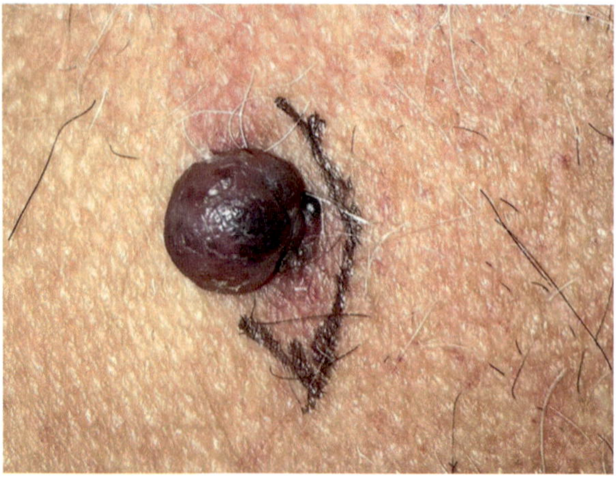

Fig. 10 Stage 2B melanoma on the neck of a 62-year-old kidney transplant male developing 4 years after transplantation. The patient developed lymph node metastases 4 years after treatment and died of progressive disease. (*Image courtesy of Dra. Carla Ferrándiz-Pulido, MD, PhD, Vall d'Hebron Hospital, Barcelona*)

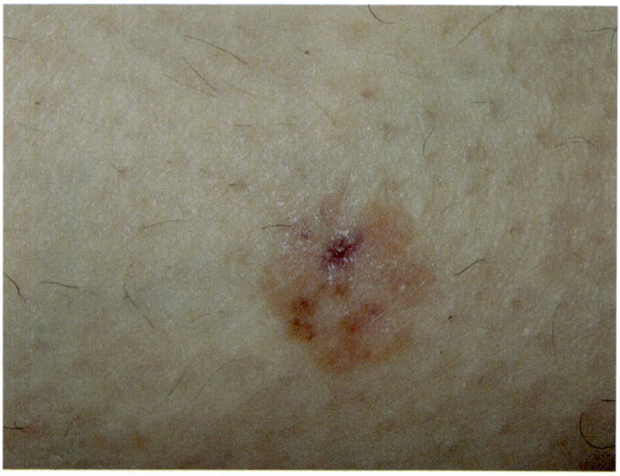

Fig. 11 A 64-year-old lung-transplanted male that developed a Stage 1A amelanotic melanoma on the thigh 2 years after transplantation. (*Image courtesy of Dra. Carla Ferrándiz-Pulido, MD, PhD, Vall d'Hebron Hospital, Barcelona*)

In their analysis of a database of 10,000 SOTR, Garrett et al. calculated an incidence of 125 melanoma cases per 100,000 SOTR, compared to an incidence of 9–18/100,000 for the total population. Organ transplant recipients with a pre-transplant melanoma had a seven-fold increased risk to develop a secondary melanoma in their post-transplant period [32].

As with immunocompetent patients, the clinical course of a melanoma in an SOTR varies according to the AJCC stage. In their 2016 publication mentioned above, Arron et al. found a slightly, but not significantly increased risk for SOTR to die of a post-transplant melanoma [24]. There are four older studies on the course

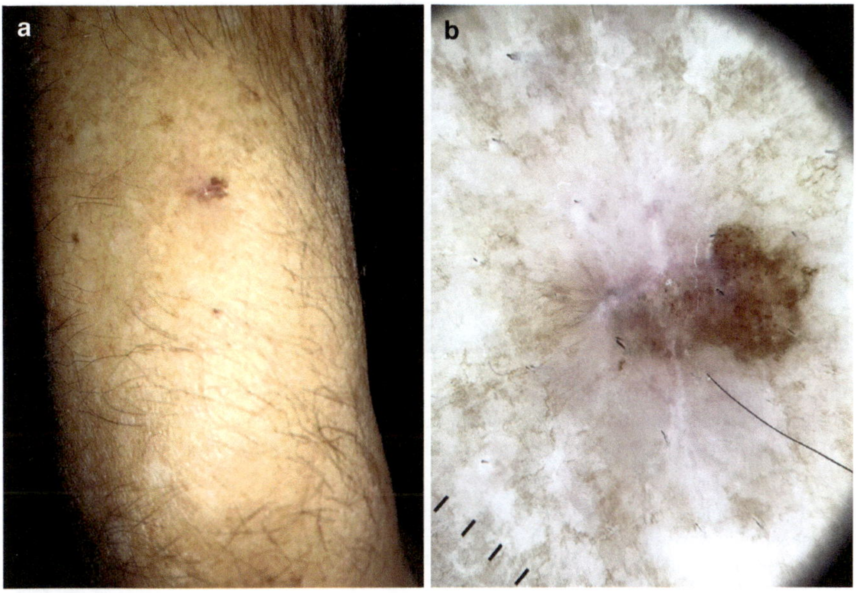

Fig. 12 A Stage 1B superficial spreading melanoma arising on a melanocytic nevus on the forearm of a 72-year-old male developed 7 years after receiving a kidney transplantation. (**a**) Clinical picture. (**b**) Dermoscopic image. (*Image courtesy of Dra. Carla Ferrándiz-Pulido, MD, PhD, Vall d'Hebron Hospital, Barcelona*)

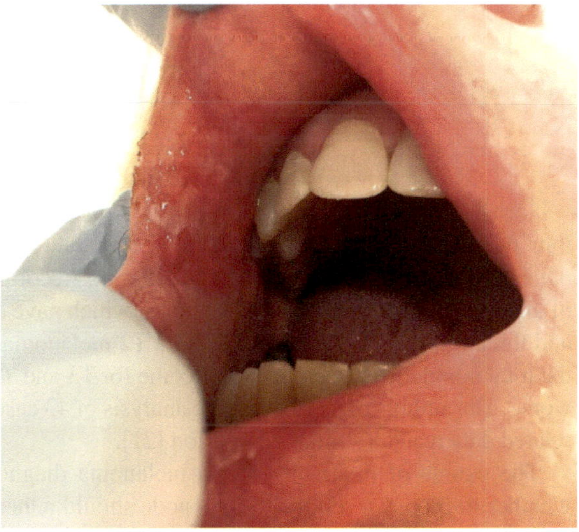

Fig. 13 A 59-year-old female developing a Stage IIIA amelanotic mucosal melanoma on the inner part of the upper lip and yugal mucosa 18 months after receiving a double lung transplantation. The patient was initially treated with surgical removal and lymphadenectomy and adjuvant radiotherapy. She presented with distant metastasis 15 months later and died of progressive disease. (*Image courtesy of Dra. Carla Ferrándiz-Pulido, MD, PhD, Vall d'Hebron Hospital, Barcelona*)

of a de novo melanoma in SOTR, but they offer only limited clinical data. Therefore, it is impossible to make definite statements on the actual mortality rate of SOTR in connection with melanoma. The prognosis for SOTR with in situ melanomas and

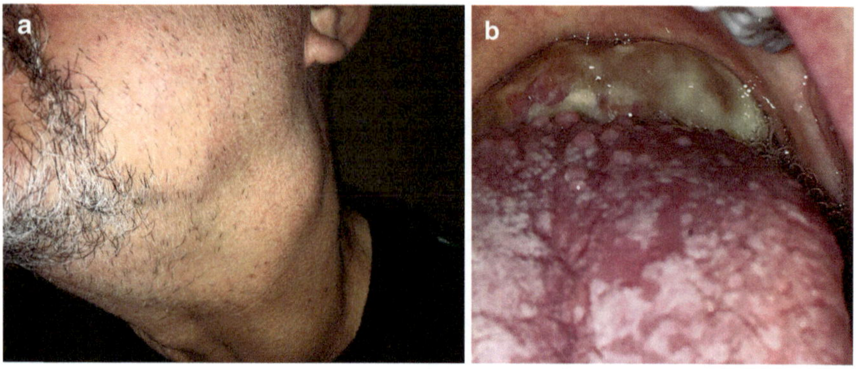

Fig. 14 A 63-year-old lung-transplanted patient presented with lymph node metastatic melanoma 10 years after transplantation (**a**). The primary melanoma was located on the dorsum of the tongue (**b**). (*Image courtesy of Dra. Carla Ferrándiz-Pulido, MD, PhD, Vall d'Hebron Hospital, Barcelona*)

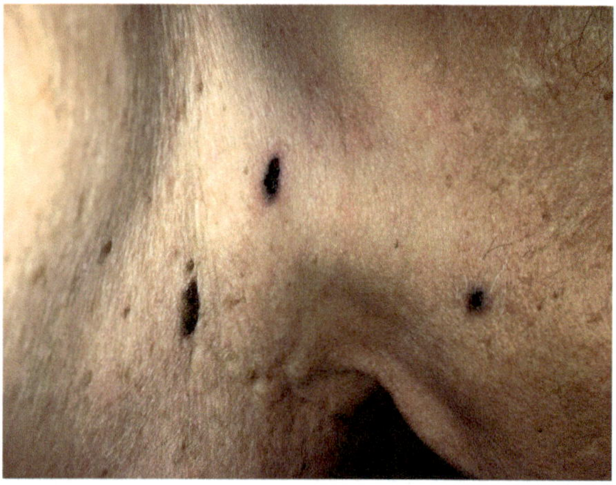

Fig. 15 Multiple cutaneous metastasis of melanoma in a kidney transplant recipient. (*Image courtesy of Dra. Carla Ferrándiz-Pulido, MD, PhD, Vall d'Hebron Hospital, Barcelona*)

thin melanomas of <0.75 mm seems comparable to that of immunocompetent patients; in contrast to melanomas >0.75 mm. According to a multicentre analysis of almost 100 post-transplant melanomas, which gave details with regard to staging and thickness, the prognosis for T1 and T2 melanomas (≤2 mm) is comparable to the total population, whereas the outcome for T3 and T4 melanomas (>2 mm) is far worse. The authors of a retrospective analysis of 43 cases with sufficient melanoma-related data reach a similar conclusion [21].

The course of treatment after a melanoma diagnosis as well as the decision whether to biopsy a sentinel lymph node should adhere to the same criteria as for an immunocompetent patient. A wide excision should suffice; the area and margins depend on the thickness of the melanoma. The IS regime should be re-assessed and/or reduced/limited to the necessary minimum to insure the survival of the transplant.

5 New Melanoma Therapies in Connection with Organ Transplantation

There has been something of a revolution in recent years with regard to therapy options and adjuvant therapies for advanced melanomas: for patients after a complete excision of regional metastases as well as for patients with inoperable metastasis, we can now offer therapies, which have a proven effect on a patient's survival—people live longer. One option is immunotherapy with immune checkpoint inhibitors (ICI), either as monotherapy with anti-programmed cell death protein 1 (PD-1) antibodies (Nivolumab or Pembrolizumab), or a combination of a PD-1 antibody, e.g. Nivolumab, and a cytotoxic lymphocyte antigen-4 (CTLA-4) antibody like Ipilimumab (Table 1). For patients with BRAF V600E or V600K metastatic melanoma, targeted therapy with BRAF and MEK Inhibitors, like Encorafenib and Binimetinib, Dabrafenib and Trametinib and Vemurafenib and Cobimetinib, present a further treatment option (Table 1).

Under a first-line therapy with Nivolumab and Pembrolizumab, we see a 5-year overall survival (OS) of 43.2–44% and for the combination of Nivolumab and Ipilimumab a 5-year OS of 52% [33]. For patients with BRAF V600E or V600K metastatic melanoma and first-line therapy with BRAF and MEK inhibitors, like Dabrafenib and Trametinib, the 5-year OS is 34% [34].

Table 1 Systemic therapies for the treatment of metastatic melanoma. Current treatment options are checkpoint inhibitors like the programmed cell death-1 (PD-1) checkpoint inhibitors Nivolumab and Pembrolizumab, the cytotoxic t-lymphocyte-associated protein 4 (CTLA-4) checkpoint inhibitor Ipilimumab as monotherapy or in combination with Nivolumab. In case of a BRAF-mutated melanoma-targeted therapy with BRAF and MEK inhibitors, like Encorafenib, Binimetinib and Dabrafenib, Trametinib and Vemurafenib and Cobimetinib, present a further treatment option

Checkpoint inhibitors		
PD-1 inhibitors	**CTLA-4 inhibitor**	**PD-1 + CTLA-4 inhibitor**
Nivolumab 480 mg i.v. every 4 weeks or Nivolumab 240 mg i.v. every 2 weeks	Ipilimumab 3 mg/kg i.v. every 3 weeks	4 cycles Nivolumab 1 mg/kg 3 mg/kg Ipilimumab i.v.
Pembrolizumab 200 mg i.v. every 3 weeks or Pembrolizumab 400 mg i.v. every 6 weeks		
Targeted therapies		
BRAF and MEK inhibitors		
Encorafenib 75 mg 6-0-0 p.o. Binimetinib 15 mg 3-0-3 p.o.	Dabrafenib 75 mg 2-0-2 p.o. Trametinib 2 mg 1-0-0 p.o.	Vemurafenib 240 mg 2-0-2 p.o. Cobimetinib 20 mg 3-0-0 p.o.

i.v. intravenously, *p.o.* per os

For the locally advanced, unresectable metastatic melanoma, AJCC stage IIIB-IV M1a, without organ involvement, the oncolytic virus—Talimogene laherparepvec (T-VEC)—is licensed (Fig. 16a–c). It is a genetically modified herpes simplex virus 1 (HSV-1) with an insertion of 2 genes copy of human granulocyte macrophage colony-stimulating factor (hGM-CSF) and a deletion of the infected cell protein (ICP) 34.5 and ICP 47 [35, 36]. T-VEC is injected intralesionally, the injection volume is dependent on the lesion size (Table 2) and leads to local and systemic anti-tumour effects. For the stage IIIB-IV M1a metastatic melanoma, this treatment leads to a 5-year OS of 48.9% [37].

For SOTR with inoperable metastases in the area of the primary tumour, a therapy with the oncolytic virus T-VEC might be under special consideration a treatment option. In our clinic, we were able to treat a patient successfully and—above all—without any complications with T-VEC, who had received both a heart and a kidney transplantation, and who had developed in-transit metastases on his arm (Fig. 17a, b) [38]. There are few other case reports of successful and safe T-VEC

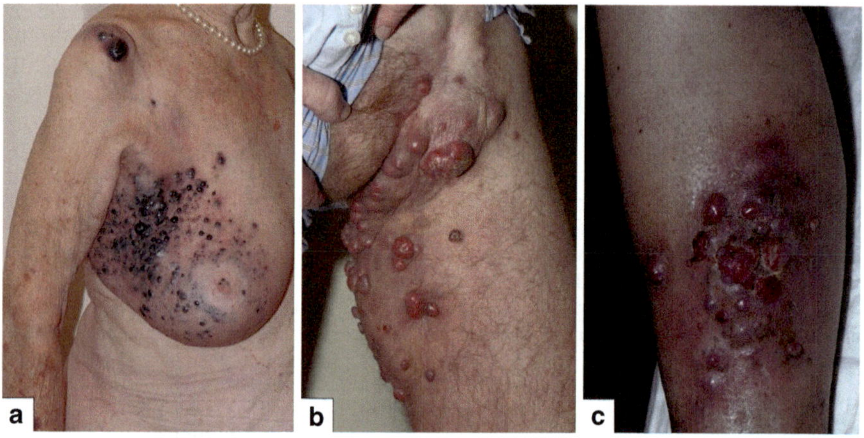

Fig. 16 Clinical images of locally advanced metastatic melanoma. (**a**) Multiple cutaneous melanoma metastases on the right chest; (**b**) advanced melanoma metastases on the left inguinal lymph nodes and the surrounding skin; (**c**) cutaneous melanoma metastases on the left leg. (*Image courtesy of the Department of Dermatology, Medical University of Vienna*)

Table 2 Application of the oncolytic virotherapy Talimogene laherparepvec (T-VEC) in locally advanced unresectable metastatic melanoma. The injectable dosage is dependent on the lesion size of the tumour, with a maximum volume of up to 4 mL

Application of T-VEC	
Lesion size of metastatic lesions	Injection volume of T-VEC
>5 cm	Up to 4 mL
>2.5–5 cm	Up to 2 mL
>1.5–2.5 cm	Up to 1 mL
>0.5–1.5 cm	Up to 0.5 mL
≤0.5 cm	Up to 0.1 mL

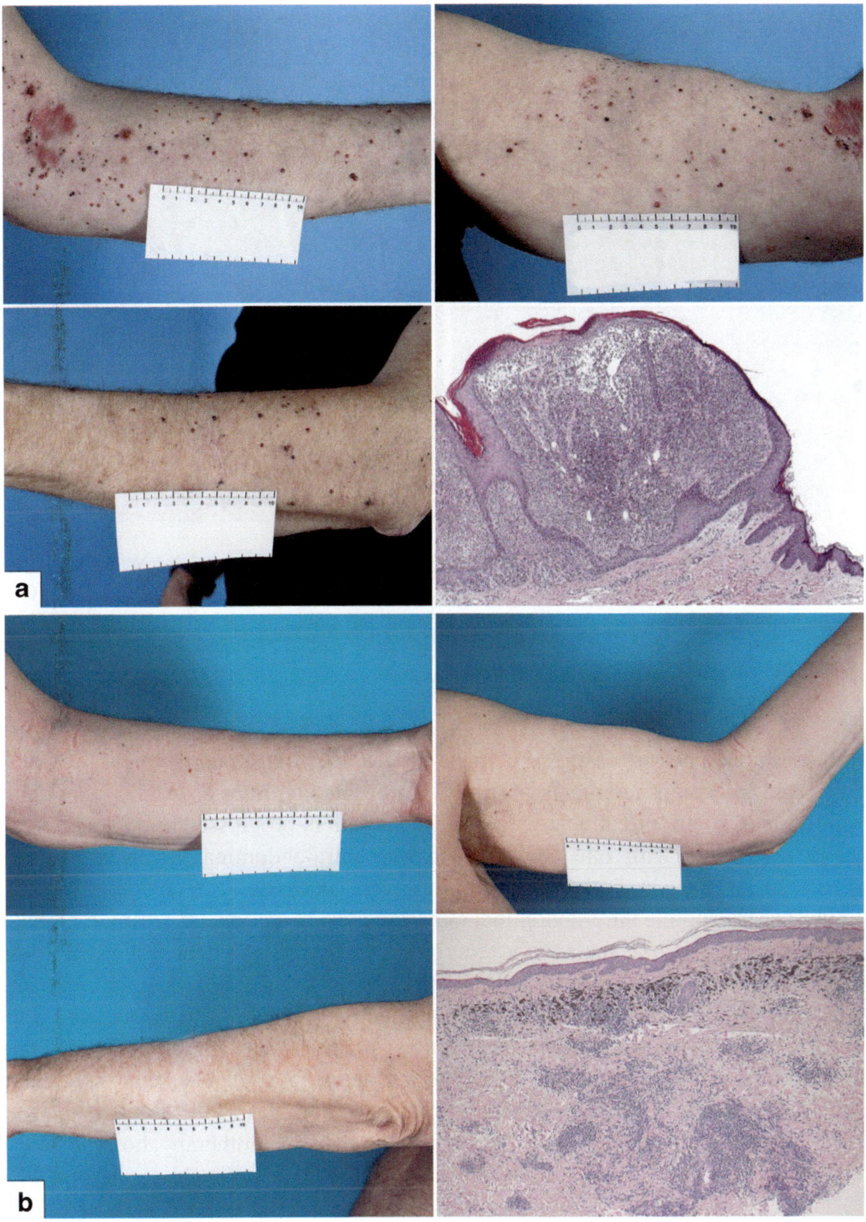

Fig. 17 A heart and kidney transplant recipient with a locally advanced, metastatic unresectable melanoma treated successfully with Talimogene laherparepvec (T-VEC) . (**a**) Before the first treatment with T-VEC, there were multiple metastatic lesions on the left arm. Histopathology showed atypical melanoma cells limited to the epidermis; (**b**) eight months after 11 cycles of T-VEC there was a complete regression of all melanoma metastases on the patient's left arm. Histopathology showed melanophages and plasma cells, with no sign of melanoma residua. (*Courtesy of Christoph Höller and Julia Maria Ressler, Department of Dermatology, Medical University of Vienna*)

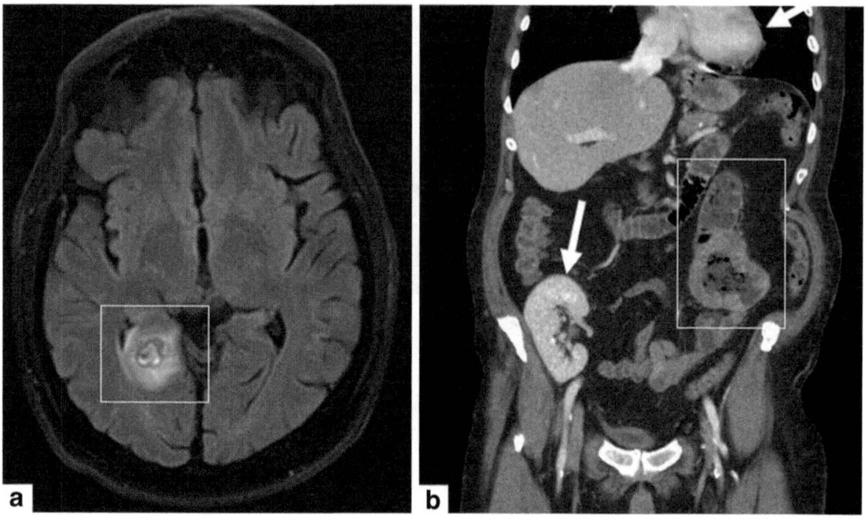

Fig. 18 Stage IV metastatic melanoma in a heart and kidney transplant recipient. (**a**) Magnetic resonance imaging (MRI) of one cerebral metastatic lesion; (**b**) Computed tomography (CT) shows an intraabdominal metastatic lesion and the kidney and heart transplant. *CT and MRI pictures provided by Prof. Füger Barbara, MD, Department of Biomedical Imaging and Image-guided Therapy, Medical University of Vienna*

application in a heart-transplant recipient [39], a liver-transplant recipient [40], and two renal-transplant recipients [41, 42]. Unfortunately, after 2 years of complete remission (CR) after treatment with T-VEC the patient progressed to stage IV metastatic melanoma with one cerebral and one intra-abdominal metastatic lesion (Fig. 18a, b). The cerebral metastatic lesion was successfully treated with gamma knife surgery and the intra-abdominal metastatic lesion was excised. Still, 6 months following surgery, the melanoma recurred with disseminated metastatic lesions. Since the tumour showed no BRAF mutation, we considered a systemic treatment with ICI. Due to the double transplantation (heart and kidney) and the reduced general condition of the patient with increasing systemic lactate dehydrogenase (LDH) levels, together with the patient we made the decision against systemic treatment with ICI; the risk of a life-threatening organ rejection was estimated as being too high. On the patient's request, we initiated a palliative chemotherapy; however, only after one cycle the patient sadly died.

Few cases of BRAF/MEK inhibitor therapy have been published so far in SOTR with stage IV BRAF V600E or V600K positive metastatic melanoma; however, they all show a course similar to that seen in patients with no transplants [43]. While the BRAF/MEK inhibitor therapy can be used to treat SOTR, immunotherapies are not usually recommended, considering the risk of organ rejection. In certain cases, organ rejection can be considered acceptable, e.g. if the transplanted organ is a kidney, and its loss could be compensated by dialysis [43].

Often, it is a mere choice between trying a treatment or accepting a patient's certain death; and there are some hopeful individual case reports of SOTR who have been treated in this way with some success, certainly with regard to the initial response and the length of a period of remission. Lipson et al. describe the use of Ipilimumab in kidney transplant patients with a metastasized melanoma, where the organ was not rejected [44]. Similarly, in other case series using Ipilimumab as the drug of choice, there were only a few individual cases of organ rejection.

A retrospective multicentre analysis from France describes the use of Ipilimumab in six SOTR with metastasizing melanoma. In one patient, the organ was rejected after the first injection; probably caused by the injection in combination with the drastic reduction of his IS. After a median period of observation of 4.5 months (ranging from 3 to 20 months), only one patient achieved a partial response and a stable disease. Four patients suffered a progression of their melanoma. Ultimately, all six patients died of their melanoma. The authors of the study see little benefit in reducing the IS, certainly not in combination with tumour immunotherapy [45].

In clinical practice, the Ipilimumab monotherapy has been replaced by the therapy with the PD-1 antibodies Nivolumab and Pembrolizumab and the combination of Ipilimumab and Nivolumab, respectively—both have proven to be much more effective. One of the reasons for this is that anti-PD-1 antibodies act mainly in the effector phase of the immune response and not—like the CTLA-4 antibody Ipilimumab in the priming phase. This may—in theory—lead to a higher rate of organ rejection. The use of ICI immunotherapy for immunosuppressed patients with melanoma is restricted to case reports and case series. Specific considerations include the potential risk of graft rejection and relevant immune-related adverse events on graft function, e.g. acute interstitial nephritis, as well as possible reduced anti-tumour activity in the presence of immunosuppressive drugs. Recent evidence—much of it from experience in advanced melanoma—suggests that the PD-1/PD-L1 axis is critical for maintaining organ tolerance, whereas CTLA-4 blockade after induction of graft tolerance does not appear to affect allograft. Tolerance of donor transplanted cells is achieved when T cells are inhibited due to binding of its PD-1 receptor with the PD-L1 expressed by donor cell; hence, the PD1/PD-L1 interaction within peripheral tissues has a critical role for maintaining allograft tolerance [46].

A retrospective multicentre analysis focussed on five kidney transplant patients and one liver transplant patient, who were treated with PD-1 inhibitors: in two patients, the donor organ was rejected, resulting in the death of the liver transplant patient; two other patients showed at least a partial response [47]. A series of seven liver transplant recipients of the Mayo Clinic were also treated with PD-1 inhibitors; one reached complete remission; two patients suffered a rejection of the donor organ, and another died of multiple organ failure, probably in connection with a rejection [48].

Aguirre et al. give a summary of several case series; out of a total of 20 patients, 12 suffered an organ rejection. The rejection rate for Nivolumab was 73%, for Pembrolizumab and Ipilimumab and Nivolumab 100%. None of the four patients treated with Ipilimumab alone suffered a rejection [49]. Due to the small samples, the exact rejection ratios vary greatly between the different studies; besides, not all published cases have been included in the analysis. But there is an obviously higher rate of organ rejections under therapies using PD-1 inhibitors. This suggests that there is an absolute contraindication for the use of PD-1 inhibitors in SOTR with vital donor organs.

A systematic search in the Google Scholar and PubMed databases was recently carried out by Kumar and co-workers to include all the published cases of organ transplant patients who received treatment with ICI including PD-1-, PD-L1-, or CTLA4 inhibitors [50]. This pooled analysis of 64 patients published in literature showed that overall allograft rejection rate is 41% in SOTR following ICI therapy. The graft rejection rate was 44% (17/39) for renal, 39% (7/19) for liver and 20% (1/5) for cardiac allografts. The highest risk for rejection was seen among patients who were treated with PD-1 inhibitors, 48–54% on nivolumab, and 39% on pembrolizumab. For all CPI and all indications, the risk was lowest with ipilimumab, namely 23%. The overall response rate was 20% with ipilimumab, 26% with nivolumab, and 53% with pembrolizumab. None of the variables including age, gender, type of cancer, type of allograft, type of immunosuppression, time since transplantation to initiation of ICI, and prior history of rejection were significantly associated with the transplant rejection on univariate analysis. The efficacy of ICI among SOTR appears promising; however, due to the risk of organ rejection alternative forms of therapies have to be discussed thoroughly with the patients prior to therapy [50–53].

In conclusion, besides treatment with BRAF and MEK inhibitors for SOTR suffering from a melanoma with a BRAF mutation, oncolytic virotherapy and immunotherapy may be an option—after a careful evaluation of the benefits, risks and costs, an in-depth interdisciplinary discussion by a tumour board, and a thorough discussion with the patient, especially with regard to the significant risk of organ rejection. While dialysis—which means a reduced quality of life as well as a reduced life expectancy—presents a fall-back option for kidney-transplant patients, when eventually the organ is sacrificed for a potentially lifesaving therapy, all other patients are faced with a potentially lethal rejection.

References

1. Green AC, Olsen CM. Increased risk of melanoma in organ transplant recipients: systematic review and meta-analysis of cohort studies. Acta Derm Venereol. 2015;95(8):923–7.
2. Dahlke E, et al. Systematic review of melanoma incidence and prognosis in solid organ transplant recipients. Transplant Res. 2014;3:10.
3. Hollenbeak CS, et al. Increased incidence of melanoma in renal transplantation recipients. Cancer. 2005;104(9):1962–7.
4. González-Cruz C, Ferrándiz-Pulido C, García-Patos Briones V. Melanoma in solid organ transplant recipients. Actas Dermosifiliogr. 2020; https://doi.org/10.1016/j.ad.2020.11.005.
5. https://gco.iarc.fr.

6. Abbas O, Miller DD, Bhawan J. Cutaneous malignant melanoma: update on diagnostic and prognostic biomarkers. Am J Dermatopathol. 2014;36(5):363–79.
7. Gershenwald JE, Scolyer RA. Melanoma staging: American Joint Committee on Cancer (AJCC) 8th edition and beyond. Ann Surg Oncol. 2018;25(8):2105–10.
8. Transplant-observatory.org.
9. Chen KT, Olszanski A, Farma JM. Donor transmission of melanoma following renal transplant. Case Rep Transplant. 2012;2012:764019.
10. Morris-Stiff G, et al. Transmission of donor melanoma to multiple organ transplant recipients. Am J Transplant. 2004;4(3):444–6.
11. Strauss DC, Thomas JM. Transmission of donor melanoma by organ transplantation. Lancet Oncol. 2010;11(8):790–6.
12. Penn I. Transmission of cancer from organ donors. Ann Transplant. 1997;2(4):7–12.
13. https://ipittr.uc.edu.
14. Birkeland SA, Storm HH. Risk for tumor and other disease transmission by transplantation: a population-based study of unrecognized malignancies and other diseases in organ donors. Transplantation. 2002;74(10):1409–13.
15. Juszczak H, et al. Potential for overlooked melanoma in solid organ donors with a severely dysplastic nevus. JAAD Case Rep. 2018;4(7):682–3.
16. Xiao D, et al. Donor cancer transmission in kidney transplantation: a systematic review. Am J Transplant. 2013;13(10):2645–52.
17. Boyle SM, et al. Donor-derived metastatic melanoma and checkpoint inhibition. Transplant Proc. 2017;49(7):1551–4.
18. Dabek RJ, et al. Development of a primary melanoma in situ within a full-thickness skin graft overlying a free muscle flap: a case report. Case Rep Plast Surg Hand Surg. 2018;5(1):23–6.
19. Penn I. Malignant melanoma in organ allograft recipients. Transplantation. 1996;61(2):274–8.
20. Colegio OR, et al. Prognosis of pretransplant melanoma. Am J Transplant. 2009;9(4):862.
21. Dapprich DC, et al. Outcomes of melanoma in recipients of solid organ transplant. J Am Acad Dermatol. 2008;59(3):405–17.
22. Matin RN, et al. Melanoma in organ transplant recipients: clinicopathological features and outcome in 100 cases. Am J Transplant. 2008;8(9):1891–900.
23. Puza CJ, Barbas AS, Mosca PJ. Outcomes of patients with a pretransplant history of early-stage melanoma. Melanoma Res. 2018;28(5):471–4.
24. Arron ST, et al. Melanoma outcomes in transplant recipients with pretransplant melanoma. Dermatol Surg. 2016;42(2):157–66.
25. Zwald F, et al. Recommendations for solid organ transplantation for transplant candidates with a pretransplant diagnosis of cutaneous squamous cell carcinoma, Merkel cell carcinoma and melanoma: a consensus opinion from the International Transplant Skin Cancer Collaborative (ITSCC). Am J Transplant. 2016;16(2):407–13.
26. Landow SM, Gjelsvik A, Weinstock MA. Mortality burden and prognosis of thin melanomas overall and by subcategory of thickness, SEER registry data, 1992-2013. J Am Acad Dermatol. 2017;76(2):258–63.
27. Whiteman DC, Baade PD, Olsen CM. More people die from thin melanomas (⩽1 melanoma) than from thick melanomas (>4 melanoma) in Queensland, Australia. J Invest Dermatol. 2015;135(4):1190–3.
28. Mocellin S, et al. The prognostic value of circulating tumor cells in patients with melanoma: a systematic review and meta-analysis. Clin Cancer Res. 2006;12(15):4605–13.
29. Kim C, Cheng J, Colegio OR. Cutaneous squamous cell carcinomas in solid organ transplant recipients: emerging strategies for surveillance, staging, and treatment. Semin Oncol. 2016;43(3):390–4.
30. Lindelöf B, et al. Incidence of skin cancer in 5356 patients following organ transplantation. Br J Dermatol. 2000;143(3):513–9.
31. Zwald FO, et al. Melanoma in solid organ transplant recipients. Am J Transplant. 2010;10(5):1297–304.

32. Garrett GL, et al. Incidence of and risk factors for skin cancer in organ transplant recipients in the United States. JAMA Dermatol. 2017;153(3):296–303.
33. Larkin J, et al. Five-year survival with combined nivolumab and ipilimumab in advanced melanoma. N Engl J Med. 2019;381(16):1535–46.
34. Robert C, et al. Five-year outcomes with dabrafenib plus trametinib in metastatic melanoma. N Engl J Med. 2019;381(7):626–36.
35. Harrington KJ, et al. Clinical development of talimogene laherparepvec (T-VEC): a modified herpes simplex virus type-1-derived oncolytic immunotherapy. Expert Rev Anticancer Ther. 2015;15(12):1389–403.
36. Andtbacka RH, et al. Talimogene laherparepvec improves durable response rate in patients with advanced melanoma. J Clin Oncol. 2015;33(25):2780–8.
37. Andtbacka RHI, et al. Final analyses of OPTiM: a randomized phase III trial of talimogene laherparepvec versus granulocyte-macrophage colony-stimulating factor in unresectable stage III-IV melanoma. J Immunother Cancer. 2019;7(1):145.
38. Ressler J, et al. Talimogene laherparepvec (T-VEC) in advanced melanoma: complete response in a heart and kidney transplant patient. A case report. Br J Dermatol. 2019;181(1):186–9.
39. Schvartsman G, et al. Safe and effective administration of T-VEC in a patient with heart transplantation and recurrent locally advanced melanoma. J Immunother Cancer. 2017;5:45.
40. Lehner GM, et al. Successful treatment of a metastatic melanoma with Talimogen laherparepvec (T-VEC) in a liver transplant patient. J Dtsch Dermatol Ges. 2020;18(12):1495–7.
41. Sunshine JC, et al. Successful treatment of in-transit metastatic melanoma in a renal transplant patient with combination T-VEC/imiquimod immunotherapy. J Immunother. 2020;43(4):149–52.
42. Gupta M, Brennan DC, Alhamad T. Talimogene laherparepvec use in kidney transplant recipient. Transplantation. 2020;104(4):e109–10.
43. Garrett GL, et al. Combined dabrafenib and trametinib therapy in metastatic melanoma and organ transplantation: case report and review of the literature. JAAD Case Rep. 2015;1(6):S23–5.
44. Lipson EJ, et al. Successful administration of ipilimumab to two kidney transplantation patients with metastatic melanoma. J Clin Oncol. 2014;32(19):e69–71.
45. Zehou O, et al. Ipilimumab for the treatment of advanced melanoma in six kidney transplant patients. Am J Transplant. 2018;18(12):3065–71.
46. De Bruyn P, et al. Immune checkpoint blockade for organ transplant patients with advanced cancer: how far can we go? Curr Opin Oncol. 2019;31(2):54–64.
47. Tio M, et al. Anti-PD-1/PD-L1 immunotherapy in patients with solid organ transplant, HIV or hepatitis B/C infection. Eur J Cancer. 2018;104:137–44.
48. DeLeon TT, et al. Pilot evaluation of PD-1 inhibition in metastatic cancer patients with a history of liver transplantation: the Mayo Clinic experience. J Gastrointest Oncol. 2018;9(6):1054–62.
49. Aguirre LE, et al. Immune checkpoint inhibitors and the risk of allograft rejection: a comprehensive analysis on an emerging issue. Oncologist. 2019;24(3):394–401.
50. Kumar V, et al. The safety and efficacy of checkpoint inhibitors in transplant recipients: a case series and systematic review of literature. Oncologist. 2020;25(6):505–14.
51. Abdel-Wahab N, et al. Checkpoint inhibitor therapy for cancer in solid organ transplantation recipients: an institutional experience and a systematic review of the literature. J Immunother Cancer. 2019;7(1):106.
52. Fisher J, et al. Immune checkpoint inhibitor therapy in solid organ transplant recipients: a patient-centered systematic review. J Am Acad Dermatol. 2020;82(6):1490–500.
53. Owoyemi I, et al. Clinical outcomes of solid organ transplant recipients with metastatic cancers who are treated with immune checkpoint inhibitors: a single-center analysis. Cancer. 2020;126(21):4780–7.

Kaposi Sarcoma

Christina Lee Chung and Carla Ferrándiz-Pulido

1 Introduction

Kaposi sarcoma was first described by Moritz Kaposi in 1872 as a multicentric, cutaneous, and extracutaneous neoplasm, predominantly affecting older individuals with a protracted clinical course. There are four recognized clinical subsets: (1) classical, appearing mostly in elderly individuals; (2) endemic, observed in black Africans; (3) AIDS-associated infection; and (4) iatrogenic, appearing in patients treated with immunosuppressants [1, 2]. For over a half century, Kaposi sarcoma, in Western populations, was known as a non-aggressive neoplastic phenomenon with no significant effect on life expectancy. The onset of the AIDS epidemic and increasing number of immunosuppressed persons has since garnered the attention of the medical community [2].

Posttransplant Kaposi sarcoma corresponds to the iatrogenic subtype and ranks among the most common cancers affecting kidney transplant recipients in developing countries. Its course may vary from indolent and chronic to rapidly progressive. Development of posttransplant Kaposi sarcoma is directly related to the chronic immunosuppressive therapy required for graft maintenance. Data support posttransplant Kaposi sarcoma to arise from reactivation of latent Kaposi sarcoma herpesvirus (or human herpesvirus type 8 [HHV-8]) infection with disease regression observed upon decreasing or removal of immunosuppression [3].

C. L. Chung
Lankenau Institute for Medical Research, Wynnewood, PA, USA

Schweiger Dermatology Group, Philadelphia, PA, USA

C. Ferrándiz-Pulido (✉)
Department of Dermatology, Hospital Universitari Vall d'Hebron, Universitat Autònoma de Barcelona, Barcelona, Spain
e-mail: carla.ferrandiz@vallhebron.cat

J. Tomimori et al. (eds.), *Atlas of Dermatologic Diseases in Solid Organ Transplant Recipients*, https://doi.org/10.1007/978-3-031-13335-0_15

2 Epidemiology

The incidence of Kaposi sarcoma in immunosuppressed transplant recipients has been reported between 54× and as high as 400–500× greater than that of the general population [4]. The mean time of onset of Kaposi sarcoma after organ transplantation is 13 months and has been reported to range from a few weeks to 18 years [5–7]. Peak onset of disease peaks is 0–2 years posttransplant and decreases thereafter. Individual risk factors for the development of Kaposi sarcoma in transplant recipients include increased age at transplantation, more aggressive immunosuppressive therapy, and greater mismatches at the HLA-B locus [8–10]. The male to female ratio has been reported to range from 2 to 40 times though one recent study found no significant difference after correcting for the increased rate of transplantation in men [11].

In 1962, George Oettle noted striking racial differences in the frequency of endemic Kaposi sarcoma [12]. Since that time, this contrast has also been observed in the transplant population with disease varying geographically and displaying significant ethnic differences in prevalence. Rates of disease are lower, less than 0.5%, among transplant recipients in the US and Western Europe but markedly increased in areas with a high endemic seroprevalence of HHV-8 [13]. The incidence among renal transplant recipients in Saudi Arabia has been reported to be 5.3% and constitutes over 80% of posttransplant neoplasms and cancers in Saudi Arabia and Turkey, respectively [14, 15]. In diverse transplant populations with high variability in geographic origin, racial differences in susceptibility to Kaposi sarcoma have been profound. Data regarding skin cancer development in transplant patients of color is scarce and the frequency of Kaposi sarcoma is variable. A single-center study from South Africa found Kaposi sarcoma to account for 79% of cancers in transplant recipients of color [11]. Subsequently, a multicenter study of 1766 transplant recipients in the USA and the UK found 15 cases of Kaposi sarcoma in 742 SOTR of color and one case among 1024 white transplant recipients. Kaposi sarcoma accounted for 26% of cutaneous malignancies diagnosed in the cohort of color but 48% of black transplant recipients [16].

The stark racial differences displayed in the frequency of Kaposi sarcoma after organ transplantation, though yet to be elucidated, may be attributed to genetic variation. The prevalence of posttransplant Kaposi sarcoma mirrors that of the prevalence of HHV-8 in a given population, with the highest rates observed in sub-Saharan Africa, intermediate frequency in the Mediterranean, West Africa, and South American, and the lowest rates seen in the USA, Northern Europe, and Asia. The prevalence of pre-transplant HHV-8 in Europe is reported as high as 80% and studies have found the rate of Kaposi sarcoma development in these patients after transplantation to range from 14% to 100% [17, 18].

While the seroprevalence of HHV-8 antibodies in developing countries is higher than in the USA and Europe, studies reveal disparate results between racial groups in South Africa. One study demonstrated a four-fold increase in HHV-8 antibody positivity in Black blood donors compared to White blood donors [19]. Another found renal transplant recipients to have higher levels of HHV-8 antibodies than the general population and significant racial differences of adjusted seroprevalence of "medium to high" titers with only 1.8% of White recipients but 7.4% of Black, 9.5% of Asian/Indian, 12.5% of transplant recipients of color of mixed race demonstrating high antibody levels [20].

3 Pathogenesis

It is now known that infection by HHV-8 is necessary for the development of Kaposi sarcoma [3]. HHV-8 is not only responsible for the development of Kaposi sarcoma but also other diseases including multicentric Castleman's disease and some cases of plasmablastic lymphoma [21]. It is a phylogenetically old human virus that co-evolved with human populations, but is now only endemic in sub-Saharan Africa, around the Mediterranean Sea, parts of South America and in a few ethnic communities, where the seroprevalence is greater than 10% [21].

Chang et al. identified and sequenced fragments belonging to a new human herpesvirus in biopsy specimens of AIDS-associated Kaposi sarcoma in 1994 [22]. Detailed epidemiological analysis of behavioral risk factors among people with HIV/AIDS concluded that Kaposi sarcoma was most likely caused by a new sexually transmissible infectious agent that appeared to be transmitted independently of HIV [21].

The origin of Kaposi sarcoma lies in endothelial cells that transform into proliferating Kaposi sarcoma spindle tumor cells. In this sense, circulating blood mononuclear and endothelial "progenitor cells" are believed to be the source of early Kaposi sarcoma lesions. Infection with HHV-8 is necessary to transform endothelial cells to lymphatic-endothelium-like cells, upregulating several lymphatic-associated genes such as lymphatic vessel endothelial receptor 1 (*LYVE1*), podoplanin, and vascular endothelial growth factor receptor 3 (*VEGFR3*) [23]. However, as HHV-8 has colonized humans physiologically for many thousands of years, HHV-8 infection alone appears to be insufficient for disease development and cofactors such as immunosuppression are needed to allow it to unfold its pathogenic potential [21]. Kaposi sarcoma progression also relies on a degree of host immune dysfunction and the local inflammatory milieu [1]. Kaposi sarcoma growth involves the upregulation of many key HHV-8 gene products, such as the latency-associated nuclear antigen (LANA-1) [23]. The virus remains latent within cells and has developed a variety of mechanisms to evade the host immune system. Clinical, histopathological, and experimental observations indicate that the continued presence of HHV-8 in tumor cells is required to maintain tumor growth [24].

There are several contributing factors associated with increased risk of Kaposi sarcoma in the transplant population including (1) uncontrolled viral replication in HHV-8-infected cells prompted by immunosuppressive medications, (2) infection through an infected donor graft, (3) seroconversion after transplantation, and (4) type and duration of immunosuppression. The decreasing risk for Kaposi sarcoma after the 2-year mark after transplantation is thought to be related to immune recovery upon tapering immunosuppression. Though infrequent, Kaposi sarcoma may occur from an HHV-8-infected donor graft, with cells seeding and proliferating in the transplant recipient. Disseminated primary Kaposi sarcoma with a fatal outcome has been reported after liver transplantation [25]. The rate of seroconversion after transplantation has been reported between 0% and 50% [25–27]. Posttransplant Kaposi sarcoma has been associated with a spectrum of immunosuppressive therapies, including corticosteroids, calcineurin inhibitors (CNI), and purine synthesis inhibitors. When compared with azathioprine-only immunosuppressive regimens, CNIs have resulted in increased rates and shorter time to onset of Kaposi sarcoma [13, 28]. Notably, increased rates of Kaposi sarcoma have been observed with anti-thymocyte globulin and regression of disease has been reported upon changing from CNIs to mycophenolate mofetil [27, 29, 30].

4 Diagnosis

4.1 Clinical Presentation

Posttransplant Kaposi sarcoma most commonly presents within 2–3 years after transplantation, when levels of immunosuppression are traditionally higher [3]. It may affect the skin as well as mucosal surfaces such as the mouth and genitalia and, less frequently, there may also be visceral involvement.

Cutaneous lesions are present in over 90% of patients. It most often develops first on the lower legs or feet although they may also affect upper limbs, the trunk, or even the face although this last location is less frequently seen in the posttransplant subtype of Kaposi sarcoma [2, 3]. Typical lesions are violaceous or purplish papules that may be difficult to identify in skin of color, where they usually have a black color that is darker than the surrounding skin (Figs. 1 and 2). Kaposi sarcoma begins as macules or papules that progress and may coalesce to form large plaques, nodules, or tumors that may ulcerate and bleed easily (Figs. 3, 4, 5, 6, 7, 8, and 9). In some cases, the lesions may have a verrucous presentation (Fig. 10) [5]. The skin lesions range in size from very small to several centimeters in diameter, and they can remain unchanged for months to years, or grow rapidly within a few weeks and disseminate becoming a generalized eruption or a diffuse infiltration of the skin (Figs. 11a–c, 12, 13, and 14). Edema may also be a consequence of extensive

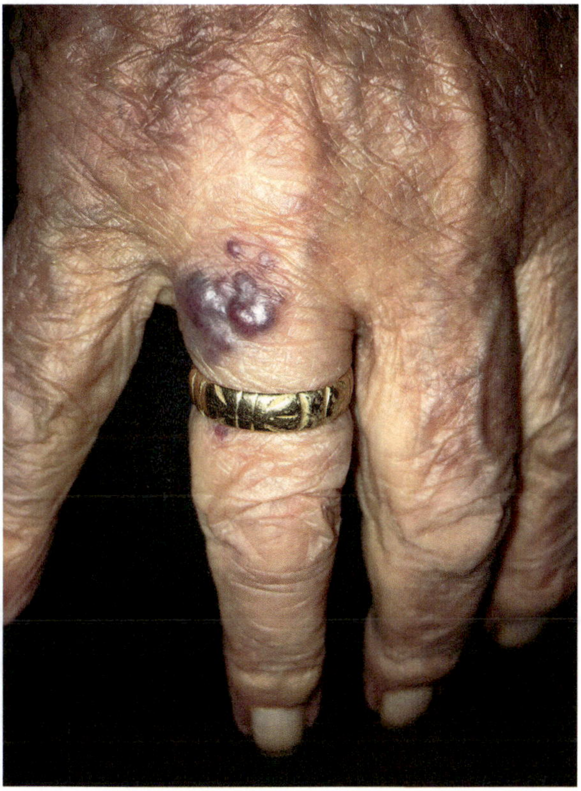

Fig. 1 A multinodular lesion of Kaposi sarcoma on the finger of a kidney transplant recipient. Note the violaceous or purple color

cutaneous disease (Fig. 15). Other secondary complications include superinfection of ulcerated lesions and the presence of dysesthesias due to the involvement of distal nerves (Fig. 16).

Mucosal involvement often affects the mouth and most commonly presents as a violaceous plaque on the palate, which may also herald disease onset (Figs. 17 and 18). Gingival hyperplasia may also occur and may be confused with the drug induced-hyperplasia associated with cyclosporine. Genital mucosa can also be affected, involving the glans or the scrotum (Fig. 19). Less frequently, Kaposi sarcoma may be observed in the ocular mucosa [2].

Visceral involvement has been reported in 50% of cases [3]. The most frequently affected organs are the lymph nodes, the gastrointestinal tract, the stomach and duodenum, and the lungs. Gastrointestinal lesions are generally asymptomatic but may progress and result in hemorrhage, perforation, or obstruction. Gastrointestinal lesions often present as infiltrated red spots on endoscopic examination. Pulmonary involvement is less frequent and may induce dyspnea, hypoxemia, and hypocapnia. Such lesions may be identified by CT scan or a bronchoscopy [2].

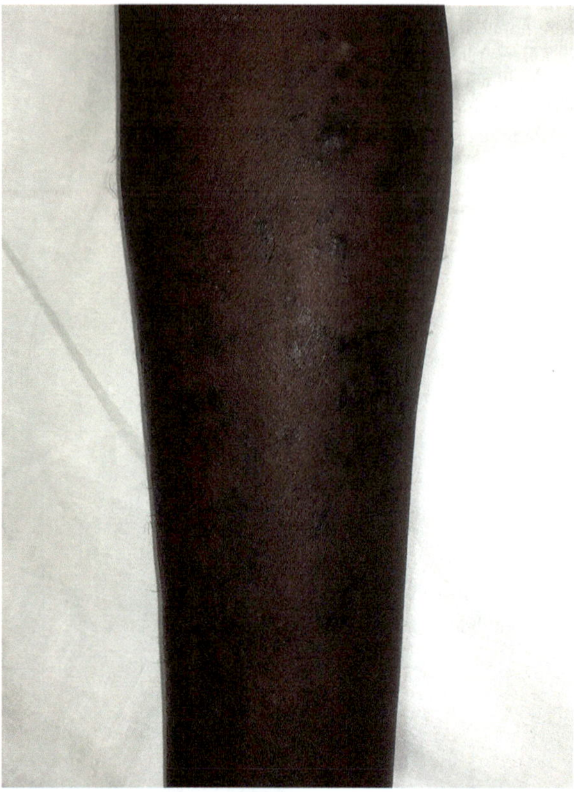

Fig. 2 Multiple macules and papular lesions on the leg difficult to diagnose because of the absence of violaceous color on black skin

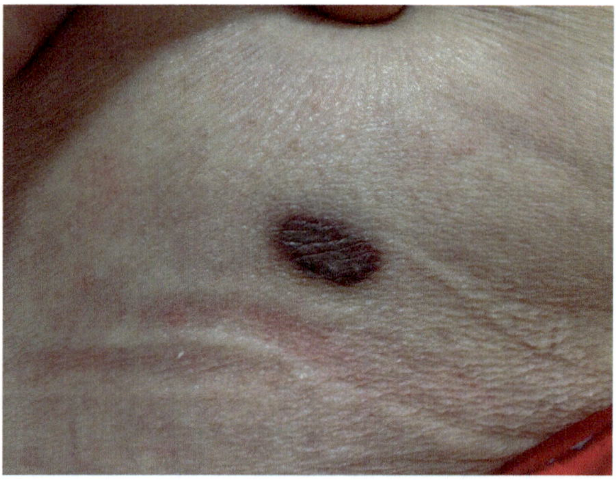

Fig. 3 Macular lesion of purplish color corresponding to a Kaposi sarcoma on the abdomen

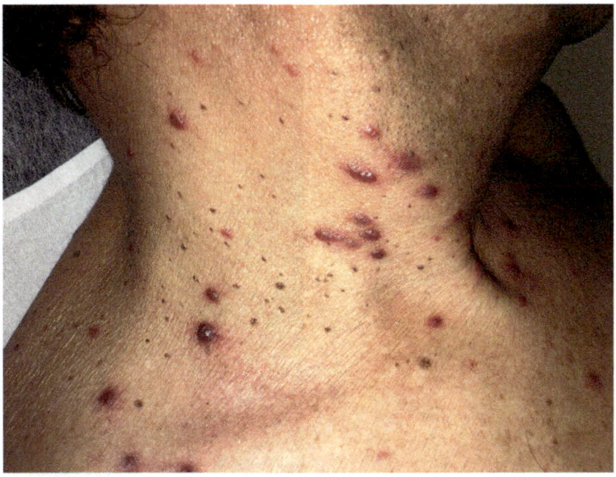

Fig. 4 Violaceous indurated papules of Kaposi sarcoma on the neck of a liver transplant recipient

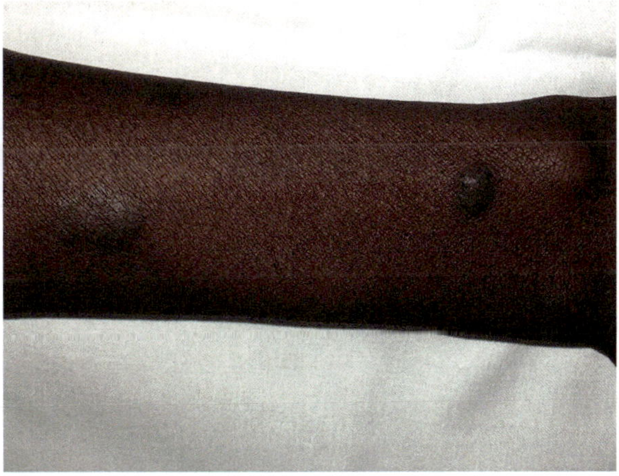

Fig. 5 Papular lesions of Kaposi sarcoma on phototype VI skin of a kidney transplant recipient

4.2 Histopathology

Histologically, Kaposi sarcoma is characterized by the presence of multiple ectatic, irregularly shaped capillaries and vascular spaces with spindle-like endothelium lines surrounded by a mixed inflammatory infiltrate. Hemosiderin and extravasated erythrocytes are often noted within the infiltrate. Initial macular lesions may be difficult to observe. LANA-1 is the most specific immunohistochemical marker available to help distinguish Kaposi sarcoma from others in the differential diagnosis; as tumor cells express LANA-1 and it serves as a surrogate marker of HHV-8 infection (Figs. 20a–c and 21a–c) [24]. Other immunostains that aid in the diagnosis are the endothelium-specific CD34 or Factor VIII. Newer histologic variants include

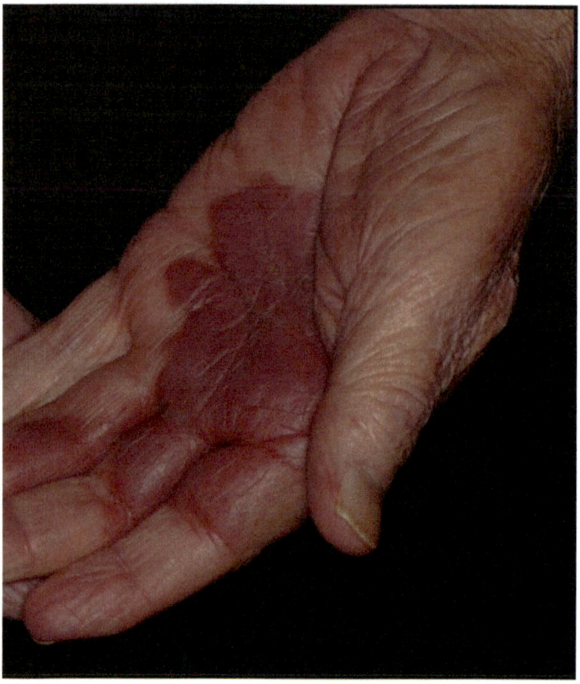

Fig. 6 Plaque-like Kaposi sarcoma affecting the palms

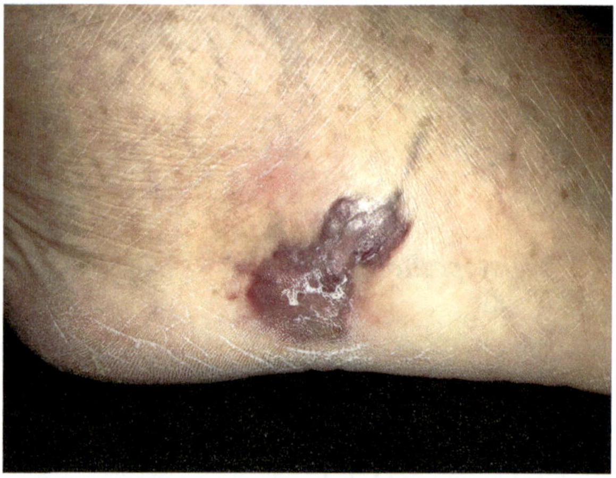

Fig. 7 Plaque-like Kaposi sarcoma on the lateral of the foot of a lung transplant recipient

anaplastic, hyperkeratotic, lymphangioma-like, bullous, telangiectatic, ecchymotic, keloidal, pyogenic granuloma-like, micronodular, intravascular, glomeruloid, and pigmented Kaposi sarcoma, as well as Kaposi sarcoma with sarcoid-like granulomas and Kaposi sarcoma with myoid nodules [24].

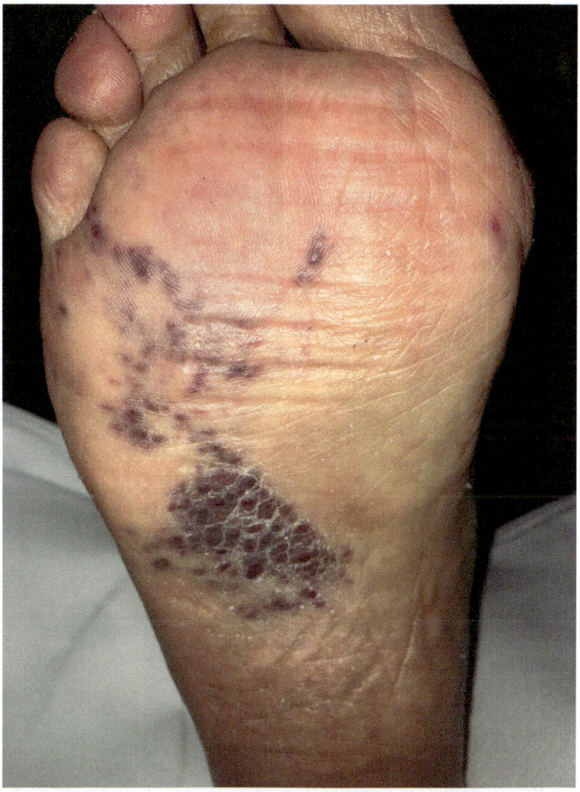

Fig. 8 Plaque-like Kaposi sarcoma affecting the sole of a lung transplant recipient

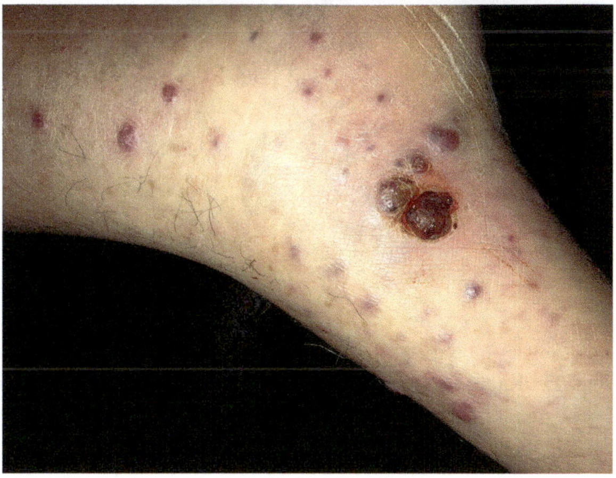

Fig. 9 Ulcerated papule of Kaposi sarcoma in a lung transplant recipient

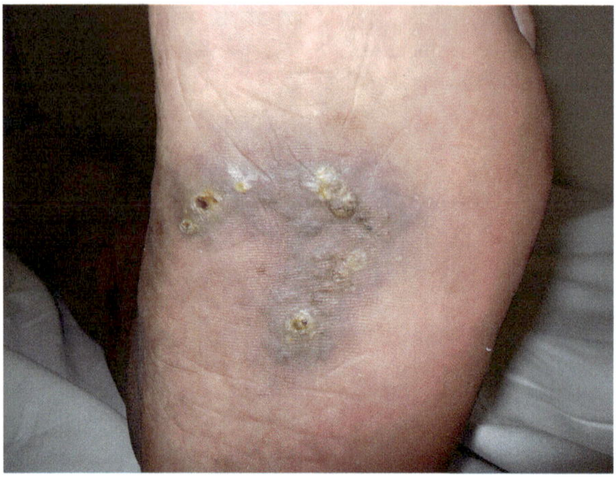

Fig. 10 First presentation of Kaposi sarcoma 8 months after receiving a lung transplantation. The patient presented with hyperkeratotic papules on a brown-violaceous dark macule on the background on the sole

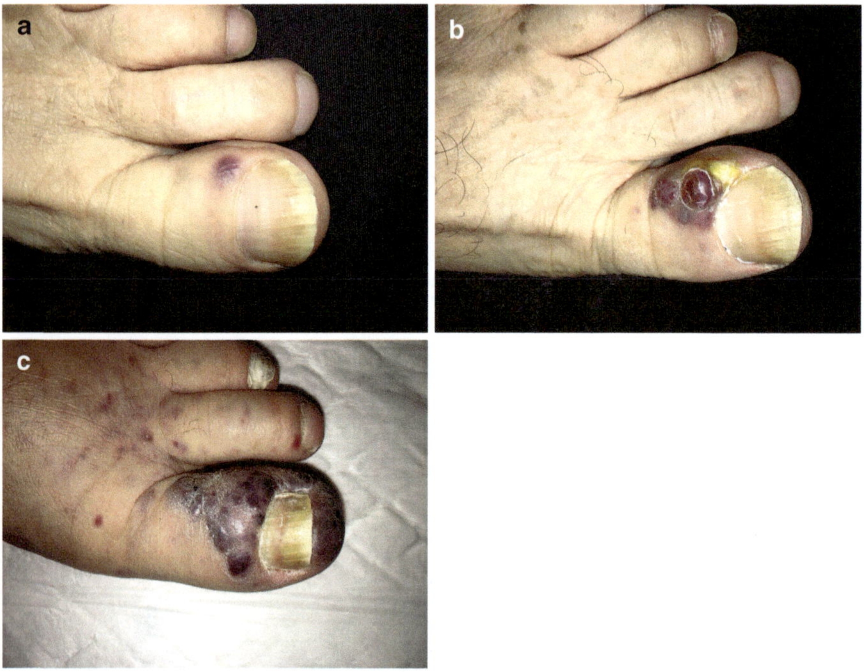

Fig. 11 Kaposi sarcoma affecting the first toe of a lung transplant recipient. (**a**) Presenting lesion as a papule. (**b**) Progression of the lesion instead of reducing immunosuppression and conversion to mTOR inhibitor. (**c**) Progression to a large plaque affecting 60% of the dorsum of the toe and satellite lesions on the dorsum of the foot

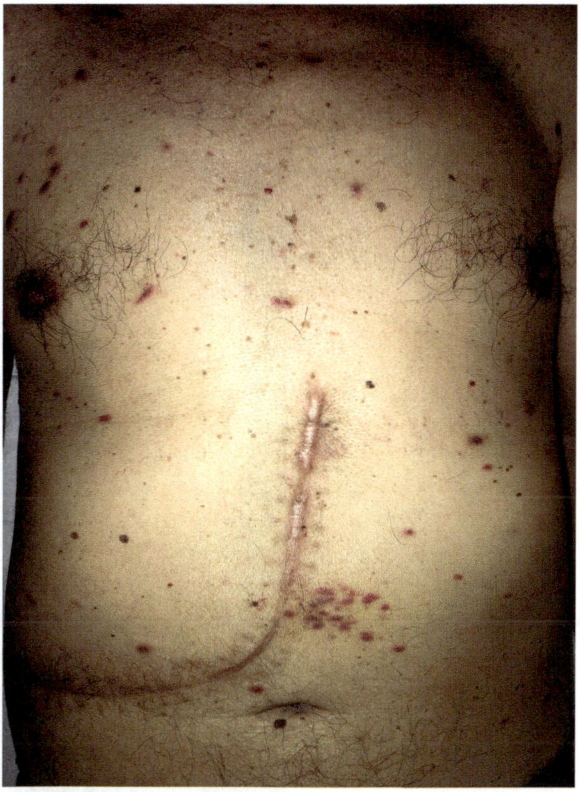

Fig. 12 Generalized papular Kaposi sarcoma in a liver transplant recipient

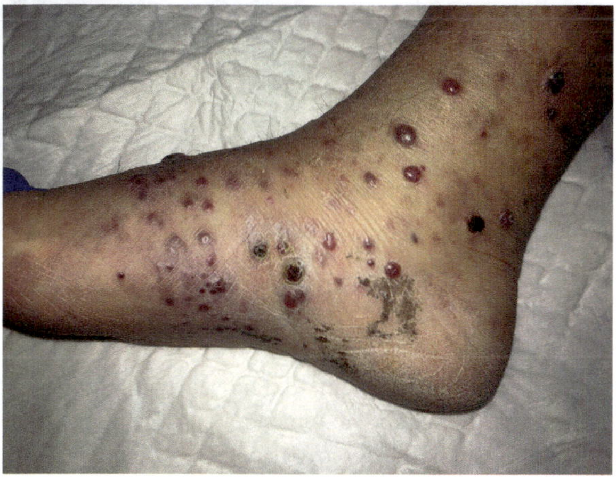

Fig. 13 Multiple papular lesions of Kaposi sarcoma progressing along the lower leg in a lung transplant recipient

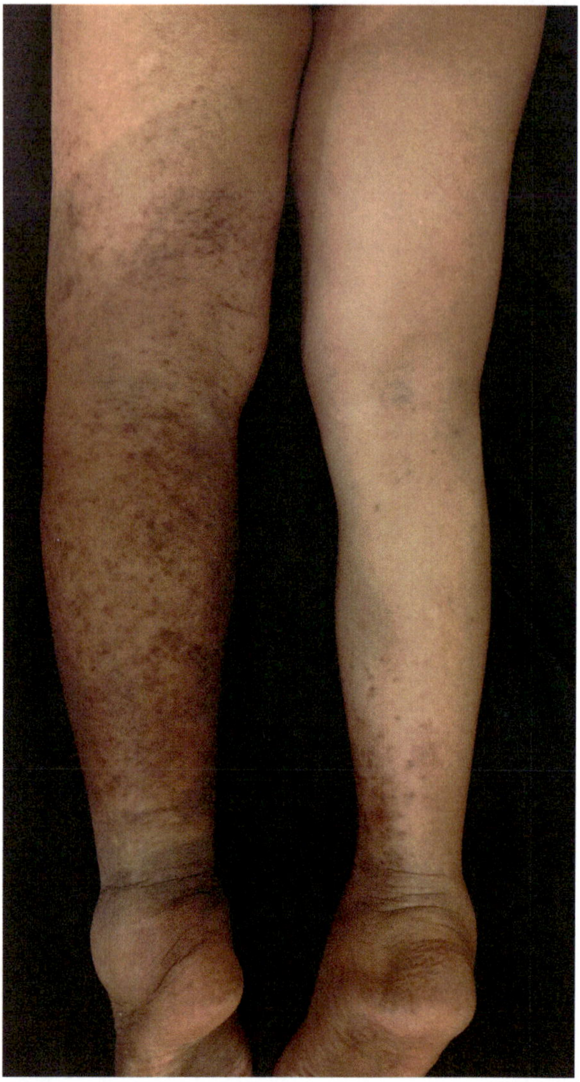

Fig. 14 Diffuse Kaposi sarcoma affecting both lower limbs in a lung transplant recipient that required treatment with liposomal doxorubicin

4.3 Radiology

Organ transplant recipients diagnosed with Kaposi sarcoma should undergo both CT scan of thorax and abdomen and esophagogastroduodenoscopy/colonoscopy to rule out the possibility of visceral involvement. Suspicious pulmonary lesions require bronchoscopy and subsequent biopsy to evaluate for lung involvement and, then, fine needle aspiration for lymph node involvement if warranted [3, 5].

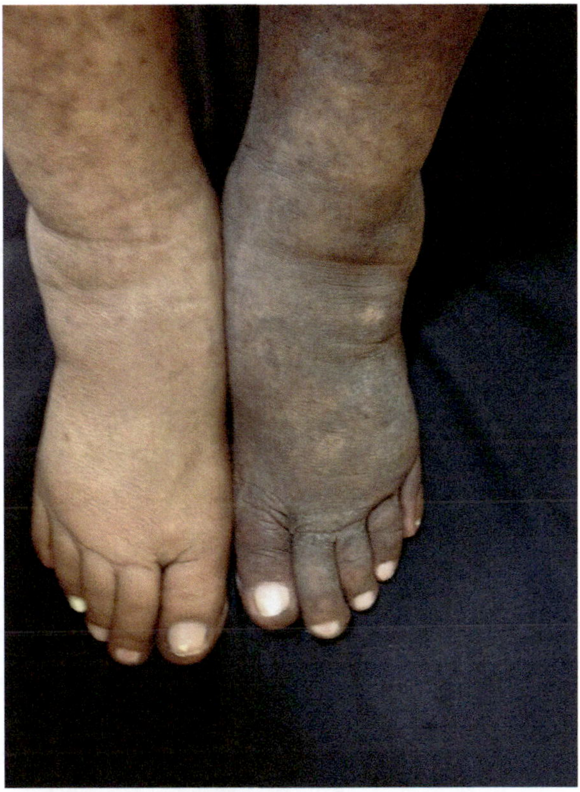

Fig. 15 Diffuse lymphedema secondary to the presence of diffuse Kaposi sarcoma on the leg

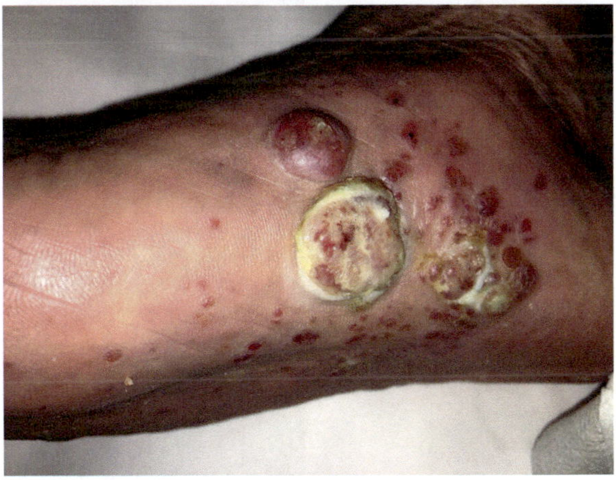

Fig. 16 Tumoral ulcerated Kaposi sarcoma on the sole of a kidney transplant recipient superinfected by *Pseudomonas aeruginosa*

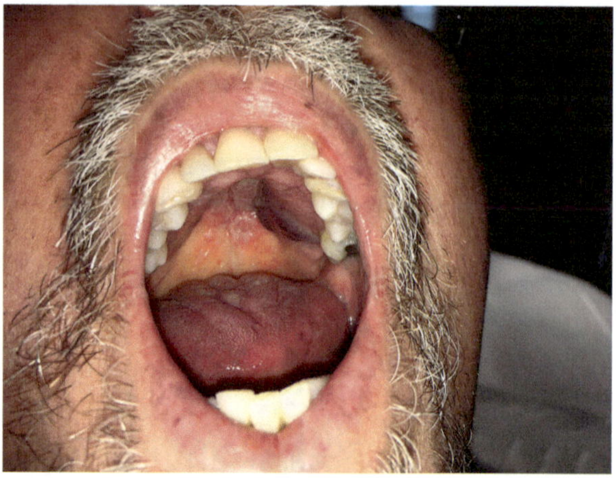

Fig. 17 Mucosal plaque of Kaposi sarcoma on the palate of a kidney transplant recipient

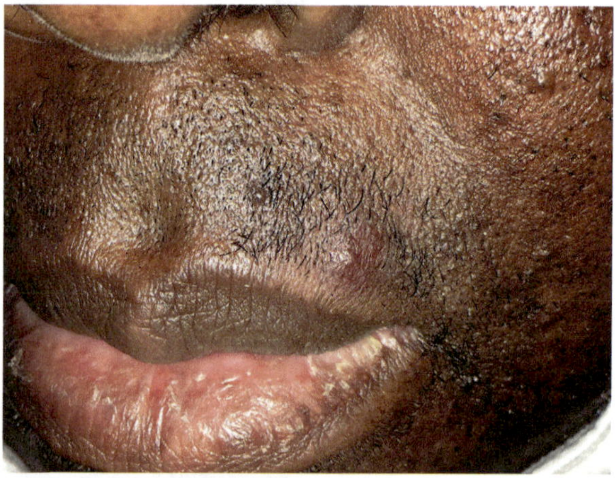

Fig. 18 Isolated violaceous papule as presenting sign of Kaposi sarcoma in a lung transplant recipient

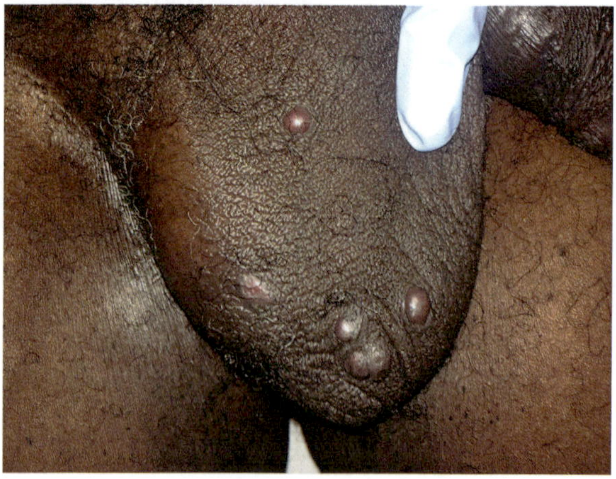

Fig. 19 Papular lesions of Kaposi sarcoma on the scrotum

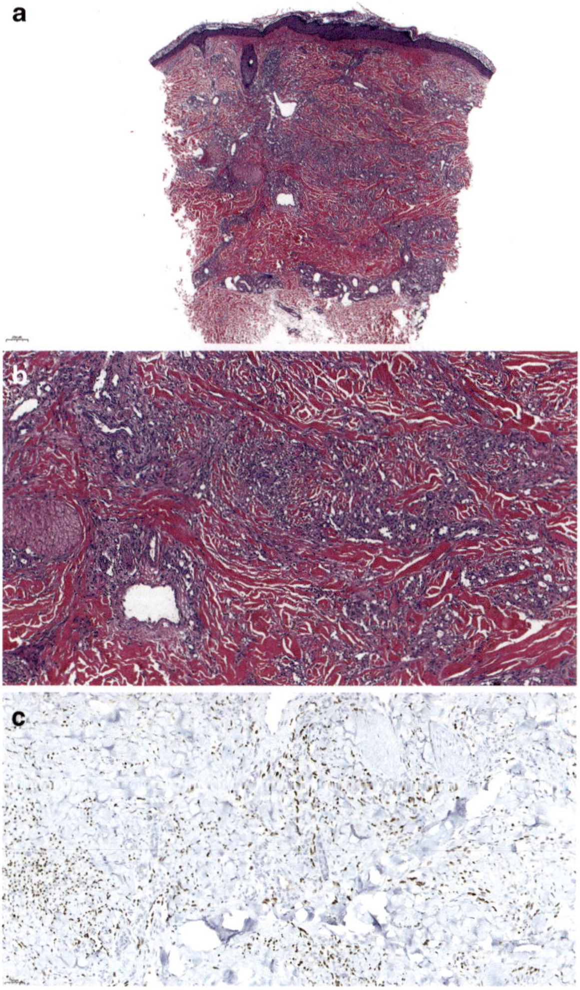

Fig. 20 Histology of early patch-stage lesion of Kaposi sarcoma. (**a**) Hypercellularity around *adnexae* and blood vessels. Increased cellularity consists of both Kaposi sarcoma cells and inflammatory cells (Hematoxylin-eosin, magnification 10×). (**b**) Angulated enlarged and ectatic vessels in the dermis with spindle-cell proliferation (Hematoxylin-eosin, magnification 40×). (**c**) Immunohistochemistry staining for LANA-1, showing tumor cells with a latent HHV-8 infection (magnification 100×). (*Images courtesy of Berta Ferrer Fàbregas, MD, Dermatopathologist, Vall d'Hebron Hospital, Barcelona*)

4.4 Other HHV-8 Diagnostic Tools

Apart from immunohistochemistry using a monoclonal antibody against LANA-1 on paraffin-embedded sections, no other specific HHV-8 tool is routinely used [2]. The utility of quantification of HHV-8 load in peripheral blood mononuclear cells by polymerase chain reaction at diagnosis or during follow-up is controversial. Some studies have found a correlation to the risk of progression while others did not find any clinical usefulness for clinical practice [5].

The only validated staging classification is for AIDS-associated Kaposi sarcoma. Patient management should distinguish three situations: localized non-aggressive, locally aggressive, and disseminated Kaposi sarcoma [2].

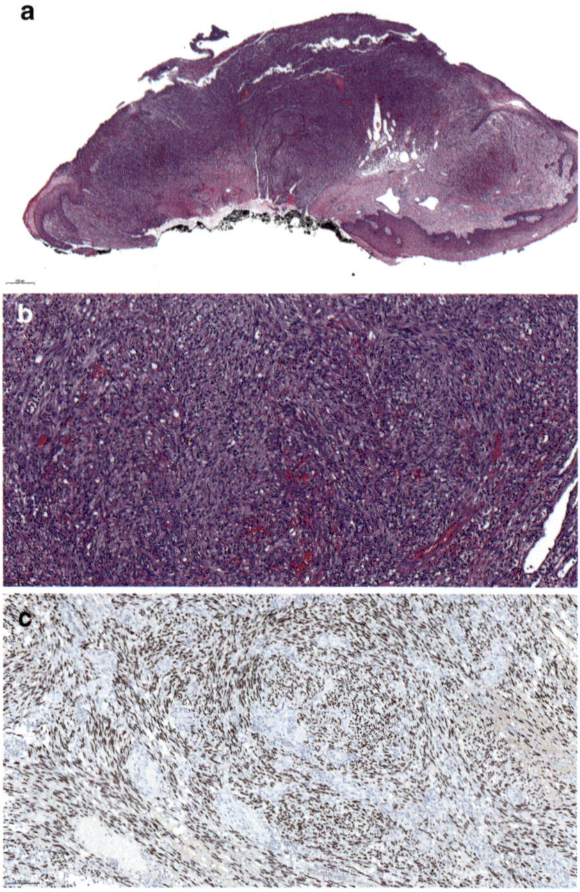

Fig. 21 Histology of tumoral lesion of Kaposi sarcoma. (**a**) Dense hypercellular infiltrate affecting the whole dermis with superficial ulceration (Hematoxylin-eosin, magnification 10×). (**b**) Very dense infiltrate of elongated spindle-cells, abnormal vessels with thinned epithelium, extravasated erythrocytes, and scattered chronic inflammatory cells (Hematoxylin-eosin, magnification 100×). (**c**) Immunohistochemistry staining for LANA-1, showing tumor cells with a latent HHV-8 infection (magnification 100×). (*Images courtesy of Berta Ferrer Fàbregas, MD, Dermatopathologist, Vall d'Hebron Hospital, Barcelona*)

5 Treatment

The management of posttransplant Kaposi sarcoma differs from the classical and HIV-associated variants. Therapeutic management is still a challenge because it requires controlling the disease while concomitantly attempting to maintain allograft function, which is critically important in case of liver, lung, or heart transplantation. Thus, the goal of treatment is to achieve a vital balance between minimizing immunosuppression and averting graft rejection. However, it is important to note complete regression of Kaposi sarcoma lesions is not necessarily the gold standard in therapy. Transplant recipients and providers may prefer to preserve adequate graft function and accept that a few stable and asymptomatic cutaneous lesions will persist. Further, remission after decreasing immunosuppression alone is achieved in 30–50% of cases based on retrospective series [31].

Mammalian Target of Rapamycin (mTOR) inhibitors (sirolimus and everolimus) are a group of immunosuppressants with antiproliferative and antiangiogenic properties [32]. These agents have been associated with a lower risk of skin cancer, including keratinocyte cancers and Kaposi sarcoma [7, 33]. Since the arrival of these new drugs at the beginning of the twenty-first century, the management of posttransplant Kaposi sarcoma has changed significantly. In 2005, conversion to mTOR inhibitors was shown to have a therapeutic effect with conversion from CNIs or purine antagonists to sirolimus inducing responses in 72–100% of patients [34, 35]. Stallone et al. demonstrated, in 15 patients with posttransplant Kaposi sarcoma, complete remission of all cutaneous lesions 3 months after sirolimus therapy was begun and cyclosporine therapy was stopped. No acute episodes of rejection or changes in kidney-graft function were reported [34]. Further studies confirmed the efficacy of CNIs withdrawal and switch to mTOR inhibitors in the management of posttransplant Kaposi sarcoma [3, 33, 36, 37]. However, relapse and the apparent absence of remission in patients with visceral Kaposi sarcoma were reported in a significant proportion of patients treated with sirolimus [38]. The switch from CNIs to sirolimus was performed either immediately after Kaposi sarcoma diagnosis concomitant with withdrawal of other immunosuppressive drugs, or less often, after several months of tapering immunosuppressive therapy to the lowest possible level. The benefit of conversion to an mTOR inhibitor is likely higher when performed soon after onset of lesions.

A recent multicenter retrospective cohort study including 145 solid organ transplant recipients from Europe reported response rate of 80% of patients treated only with immunosuppression reduction and conversion to mTOR inhibitors, with low rates of Kaposi sarcoma-related deaths [3]. Though the switch to mTOR inhibitors has become part of the standard management of posttransplant Kaposi sarcoma, Lebbe et al. noted in 2006 that this strategy could prove either transiently or ineffective in a subset of patients with severe disease [35]. Additionally, Delyon et al. also observed a significantly higher long-term risk of disease progression in SOTR who received mTOR inhibitors [3]. Immunosuppression was also minimized in almost all cases included in this study and 50% of complete remission were achieved solely by a decrease of immunosuppression [3].

When SOTR with Kaposi sarcoma fails to respond to reduction of immunosuppression or conversion to an mTOR inhibitor, or changes in immunosuppressive therapy are contraindicated, it may then be managed similarly to classic Kaposi sarcoma. Following an insufficient response to modification of immunosuppression, next steps include systemic chemotherapy, particularly in cases of extensive, symptomatic visceral Kaposi sarcoma or rapidly progressing disease [35]. Higher response rates have been observed when combining short-term chemotherapy with mTOR inhibitors conversion [3]. Chemotherapy including single agent or combinations has been proposed, with none notably superior to another, including liposomal anthracycline (doxorubicin, daunorubicin) or taxanes (paclitaxel or docetaxel). Importantly, interferon alfa is generally not recommended after organ transplantation because its use is associated with higher rejection risk [2].

Local treatments with surgical or laser removal or cryotherapy may be indicated for sporadic, well-defined, limited, and superficial lesions. As Kaposi sarcoma affects predominantly transplant recipients of color, patients must be counselled regarding the risk of hypopigmentation after cryotherapy. Intralesional chemotherapy, including intralesional vincristine or vinblastine, has demonstrated partial response rates, with recurrences 5–6 months after [39]. Electrochemotherapy is another procedure, which combines intralesional or intravenous low-dose chemotherapy, usually bleomycin, and electroporation, enhancing drug uptake into tumoral cells. In several prospective trials, complete response in about 65–89% of cases after 1–3 sessions have been observed although iatrogenic Kaposi sarcoma were excluded from the trials [40, 41].

Finally, radiotherapy ranks among the most effective treatments for all forms of localized Kaposi sarcoma [2]. It requires, however, a careful balance as it induces rapid regression of the lesions but also increases the long-term risk of developing cutaneous carcinomas and chronic lymphedema. The latter may create clinical challenges in the diagnosis of a recurrent disease and also confounds the application of further treatments in these cases.

Anecdotally, other treatments have been tried in SOTR with partial responses. Topical 5% imiquimod achieved complete response in 1 of 2 treated patients. The second had a clinical response but histology showed persistence of disease [42]. Topical 9-cis-retinoid acid (alitretinoin gel 0.1%) has also been used in Kaposi sarcoma with responses in one-third to one-half of patients [43]. Local irritation and inflammation are common side effects of both treatments.

6 Prognosis

Treatment of posttransplant Kaposi sarcoma is likely to result in an improved prognosis of Kaposi sarcoma. Initial registries of transplant recipients with Kaposi sarcoma reported disease-associated death of 11% in patients with only cutaneous lesions and as high as 57% in patients with visceral involvement [31]. Now, with the introduction of mTOR inhibitors, Kaposi sarcoma-associated mortality has decreased significantly.

References

1. Douglas JL, Gustin JK, Dezube B, Pantanowitz JL, Moses AV. Kaposi's sarcoma: a model of both malignancy and chronic inflammation. Panminerva Med. 2007;49(3):119–38.
2. Lebbe C, Garbe C, Stratigos AJ, et al. Diagnosis and treatment of Kaposi's sarcoma: European consensus-based interdisciplinary guideline (EDF/EADO/EORTC). Eur J Cancer (Oxford, England). 1990;2019(114):117–27. https://doi.org/10.1016/j.ejca.2018.12.036.
3. Delyon J, Rabate C, Euvrard S, et al. Management of Kaposi sarcoma after solid organ transplantation: a European retrospective study. J Am Acad Dermatol. 2019;81(2):448–55. https://doi.org/10.1016/j.jaad.2019.03.028.

4. Zavos G, Bokos J, Papaconstantinou I, et al. Clinicopathological aspects of 18 Kaposi's sarcoma among 1055 Greek renal transplant recipients. Artif Organs. 2004;28(6):595–9. https://doi.org/10.1111/j.1525-1594.2004.00019.x.
5. González-Cruz C, Ferrándiz-Pulido C, Ferrer Fàbregas B, García-Patos Briones V. Posttransplant Kaposi sarcoma: analysis of a series of 13 patients. Med Clin (Barc). 2021. Published online Jul 7. pii: S0025-7753(21)00335-3. https://doi.org/10.1016/j.medcli.2021.04.030.
6. Woodle ES, Hanaway M, Buell J, et al. Kaposi sarcoma: an analysis of the US and international experiences from the Israel Penn International Transplant Tumor Registry. Transplant Proc. 2001;33(7–8):3660–1. https://doi.org/10.1016/s0041-1345(01)02577-5.
7. Euvrard S, Kanitakis J, Claudy A. Skin cancers after organ transplantation. N Engl J Med. 2003;348(17):1681–91. https://doi.org/10.1056/NEJMra022137.
8. Mbulaiteye SM, Pfeiffer RM, Engels EA, et al. Detection of Kaposi sarcoma-associated herpesvirus DNA in saliva and buffy-coat samples from children with sickle cell disease in Uganda. J Infect Dis. 2004;190(8):1382–6. https://doi.org/10.1086/424489.
9. Engels EA, Pfeiffer RM, Fraumeni JF, et al. Spectrum of cancer risk among US solid organ transplant recipients. JAMA. 2011;306(17):1891–901. https://doi.org/10.1001/jama.2011.1592.
10. Tessari G, Naldi L, Boschiero L, et al. Incidence and clinical predictors of a subsequent nonmelanoma skin cancer in solid organ transplant recipients with a first nonmelanoma skin cancer: a multicenter cohort study. Arch Dermatol. 2010;146(3):294–9. https://doi.org/10.1001/archdermatol.2009.377.
11. Moosa MR. Kaposi's sarcoma in kidney transplant recipients: a 23-year experience. QJM Mon J Assoc Physicians. 2005;98(3):205–14. https://doi.org/10.1093/qjmed/hci028.
12. Oettle AG. Geographical and racial differences in the frequency of Kaposi's sarcoma as evidence of environmental or genetic causes. Acta Unio Int Contra Cancrum. 1962;18:330–63.
13. Farge D. Kaposi's sarcoma in organ transplant recipients. The Collaborative Transplantation Research Group of Ile de France. Eur J Med. 1993;2(6):339–43.
14. Duman S, Töz H, Aşçi G, et al. Successful treatment of post-transplant Kaposi's sarcoma by reduction of immunosuppression. Nephrol Dial Transplant. 2002;17(5):892–6. https://doi.org/10.1093/ndt/17.5.892.
15. Qunibi W, Akhtar M, Sheth K, et al. Kaposi's sarcoma: the most common tumor after renal transplantation in Saudi Arabia. Am J Med. 1988;84(2):225–32. https://doi.org/10.1016/0002-9343(88)90418-4.
16. Kentley J, Allawh R, Rao S, et al. The burden of cutaneous disease in solid organ transplant recipients of color. Am J Transplant. 2021;21(3):1215–26. https://doi.org/10.1111/ajt.16210.
17. Andreoni M, Goletti D, Pezzotti P, et al. Prevalence, incidence and correlates of HHV-8/KSHV infection and Kaposi's sarcoma in renal and liver transplant recipients. J Infect. 2001;43(3):195–9. https://doi.org/10.1053/jinf.2001.0899.
18. Aseni P, Vertemati M, Minola E, et al. Kaposi's sarcoma in liver transplant recipients: morphological and clinical description. Liver Transplant. 2001;7(9):816–23. https://doi.org/10.1053/jlts.2001.26925.
19. Sitas F, Carrara H, Beral V, et al. Antibodies against human herpesvirus 8 in black South African patients with cancer. N Engl J Med. 1999;340(24):1863–71. https://doi.org/10.1056/NEJM199906173402403.
20. Stein L, Carrara H, Norman R, Alagiozoglou L, Morris L, Sitas F. Antibodies against human herpesvirus 8 in South African renal transplant recipients and blood donors. Transplant Infect Dis. 2004;6(2):69–73. https://doi.org/10.1111/j.1399-3062.2004.00061.x.
21. Mariggiò G, Koch S, Schulz TF. Kaposi sarcoma herpesvirus pathogenesis. Philos Trans R Soc Lond Ser B Biol Sci. 2017;372(1732):20160275. https://doi.org/10.1098/rstb.2016.0275.
22. Chang Y, Cesarman E, Pessin MS, et al. Identification of herpesvirus-like DNA sequences in AIDS-associated Kaposi's sarcoma. Science. 1994;266(5192):1865–9. https://doi.org/10.1126/science.7997879.

23. Hong Y-K, Foreman K, Shin JW, et al. Lymphatic reprogramming of blood vascular endothelium by Kaposi sarcoma-associated herpesvirus. Nat Genet. 2004;36(7):683–5. https://doi.org/10.1038/ng1383.
24. Radu O, Pantanowitz L. Kaposi sarcoma. Arch Pathol Lab Med. 2013;137(2):289–94. https://doi.org/10.5858/arpa.2012-0101-RS.
25. Marcelin A-G, Roque-Afonso A-M, Hurtova M, et al. Fatal disseminated Kaposi's sarcoma following human herpesvirus 8 primary infections in liver-transplant recipients. Liver Transplant. 2004;10(2):295–300. https://doi.org/10.1002/lt.20058.
26. Regamey N, Tamm M, Wernli M, et al. Transmission of human herpesvirus 8 infection from renal-transplant donors to recipients. N Engl J Med. 1998;339(19):1358–63. https://doi.org/10.1056/NEJM199811053391903.
27. Hussein MM, Mooij JM, Roujouleh HM. Regression of post-transplant Kaposi's sarcoma after replacing cyclosporine with mycophenolate mofetil. Saudi J Kidney Dis Transplant. 2001;12(1):42–4.
28. Montagnino G, Bencini PL, Tarantino A, Caputo R, Ponticelli C. Clinical features and course of Kaposi's sarcoma in kidney transplant patients: report of 13 cases. Am J Nephrol. 1994;14(2):121–6. https://doi.org/10.1159/000168700.
29. Milliancourt C, Barete S, Marcelin AG, et al. Human herpesvirus-8 seroconversions after renal transplantation. Transplantation. 2001;72(7):1319–20. https://doi.org/10.1097/00007890-200110150-00023.
30. Vella JP, Mosher R, Sayegh MH. Kaposi's sarcoma after renal transplantation. N Engl J Med. 1997;336(24):1761. https://doi.org/10.1056/nejm199706123362416.
31. Penn I. Kaposi's sarcoma in transplant recipients. Transplantation. 1997;64(5):669–73. https://doi.org/10.1097/00007890-199709150-00001.
32. Geissler EK, Schlitt HJ, Thomas G. mTOR, cancer and transplantation. Am J Transplant. 2008;8(11):2212–8. https://doi.org/10.1111/j.1600-6143.2008.02391.x.
33. Campistol JM, Schena FP. Kaposi's sarcoma in renal transplant recipients—the impact of proliferation signal inhibitors. Nephrol Dial Transplant. 2007;22(Suppl 1):i17–22. https://doi.org/10.1093/ndt/gfm089.
34. Stallone G, Schena A, Infante B, et al. Sirolimus for Kaposi's sarcoma in renal-transplant recipients. N Engl J Med. 2005;352(13):1317–23. https://doi.org/10.1056/NEJMoa042831.
35. Lebbé C, Euvrard S, Barrou B, et al. Sirolimus conversion for patients with posttransplant Kaposi's sarcoma. Am J Transplant. 2006;6(9):2164–8. https://doi.org/10.1111/j.1600-6143.2006.01412.x.
36. Gutiérrez-Dalmau A, Sánchez-Fructuoso A, Sanz-Guajardo A, et al. Efficacy of conversion to sirolimus in posttransplantation Kaposi's sarcoma. Transplant Proc. 2005;37(9):3836–8. https://doi.org/10.1016/j.transproceed.2005.10.076.
37. Hernández-Sierra A, Rovira J, Petit A, et al. Role of HHV-8 and mTOR pathway in post-transplant Kaposi sarcoma staging. Transplant Int. 2016;29(9):1008–16. https://doi.org/10.1111/tri.12800.
38. Monaco AP. The role of mTOR inhibitors in the management of posttransplant malignancy. Transplantation. 2009;87(2):157–63. https://doi.org/10.1097/TP.0b013e318193886e.
39. Brambilla L, Bellinvia M, Tourlaki A, Scoppio B, Gaiani F, Boneschi V. Intralesional vincristine as first-line therapy for nodular lesions in classic Kaposi sarcoma: a prospective study in 151 patients. Br J Dermatol. 2010;162(4):854–9. https://doi.org/10.1111/j.1365-2133.2009.09601.x.
40. Di Monta G, Caracò C, Benedetto L, et al. Electrochemotherapy as "new standard of care" treatment for cutaneous Kaposi's sarcoma. Eur J Surg Oncol. 2014;40(1):61–6. https://doi.org/10.1016/j.ejso.2013.09.002.
41. Curatolo P, Quaglino P, Marenco F, et al. Electrochemotherapy in the treatment of Kaposi sarcoma cutaneous lesions: a two-center prospective phase II trial. Ann Surg Oncol. 2012;19(1):192–8. https://doi.org/10.1245/s10434-011-1860-7.

42. Prinz Vavricka BM, Hofbauer GFL, Dummer R, French LE, Kempf W. Topical treatment of cutaneous Kaposi sarcoma with imiquimod 5% in renal-transplant recipients: a clinicopathological observation. Clin Exp Dermatol. 2012;37(6):620–5. https://doi.org/10.1111/j.1365-2230.2011.04278.x.
43. Bodsworth NJ, Bloch M, Bower M, Donnell D, Yocum R, International Panretin Gel KS Study Group. Phase III vehicle-controlled, multi-centered study of topical alitretinoin gel 0.1% in cutaneous AIDS-related Kaposi's sarcoma. Am J Clin Dermatol. 2001;2(2):77–87. https://doi.org/10.2165/00128071-200102020-00004.

Lymphoproliferative Diseases

Adriana Maria Porro and Camila Arai Seque Ouki

1 Introduction

The increased risk of malignancy, including lymphoid tumors, in solid organ transplant recipients (SOTR) has been recognized for many years [1–3]. Posttransplant lymphoproliferative disorders (PTLD) represent immunosuppression-related lymphoid proliferation that occur in the setting of solid organ transplantation (SOT) and bone marrow transplantation [4]. PTLD represents a heterogeneous group of abnormal lymphoid proliferations, generally of B cells, that occur in the setting of ineffective T-cell function because of pharmacologic immunosuppression after organ transplantation [5]. It is one of the most serious complications among SOTR, reducing both patient and organ survival [6]. Although most cases are due to Epstein Barr virus (EBV) infection, as manifested by the presence of EBV within the malignant tissue, EBV-negative disease is becoming increasingly common [4, 7].

2 Epidemiology

PTLD is the most common non-skin cancer in SOTR, comprising approximately 20% of all cancers after transplantation [8–10]. The incidence varies by type of transplant, age of the patient, and degree of immunosuppression. It is more common in pediatric patients owing to high rates of EBV seronegativity at the time of transplantation although there appears to be a decline in rates that may be attributed to factors such as changes in immunosuppression and increased monitoring of EBV

A. M. Porro · C. A. S. Ouki (✉)
Department of Dermatology, Escola Paulista de Medicina, Universidade Federal de São Paulo, São Paulo, Brazil

J. Tomimori et al. (eds.), *Atlas of Dermatologic Diseases in Solid Organ Transplant Recipients*, https://doi.org/10.1007/978-3-031-13335-0_16

viral loads with preemptive reduction of immunosuppression [11]. The incidence of PTLD is higher after intestinal, lung and heart-lung transplantation, whereas lower rates are reported after liver and kidney transplantation [12]. The incidence density for PTLD according to the U.S. National Transplant Database ranged in 2012 from 1.58 per 1000 person-years (kidney) to 2.24 (heart), 2.44 (liver), and 5.72 (lung) [13]. In the French PTLD registry, cumulative incidence was 1% by 5 years and 2.1% by 10 years [14]. In adults, the incidence rates in kidney and liver transplant recipients are approximately 1–3% [4] and continues to decrease with age [10]. PTLD is most likely to develop during the first year after transplantation. The incidence in the first year is 224 per 100,000 but decreases to 54 per 100,000 in the second year and continues to decrease [15]. In kidney transplant patients, early PTLD (occurring within the first-year posttransplantation) has been reported in 0.46 per 100 person years [16].

The main risk factors for the development of early PTLD are the EBV serostatus of the recipient and the degree of T-cell immunosuppression. The incidence of PTLD in EBV-seronegative recipients is higher than for EBV-seropositive recipients because patients who were not exposed to EBV before transplantation usually acquire the infection from the donor [17]. This likely accounts for the observation that PTLD is more common in children than in adults, as already mentioned [18]. The degree of immunosuppression is also an important factor in the development of PTLD, with the degree of T-cell immunosuppression being of greater importance than the degree of B-cell immunosuppression [4]. The role of each immunosuppressive drug is difficult to assess in terms of risk of PTLD development [19], especially as transplant recipients receive a combination of drugs for induction, maintenance, and sometimes rejection treatment. The role of maintenance immunosuppression drugs (tacrolimus, mycophenolate, azathioprine, cyclosporine, and mTOR inhibitors) is not clear and data are partly contradictory [12]. Older age (>60 years) and long-term immunosuppression are the most recognized risk factors for late PTLD (1 year after transplantation) [14, 20].

3 Pathogenesis

The majority of PTLD are related to EBV infection. EBV is a member of the herpesvirus family first implicated as a cause for malignancy in 1964, in Burkitt's lymphoma [21]. Since then, it has also been implicated as a causative factor in nasopharyngeal carcinoma and Hodgkin's disease, as well as PTLD. EBV infects and immortalizes B cells in more than 90% of humans, persisting for the lifetime. It is transmitted via oral secretions, blood, transplanted allogeneic hematopoietic cells, or solid donor organs [22]. EBV infection is generally asymptomatic in children but occurring during adolescence or adulthood results in infectious mononucleosis, characterized by the triad of fever, lymphadenopathy, and pharyngitis [23]. During primary EBV infection in immunocompetent people, the EBV genome forms an episome that remains latent in resting memory B cells, and these latently infected B lymphocytes are controlled by cytotoxic T cells (CTLs) [23]. However, in certain immunocompromised patients, the critical T-cell control of B-cell growth is lacking, with proliferation of EBV-infected B cells, resulting in hyperplasia or malignancy, including PTLD [23]. After solid organ transplantation, the EBV-infected cells that give rise to PTLD are typically of host origin, representing reactivation of a latent EBV infection and manifesting as a multisystem disease. Primary EBV infection may also cause PTLD, but this more commonly occurs in children who have not had prior EBV infection [24].

Most cases of PTLD are associated with EBV infection, but there are cases with no evidence of EBV involvement. A study of 176 SOTR with PTLD demonstrated that the proportion of EBV-negative PTLD cases is increasing [7]. This subtype has distinct characteristics from the EBV-positive PTLD: a later onset of disease (median of 50 months posttransplant), monomorphic histology, and a more aggressive course (reported median survival of 1 month) [7, 25, 26].

4 Clinical Presentation

PTLD can develop at any time after transplantation, but approximately 60% of patients present with early PTLD, within 1 year after transplantation. The median onset of disease in the solid organ transplant population is 6 months. However, cases have been reported as early as 1 week and as late as 17 years posttransplantation [27–30].

The clinical presentation of PTLD is highly variable. Symptoms may be related to viral infection, mass effect, organ dysfunction, or lymphoma-related B symptoms, depending on the type of PTLD, rate of progression, and involved organs. Some patients are asymptomatic while others can present nonspecific systemic symptoms (fever, weight loss, malaise, anemia, allograft dysfunction), or reflecting the localization of the mass (lymph node enlargement across one or several sites externally or internally) (Table 1). In more than one-half of cases, PTLD involves sites outside lymphoid tissue (i.e., extranodal), as the gastrointestinal tract, lungs, skin, liver, central nervous system (CNS), and the allograft itself. Involvement of the allograft can lead to allograft dysfunction (renal failure, heart failure, or respiratory dysfunction). PTLD may be difficult to distinguish from organ rejection and infections [4, 5, 31–33].

Table 1 PTLD systemic symptoms

Fever
Weight loss
Malaise
Anemia
Allograft dysfunction
Lymph node enlargement

4.1 PTLD and Skin

Cutaneous involvement in PTLD is relatively rare. Until 2004, there were only 19 cases reported and Beynet et al. published four additional patients, two after renal, one heart-lung, and one cardiac transplantation. In this report, all patients had late B-cell PTLD with a median of 8 years from organ allograft to tumor diagnosis. The extent, number, and anatomic location of skin lesions varied from a localized patch to widespread nodules. None of the patients exhibited systemic symptoms at the time of PTLD diagnosis. In situ hybridization detected EBV messenger RNA in three cases. The lesions responded to therapy in all patients, with a median follow-up of 2.5 years [34].

Another patient reported in 2004 had an EBV-positive B-cell PTLD 2 years after kidney transplant, confined to the skin. He presented multiple well-demarcated, violaceous, round to oval plaques of 0.5–3.0 cm diameter on the lower leg and had favorable outcome [35].

In 2010, Salama et al. reported four other patients with cutaneous PTLD after renal transplantation, three with B-cell lymphoma (all of them EBV-positive) and one with T-cell lymphoma. In three patients, PTLD was restricted to the skin and the fourth had a systemic B-cell lymphoma with primary cutaneous presentation. This last patient had an abdominal lymphoma and died of sepsis and the other three had favorable outcome. The patient's lesions were mostly erythematous nodules on the legs and abdominal skin [36].

Multicenter European case series published in 2013 by Seçkin et al. analyzed retrospectively 35 cases of primary cutaneous PTLD. The median interval between transplantation and diagnosis was 85 months. Fifty-seven percent of patients had a kidney transplant. Unlike other published cases, in this case series primary cutaneous T-cell PTLD (68.6%, 50% being mycosis fungoides) were more common than primary cutaneous B-cell PTLD (31.4%). Among the 11 cutaneous B-cell PTLD cases, 90.9% were classified as EBV-associated B-cell lymphoproliferations. Sixteen (45.7%) patients died after a median follow-up of 19.5 months [37].

In 2021, our group published four additional PTLD patients, two of them primarily cutaneous, and two systemic with secondary cutaneous manifestations. All had late onset: two patients 6 years after transplantation, one patient 15 years and the other 17 years after kidney transplantation. Two of these patients had monomorphic B-cell type PTLD, one monomorphic T-cell, and the other plasmacytic hyperplasia. The cutaneous lesions were a nodule on the scalp (Fig. 1a, b), a verrucous nodule on the face (Fig. 2a, b), a cellulitis-like plaque on the trunk (Fig. 3), and erythematous papules and nodules on the leg (Fig. 4). EBV was detected in two patients. Both patients with systemic disease had fatal outcome, and those with primary cutaneous involvement responded to treatment [30]. In sum, the main clinical characteristics of cutaneous PTLD seen in these most recently published case series were kidney transplant recipients, developing a late onset PTLD, with EBV positivity (in B-cell PTLD), and the cutaneous lesions presenting as erythematous and/or violaceous papules, nodules, and patches occurring in any part of the skin (Table 2). Prognosis depended on the presence of systemic disease, observed in the minority of these cases.

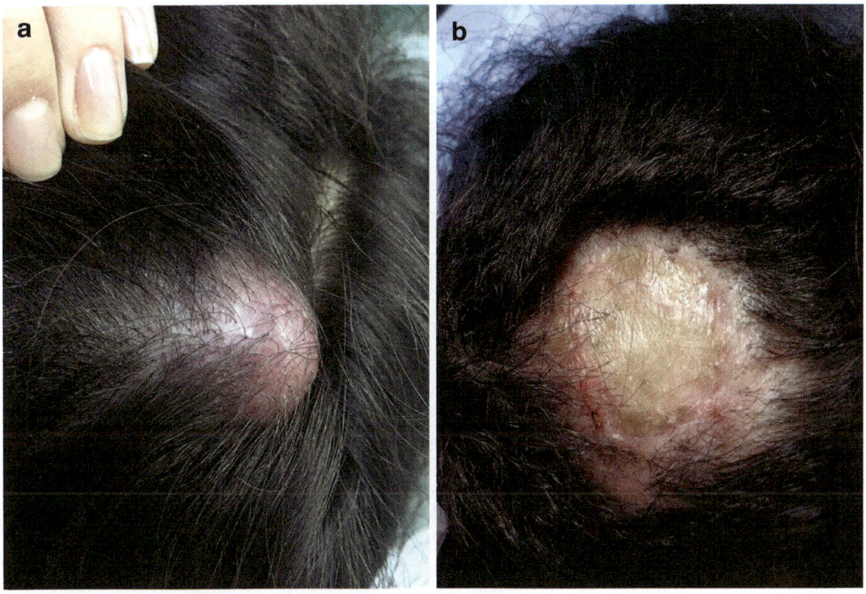

Fig. 1 (**a**) Erythematous indurated single nodule on the scalp corresponding to an early plasmacytic hyperplasia PTLD lesion (EBV-positive plasmocytoma-like PTLD) in a 51-year-old female with a history of 17-years kidney transplantation. Scalp computed tomography was unremarkable. Surgical removal and reduction of immunosuppression were performed. (**b**) Skin graft after surgical excision showing no recurrence after a 2-year follow-up

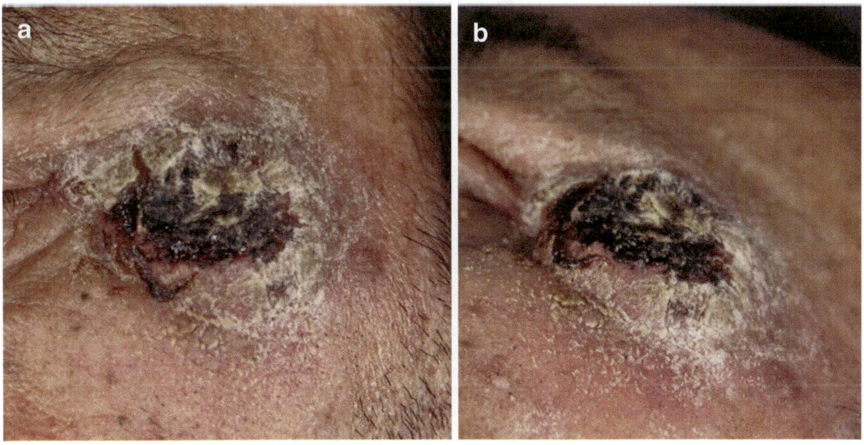

Fig. 2 (**a**) Periocular crusted ulcerated nodule with a rapid growth corresponding to a monomorphic CD30+ anaplastic T-cell PTLD in a 56-year-old male with a history of 6-years kidney transplantation. Imaging staging was unremarkable. Immunosuppression was discontinued and chemotherapy + radiotherapy were performed. Five months later, everolimus was introduced. There was no evidence of recurrence after 1-year follow-up. (**b**) Protuberance view of the same lesion

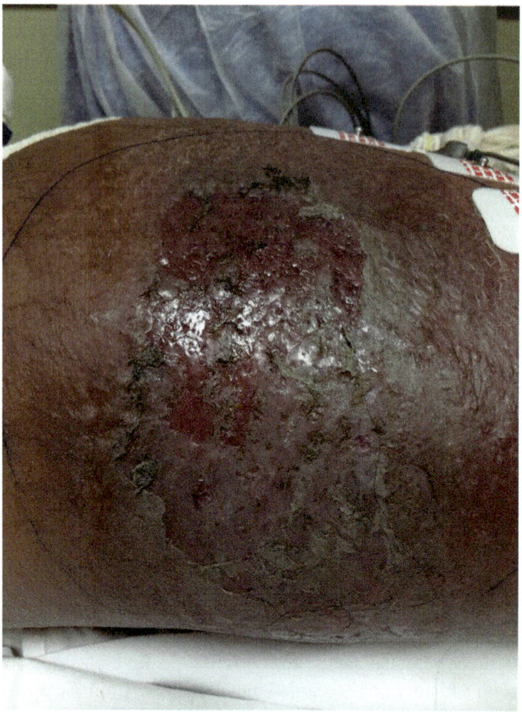

Fig. 3 Ulcerated cellulitis-like plaque on the lateral trunk corresponding to a secondary contiguous cutaneous involvement 2 months after primary gastrointestinal PTLD diagnosis in a 51-year-old female with a history of 6-years kidney transplantation. Chemotherapy was started but patient had a fatal outcome 12 days later

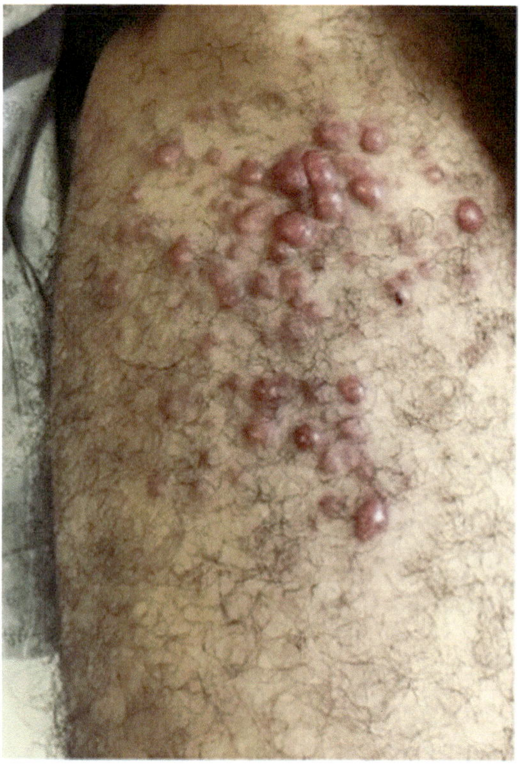

Fig. 4 Multiple erythematous papules and nodules associated with right inguinal hardened lymph node enlargement corresponding to monomorphic PTLD with secondary cutaneous involvement in a 43-year-old male with a history of 15-years kidney transplantation. Staging also revealed mediastinal, inguinal lymph nodes, and bone marrow impairment by lymphoma. There was no time to start treatment since patient died a few days after diagnosis

Table 2 PTLD cutaneous manifestations

Erythematous and/or violaceous: • Patches • Papules • Plaques (including cellulitis-like) • Nodules

Table 3 WHO classification for PTLD

Subtype		Clonal status	EBV status
Early lesions	Plasmacytic hyperplasia Infectious mononucleosis-like Florid follicular hyperplasia	Polyclonal	Generally EBV+
Polymorphic		Monoclonal	Generally EBV+
Monomorphic	B-cell lymphomas T/NK cell lymphomas	Monoclonal	Frequently EBV+ Rarely EBV+
Classic Hodgkin lymphoma-like		Monoclonal	Frequently EBV+

5 Classification

The World Health Organization classifies PTLD into six main categories according to histologic, immunophenotypic, genetic, and clinical features (Table 3) [38].

5.1 *Plasmacytic Hyperplasia and Infectious Mononucleosis-Like PTLDs*

Early lesions occur in children and adult SOTR without a prior EBV infection, mimicking plasmacytic hyperplasia and infectious mononucleosis-like features. Polyclonal B cells, plasma cells, and T cells form masses and the architecture of the underlying tissue is preserved (Fig. 5a–d). EBV is present in most cases. Extent of proliferation, clinical situation, and EBV status can differentiate early lesions of PTLD from reactive lymphoid hyperplasia, as they are both benign polyclonal lymphoproliferations.

5.2 *Florid Follicular Hyperplasia PTLD*

In 2016, WHO histological classification for PTLD incorporated florid follicular hyperplasia as a new form of early lesions based on chromosomal abnormalities that may lead to uncontrolled lymphoid proliferation [39]. Histology consists of polyclonal B cells merged in T cells and apparent hyperplastic germinal centers. EBV presence is variable.

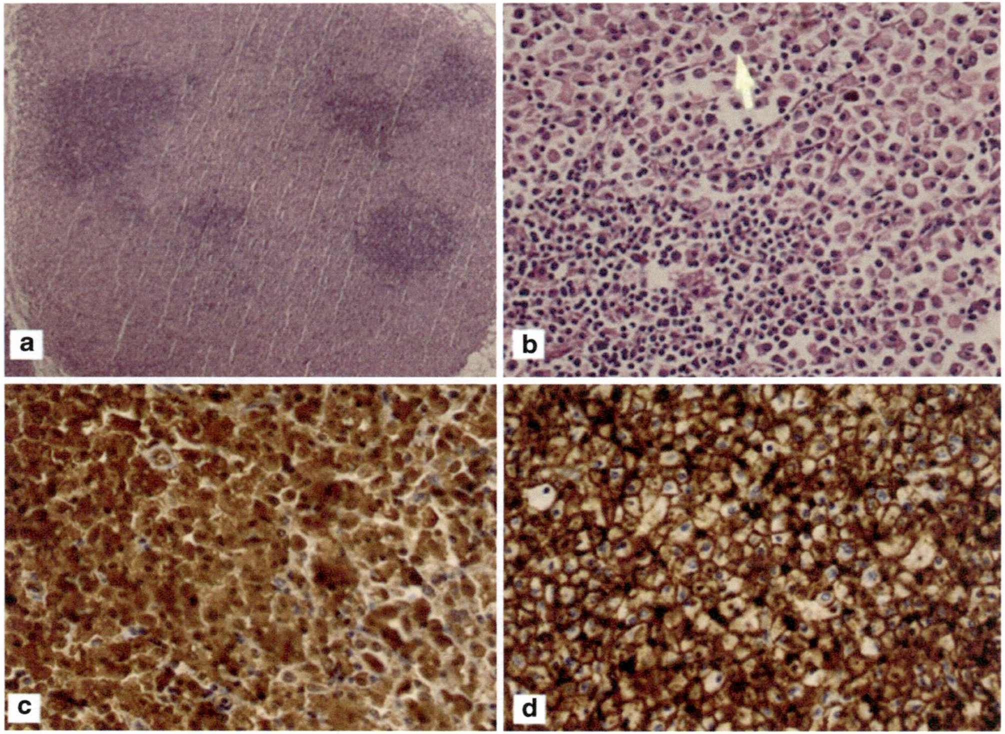

Fig. 5 Plasmacytic hyperplasia PTLD. (**a**) Scalp biopsy with diffuse proliferation of mature plasma cells, with lymphocyte aggregates (HE 40×). (**b**) In detail, the large amount of mature plasma cells (arrow) permeated by small lymphocytes (HE 400×). (**c**) Immunohistochemistry with intense Kappa marker immunoexpression (400×). (**d**) Immunohistochemistry with intense Lambda marker immunoexpression (400×), compatible with benign polyclonal lymphoproliferation and removing the possibility of plasmacytoma or myeloma—which are characterized by only one chain (kappa or lambda) immunoexpression

5.3 *Polymorphic PTLD*

Polymorphic PTLD demonstrates a polyclonal infiltrate composed of cells all along the spectrum of B-cell maturation (immunoblasts, plasma cells, and lymphoid cells) that disrupt the normal architecture of surrounding tissue and do not fulfill the criteria for any type of B-cell or T/NK (natural killer)-cell lymphomas recognized in immunocompetent patients. EBV is usually present. Polymorphic PTLD is the most common form of PTLD in children.

5.4 *Monomorphic PTLD*

Monomorphic PTLD is an heterogeneous group composed of monoclonal malignant B-cell or T-cell origin that must fulfill criteria for one of the B-cell or T/NK cell lymphomas recognized in immunocompetent hosts. Particularly, small B-cell lymphoid neoplasms (follicular lymphoma, small lymphocytic lymphoma) and marginal zone lymphomas (MALT) arising in the posttransplant setting are not considered PTLD. Histology of monomorphic lesions shows a lymphoid infiltrate and effacement of normal tissue architecture (Fig. 6a–d). Monomorphic PTLD is

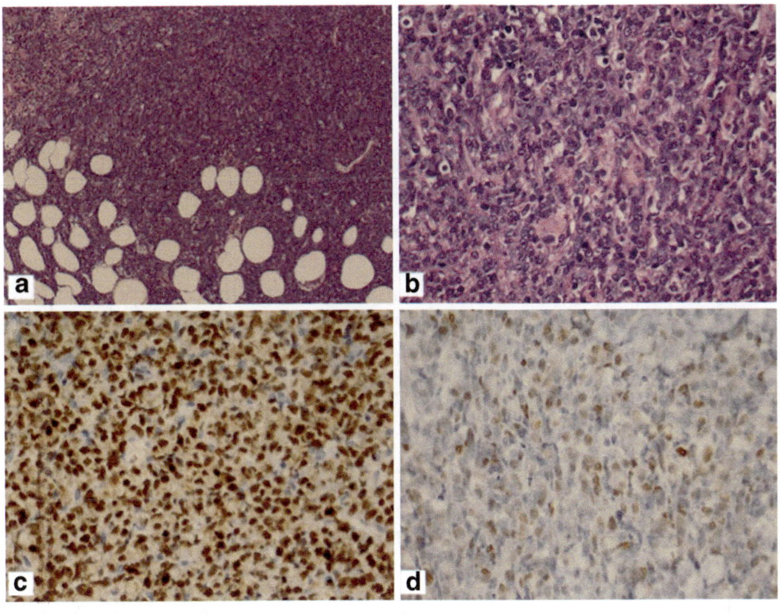

Fig. 6 Monomorphic B-cell PTLD. (**a**) Non-epidermotropic diffuse lymphocytic proliferation (HE 40×). (**b**) In detail, a mitotic figure in an area with intense diffuse atypical lymphoid proliferation (HE 400×). (**c**) Immunohistochemistry with positivity for MUM1, characterizing diffuse atypical lymphoid proliferation of B cells (400×). (**d**) In situ hybridization with immunoexpression of EBV marker (400×)

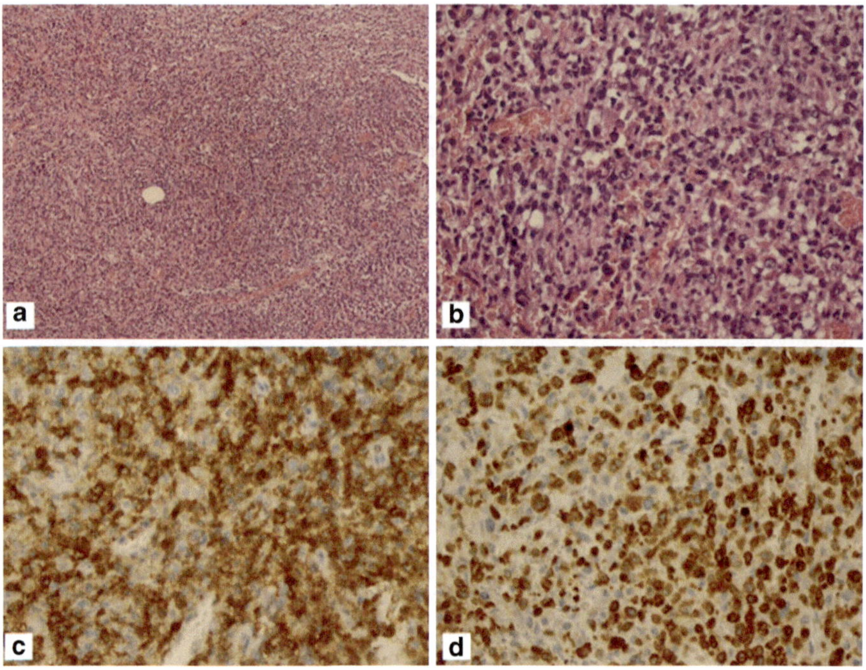

Fig. 7 Monomorphic CD30+ anaplastic T-cell PTLD. (**a**) Non-epidermotropic diffuse lymphocytic proliferation (HE 40×). (**b**) Diffuse atypical lymphoid proliferation (HE 400×). (**c**) Immunohistochemistry with positivity for CD4 (400×). (**d**) Immunohistochemistry with positivity for CD30 (400×), compatible with CD30+ anaplastic T-cell lymphoma

further classified based on the subtype of lymphoma. The vast majority resembles B-cell lymphomas, especially diffuse large B-cell lymphoma and less commonly Burkitt lymphoma or plasma cell neoplasm (e.g., myeloma or extramedullary plasmacytoma) [40]. Lymphomas of T/NK cell origin are uncommon, but when seen are usually classified as peripheral T-cell lymphoma not otherwise specified or EBV-positive T/NK cell lymphoma. T-cell PTDL is rarely reported [41] (Fig. 7a–d) although a European multicenter case series suggests that primary cutaneous T-cell PTLD are more common than primary cutaneous B-cell PTLD, similarly to the general population [37].

5.5 Classical Hodgkin Lymphoma-Like PTLD

Classical Hodgkin lymphoma-like is the least common form of PTLD, but when occurs, it is more frequent in renal transplant recipients. Histological criteria and EBV positivity fulfill the diagnosis of classic Hodgkin lymphoma, including

CD15 and CD30 expression, CD20 variable expression, and do not express CD3 or CD45.

Of note, indolent small B-cell lymphomas arising in transplant recipients are not included among the PTLDs.

6 Diagnosis and Staging

The diagnosis of PTLD relies on tissue biopsy, laboratory evaluation, and radiographic imaging (Table 4). There is no specific staging system for PTLD.

As in all lymphomas, diagnosis of PTLD requires tumor tissue histologic examination. Biopsy tissue should be reviewed by an expert hematopathologist for morphology, immunohistochemical, immunophenotyping evaluation, EBV presence, cytogenetics, and gene rearrangement studies [42].

Abnormal laboratory results in patients with suspected PTLD are similar to non-transplant patients with lymphoproliferative disorders and include unexplained anemia, thrombocytopenia and/or leukopenia, elevated lactate dehydrogenase levels (LDH), hyperuricemia, and the presence of monoclonal protein in serum or urine protein electrophoresis [43].

Contrast-enhanced computed tomography (CT) of the neck, chest, abdomen, and pelvis should be performed for disease extension measurement and is useful in monitoring treatment response. When available, a combined positron emission tomography (PET/CT) can identify metabolically active sites of disease that have not yet increased in size, and it is also better in detecting bone marrow involvement. Magnetic resonance imaging (MRI) is recommended to assess central nervous system disease if symptoms are present [44].

Table 4 Initial work up for PTLD diagnosis and staging

Tissue biopsy	Morphology Immunohistochemistry Immunophenotyping EBV presence Cytogenetics
Laboratorial evaluation	Complete blood count LDH Serum uric acid Serum or urine protein electrophoresis
Imaging	CT of the neck, chest, abdomen, pelvis PET/CT if available MRI if assess to central nervous system needed

LDH lactate dehydrogenase levels, *CT* contrast-enhanced computed tomography, *PET/CT* combined positron emission computed tomography, *MRI* magnetic resonance imaging

7 Treatment

The two main goals of therapy are eradication of the PTLD and preservation of graft function. Usually, these goals conflict and one must be prioritized. The main PTLD initial therapies are reduction of immunosuppression, rituximab, cytotoxic chemotherapy, surgery for localized disease, or a combination of these. Reducing immunosuppression and targeting B-cell proliferation with rituximab alone or in combination with chemotherapy drugs are commonly used strategies to treat PTLD. Other treatments as adoptive immunotherapy with EBV-specific T cells are reserved for unresponsive disease. There are no randomized trials comparing these treatment options and data largely come from expert opinion, retrospective analyses, and uncontrolled prospective case series. Therefore, management of PTLD varies according to PTLD subtype, type of transplant and from institution to institution. Aggressiveness of PTLD, risk of allograft loss, CD20 positivity or not, expected response time, and drug toxicities must be taken into consideration for therapy choice [45, 46].

Besides laboratorial and image evaluation, pretreatment assessment should include assessment of transplanted organ function, study of cardiac function pre-anthracycline-based chemotherapy and fertility-preserving measures.

7.1 Reduction of Immunosuppression

Reduction of immunosuppression is the first step in therapy and should be incorporated into the initial management of all patients with PTLD, unless concern regarding graft rejection makes this approach unfeasible. Recovery of the host's immune system will allow for EBV-specific T cells to proliferate and control the disease. As known, reduction of immunosuppression increases the risk of allograft rejection and the minimum reduction of immunosuppression to control the PTLD while preserving the allograft is unknown. A careful decrease in immunosuppressive therapy, often a reduction of 25–50% from baseline is used if alternative organ support is available (e.g., renal transplant) and should be reduced to the lowest tolerated level. The majority of early lesions either resolve completely or improve significantly within 3–5 weeks. Complete responses are less common in other types of PTLD. Predictors of lack of response to reduction of immunosuppression include a serum LDH >2.5 times the upper limit of normal, organ dysfunction, and multiple visceral sites of disease [28, 47, 48].

7.2 *Rituximab*

Targeting B-cell proliferation with rituximab is a standard therapy for CD20-positive PTLD patients, despite reduction of immunosuppression, in combination with cytotoxic chemotherapy (either sequentially or concurrently) or as a single agent. Rituximab plus combination with chemotherapy seems to reduce the risk of renal graft impairment. However, disease progression can occur 1 year after an initial response to rituximab monotherapy [49, 50].

7.3 *Chemotherapy*

Cytotoxic chemotherapy should be considered for patients who do not achieve a complete response to or progress after rituximab monotherapy, those with clinically aggressive lymphoma, or patients with critical organ compromise who require a rapid response to therapy. Patients with CD20-negative PTLD who are not candidates for rituximab are treated with chemotherapy after reduction of immunosuppression. R-CHOP (rituximab plus cyclophosphamide, doxorubicin, vincristine, and prednisone) is recommended for most patients with CD20-positive PTLD, as this association increases approximately 65% remission rates. Overall response rates for anthracycline-based regimens are higher than for rituximab monotherapy and range from 42% to 100%. However, this response is at the expense of high treatment-related mortality of 25–50% [50–54].

7.4 *Surgery*

When possible, complete surgical excision of localized disease is highly effective. Localized disease treated with definitive local therapy (surgery or radiation), combined with reduction of immunosuppression, have an excellent prognosis, with PTLD-related mortality rates reported between 0% and 26% [28, 32].

7.5 *Adoptive Immunotherapy*

Adoptive immunotherapy uses EBV-specific cytotoxic T lymphocytes or donor lymphocyte infusion in an attempt to eliminate dividing B cells in EBV-associated PTLD. Prevention and remission of EBV-induced PTLD can be up to 90%. The main complication is acute and chronic graft-versus-host disease [55, 56].

7.6 *Initial Management According to PTLD Subtype* (Table 5)

7.6.1 Early Lesions

For most patients reduction of immunosuppression alone is recommended, rather than in combination with other therapies (rituximab, chemotherapy, antiviral). Rituximab may be reserved for residual disease despite reduction of immunosuppression or for those who cannot tolerate it.

7.6.2 Polymorphic PTLD

The use of rituximab for CD20-positive PTLD in addition to reduction of immunosuppression is recommended, rather than combination with chemotherapy. CD20-negative PTLDs are not candidates for rituximab and are treated with chemotherapy plus reduction of immunosuppression.

7.6.3 Monomorphic PTLD

For patients with monomorphic CD20-positive PTLD, the use of rituximab, either alone or in combination with chemotherapy, in addition to reduction of immunosuppression is recommended. CD20-negative PTLD patients can be treated with chemotherapy and reduction of immunosuppression.

Table 5 Therapies in PTLD subtypes

Subtype	Initial treatment	Combined treatment (if required)
Early lesions	Reduction of immunosuppression	Rituximab
Polymorphic	Reduction of immunosuppression for all Rituximab for CD20-positive PTLD Chemotherapy for CD20-negative PTLD	Chemotherapy for CD20-positive PTDL
Monomorphic	Reduction of immunosuppression for all Rituximab + chemotherapy for CD20-positive PTLD Chemotherapy for CD20-negative PTLD	
Classic Hodgkin lymphoma-like	Reduction of immunosuppression Chemotherapy	Radiotherapy

7.6.4 Classical Hodgkin Lymphoma-Like PTLD

In these cases, management with chemotherapy with or without radiation therapy according to protocols used for classic Hodgkin lymphomas.

8 Surveillance and Prevention

8.1 EBV Viral Load

The vast majority of EBV-positive PTLD cases present a marked EBV viral load elevation. Recipient EBV-serostatus is the most important risk factor in PTLD development. Recipient EBV seronegativity was associated with a 5–12-fold higher risk of PTLD in adult cohorts. This observation suggests that monitoring EBV viral load levels by quantitative polymerase chain reaction (PCR) in high-risk patients could allow PTLD early detection. EBV monitoring of high-risk PTLD patients have been incorporated in many transplant centers although they differ about high-risk patient definition and cutoff to determine EBV positivity. Since most of EBV-positive PTLD occurs in the first-year posttransplantation, high-risk patients should be monitored at least during this period. A kidney transplant recipient may begin the screening within the first week after transplant, followed by monthly monitoring for the next 3–6 months, and then every 3 months until completing 1 year of follow-up. If EBV loads significantly increases, a careful clinical and radiological examination should be performed to search for lymphadenopathy, mass lesions, and other compatible signs of PTLD, as reducing immunosuppression should be considered. Most centers administer preemptive rituximab therapy and some experts would also consider the use of antivirals [12, 57–59].

8.2 Antiviral Agents

Initial attempts to prevent PTLD in SOTR used antiviral therapies, such as thymidine kinase inhibitors (ganciclovir or acyclovir) to eradicate or control EBV for high-risk patients. Although ganciclovir inhibits EBV replication in vitro, thymidine kinase inhibitors are ineffective against EBV in vivo. Data regarding antiviral efficacy in preventing PTLD in SOTR is also limited. Support for the use of antiviral prophylaxis comes only from retrospective and single-arm prospective studies, as meta-analysis do not support the routine use of antivirals for preemptive therapy of EBV viremia for prevention of PTLD in high-risk patients [60–62].

Immunoglobulin preparations containing anti-EBV antibodies have also been considered. A kidney transplantation induction therapy using the combination of basiliximab and low-dose thymoglobulin led to an absence or a very low rate of PTLD. Data supporting the rationale for the use of mTOR inhibitors for reducing the incidence of PTLD remains controversial, raising the question whether the overall intensity of clinical immunosuppression rather than the use of one particular drug may be the critical factor in the onset of PTLD [63–65].

9 Prognosis

PTLD prognosis varies with clonality and disease extension. Published series suggest overall survival rates between 25% and 35%. Monomorphic PTDL mortality can be as high as 80%. T-cell PTLDs also have an extremely poor prognosis. PTLD with primary skin presentation seems to have a favorable outcome in comparison to extranodal disease PTLD [66–68].

Of importance, many of these studies were prior to rituximab availability, which appears to improve outcomes in CD20-positive PTLD, as well as the use of cytotoxic EBV-specific T cells. Presently, many other drugs are being tested for PTLD, such as leflunomide and its active metabolite teriflunomide, checkpoint inhibitor blockade, especially the PD1/PDL1 pathway, and anti-CD30 monoclonal antibody (brentuximab) for CD30-positive PTLD [69–72].

Graft-specific concerns include the increase of graft failure risk due to reduction of immunosuppression and drug toxicity required for PTLD treatment, and in cases of allograft loss, the risk of repeat such malignance in the received retransplant. Fortunately, recurrence of PTLD in patients having undergone retransplantation is a rare event [73, 74].

References

1. Starzl TE, Discussion of Murray JE, Wilson RE, Tilney NL, et al. Five years' experience in renal transplantation with immunosuppressive drugs: survival, function, complications and the role of lymphocyte depletion by thoracic duct fistula. Ann Surg. 1968;168:416–35.
2. Penn I, Hammond W, Brettschneider L, et al. Malignant lymphomas in transplantation patients. Transplant Proc. 1969;1:106–12.
3. Bhatia S, Ramsay NK, Steinbuch M, et al. Malignant neoplasms following bone marrow transplantation. Blood. 1996;87:3633–9.
4. Nagle SJ, Reshef R, Tsai DE. Posttransplant lymphoproliferative disorder in solid organ and hematopoietic stem cell transplantation. Clin Chest Med. 2017;38:771–83.
5. Loren AW, Porter DL, Stadtmauer EA, Tsai DE. Post-transplant lymphoproliferative disorder: a review. Bone Marrow Transplant. 2003;31:145–55.
6. Mahale P, Shiels MS, Lynch CF, Engels EA. Incidence and outcomes of primary central nervous system lymphoma in solid organ transplant recipients. Am J Transplant. 2018;18:453–61.
7. Luskin MR, Heil DS, Tan KS, et al. The impact of EBV status on characteristics and outcomes of posttransplantation lymphoproliferative disorder. Am J Transplant. 2015;15:2665–73.
8. Penn I. Cancers complicating organ transplantation. N Engl J Med. 1990;323(25):1767–9.

9. Adami J, Gabel H, Lindelof B, et al. Cancer risk following organ transplantation: a nationwide cohort study in Sweden. Br J Cancer. 2003;89(7):1221–7.
10. Hall EC, Pfeiffer RM, Segev DL, Engels EA. Cumulative incidence of cancer after solid organ transplantation. Cancer. 2013;119(12):2300–8.
11. Martin-Moreno PL, Panizo C. Update on posttransplant lymphoproliferative disease. Curr Opin Nephrol Hypertens. 2018;27:1–5.
12. San-Juan R, Comoli P, Caillard S, et al. Epstein-Barr virus-related post-transplant lymphoproliferative disorder in solid organ transplant recipients. Clin Microbiol Infect. 2014;20(Suppl. 7):109–18.
13. Sampaio MS, Cho YW, Qazi Y, Bunnapradist S, Hutchinson IV, Shah T. Posttransplant malignancies in solid organ adult recipients: an analysis of the U.S. National Transplant Database. Transplantation. 2012;94(10):990–8.
14. Caillard S, Lamy FX, Quelen C, et al. Epidemiology of posttransplant lymphoproliferative disorders in adult kidney and kidney pancreas recipients: report of the French registry and analysis of subgroups of lymphomas. Am J Transplant. 2012;12(3):682–93.
15. Opelz G, Dohler B. Lymphomas after solid organ transplantation: a collaborative transplant study report. Am J Transplant. 2004;4(2):222–30.
16. Caillard S, Lelong C, Pessione F, Moulin B. Post-transplant lymphoproliferative disorders occurring after renal transplantation in adults: report of 230 cases from the French registry. Am J Transplant. 2006;6:2735–42.
17. Walker RC, Marshall WF, Strickler JG, et al. Pretransplantation assessment of the risk of lymphoproliferative disorder. Clin Infect Dis. 1995;20(5):1346–53.
18. McDonald RA, Smith JM, Ho M, et al. Incidence of PTLD in pediatric renal transplant recipients receiving basiliximab, calcineurin inhibitor, sirolimus and steroids. Am J Transplant. 2008;8(5):984–9.
19. Birkeland AS, Hamilton-Dutoit S. Is post-transplant lymphoproliferative disorder (PTLD) caused by any specific immunosuppressive drug or by the transplantation per se? Transplantation. 2003;76:984–8.
20. van Leeuwen MT, Grulich AE, Webster AC, et al. Immunosuppression and other risk factors for early and late non-Hodgkin lymphoma after kidney transplantation. Blood. 2009;114:630–7.
21. Epstein MA, Achong BG, Barr YM. Virus particles in cultured lymphoblasts from Burkitt's lymphoma. Lancet. 1964;1:702–3.
22. Odumade OA, Hogquist KA, Balfour HHJ. Progress and problems in understanding and managing primary Epstein-Barr virus infections. Clin Microbiol Rev. 2011;24(1):193–209.
23. Cohen JI. Epstein-Barr virus infection. N Engl J Med. 2000;343(7):481–92.
24. Zutter MM, Martin PJ, Sale GE, et al. Epstein–Barr vírus lymphoproliferation after bone marrow transplantation. Blood. 1988;72:520–9.
25. Leblond V, Davi F, Charlotte F, et al. Posttransplant lymphoproliferative disorders not associated with Epstein–Barr virus: a distinct entity? J Clin Oncol. 1998;16:2052–9.
26. Nelson BP, Nalesnik MA, Bahler DW, et al. Epstein–Barr virus-negative post-transplant lymphoproliferative disorders: a distinct entity? Am J Surg Pathol. 2000;24:375–85.
27. Nalesnik MA. Posttransplantation lymphoproliferative disorders (PTLD): current perspectives. Semin Thorac Cardiovasc Surg. 1996;8:139–48.
28. Tsai DE, Hardy CL, Tomaszewski JE, et al. Reduction in immunosuppression as initial therapy for posttransplant lymphoproliferative disorder: analysis of prognostic variables and long-term follow-up of 42 adult patients. Transplantation. 2001;71(8):1076–88.
29. Dotti G, Fiocchi R, Motta T, et al. Lymphomas occurring late after solid-organ transplantation: influence of treatment on the clinical outcome. Transplantation. 2002;74(8):1095–102.
30. Ferreira MCS, Seque CA, Enokihara MMSS, et al. Post-transplant lymphoproliferative disorder with cutaneous involvement: a series of four cases. Clin Transpl. 2021;35:e14162.
31. Allen UD, Preiksaitis JK. Epstein-Barr virus and posttransplant lymphoproliferative disorder in solid organ transplantation. Am J Transplant. 2013;13(Suppl 4):107–20.

32. Benkerrou M, Durandy A, Fischer A. Therapy for transplant related lymphoproliferative diseases. Hematol Oncol Clin North Am. 1993;7:467–75.
33. Dharnidharka VR. Comprehensive review of post-organ transplant hematologic cancers. Am J Transplant. 2018;18:537–49.
34. Beynet DP, Wee SA, Horwitz SS, et al. Clinical and pathological features of posttransplantation lymphoproliferative disorders presenting with skin involvement in 4 patients. Arch Dermatol. 2004;140:1140–6.
35. Capaldi L, Robinson-Bostom L, Kerr P, Gohh R. Localized cutaneous posttransplant Epstein-Barr virus-associated lymphoproliferative disorder. J Am Acad Dermatol. 2004;51:778–80.
36. Salama S, Todd S, Cina DP, Margetts P. Cutaneous presentation of post-renal transplant lymphoproliferative disorder: a series of four cases. J Cutan Pathol. 2010;37:641–53.
37. Seçkin D, Barete S, Euvrard S, et al. Primary cutaneous posttransplant lymphoproliferative disorders in solid organ transplant recipients: a multicenter European case series. Am J Transplant. 2013;13:2146–53.
38. Swerdlow SH, Campo E, Harris NL, et al., editors. WHO classification of tumours of haematopoietic and lymphoid tissues. Revised 4th ed. Lyon: International Agency for Research on Cancer (IARC); 2017.
39. Vakiani E, Nandula SV, Subramaniyam S, et al. Cytogenetic analysis of B-cell posttransplant lymphoproliferations validates the World Health Organization classification and suggests inclusion of florid follicular hyperplasia as a precursor lesion. Hum Pathol. 2007;38(2):315–25.
40. Caillard S, Agodoa LY, Bohen EM, et al. Myeloma, Hodgkin disease, and lymphoid leukemia after renal transplantation: characteristics, risk factors and prognosis. Transplantation. 2006;81(6):888–95.
41. Rajakariar R, Bhattacharyya M, Norton A, et al. Post-transplant T-cell lymphoma: a case series of four patients from a single unit and review of the literature. Am J Transplant. 2004;4(9):1534–8.
42. Parker A, Bowles K, Bradley JA, et al. Diagnosis of post-transplant lymphoproliferative disorder in solid organ transplant recipients—BCSH and BTS guidelines. Br J Haematol. 2010;149(5):675–92.
43. Lemoine A, Pham P, Azoulay D, et al. Detection of gammopathy by serum protein electrophoresis for predicting and managing therapy of lymphoproliferative disorder in 911 recipients of liver transplants. Blood. 2001;98(5):1332–8.
44. Cheson BD, Fisher RI, Barrington SF, et al. Recommendations for initial evaluation, staging, and response assessment of Hodgkin and non-Hodgkin lymphoma: the Lugano classification. J Clin Oncol. 2014;32(27):3059–68.
45. EBPG Expert Group on Renal Transplantation. European best practice guidelines for renal transplantation. Section IV: long-term management of the transplant recipient. IV.11 Paediatrics (specific problems). Nephrol Dial Transplant. 2002;17(Suppl 4):55–8.
46. Parker A, Bowles K, Bradley JA, et al. Management of post-transplant lymphoproliferative disorder in adult solid organ transplant recipients—BCSH and BTS guidelines. Br J Haematol. 2010;149(5):693–705.
47. Paya CV, Fung JJ, Nalesnik MA, et al. Epstein-Barr virus-induced posttransplant lymphoproliferative disorders. ASTS/ASTP EBV-PTLD Task Force and the Mayo Clinic Organized International Consensus Development meeting. Transplantation. 1999;68(10):1517–25.
48. Reshef R, Vardhanabhuti S, Luskin MR, et al. Reduction of immunosuppression as initial therapy for posttransplantation lymphoproliferative disorder (bigstar). Am J Transplant. 2011;11(2):336–47.
49. Choquet S, Oertel S, LeBlond V, et al. Rituximab in the management of post-transplantation lymphoproliferative disorder after solid organ transplantation: proceed with caution. Ann Hematol. 2007;86(8):599–607.
50. Trappe R, Oertel S, Leblond V, et al. Sequential treatment with rituximab followed by CHOP chemotherapy in adult B-cell post-transplant lymphoproliferative disorder (PTLD): the prospective international multicentre phase 2 PTLD-1 trial. Lancet Oncol. 2012;13(2):196–206.

51. Trappe RU, Dierickx D, Zimmermann H, et al. Response to rituximab induction is a predictive marker in B-cell post-transplant lymphoproliferative disorder and allows successful stratification into rituximab or R-CHOP consolidation in an international, prospective, multicenter phase II trial. J Clin Oncol. 2017;35(5):536–43.
52. Taylor AL, Bowles KM, Callaghan CJ, et al. Anthracycline-based chemotherapy as first-line treatment in adults with malignant posttransplant lymphoproliferative disorder after solid organ transplantation. Transplantation. 2006;82(3):375–81.
53. Elstrom RL, Andreadis C, Aqui NA, et al. Treatment of PTLD with rituximab or chemotherapy. Am J Transplant. 2006;6(3):569–76.
54. Mamzer-Bruneel MF, Lome C, Morelon E, et al. Durable remission after aggressive chemotherapy for very late post-kidney transplant lymphoproliferation: a report of 16 cases observed in a single center. J Clin Oncol. 2000;18(21):3622–32.
55. Haque T, Wilkie GM, Taylor C, et al. Treatment of Epstein-Barr-virus-positive post-transplantation lymphoproliferative disease with partly HLA-matched allogeneic cytotoxic T cells. Lancet. 2002;360(9331):436–42.
56. Heslop HE, Slobod KS, Pule MA, et al. Long-term outcome of EBV-specific T-cell infusions to prevent or treat EBV-related lymphoproliferative disease in transplant recipients. Blood. 2010;115(5):925–35.
57. Stevens SJ, Verschuuren EA, Pronk I, et al. Frequent monitoring of Epstein-Barr virus DNA load in unfractionated whole blood is essential for early detection of posttransplant lymphoproliferative disease in high-risk patients. Blood. 2001;97(5):1165–71.
58. Tsai DE, Douglas L, Andreadis C, et al. EBV PCR in the diagnosis and monitoring of post-transplant lymphoproliferative disorder: results of a two-arm prospective trial. Am J Transplant. 2008;8(5):1016–24.
59. EBPG Expert Group on Renal Transplantation. European best practice guidelines for renal transplantation. Section IV: long-term management of the transplant recipient. IV.6.1. Cancer risk after renal transplantation. Post-transplant lymphoproliferative disease (PTLD): prevention and treatment. Nephrol Dial Transplant. 2002;17(Suppl 4):31–6.
60. Funch DP, Walker AM, Schneider G, et al. Ganciclovir and acyclovir reduce the risk of post-transplant lymphoproliferative disorder in renal transplant recipients. Am J Transplant. 2005;5(12):2894–900.
61. Opelz G, Daniel V, Naujokat C, et al. Effect of cytomegalovirus prophylaxis with immunoglobulin or with antiviral drugs on post-transplant non-Hodgkin lymphoma: a multicenter retrospective analysis. Lancet Oncol. 2007;8(3):212–8.
62. Al-Dabbagh MA, Gitman MR, Kumar D, et al. The role of antiviral prophylaxis for the prevention of Epstein-Barr virus-associated posttransplant lymphoproliferative disease in solid organ transplant recipients: a systematic review. Am J Transplant. 2017;17:770–81.
63. Humar A, Hebert D, Davies HD, et al. A randomized trial of ganciclovir versus ganciclovir plus immune globulin for prophylaxis against Epstein-Barr virus related posttransplant lymphoproliferative disorder. Transplantation. 2006;81(6):856–61.
64. Ciancio G, Gaynor JJ, Guerra G, et al. Randomized trial of rATg/Daclizumab vs. rATg/Alemtuzumab as dual induction therapy in renal transplantation: results at 8 years of follow-up. Transpl Immunol. 2017;40:42–50.
65. Spagnoletti G, Salerno MP, Calia R, et al. Thymoglobulin plus basiliximab mixed cocktail to start? Transpl Immunol. 2017;43–44:1–2.
66. Caillard S, Porcher R, Provot F, et al. Post-transplantation lymphoproliferative disorder after kidney transplantation: report of a nationwide French registry and the development of a new prognostic score. J Clin Oncol. 2013;31(10):1302–9.
67. Evens AM, David KA, Helenowski I, et al. Multicenter analysis of 80 solid organ transplantation recipients with post-transplantation lymphoproliferative disease: outcomes and prognostic factors in the modern era. J Clin Oncol. 2010;28(6):1038–46.
68. Mraz-Gernhard SHS, Kohler S, Hoppe RT, et al. Cutaneous B-cell lymphoma: superior prognosis for patients with disease limited to the skin. J Invest Dermatol. 2001;117:536.

69. Bilger A, Plowshay J, Ma S, et al. Leflunomide/teriflunomide inhibit Epstein-Barr virus (EBV) induced lymphoproliferative disease and lytic viral replication. Oncotarget. 2017;8:44266–80.
70. Dierickx D, Habermann TM. Posttransplantation lymphoproliferative disorders in adults. N Engl J Med. 2018;378:549–62.
71. Barnett R, Barta VS, Jhaveri KD. Preserved renal-allograft function and the PD-1 pathway inhibitor nivolumab. N Engl J Med. 2017;376:191–2.
72. Hartley C, Vaughan JW, Jarzembowski J, et al. CD30 expression in monomorphic posttransplant lymphoproliferative disorder, diffuse large B-cell lymphoma correlates with greater regulatory T-cell infiltration. Am J Clin Pathol. 2017;148:485–93.
73. Caillard S, Cellot E, Dantal J, et al. A French cohort study of kidney retransplantation after post-transplant lymphoproliferative disorders. Clin J Am Soc Nephrol (CJASN). 2017;12(10):1663–70.
74. Caillard S, Cellot E, Dantal J, et al. A French cohort study of kidney retransplantation after posttransplant lymphoproliferative disorders. Clin J Am Soc Nephrol. 2017;12:1663–70.

Other Rare Cancers

Jane Tomimori, Anamaria da Silva Facina, and Milvia Maria Simões e Silva Enokihara

1 Introduction

In this chapter, we present rare malignant neoplasms diagnosed in solid organ transplant recipients (SOTRs). We include neoplasms that had been described among SOTRs in the literature: follicular origin carcinoma, eccrine carcinoma, sebaceous carcinoma, dermatofibrosarcoma protuberans, angiosarcoma, Merkel cell carcinoma, and carcinosarcoma.

2 Follicular Carcinoma

2.1 Epidemiology

There are few reports of follicular carcinomas in SOTRs. This tumor is commonly found in elderly on sun-exposed areas (face, scalp, neck, and dorsum of the hand) and presents low malignancy [1].

There are four reports of trichilemmal carcinoma in three renal transplant recipients (RTRs) and in one heart transplant recipient [2–4].

J. Tomimori (✉) · A. da Silva Facina
Department of Dermatology, Escola Paulista de Medicina, Universidade Federal de São Paulo, São Paulo, SP, Brazil
e-mail: jane.tomimori@unifesp.br; Anamaria.facina@unifesp.br

M. M. Simões e Silva Enokihara
Department of Pathology, Escola Paulista de Medicina, Universidade Federal de São Paulo, São Paulo, SP, Brazil

J. Tomimori et al. (eds.), *Atlas of Dermatologic Diseases in Solid Organ Transplant Recipients*, https://doi.org/10.1007/978-3-031-13335-0_17

2.2 *Pathogenesis*

The cellular origin of this carcinoma is hair follicle cell, so the differential diagnosis includes skin carcinomas. There is a long latency period for lesion development that is related to sun exposure or radiotherapy [1].

2.3 *Clinical Presentation*

Usually, it is a solitary carcinoma that can manifest as an exophytic or polypoid nodule. Ulceration and keratotic surface could also be observed. In immunocompetent patients, trichilemmal carcinoma is an indolent neoplasm with low aggressiveness, whereas the iatrogenic immunosuppression can lead to lymph node, pulmonary, and hepatic metastases [3].

2.4 *Histopathology*

The tumors are multilobulated with infiltrative growths connected to the epidermis and pilosebaceous structures. These structures present reminiscent features of the outer root sheath, which may extend to the deep dermis or into subcutaneous fat. The tumor is composed of glycogen-containing clear cells. Basement membrane may be evidenced by PAS-stain, particularly near the clear cell proliferation and a high mitotic rate is often present [5]. By immunohistochemistry, there are CD34-positive cells, CK5/6 (++), p63 (++), p40 (++), CD10 (−), Ki-67 (+) [6, 7]. EMA (epithelial membrane antigen) and CEA (carcinoembryonic antigen) are negatives. The differential diagnoses are: squamous cell carcinoma, basal cell carcinoma, and keratoacanthomas [8].

2.5 *Treatment*

Mohs micrographic surgery should always be considered for this cancer treatment [1, 2].

3 Eccrine Carcinoma

3.1 *Epidemiology*

Eccrine carcinoma is a very rare malignant skin appendageal tumor that is derived from sweat glands [9]. This neoplasm is highly invasive and metastatic. The incidence is approximately 0.005% of all cutaneous epithelial tumors [10]. It could occur among individuals with low skin phototype, in the fourth or fifth decades of life and do not present gender preference [9].

3.2 *Pathogenesis*

The etiology is not well established. Local skin injury and X-ray radiation may be its cause. A rare squamous variant of eccrine porocarcinoma was described and must be related to ultraviolet radiation and chronic immunosuppression. The adnexal carcinomas may have apocrine or eccrine cell origin.

The classification of malignant eccrine tumors is still very confusing with identical tumors reported in the literature under three or more designations. Some of the ductal adenocarcinomas are high-grade tumors. The malignant eccrine poroma (porocarcinoma) is of intermediate malignancy. The low malignancy group includes microcystic adnexal carcinoma and eccrine epithelioma [9].

3.3 *Clinical Presentation*

The most common location is head and neck area (Fig. 1a–c), with predilection for the central region of the face (upper and lower lip). The other sites affected are nasolabial folds, nose, cheek, scalp, chin, periorbital area (Fig. 2), and extremities [11, 12]. The lesion is solitary, firm, pale, nodule, or plaque. The epidermis could be normal, atrophic, or ulcerated (Figs. 3 and 4). As it is a rare tumor, it could be mistaken for basal cell carcinoma, amelanotic melanoma, and squamous cell carcinoma [13]. The tumor recurrence is more frequent in other sites compared to recurrence

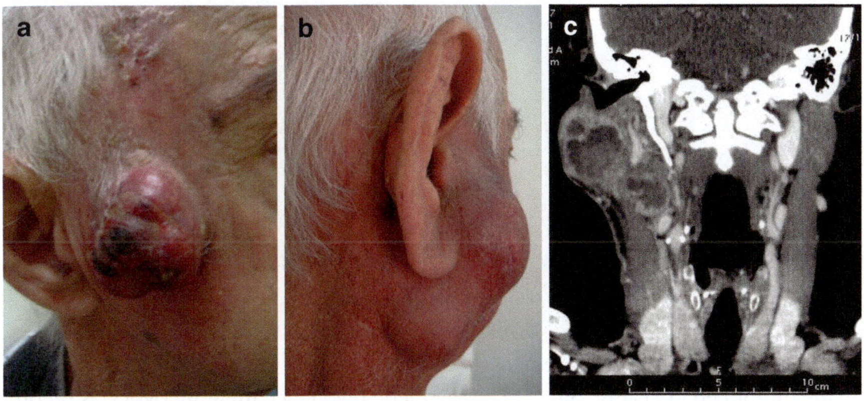

Fig. 1 Eccrine carcinoma in kidney transplant recipient: (**a**) one month of cutaneous lesion evolution, (**b**) tumoral mass, 2 weeks after excisional surgery, (**c**) computed tomography shows tumor infiltration, 2 weeks after excisional surgery. (Reproduced from Higashi et al. 2015)

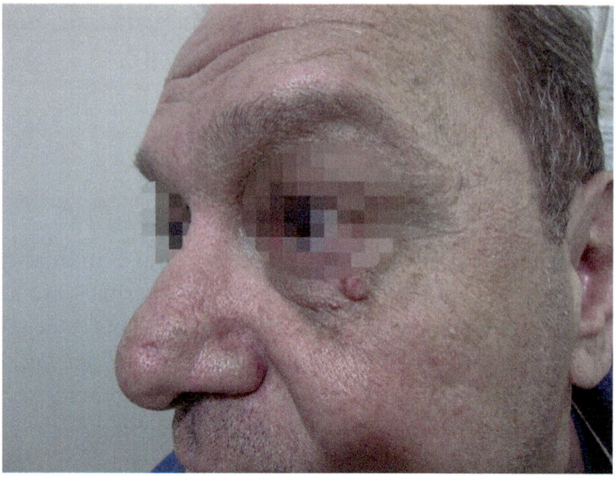

Fig. 2 Eccrine carcinoma on infrapalpebral region in kidney transplant recipient

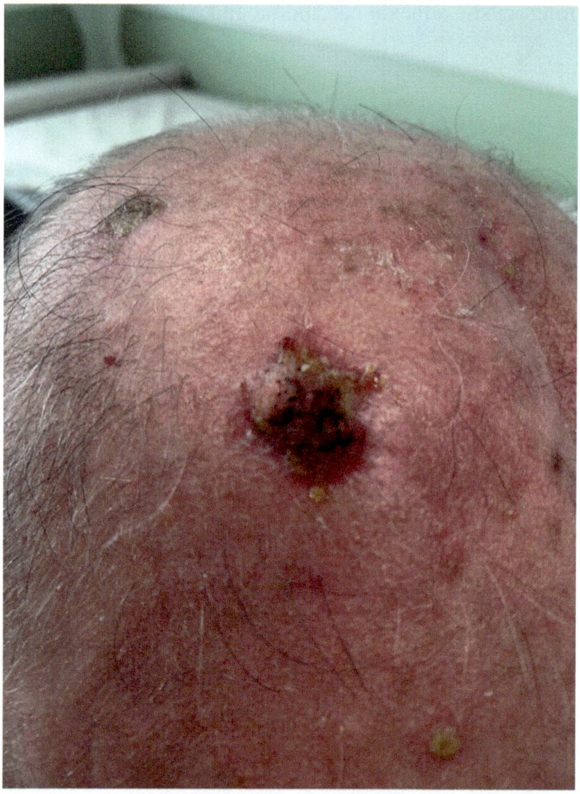

Fig. 3 Ulcerated porocarcinoma on scalp in kidney transplant recipient

in the tumor bed [12] (Fig. 5a–c). The magnetic resonance imaging (MRI) is recommended for tumor extent evaluation and positron emission tomography/computed tomography (PET/CT) for metastasis detection [12].

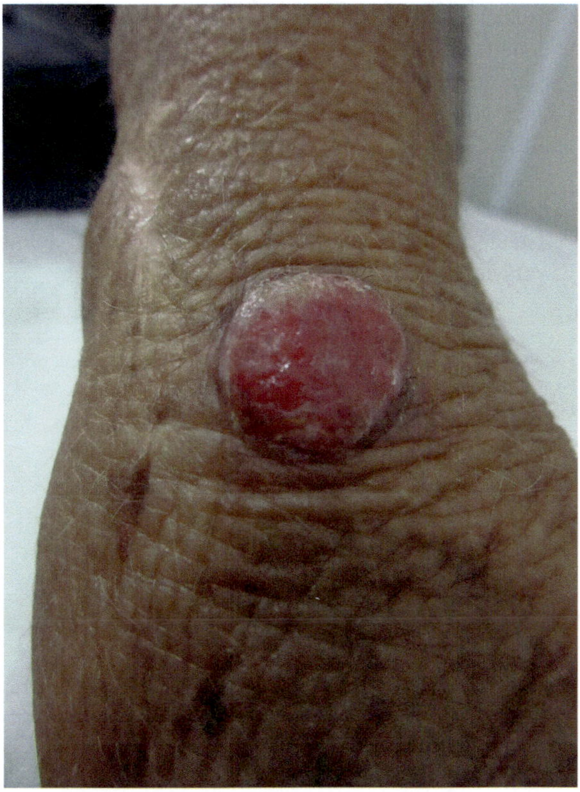

Fig. 4 Porocarcinoma as ulcerated vegetation on hand in kidney transplant recipient

Among immunosuppressed patients, this tumor grows very fast [14]. The metastases may develop in the lungs, retroperitoneum, bone, liver, breast, bladder, or ovary [12].

3.4 Histopathology

In histopathology, it is observed the presence of cords, cysts, nests, and islands of small basaloid cells, sharply demarcated from the adjacent keratinocytes. Tubules of tumor can invade the dermis and subjacent muscle. Clear cell areas, squamous differentiation, melanin pigment, and focal necrosis may be present in the dermal nests. Ductal structures are also found. Perineural and intraneural infiltration could be observed (Fig. 6a) [7]. The cuboidal and uniform squamous cells are dispersed in a dense collagenous stroma [9].

In immunohistochemical analysis, there is positivity for EMA (Fig. 6b) and CEA (Fig. 6c), AE1/AE3 (cytokeratins), CK 5–6, p63, and S100 protein. They are useful markers for eccrine sweat glands diagnosis [9]. Ki-67 antigen is overexpressed in

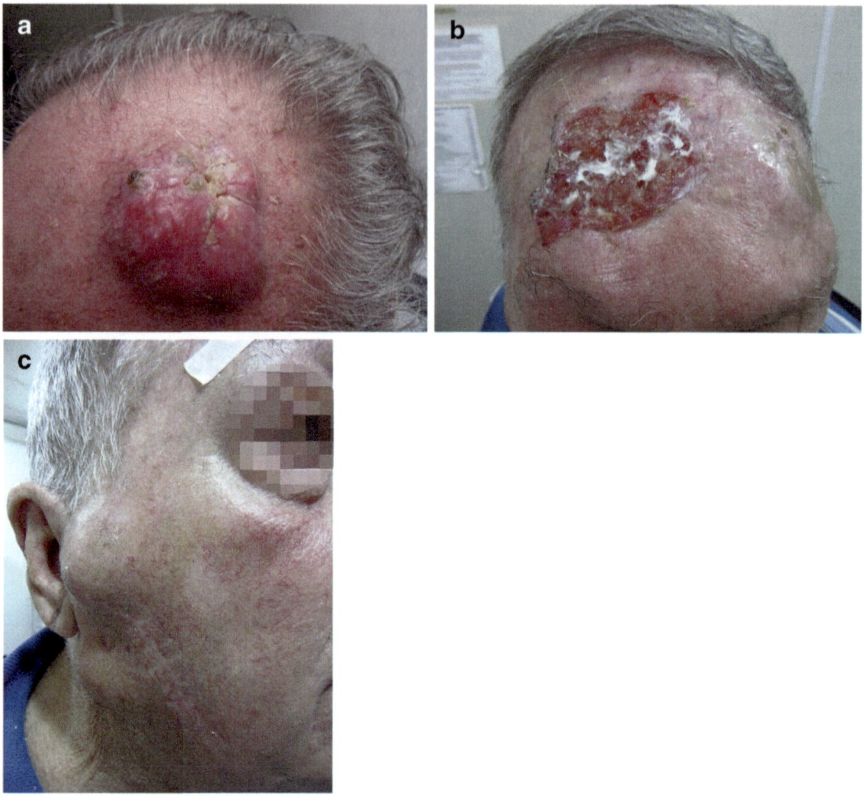

Fig. 5 Eccrine carcinoma in kidney transplant recipient: (**a**) primary tumor on left side of frontal region; (**b**) relapse of cutaneous metastasis on right side of frontal region, after 2 years. Previously, the patient was submitted to surgery after 1 year evolution; (**c**) relapse of parotid and cervical lymph node on right side, after 2 years. Previous parotid and lymph nodes surgery after 1 year evolution

malignant soft tissue tumors. It is a useful antibody to evaluate metastasis, tumor development, tumor recurrence, and prognosis. Its index increases progressively with neoplasm invasion [15]. When estrogen receptor is positive; tamoxifen, a selective estrogen receptor modulator, can be recommended as an adjuvant therapy [12].

3.5 Treatment

Surgical excision is the recommended treatment for eccrine carcinoma. For adnexal carcinomas, the lymph node biopsy is not a good predictor for survival evaluation in advanced stage [16] although some authors recommend the lymphadenectomy [12, 15]. Radiation therapy and chemotherapy are not efficient [11, 13]. There are some

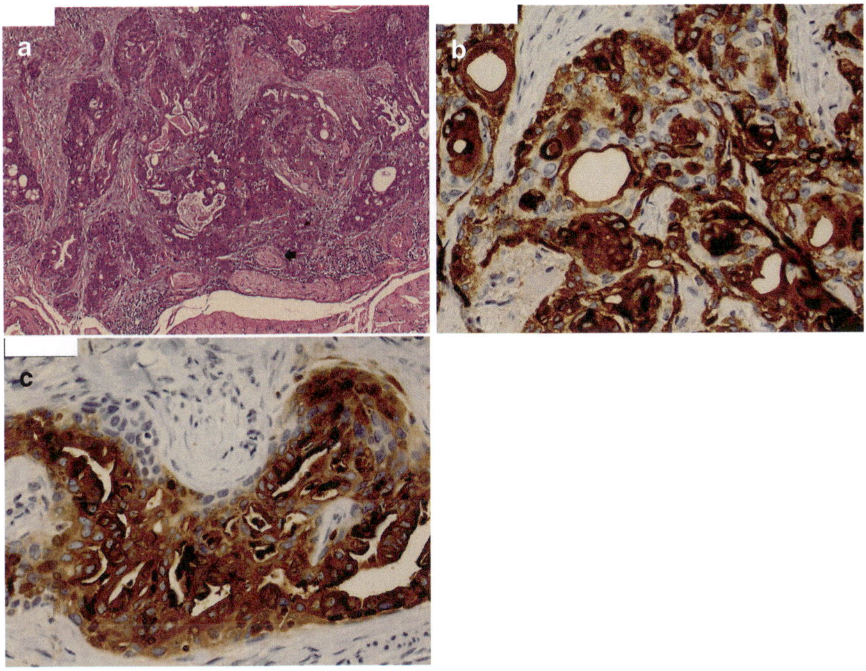

Fig. 6 Eccrine carcinoma: (**a**) groups of small basaloid cells that infiltrate the stroma and invade into dermis and muscle. Ductal structures are also found. Perineural and intraneural infiltration is observed (arrow) (H&E, 100×); (**b**) positivity for EMA in cells' cytoplasm (immunochemistry, 400×); (**c**) positivity for CEA (immunochemistry, 400×)

reports about the use of taxoid group (paclitaxel and docetaxel) [13], tamoxifen [17], 5-fluorouracil [13], and topical aminolevulinic acid photodynamic therapy [18].

4 Sebaceous Carcinoma

4.1 Epidemiology

Sebaceous carcinoma is a rare appendageal neoplasm that affects ocular or extra-ocular sites. The risk factors are advanced age and history of irradiation [19]. This skin tumor may be associated with Muir-Torre syndrome (MTS), a genetical disorder. The prevalence is 0.2–4.6% of all cutaneous neoplasms in the immunocompetent population, and it is the third palpebral cancer in frequency [19].

The higher prevalence is described among SOTRs being estimated at 0.09% [20], representing an increased incidence of 25 folds [21]. In these population, it is more frequent in male and elderly individuals, with low skin phototypes. There is an association with squamous cell carcinoma (SCC) [22]. It is more frequent in lung transplant recipients [21].

4.2 Pathogenesis

Probably, this tumor arises from sebaceous glands of the eyelid, explaining the high incidence on periorbital area. Sebaceous carcinoma is the third most common neoplasm on the eyelid area, after basal cell carcinoma and squamous cell carcinoma. Multiple sebaceous neoplasms may be related to Muir-Torre syndrome. It is an autosomal dominant genodermatosis, with increased risk of multiple neoplasia. The patient develops cutaneous neoplasia as epitheliomas, adenomas, acanthomas, and carcinomas; associated with internal malignancy, such as hereditary nonpolyposis colorectal cancer and other cancers: endometrium, stomach, small bowel, pancreas, urogenital tract, and larynx [22]. Stone et al. reported a patient with known Muir-Torre syndrome, who developed multiple sebaceous adenomas after cyclosporine and prednisolone therapy [23]. The appearance of sebaceous adenomas and sebaceous carcinoma may be associated with microsatellite instability (MSI) in patients with Muir-Torre syndrome [24]. The MSI is due to the accumulation of numerous mutations across the genome, especially in repetitive sequences (microsatellites) [25]. This sign may be useful for the diagnosis of MTS in patients receiving solid organ transplants. The MSI may play a predominant role in the development of a specific range of tumor types. The MSI in neoplasms among renal transplant recipients is associated with loss of hMSH2 expression by immunohistochemistry [22].

4.3 Clinical Presentation

The sebaceous carcinoma can manifest as a papule or erythematous nodule, slightly yellowish with a central ulceration [19] (Fig. 7). The lesion is very similar to non-melanoma skin cancer. The most common location in the immunocompetent

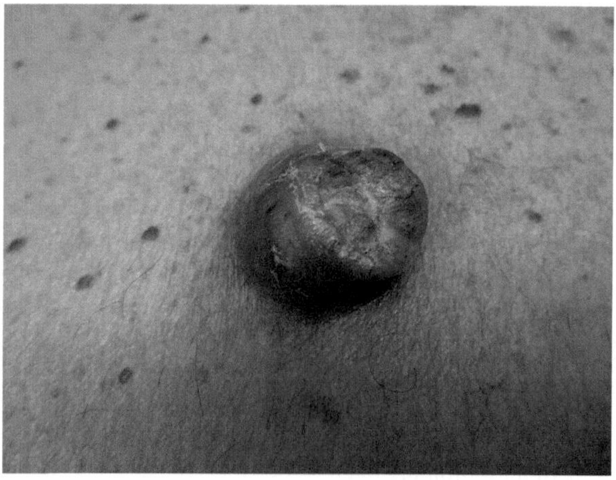

Fig. 7 Sebaceous carcinoma on posterior thoracic region in kidney transplant recipient

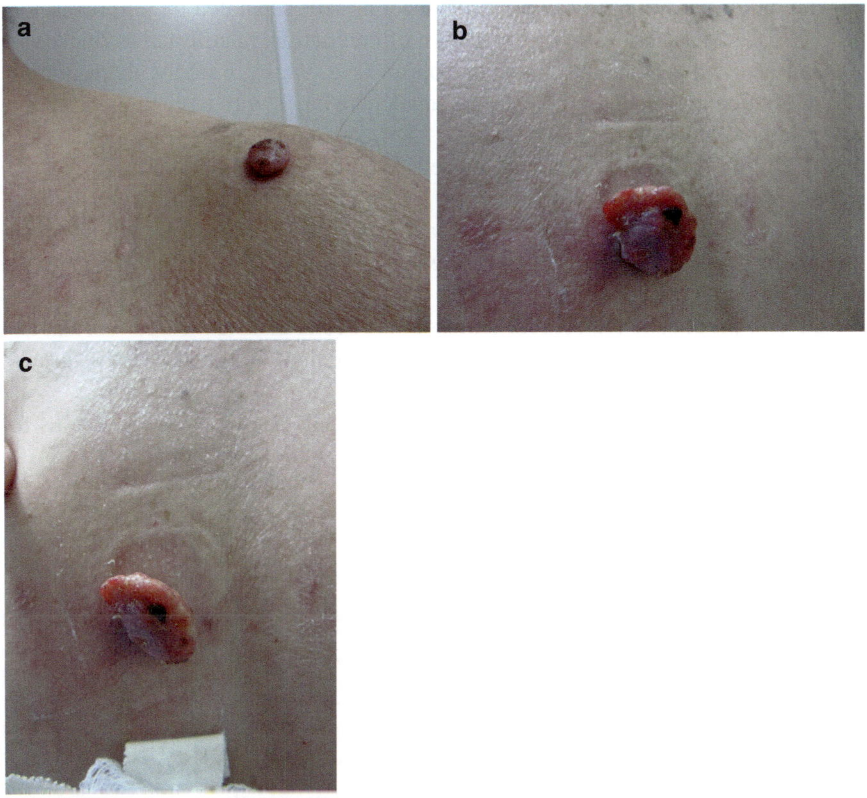

Fig. 8 Association of sebaceous origin tumor in kidney transplant recipient: (**a**) sebaceous adenoma on left shoulder; (**b**, **c**) pedunculated and ulcerated sebaceous carcinoma on posterior thoracic region

individuals is the periorbital region (about 75%), which is not a rule in immunosuppressed patients. They can be located in the head and neck region, as well as in the trunk, upper and lower limbs, shoulder, and genitalia [19]. It could appear about 5–7 years after the solid organ transplantation [20]. Figure 8a–c shows a renal transplant recipient with two tumors: a sebaceous adenoma on the left shoulder and sebaceous carcinoma on his back.

4.4 Histopathology

Sebaceous carcinomas can be classified in two groups: those arising in the ocular adnexa, particularly the Meibomian and Zeiss glands and tumors arising in extraocular sites (20% of all sebaceous carcinomas are found on the head and neck area of elderly individuals).

The tumor is composed of lobules or sheet of cells separated by a fibrovascular stroma. The cells show variable sebaceous differentiation, manifested as finely vacuolated or foamy rather than clear cytoplasm (Fig. 9a, b). Usually, there is more differentiation at the center of nests. The nuclei are large, with large nucleoli. There are scattered mitoses. Focal necrosis is not uncommon, and this may have a "comedo-like" pattern. The vacuolated cells show abundant lipid if a frozen section is stained with Sudan [25, 26].

The periocular lesions often show a pagetoid or less commonly, a carcinoma *in situ* on the overlying conjunctiva or on the epidermis of the eyelid. Such changes are not usually seen in extraocular cases [25, 26].

Adverse prognostic features for tumors of the ocular adnexa include vascular and lymphatic invasion, orbital extension, poor differentiation, an infiltrative growth pattern, and large tumor size [25, 26].

By immunohistochemical analysis, the tumor cells show positive reactions for EMA (Fig. 10a) and androgen receptor (AR) (Fig. 10b), but not for CEA, S100

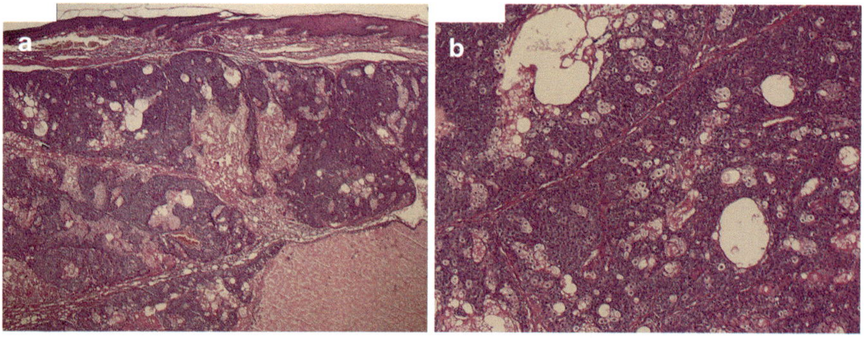

Fig. 9 Sebaceous carcinoma histopathology with sheets of cells separated by a fibrovascular stroma. The cells show variable sebaceous differentiation (H&E staining) (**a**) magnification 40×; (**b**) magnification 100×

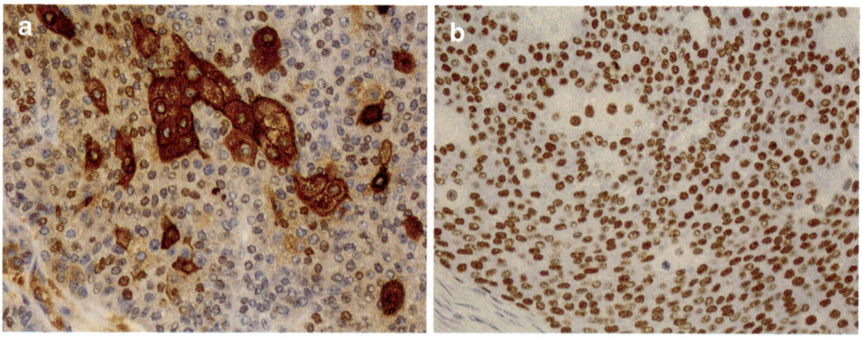

Fig. 10 Sebaceous carcinoma: (**a**) positivity for EMA in cells' cytoplasm (immunohistochemistry, 400×); (**b**) positivity for androgen receptor nuclei cells (immunochemistry, 400×)

protein. In poorly differentiated tumors, EMA staining is often absent but nuclear staining for AR is present, making it the more reliable marker. Sebaceous carcinoma expresses statistically significant increased levels of p53 and Ki67 compared to benign lesions [7].

Muir-Torre syndrome is an autosomal dominant disease. Mutations in one of the DNA mismatch repair genes MLH1, MSH2, and MSH6 have been found in these patients. Mutations in MSH2 account for the majority of cases (90%), whereas MSH6 mutations are limited to a few cases. PMS2 mutations have not been reported so far in the Muir-Torre syndrome, but they have been in the Lynch syndrome [25, 26].

4.5 *Treatment*

Early excision of tumor is recommended, as periocular lesions can evolve to enucleation. Mohs micrographic surgery is proposed [20], especially for periorbital cancers. The excision margins must be of 5–6 mm. For inoperable patients, radiotherapy is the treatment of choice and also as an adjuvant therapy [27]. The use of pembrolizumab, a humanized antibody that targets the programmed cell death protein 1 (PD-1) receptor of lymphocytes, could be used in advanced and metastatic sebaceous carcinoma [28].

5 Dermatofibrosarcoma Protuberans

5.1 *Epidemiology*

Dermatofibrosarcoma protuberans (DFSP) is the most common soft tissue sarcoma in the skin. It is a malignant tumor, whose fibroblastic origin is presumed and usually recur in the same site. The incidence per year varies from 2.6 to 6.5 per million people depending on the population analyzed. Affects men and women equally [29, 30].There are few cases of this mesenchymal tumor in SOTRs [31].

5.2 *Pathogenesis*

The pathogenesis is not well understood. Previous trauma has been connected to the development of some lesions. It is a rare skin tumor marked by infiltrative asymmetric growth and involvement of gene translocation. There are two genes engaged in growth factors, the collagen gene (COL1A1) on chromosome 17 and platelet-derived growth factor (PDGF) gene on chromosome 22. The mechanism of translocation implies a new chimeric gene present in almost 90% of DFSP [32].

5.3 Clinical Presentation

Usually appears in individuals aged 20–59 years and seems to be more frequent in high phototype. The common presentation is an asymptomatic solitary and indurated red, violaceous and/or brown plaque that can ulcerate. It can evolve from nodules to tumors (Figs. 11 and 12). The most common anatomic sites are trunk, upper and lower limbs, head, and genitals. Pain is described in around 35% of patients and history of previous trauma has been reported in almost 16.5%. Clinically, DFSP can be misdiagnosed by different lesions like scar, cyst, lipoma, basal cell carcinoma, and liposarcoma. An uncommon, pigmented variant, Bednar tumor, appears in 5% of DFSP [33].

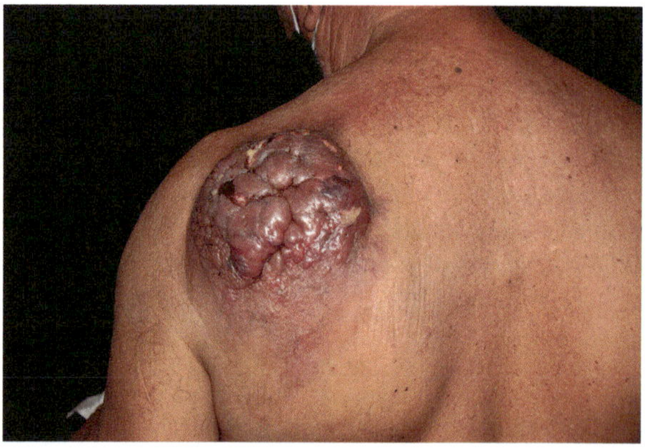

Fig. 11 Dermatofibrosarcoma protuberans on high back. (Collection of Department of Dermatology, Hospital of Clinics, University of São Paulo Medical School—HC-FMUSP)

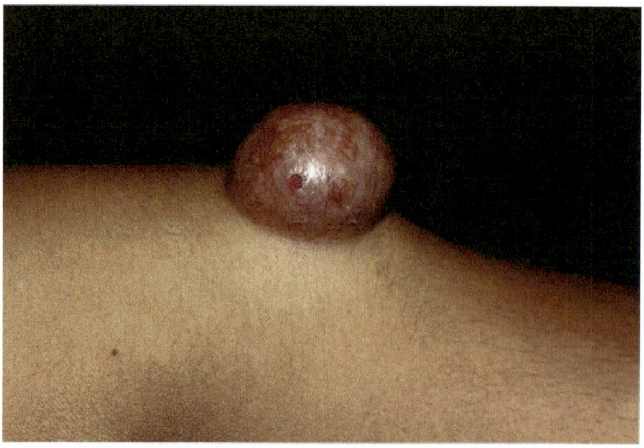

Fig. 12 Dermatofibrosarcoma protuberans on arm. (Collection of Department of Dermatology, Hospital of Clinics, University of São Paulo Medical School—HC-FMUSP)

5.4 *Histopathology*

Dermatofibrosarcoma protuberans is a dermal tumor that extends into subcutis, with atypical spindle cell proliferation. Increase of the neoplasia cellularity and more than eight mitoses per ten high power fields appear to be associated with metastasis. There are small amounts of intermingled collagen. At points of the intersection of the fascicles, there may be an acellular collagenous focus from which the fascicle appears to radiate. This referred to a storiform pattern (Fig. 13). Fibrosarcomatous change, seen particularly in recurrences, represents a form of tumor progression.

Immunohistochemical studies have shown that the tumor cells in DFSP contain vimentin, but they are negative for S100 protein. The most diagnostic marker is the human progenitor cell antigen, CD34, with stains 50–100% of the cells in DFSP (Fig. 14) [7, 32].

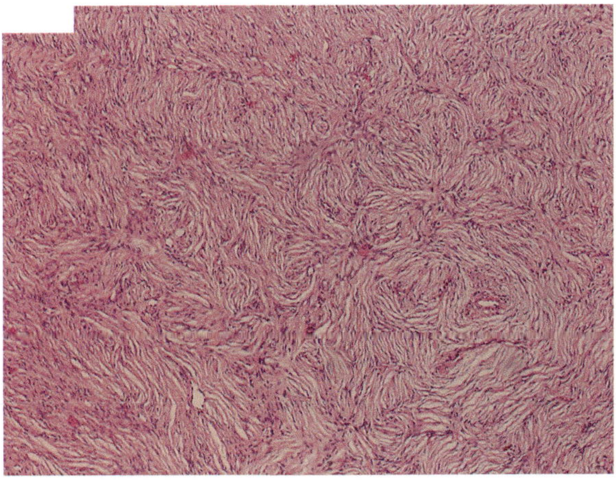

Fig. 13 Dermatofibrosarcoma protuberans: atypical spindle cell and storiform pattern (hematoxylin-eosin, 100×)

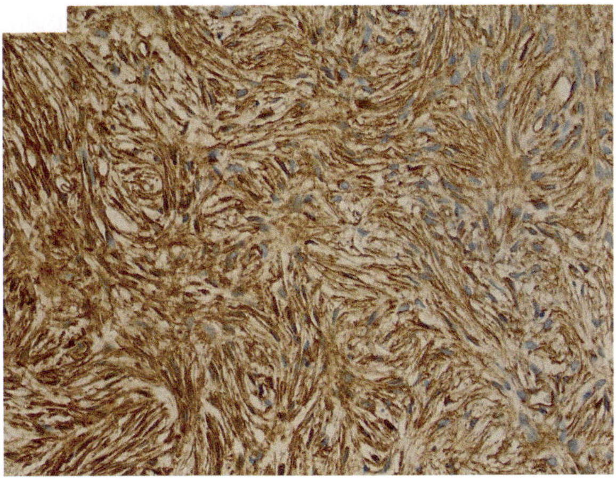

Fig. 14 Dermatofibrosarcoma protuberans: positivity for CD34 in cells' cytoplasm (immunochemistry, 400×)

5.5 *Treatment*

Surgery with wide local excision presents 20% risk of recurrence. The margins should be around 4 cm and if the tumor is large or within a difficult anatomic site, Mohs micrographic surgery (MMS) should be chosen [34]. Despite MMS being a gold standard procedure for basal cell carcinoma, it is also used for DFSP, which guarantees tumor appropriate excision margins. Adjuvant radiation therapy should be recommended in some cases to lower the recurrences. Although the risk for metastasis is low, in some cases when the malignancy is unresectable, the treatment with imatinib ought to be used [35]. The mortality is still low. The survival rate is around 99.1% in 10 years [32].

6 Angiosarcoma

6.1 *Epidemiology*

Angiosarcoma is a high-grade malignant neoplasm that occurs in adults and elderly, with a low skin phototype, mainly on the cephalic segment. It may be associated with postmastectomy and Stewart-Treves syndrome, lymphedema, and immunosuppression [36].

Among SOTRs, the development of angiosarcoma ranges from 8 months to 12 years after transplantation [37].

6.2 *Pathogenesis*

It is a malignant proliferation with endothelial differentiation. Its association with lymphedema is not well understood. In renal transplant recipients, it is frequently observed on the arteriovenous fistula, including nonfunctioning [38, 39]. There are some theories for the high occurrence on the site of arteriovenous fistula, as the oscillatory blood flow may upregulate the vascular adhesion molecules that stimulate the endothelial proliferation. The overproduction of metalloproteinase could increase the metastatic potential in sarcomas [40]. The arteriovenous fistula could reduce lymphatic drainage, reducing immune vigilance [41].

This sarcoma is not related to herpesvirus-8, as it is observed in Kaposi sarcoma [37, 39]. Immunosuppressant drugs such as calcineurin inhibitors could be the main responsible for the development and progression of angiosarcoma, as this group of drugs may facilitate cytokine production (transforming growth factor β and vascular endothelial growth factor), which promotes angiogenesis and tumor growth [42]. Radiotherapy is a risk factor, as many neoplasms develop on irradiated areas [43].

6.3 Clinical Presentation

It affects mainly elderly individuals with the primary lesion on the head and neck area. It appears as an erythematous-violaceous macule, often yellowish, similar to a contusion. More advanced cutaneous lesion is a nodule or tumor that may ulcerate in the center and bleed easily. It is an extremely aggressive neoplasm, progressing to locoregional metastasis. The prognosis is very poor and the dissemination of the tumor may occur in about 1 year [37]. Metastases are common in liver, breast, lungs, skin, spleen, and bone. More than 90% of the angiosarcoma develops after mastectomy, lymphadenectomy, and Stewart-Treves syndrome [43]. MRI with gadolinium enhancement is useful for tumor delimitation. In renal transplant recipients, the angiomatous lesions are common at the site of arteriovenous fistula (Figs. 15a, b and 16a, b).

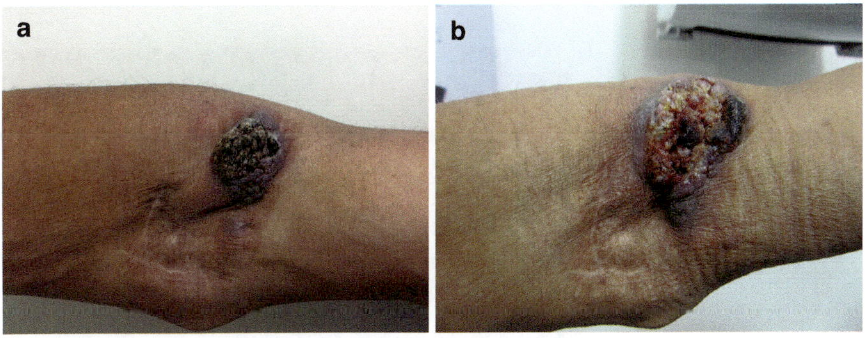

Fig. 15 Angiosarcoma in kidney transplant recipient: (**a**) angiomatous tumor with irregular surface on the arteriovenous fistula; (**b**) one month evolution with tumor necrosis

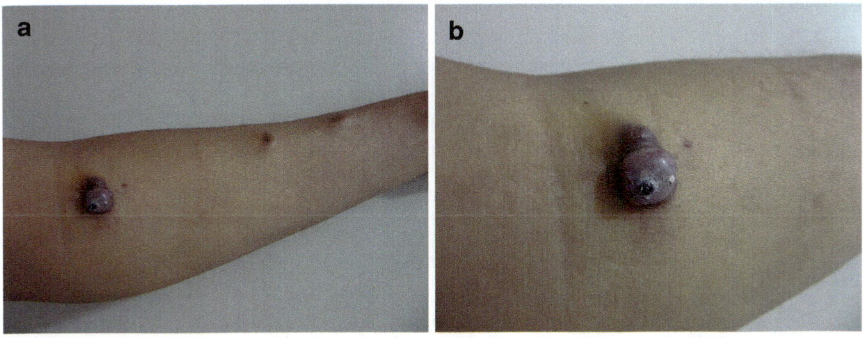

Fig. 16 Epithelioid angiosarcoma in kidney transplant recipient: (**a**) tumor on proximal portion of the left forearm on arteriovenous fistula; (**b**) angiomatous characteristics of the tumor with hematic crust

6.4 Histopathology

There is a superficial and deep dermal proliferation of vascular channels with few or absence of erythrocytes. The single layer of endothelial cells is atypical with large hyperchromatic nuclei. Papillary projection may be observed in these atypical endothelial cells. Hemorrhage, erythrocytes extravasation and hemosiderin deposition may be present. Subcutaneous tissue and perineural infiltration are observed. Tumors associated with lymphedema may retain lymphatic characteristics [43]. Although considered as a distinct vascular tumor, angiosarcoma shares many overlapping histopathological features with other vascular and epithelioid tumors such as epithelioid angiosarcoma (Fig. 17). This tumor shows aggressive behavior and carries a severe prognosis, thus early diagnosis is important to achieve the best possible outcomes.

Using immunohistochemical staining, this tumor is positive for vimentin (Fig. 18a), vascular markers CD31 (Fig. 18b) and CD34. The factor VIII, which is

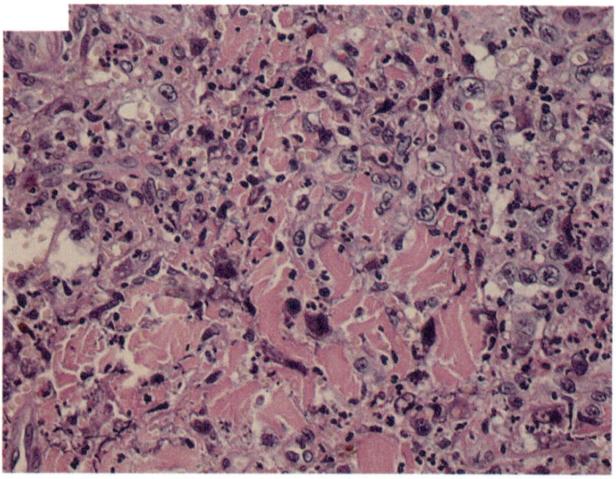

Fig. 17 Epithelioid cutaneous angiosarcoma histopathology: endothelial atypical cells with large hyperchromatic nuclei (hematoxylin-eosin, 400×)

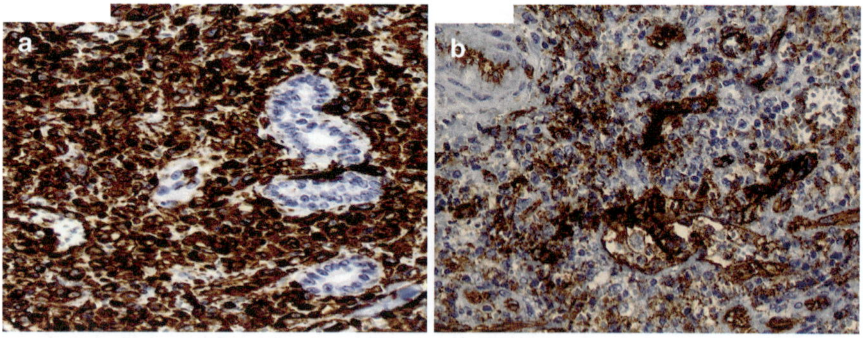

Fig. 18 Epithelioid cutaneous angiosarcoma Immunohistochemical analysis: (**a**) positivity for vimentin (400×); (**b**) positivity for CD31 (400×)

also specific for endothelial cells may present few positivity, even in well-differentiated angiosarcomas. The sensitivity for this marker is low. It is negative for human herpesvirus 8 (HHV8) [43]. Differential diagnoses are epithelioid hemangioendothelioma, epithelioid sarcoma, malignant melanoma, and anaplastic large cell lymphoma [7].

6.5 *Treatment*

Treatment is surgical excision with wide margins. The recurrence rate is extremely high, even with negative margins. Chemotherapy with paclitaxel or doxorubicin has been reported [44]. The neoplasm is not very radiosensitive, and radiotherapy must be considered as a palliative therapy. Treatment with sorafenib, an oral multiple-kinase inhibitor of KIT, FLT-3, VEGFR-1,2,3, and PDGFR-β, is reported with tumor growth reduction [45].

7 Merkel Cell Carcinoma

7.1 *Epidemiology*

Merkel cell carcinoma (MCC) is an aggressive neuroendocrine neoplasm, with various neuroectodermal-derived cells such as Merkel cells. It occurs in elderly, female, and individuals with low skin phototypes [46].

Among SOTRs, the incidence of MCC is higher in men, with a median age of 49 years. It occurs in long-term transplant recipients and the risk ranges between 10- and 24-fold higher compared to the immunocompetent individuals [7, 48]. The risk is higher in renal transplant recipients compared to heart or lung [49].

7.2 *Pathogenesis*

In 2008, the relationship between MCC and polyomavirus infection was established [50]. About 80% of these carcinomas are infected by polyomavirus. There is a viral DNA integration into the host genome, suggesting that the viral infection is an early event [46].

The pathogenesis should be like squamous cell carcinoma, as it has been reported the association of MCC with keratinocyte tumors such as actinic keratosis, Bowen's disease, and basal cell carcinoma as well as with high ultraviolet exposure.

The long-term iatrogenic immunosuppression is an important risk factor for MCC [47]. Surprisingly, a higher risk of MCC is associated with mTORi (mammalian target of rapamycin inhibitor). Probably, mTORi does not inhibit tumor cell growth [47].

7.3 Clinical Presentation

It is a non-tender, pink-red to violaceous dome-shaped, solitary nodule or tumor. The lesion may develop a central ulcer on the nodular lesion (Fig. 19). The neoplasm has an extremely aggressive behavior, with a rapid growth and frequent recurrences. About 50% of patients are diagnosed on the head and neck, followed by upper extremities, trunk, and lower extremities [47]. The tumor size at the time of diagnosis counts in determining the prognosis. Lymph nodes and distant metastases are common [46] (Fig. 20a–c).

MCC is more aggressive and deadly in immunosuppressed patients, with a mortality of 56% [48]. For suspicion of distant metastases, PET-CT scan is very useful [49].

7.4 Histopathology

The tumor is composed of small, round to oval cells of uniformed size. The nucleus is vesicular with multiple small nucleoli. Mitoses and apoptotic bodies are usually numerous. The cytoplasm is scanty (Fig. 21). There are three distinct histopathological patterns: trabecular, small cell, and intermediate. Overlap features are common.

Immunohistochemical studies show cytokeratin as paranuclear globules (dot-like) immunoreactivity, especially CK20. The neuroendocrine markers are positive such as NSE, chromogranin, and synaptophysin. It is negative for S100 protein [7, 51] (Fig. 22a–c).

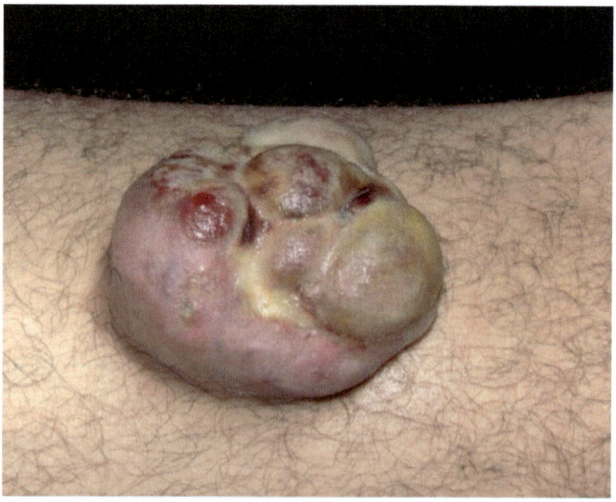

Fig. 19 Cutaneous Merkel cell carcinoma in kidney transplant recipient. (Collection of Department of Dermatology, Hospital of Clinics, University of São Paulo Medical School—HC-FMUSP)

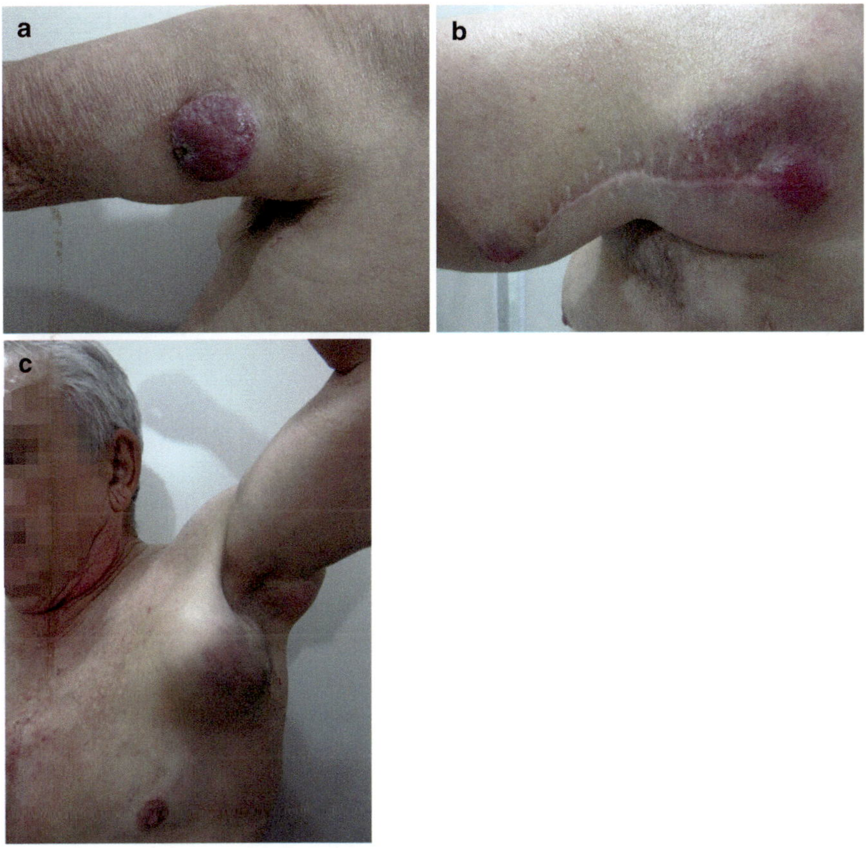

Fig. 20 Merkel cell carcinoma in kidney transplant recipient: (**a**) a rapid growth tumor on arm; (**b**) local cutaneous relapse of Merkel cell carcinoma, after 8 months of surgery; (**c**) axillary lymph node metastasis, after 8 months of surgery

Fig. 21 Merkel cell carcinoma histopathology: presence of small, round cells, with numerous mitoses and apoptotic bodies. The cytoplasm is scanty (hematoxylin-eosin, 400×)

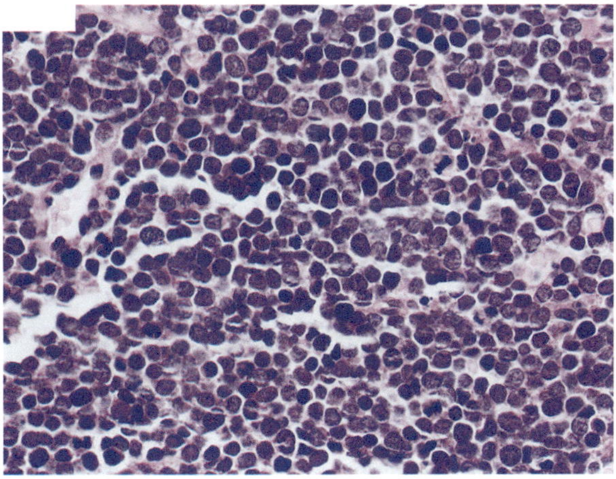

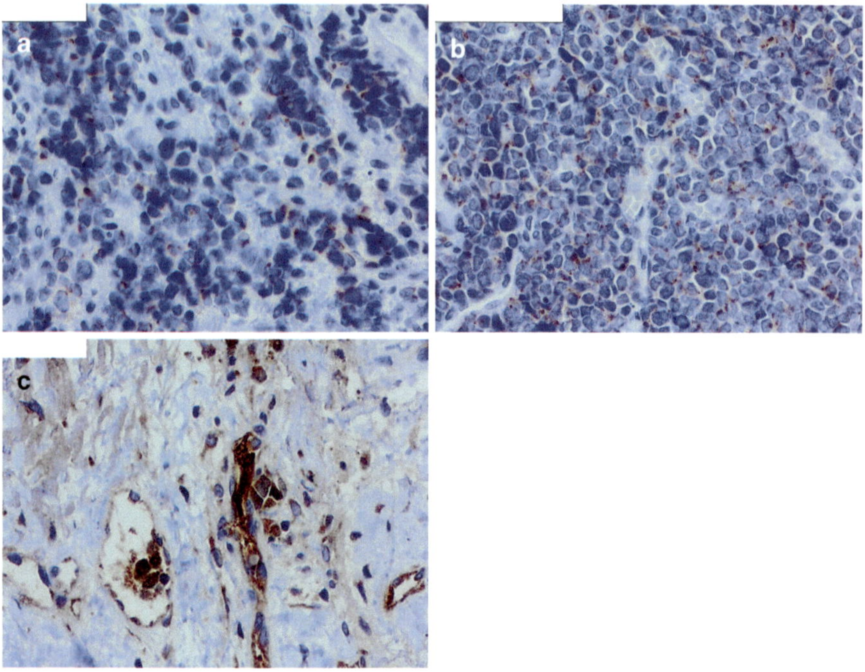

Fig. 22 Merkel cell carcinoma, immunohistochemical analysis: (**a**) positivity for CK20, as paranuclear globules (dot-like) (400×); (**b**) positivity for chromogranin, as paranuclear globules (dot-like) (400×); (**c**) positivity for NSE, showing atypical cells inside the capillary (400×)

7.5 Treatment

The current recommendations for surgical excision are based on the tumor size: ≤2 cm, excision with 1 cm margins, and >2 cm, excision with 2 cm margins [52]. Adjuvant treatment with radiotherapy decreases local recurrences and improves patient's survival [53]. Even in high-risk patients, the cure by association of surgery and radiotherapy increases 50% [53]. There are few benefits with chemotherapy (carboplatin, cisplatin, etoposide). The mortality of older patients receiving chemotherapy is about 16% [54]. Recently, anti-PD-L1 antibody (avelumab) and anti-PD-1 (pembrolizumab) seem to be useful in MCC treatment [49, 54]. It is consensus that the association of surgical excision, sentinel lymph node biopsy, and radiotherapy is the best therapy for MCC [53, 55].

8 Carcinosarcoma

8.1 Epidemiology

Carcinosarcoma is a rare and high malignant complex tumor. It occurs on sun-exposed areas, mainly on the head and neck, of elderly individuals, regardless of gender. Metastasis can affect the liver or abdominal cavity. The prognosis of cutaneous carcinosarcoma is better than those of systemic origin [56].

8.2 Pathogenesis

It is known as a mixed or biphasic tumor that is composed of epithelial and mesenchymal elements. In 1919, Meyer proposed a classification for mixed malignant tumors into three groups: (1) collision tumor: there is a simultaneous growth of two tumors with independent cellularity; (2) combination tumor: there is a growth of two different types of cells derived from a single stem cell; and (3) tumor composition: blastomatous growth occurs both in the parenchyma and in the stroma [57]. The last two hypotheses are accepted to explain the origin of the carcinosarcoma. It is also known as monoclonal theory and multiclonal theory, respectively [58]. More recently, Mondolfi et al. showed an overlapping feature of epithelial and mesenchymal differentiation, suggestive of a common clonal origin [59].

Although rare, this neoplasm is described in several organs such as genital tract, urinary bladder, gastrointestinal tract, breast, lung, liver, uterus, kidney, thyroid, head and neck, and skin. On the skin, it may appear over a burn scar, radiotherapy scarring, or over normal skin.

8.3 Clinical Presentation

The most common presentation is a nodule with ulceration in a sun-exposed area. The differential diagnoses are squamous cell carcinoma, basal cell carcinoma, keratoacanthoma, and dermatofibrosarcoma protuberans. Regional lymph nodes metastasis can be seen. Tumor recurrence is also reported. We present a 71-year-old, male, renal transplant recipient with two ulcerated lesions: (a) frontal: carcinosarcoma and (b) parietal: poorly differentiated squamous cell carcinoma. One year after the surgical excision, he presented supraclavicular lymph nodes metastasis of squamous cell carcinoma (Fig. 23a–c).

In the literature, there is no description of cutaneous carcinosarcoma in SOTRs. There is an interesting report of a renal transplant recipient, who developed multifocal urothelial carcinosarcoma which developed on the deceased donor allograft [60].

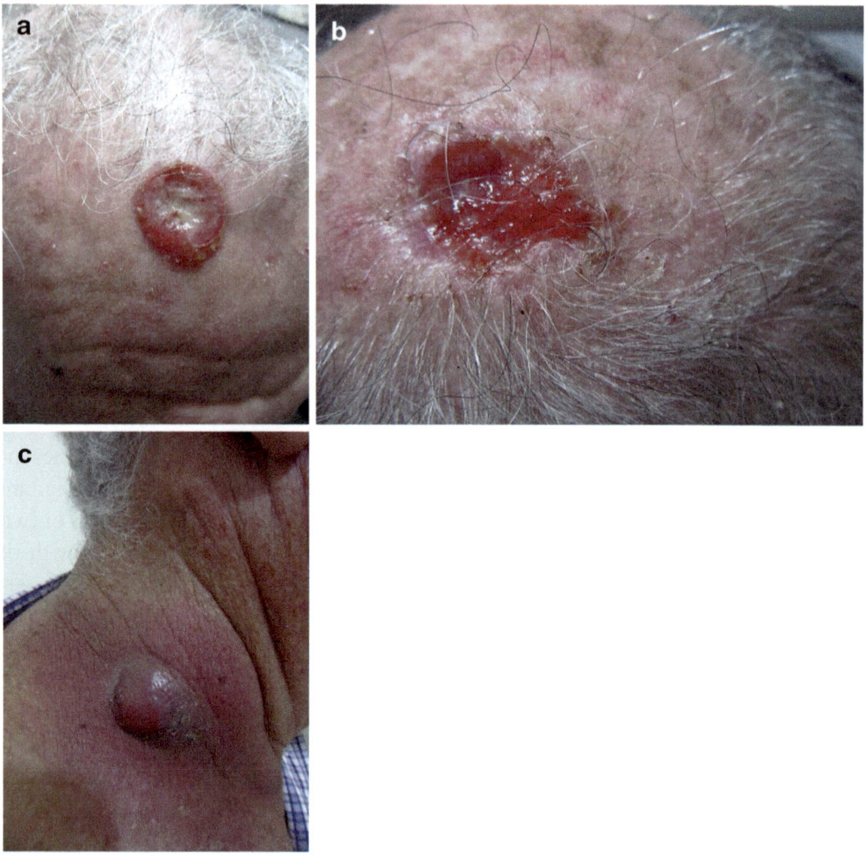

Fig. 23 Association of tumors in renal transplant recipient: (**a**) carcinosarcoma on frontal region; (**b**) poorly differentiated squamous cell carcinoma on parietal region; (**c**) one year after, supraclavicular lymph node metastasis of squamous cell carcinoma

8.4 Histopathology

For diagnosis, the tumor must contain an intimate admixture of epithelial and mesenchymal malignant elements (Fig. 24). The epithelial component can be a squamous cell carcinoma, adnexal or a basal cell carcinoma, and the mesenchymal component can be a poorly differentiated dermal sarcoma, which can be leiomyosarcoma, fibrosarcoma, osteosarcoma, chondrosarcoma or rhabdomyosarcoma [61]. When the epithelial component is a squamous cell carcinoma, it may be well or poorly differentiated. There are pleomorphic spindle cells with eosinophilic cytoplasm [56]. When the epithelial component is composed by adnexal origin carcinoma, the prognosis is worse [62].

In immunohistochemistry, it is suggested that the use of two panels of antibodies. One for epithelial cells and another for mesenchymal cells markers For epithelial cell markers, two antibodies are recommended: cytokeratin AE1/AE3, which is

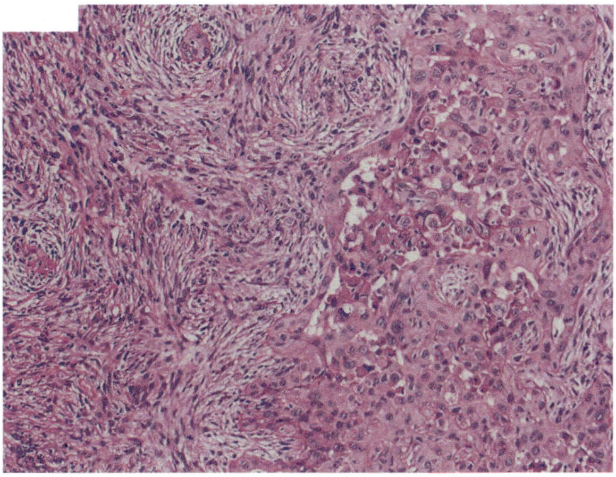

Fig. 24 Carcinosarcoma histopathology: admixture of epithelial (on the right) and mesenchymal elements with spindle cells (on the left) (100×)

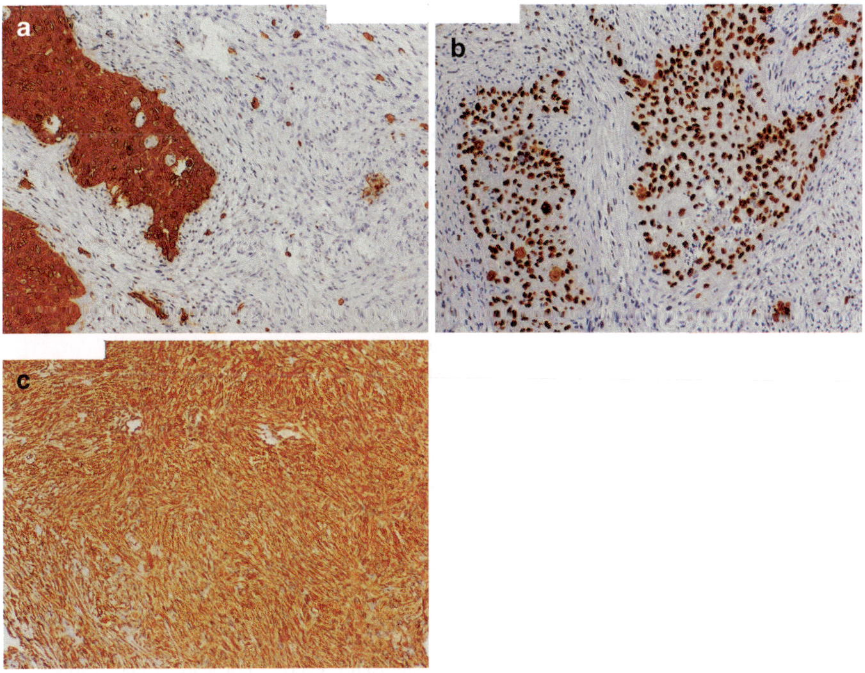

Fig. 25 Carcinosarcoma, immunohistochemical analysis: (**a**) positivity for AE1AE3 in epithelial component (400×); (**b**) positivity for p63 in epithelial component (400×); (**c**) positivity for vimentin for spindle atypical cells (400×)

positive in tumors of epithelial origin (Fig. 25a), and the p63 (Fig. 25b) homologous protein of p53, which is positive in poorly differentiated epithelial cells. Generally, they are both positive in the epithelial component and negative in the sarcomatous component. AE1/AE3 can be weakly positive or negative. The p63 protein may be positive in the transition area of this biphasic tumor. Vimentin is negative for the epithelial component and positive for the sarcomatous component (Fig. 25c). There may be a positive reaction for EMA (epithelial membrane antigen) in the epithelial component. The mesenchymal tumor can be focally positive for smooth muscle actin [63].

8.5 *Treatment*

Surgery is the treatment of choice, with complete resection. In the literature, there is no consensus regarding the recommended margin. Margins range from 5 to 35 mm [56, 64]. Tumor recurrence and metastasis are reported.

References

1. Nemetz MA, da Cunha RM, Reeck P, et al. Trichilemmal carcinoma: a case study. Rev Bras Otorrinolaringol. 2004;70:832–5.
2. Garrett AB, Azmi FH, Ogburia KS. Trichilemmal carcinoma: a rare cutaneous malignancy: a report of two cases. Dermatol Surg. 2004;30:113–5.
3. Hiramatsu K, Sasaki K, Matsuda M, et al. A case of trichilemmal carcinoma with distant metastases in a kidney transplantation patient. Transplant Proc. 2015;47:155–7.
4. Kanitakis J, Euvrard S, Sebbag L, et al. Trichilemmal carcinoma of the skin mimicking a keloid in a heart transplant recipient. J Heart Lung Transplant. 2007;26:649–51.
5. McCalmont TH. Adnexal neoplasm. In: Bolognia J, Jorizzo J, Schaffer J, editors. Dermatology. 3rd ed. Philadelphia: Elsevier Saunders; 2012. p. 1829–49.
6. Zhang QY, Ma LM, Tang ZQ. [Giant trichilemmal carcinoma of the retroauricular: a case report]. Lin Chung Er Bi Yan Hou Tou Jing Wai Ke Za Zhi. 2020;34:83–5.
7. Patterson JW, Hosler GA. Weedon's skin pathology. 4th ed. Philadelphia: Elsevier; 2016.
8. Chaichamnan K, Satayasoontorn K, Puttanupaab S, et al. Malignant proliferating trichilemmal tumors with CD34 expression. J Med Assoc Thail. 2010;93(Suppl 6):S28–34.
9. Hoppenreijs VPT, Reuser TQ, Mooy CM, et al. Syringomatous carcinoma of the eyelid and orbit: a clinical and histopathological challenge. 1997.
10. Wick MR, Goellner JR, Wolfe JT, et al. Adnexal carcinomas of the skin I. Eccrine carcinomas. Cancer. 1985;56:1147–62.
11. Hoppenreijs VPT, Reuser TTQ, Mooy CM, et al. Syringomatous carcinoma of the eyelid and orbit: a clinical and histopathological challenge. Br J Ophthalmol. 1997;81:668–72.
12. Staiger RD, Helmchen B, Papet C, et al. Spiradenocarcinoma: a comprehensive data review. Am J Dermatopathol. 2017;39:715–25.
13. Plunkett TA, Hanby AM, Miles DW, et al. Metastatic eccrine porocarcinoma: response to docetaxel (Taxotere) chemotherapy. Ann Oncol. 2001;12:411–4.
14. Higashi VS, Ogawa MM, Enokihara MMSS, et al. Aggressiveness of poorly differentiated sweat gland carcinoma in kidney transplant recipient. Int J Dermatol. 2015;54:78–80.
15. Shen J, Pan X, Lu Y, et al. A case of eccrine porocarcinoma characterized by a progressive increase in the level of Ki-67 index: case report and review of literature. BMC Surg. 2019;19:142.
16. Goyal A, Marghitu T, Goyal N, et al. Surgical management and lymph-node biopsy of rare malignant cutaneous adnexal carcinomas: a population-based analysis of 7591 patients.

Arch Dermatol Res. 313:623. Epub ahead of print 23 Sept 2020. https://doi.org/10.1007/s00403-020-02143-5.
17. Schröder U, Dries V, Wittekindt C, et al. Successful adjuvant tamoxifen therapy for estrogen receptor-positive metastasizing sweat gland adenocarcinoma: need for a clinical trial? Ann Otol Rhinol Laryngol. 2004;113:242–4.
18. He X, Yang Y, Yang Y, et al. Treatment of sweat gland carcinoma with topical aminolevulinic acid photodynamic therapy: an effective treatment method to improve surgical outcomes. Photodiagn Photodyn Ther. 2017;17:233–5.
19. Seo BF, Jung HW, Choi IK, et al. Sebaceous carcinoma of the suprapubic area in a liver transplant recipient. Ann Dermatol. 2014;26:395–8.
20. Hoss E, Nelson SA, Sharma A. Sebaceous carcinoma in solid organ transplant recipients. Int J Dermatol. 2017;56:746–9.
21. Sargen MR, Cahoon EK, Lynch CF, et al. Sebaceous carcinoma incidence and survival among solid organ transplant recipients in the United States, 1987-2017. JAMA Dermatol. 2020;156:1307–14.
22. Harwood CA, Swale VJ, Bataille VA, et al. An association between sebaceous carcinoma and microsatellite instability in immunosuppressed organ transplant recipients. J Invest Dermatol. 2001;116:246–53.
23. Stone MS, Duncan WC, McGavran MH. Torre's syndrome: exacerbation of cutaneous manifestations with immunosuppression. J Am Acad Dermatol. 1986;15:1101–3.
24. Kaminska ECN, Iyengar V, Tsoukas M, et al. Borderline sebaceous neoplasm in a renal transplant patient without Muir-Torre syndrome. J Cutan Pathol. 2013;40:336–40.
25. Tomonari M, Shimada M, Nakada Y, et al. Muir-Torre syndrome: sebaceous carcinoma concurrent with colon cancer in a kidney transplant recipient; a case report. BMC Nephrol. 2019;20:394.
26. Flux K. Sebaceous neoplasms. Surg Pathol Clin. 2017;10:367–82.
27. Hata M, Koike I, Omura M, et al. Noninvasive and curative radiation therapy for sebaceous carcinoma of the eyelid. Int J Radiat Oncol. 2012;82:605–11.
28. Domingo-Musibay E, Murugan P, Giubellino A, et al. Near complete response to Pembrolizumab in microsatellite-stable metastatic sebaceous carcinoma. J Immunother Cancer. 2018;6:58.
29. Criscione VD, Weinstock MA. Descriptive epidemiology of dermatofibrosarcoma protuberans in the United States, 1973 to 2002. J Am Acad Dermatol. 2007;56:968–73.
30. Durack A, Gran S, Gardiner MD, et al. A 10-year review of surgical management of dermatofibrosarcoma protuberans. Br J Dermatol. 2021;184:731–9.
31. Brown VL, Proby CM, Harwood CA, et al. Dermatofibrosarcoma protuberans in a renal transplant recipient. Histopathology. 2003;42:198–200.
32. Llombart B, Serra C, Requena C, et al. Sarcomas cutáneos: directrices para el diagnóstico y tratamiento. Dermatofibrosarcoma protuberans. Actas Dermosifiliogr. 2018;109:868–77.
33. Akram J, Wooler G, Lock-Andersen J. Dermatofibrosarcoma protuberans: clinical series, national Danish incidence data and suggested guidelines. J Plast Surg Hand Surg. 2014;48:67–73.
34. Kimmel Z, Ratner D, Kim JYS, et al. Peripheral excision margins for dermatofibrosarcoma protuberans: a meta-analysis of spatial data. Ann Surg Oncol. 2007;14:2113–20.
35. Navarrete-Dechent C, Mori S, Barker CA, et al. Imatinib treatment for locally advanced or metastatic dermatofibrosarcoma protuberans: a systematic review. JAMA Dermatol. 2019;155:361–9.
36. Blackmon J, Rajpara A, Patel V, et al. Primary scalp angiosarcoma with metastasis to the liver in an orthotopic liver transplant patient. Exp Clin Transplant. 2014;12:269–72.
37. Ahmed I, Hamacher KL. Angiosarcoma in a chronically immunosuppressed renal transplant recipient. Am J Dermatopathol. 2002;24:330–5.
38. Roy SF, Ghazawi FM, Alsarheed A, et al. Angiosarcoma arising within a nonfunctioning arteriovenous fistula. Int J Dermatol. 2018;57:1513–5.

39. Wehrli BM, Janzen DL, Shokeir O, et al. Epithelioid angiosarcoma arising in a surgically constructed arteriovenous fistula: a rare complication of chronic immunosuppression in the setting of renal transplantation. Am J Surg Pathol. 1998;22:1154–9.
40. Benassi MS, Gamberi G, Magagnoli G, et al. Metalloproteinase expression and prognosis in soft tissue sarcomas. Ann Oncol. 2001;12:75–80.
41. Bordea C, Cortina-Borja M, Wojnarowska F, et al. Distribution of upper limb skin cancers in relation to arteriovenous fistula side in renal transplant recipients. Transplantation. 2001;71:143–5.
42. Guba M, Graeb C, Jauch K-W, et al. Pro- and anti-cancer effects of immunosuppressive agents used in organ transplantation. Transplantation. 2004;77:1777–82.
43. North PE. Vascular neoplasms and neoplastic-like proliferations. In: Bolognia J, Jorizzo J, Schaffer J, editors. Dermatology. 3rd ed. Philadelphia: Elsevier Saunders; 2012. p. 1915–41.
44. Webster P, Wujanto L, Fisher C, et al. Malignancies confined to disused arteriovenous fistulae in renal transplant patients: an important differential diagnosis. Am J Nephrol. 2011;34:42–8.
45. Ono S, Tanioka M, Fujisawa A, et al. Angiosarcoma of the scalp successfully treated with a single therapy of sorafenib. Arch Dermatol. 2012;148:683–5.
46. Argenyi ZB. Neural and neuroendocrine neoplasms (other than neurofibromatosis). In: Bolognia J, Jorizzo J, Schaffer J, editors. Dermatology. Philadelphia: Elsevier Saunders; 2012. p. 1943–60.
47. Clarke CA, Robbins HA, Tatalovich Z, et al. Risk of Merkel cell carcinoma after solid organ transplantation. JNCI: J Natl Cancer Inst. 2015;107:dju382.
48. Penn I, First MR. Merkel's cell carcinoma in organ recipients: report of 41 cases. Transplantation. 1999;68:1717–21.
49. Mittal A, Colegio OR. Skin cancers in organ transplant recipients. Am J Transplant. 2017;17:2509–30.
50. Feng H, Shuda M, Chang Y, et al. Clonal integration of a polyomavirus in human Merkel cell carcinoma. Science. 2008;319:1096–100.
51. Cheuk W, Kwan MY, Suster S, et al. TTF-1 and CK 20 in small cell carcinomas. 2001.
52. Miller SJ, Alam M, Andersen J, et al. Merkel cell carcinoma. JNCCN: J Natl Compr Cancer Netw. 2009;7:322–32.
53. Garneski KM, Nghiem P. Merkel cell carcinoma adjuvant therapy: current data support radiation but not chemotherapy. J Am Acad Dermatol. 2007;57:166–9.
54. Uchi H. Merkel cell carcinoma: an update and immunotherapy. Front Oncol. 2018;8:6–10.
55. Zwald F, Leitenberger J, Zeitouni N, et al. Recommendations for solid organ transplantation for transplant candidates with a pretransplant diagnosis of cutaneous squamous cell carcinoma, Merkel cell carcinoma and melanoma: a consensus opinion from the International Transplant Skin Cancer Collaboration. Am J Transplant. 2016;16:407–13.
56. Kwak H-B, Park J, Kim H-U, et al. Cutaneous carcinosarcoma: a clinicopathologic and immunohistochemical analysis of 11 Korean cases. J Korean Med Sci. 2019;34:1–10.
57. Meyer R. Beitrag zur Verständigung über die Namengebung in der Geschwulstlehre. Zentralbl Allg Path Anat. 1919;30:291–6.
58. Thompson L, Chang B, Barsky SH. Monoclonal origins of malignant mixed tumors (carcinosarcomas): evidence for a divergent histogenesis. Am J Surg Pathol. 1996;20:277–85.
59. Paniz Mondolfi AE, Jour G, Johnson M, et al. Primary cutaneous carcinosarcoma: insights into its clonal origin and mutational pattern expression analysis through next-generation sequencing. Hum Pathol. 2013;44:2853–60.
60. Buzogány I, Bagheri F, Süle N, et al. Association between carcinosarcoma and the transplanted kidney. Anticancer Res. 2006;26:751–3.
61. Bigby SM, Charlton A, Miller MV, et al. Biphasic sarcomatoid basal cell carcinoma (carcinosarcoma): four cases with immunohistochemistry and review of the literature. J Cutan Pathol. 2005;32:141–7.

62. Tran TA, Muller S, Chaudahri PJ, et al. Cutaneous carcinosarcoma: adnexal vs. epidermal types define high- and low-risk tumors. Results of a meta-analysis. J Cutan Pathol. 2005;32:2–11.
63. Brasanac D, Boricic I, Todorovic V, et al. Primary cutaneous carcinosarcoma: case report with expanded immunohistochemical analysis. Int J Dermatol. 2008;47:496–501.
64. Song EY, Wallace SJ, Sheikh H, et al. Cutaneous carcinosarcoma: a small case series and review of the literature of a rare skin tumor. Cureus. 2020;12:e9569.

Index

J. Tomimori et al. (eds.), *Atlas of Dermatologic Diseases in Solid Organ Transplant Recipients*, https://doi.org/10.1007/978-3-031-13335-0

D

G

H

I

K

R

S

GPSR Compliance

The European Union's (EU) General Product Safety Regulation (GPSR) is a set of rules that requires consumer products to be safe and our obligations to ensure this.

If you have any concerns about our products, you can contact us on ProductSafety@springernature.com

In case Publisher is established outside the EU, the EU authorized representative is:

Springer Nature Customer Service Center GmbH
Europaplatz 3
69115 Heidelberg, Germany

Batch number: 10726133

Printed by Printforce, the Netherlands